Gene Therapy of Cancer

METHODS IN MOLECULAR MEDICINE™

John M. Walker, SERIES EDITOR

METHODS IN MOLECULAR MEDICINE™

Gene Therapy of Cancer

Methods and Protocols

Edited by

Wolfgang Walther

Max-Delbrück-Center for Molecular Medicine, Berlin, Germany

and

Ulrike Stein

Max-Delbrück-Center for Molecular Medicine, Berlin, Germany

Humana Press 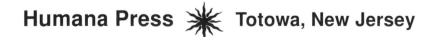 Totowa, New Jersey

Cover design by Patricia Cleary

Cover illustration taken from Fig. 3 in Chapter 24. The illustration depicts intratumoral detection of oncolytic vectors containing a reporter gene.

For additional copies, pricing for bulk purchases, and/or information about other Humana titles, contact Humana at the above address or at any of the following numbers: Tel.: 973-256-1699; Fax: 973-256-8341; E-mail: humana@humanapr.com; Website: http://humanapress.com

Printed in the United States of America. 10 9 8 7 6 5 4 3 2 1

Library of Congress Cataloging in Publication Data

Main entry under title:

Methods in molecular medicine™.

Gene therapy of cancer : methods and protocols / edited by Wolfgang
    Walther and Ulrike Stein.
        p. cm. -- (Methods in molecular medicine ; 35)
    Includes bibliographical references and index.
    ISBN 0-89603-714-2 (hard : alk. paper). --ISBN 0-89603-843-2
(comb : alk. paper)
    1. Cancer--Gene therapy Laboratory manuals. I. Walther,
Wolfgang. II. Stein, Ulrike. II. Series
    [DNLM: 1. Neoplasms--therapy. 2. Gene Therapy--methods. QZ 266
    G3259 2000]
RC271.G45G484 2000
616.99'4042--dc21
DNLM/DLC
for Library of Congress   99-38474
                                                                        CIP

Preface

Since the discovery of the molecular structure of genes and the unveiling of the molecular basis of numerous human diseases, scientists have been fascinated with the possibility of treating certain diseases by transducing foreign DNA into the affected cells. Initially, it was proposed that the foreign DNA could either replace defective nonfunctional genes, or code for therapeutic proteins. This concept has evolved into the rapidly growing field of gene therapy.

Even though surgery, radiotherapy, and chemotherapy are widely available and routinely used for cancer treatment, these therapies fail to cure approximately 50 percent of cancer patients. Therefore, since it is a disease characterized by aberrant gene expression, cancer has been a target of gene therapy research since the inception of this treatment modality. Numerous cancer gene therapy strategies are currently being investigated, including gene replacement therapy, the regulation of gene expression to modulate immunological responses to tumors, the direct killing of tumor cells, and direct interference with tumor growth. In this context, gene transfer systems, tumor-specific expression vectors, and novel therapeutic genes have been extensively studied. All these strategies aim for the selective destruction of human malignant disease while circumventing the destruction of nonmalignant cells and tissues thereby minimizing toxicity to the patient.

Rapid progress in the field of cancer gene therapy, exemplified by the vast number of publications in this area, creates a challenging situation for scientists and clinicians who need to be cognizant of the most recent advances in gene transfer techniques. This volume of *Gene Therapy of Cancer: Methods and Protocols* in the *Methods in Molecular Medicine* series will provide researchers with a broad array of methods used to study cancer gene therapy in both the laboratory and clinical trials. Moreover, several chapters are included to provide short overviews of specialized gene therapy strategies for the treatment of particular malignancies.

Gene Therapy of Cancer: Methods and Protocols does not provide comprehensive reviews of all methodologies currently used for gene therapy of cancer. Rather the topics we have selected consist of approved procedures, current trends, and representative strategies in cancer gene therapy using different classes of therapeutic genes, suppressor genes, antisense oligonucleotides, ribozymes, viral- and nonviral-vector systems, and tumor targeting approaches at the preclinical and, more importantly, at the clinical level. For cancer gene therapy to be successful in the treatment of human cancers, extensive preclinical evaluation is essential. Therefore, the first part of this book discusses relevant experiments from preclinical studies followed by clinical gene therapy protocols in the second part.

Gene Therapy of Cancer: Methods and Protocols should provide practical guidance for basic and clinical researchers, as well as graduate and postgraduate students working in the exciting and emerging field of gene therapy.

Wolfgang Walther
Ulrike Stein

Contents

Contributors

MANISH AGHI • *Molecular Neurogenetics Unit, Massachusetts General Hospital East, Charlestown, MA*

ANDREAS ALBERS • *Centrum Somatische Gentherapie at Freie Universität Berlin, Berlin, Germany*

RAMON ALEMANY • *Wallace Tumor Institute, Department of Medicine– Pulmonary and Critical Care, University of Alabama, Birmingham, AL*

K.-H. ALTMAN • *Oncology Research, Novartis Pharma, Basel, Switzerland*

DONALD D. ANTHONY • *Department of Pharmacology, Case Western Reserve University, Cleveland, OH*

DAVID BERMUDES • *VION Pharmaceuticals, New Haven, CT*

MASAMI BESSHO • *First Department of Internal Medicine, Saitama Medical School, Saitama, Japan*

GUADALUPE BILBAO • *Gene Therapy Program, University of Alabama at Birmingham, Birmingham, AL*

HANS BOJAR • *Institut für Onkologische Chemie, Heinrich Heine Universität Düsseldorf, Düsseldorf, German*

ROBERTA BONAGURO • *Institute of Microbiology, University of Padova Medical School, Padova, Italy*

KARSTEN BRAND • *Max-Delbrück-Center for Molecular Medicine, Berlin, Germany*

XANDRA O. BREAKEFIELD • *Molecular Neurogenetics Unit, Massachusetts General Hospital East, Charlestown, MA*

J. MARTIN BROWN • *Cancer Biology Research Laboratories, Department of Radiation Oncology, Stanford University School of Medicine, Stanford, CA*

PATRICIA A. BRUSO • *Department of Head and Neck Surgery, The University of Texas M.D. Anderson Cancer Center, Houston, TX*

LING CHEN • *Department of Human Genetics, Merck Research Laboratories, West Point, PA*

GARY L. CLAYMAN • *Department of Head and Neck Surgery, M.D. Anderson Cancer Center, University of Texas, Houston, TX*

FREDERICO COLOMBO • *Institute of Microbiology, University of Padova Medical School, Padova, Italy*

MARIO P. COLOMBO • *Experimental Oncology Department, Istituto Nazionale Tumori, Milano, Italy*

JUAN LUIS CONTRERAS • *Gene Therapy Program, Lurleen B. Wallace Tumor Institute, Comprehensive Cancer Center, University of Alabama at Birmingham, Birmingham, AL*

MATTHEW COOPERBERG • *Genetic Therapy Program of the Yale Cancer Center, and the Medical Oncology Section, Department of Internal Medicine, Yale University School of Medicine, New Haven, CT*

DAVID T. CURIEL • *Gene Therapy Program, University of Alabama at Birmingham, Birmingham, AL*

ALBERT DEISSEROTH • *Department of Internal Medicine, Yale University School of Medicine, New Haven, CT*

DON DIZON • *Genetic Therapy Program of the Yale Cancer Center and the Medical Oncology Section, Department of Internal Medicine, Yale University School of Medicine, New Haven, CT*

INGO DREXLER • *Institut für Molekulare Medizin, Bavarian Nordic Research Institute, Neuherberg, Germany*

VOLKER ERFLE • *Institut für Molekulare Medizin, Bavarian Nordic Research Institute, Neuherberg, Germany*

DORIANO FABBRO • *Oncology Research, Novartis Pharma, Basel, Switzerland*

FRANK FLOETH • *Neurochirurgische Klinik, Heinrich Heine Universität Dusseldorf, Germany*

MARY E. FOX • *Division of Basic Sciences, Fred Hutchinson Cancer Research Center, Seattle, WA*

DOUGLAS K. FRANK • *Department of Head and Neck Surgery, M.D. Anderson Cancer Center, University of Texas, Houston, TX*

SCOTT M. FREEMAN • *Clinical Research Oncology, Schering–Plough Research Institute, Kenilworth, NJ*

SI QING FU • *Genetic Therapy Program of the Yale Cancer Center and the Medical Oncology Section, Department of Internal Medicine, Yale University School of Medicine, New Haven, CT*

EVANTHIA GALANIS • *Division of Medical Oncology, Mayo Clinic, Rochester, MN*

THOMAS GEIGER • *Oncology Research, Novartis Pharma, Basel, Switzerland*

AMATO J. GIACCIA • *Cancer Biology Research Laboratories, Department of Radiation Oncology, Stanford University School of Medicine, Stanford, CA*

JESUS GOMEZ-NAVARRO • *Gene Therapy Program, University of Alabama at Birmingham, Birmingham, AL*

WALTER GÜNZBURG • *Institute of Virology, University of Veterinary Sciences, Vienna, Austria*

XIANG YANG DAVID GUO • *Genetic Therapy Program of the Yale Cancer Center and the Medical Oncology Section, Department of Internal Medicine, Yale University School of Medicine, New Haven, CT*

NAGY B. HABIB • *Liver Surgery Section, Imperial College School of Medicine Hammersmith Hospital Campus, London, UK*

JODI E. D. HECHT • *Department of Biology, Boston University, Boston, MA*

KARL HELLER • *Institut für Molekulare Medizin, Bavarian Nordic Research Institute, Neuherberg, Germany*

ULRICH HERRLINGER • *Neurologische Universitätsklinik Tübingen, Tübingen, Germany*

JEFFREY T. HOLT • *Department of Cell Biology, Vanderbilt University, Nashville, TN*

AKIO IDO • *Second Department of Internal Medicine, Miyazaki Medical College, Miyazaki, Japan*

ANDREAS JACOBS • *Molecular Neurogenetics Unit, Massachusetts General, Hospital East, Charlestown, MA*

YOUSSEF JOUNAIDI • *Department of Biology, Boston University, Boston, MA*

KEIZO KAZANO • *Gene Therapy Program, University of Alabama at Birmingham, Birmingham, AL*

DAVID H. KIRN • *Onyx Pharmaceuticals, Richmond, CA*

HIROYUKI KOBAYASHI • *Division of Neoplastic Diseases, Department of Medicine, Mount Sinai School of Medicine, New York, NY*

WEN-HWA LEE • *Department of Molecular Medicine, Institute of Biotechnology, The University of Texas Health Science Center, San Antonio, TX*

MARILYN J. LEMMON • *Cancer Biology Research Laboratories, Department of Radiation Oncology, Stanford University School of Medicine, Stanford, CA*

NICHOLAS R. LEMOINE • *Imperial Cancer Research Fund Oncology Group, Imperial College School of Medicine at Hammersmith, Hammersmith Hospital, London, UK*

DEBBIE LIN • *Genetic Therapy Program of the Yale Cancer Center and the Medical Oncology Section, Department of Internal Medicine, Yale University School of Medicine, New Haven, CT*

BROOKS LOW • *Therapeutic Radiology, Yale University School of Medicine, New Haven, CT*

SELINA LUGER • *Bone Marrow Transplant Program, Division of Hematology and Oncology, Hospital of the University of Pennsylvania, Philadelphia, PA*

KATALIN V. LUKACS • *National Heart and Lung Institute, Imperial College, London, UK*

AIZEN J. MARROGI • *Department of Surgery, Louisiana State University School of Medicine, New Orleans, LA*

NIGEL P. MINTON • *Centre for Applied Microbiology and Research, Porton Down, Salisbury, Wiltshire, UK*

RAGAI R. MITRY • *Liver Surgery Section, Imperial College School of Medicine, Hammersmith Hospital Campus, London, UK*

B. P. MONIA • *Department of Molecular Pharmacology, Carlsbad Research Center, ISIS Pharmaceuticals, Carlsbad, CA*

ANUPAMA MUNSHI • *Department of Surgery, Louisiana State University School of Medicine, New Orleans, LA*

SHIGENOBU NAGATAKI • *Radiation Effects Research Foundation, Hiroshima, Japan*

ARTIT NAKAKES • *National Heart and Lung Institute, Imperial College, London, UK*

THONG NANAKORN • *Genetic Therapy Program of the Yale Cancer Center and the Medical Oncology Section, Department of Internal Medicine, Yale University School of Medicine, New Haven, CT*

JOHN NEMUNAITIS • *Mary C. Crowley Cancer Research Program, Baylor Research Institute, Baylor University Medical Center, Dallas, TX*

PATRICE S. OBERMILLER • *Department of Cell Biology, Vanderbilt University, Nashville, TN*

MARION OHLMANN • *Institut für Molekulare Medizin, Bavarian Nordic Research Institute, Neuherberg, Germany*

TAKAO OHNUMA • *Division of Neoplastic Diseases, Department of Medicine, Mount Sinai School of Medicine, New York, NY*

GIORGIO PALÙ • *Institute of Microbiology, University of Padova Medical School, Padova, Italy*

YUE XIN PAN • *Department of Pharmacology, School of Medicine, Case Western Reserve University, Cleveland, OH*

HARDEV S. PANDHA • *Department of Medicine, Royal Marsden Hospital, Surrey, UK*

JOHN M. PAWELEK • *Departments of Dermatology and Pharmacology, Yale University School of Medicine, New Haven, CT*

LENE PEDERSEN • *Department of Molecular and Structural Biology, University of Aarhus, Aarhus, Denmark*

Xue Yan Peng • *Genetic Therapy Program of the Yale Cancer Center and the Medical Oncology Section, Department of Internal Medicine, Yale University School of Medicine, New Haven, CT*

Massimo Pizzato • *Institute of Microbiology, University of Padova Medical School, Padova, Italy*

Alexander L. Rakhmilevich • *Department of Human Oncology, University of Wisconsin Medical School, Madison, WI*

Rajagopal Ramesh • *Department of Thoracic and Cardiovascular Surgery, M.D. Anderson Cancer Center, Houston, TX*

Daniel J. Riley • *Department of Medicine, Division of Nephrology, University of Texas Health Center, San Antonio, TX*

Monica Rodolfo • *Department of Experimental Oncology, Istituto Nazionale Tumori, Milano, Italy*

Joseph Rubin • *Division of Medical Oncology, Mayo Clinic, Rochester, MN*

Volker Sandig • *Max-Delbrück-Center for Molecular Medicine, Berlin, Germany*

Kevin J. Scanlon • *Berlex Biosciences, Richmond, CA*

Dirk Schadendorf • *Clinical Cooperation Unit for Dermatology at the Department of Dermatology Clinics, Mannheim Universität Heidelberg, Mannheim, Germany*

Pamela Schreiber Schwartz • *Department of Biology, Boston University, Boston, MA*

Peter M. Schlag • *Departments of Surgery and Surgical Oncology, Robert-Rössle-Clinic, Charité at the Humboldt University, Berlin Germany*

Deborah E. Schuback • *Molecular Neurogenetics Unit, Massachusetts General Hospital East, Charlestown, MA*

Robert H. Shoemaker • *Antiviral Evaluations Branch, Developmental Therapeutics Program, National Cancer Institute, Rockville, MD*

Shrinavassan Shrimdkandada • *Genetic Therapy Program of the Yale Cancer Center and the Medical Oncology Section, Department of Internal Medicine, Yale University School of Medicine, New Haven, CT*

Kyonghee Kay Son • *Department of Pharmaceutics, College of Pharmacy, Rutgers, The State University of New Jersey, Piscataway, NJ*

Ulrike Stein • *Max-Delbrück-Center of Molecular Medicine, Robert-Rössle Strasse, Berlin, Germany*

Wolfram Sterry • *Department of Dermatology Charité, Humboldt University Berlin, Berlin, Germany*

Michael Strauss • *Max-Delbrück-Center for Molecular Medicine, Berlin, Germany*

Gerd Sutter • *Institut für Molkulare Medizin, Bavarian Nordic Research Institute, Neuherberg, Germany*

TOSHIYA SUZUKI • *First Department of Internal Medicine, Saitama Medical School, Saitama, Japan*

ALEX W. TONG • *Mary C. Crowley Cancer Research Program, Baylor Research Institute, Baylor University Medical Center, Dallas, TX*

UWE TREFZER • *Department of Dermatology, Medical Faculty Charité, Humboldt-University Berlin, Berlin, Germany*

SHOTARO TSURUTA • *The First Department of Internal Medicine, Nagasaki University School of Medicine, Nakgasaki, Japan*

THOMAS TÜTING • *Department of Dermatology, University of Mainz, Mainz, Germany*

WOLFGANG UCKERT • *Max-Delbrück-Center for Molecular Medicine, Berlin, Germany*

PETER WALDEN • *Department of Dermatology, Medical Faculty Charité, Humboldt-University Berlin, Berlin, Germany*

WOLFGANG WALTHER • *Max-Delbrück-Center of Molecular Medicine, Robert-Rössle-Strasse, Berlin, Germany*

FU-SHENG WANG • *Department of Medicine, Division of Neoplastic Diseases, Mount Sinai School of Medicine, New York, NY*

DAVID J. WAXMAN • *Department of Biology, Boston University, Boston, MA*

FRIEDRICH WEBER • *Neurochirurgische Klinik, Heinrich Heine Universität Düsseldorf, Düsseldorf, Germany*

GUIDO WEINGART • *Department of Dermatology, Medical Faculty Charité, Humboldt-University Berlin, Berlin, Germany*

JONG HO WON • *Genetic Therapy Program of the Yale Cancer Center and the Medical Oncology Section, Department of Internal Medicine, Yale University School of Medicine, New Haven, CT*

LIAN HUA YIN • *Genetic Therapy Program of the Yale Cancer Center and the Medical Oncology Section, Department of Internal Medicine, Yale University School of Medicine, New Haven, CT*

JINGPING YANG • *Genetic Therapy, Gaithersburg, MD*

NING-SUN YANG • *Comprehensive Cancer Center, University of Wisconsin Medical School, Madison, WI*

WEI-WEI ZHANG • *GenStar Therapeutics, San Diego, CA*

YU-AN ZHANG • *Mary C. Crowley Cancer Research Program, Baylor Research Institute, Baylor University Medical Center, Dallas, TX*

I

EXPERIMENTAL APPROACHES IN CANCER GENE THERAPY

A: Immunotherapy/Tumor Vaccination

1

Immunizing Potential of Cytokine-Transduced Tumor Cells

Mario P. Colombo and Monica Rodolfo

1. Introduction

1.1. Cytokine-Gene-Modified Tumor Cell Vaccines for Cancer Immunotherapy: Concepts, Rationale, and Prospective

The molecular definition of tumor antigens, costimulatory signals, and the possibility to genetically engineer tumor cells as well as simple protocols for efficient isolation and preparation of dendritic cells (DC) renew the interest in tumor immunotherapy and vaccination, in particular. Engineering of tumor cells with the gene of a particular cytokine is a way of releasing that cytokine at the tumor site. In contrast to bolus administration, it provides a constant supply of cytokine. If live-engineered tumor cells are injected, their proliferation results in both the provision of antigen and an increase of cytokine concentration until a physiological or a pharmacological threshold is reached, and its biological activity begins. The following inflammatory reaction is then responsible for tumor destruction, thus, turning off the initial trigger. The efficacy of this feedback action is determined by the type of cytokine, its quantity and activity, the histotype of the tumor and the molecules it releases, and its extracellular matrix *(1)*. However, the relevant point is that a cascade of events other than tumor debulking are initiated by the transduced cytokines. Infiltration of different leukocyte types, including antigen-presenting cells (APC), and the release of secondary cytokines contribute to the induction of a systemic and memory response. Also, injection of replication in competent cells because of irradiation can exert the same effect, in this case the amount of cytokine to be released *in situ* to trigger the system, should be predetermined.

From: *Methods in Molecular Medicine, Vol. 35: Gene Therapy: Methods and Protocols*
Edited by: W. Walther and U. Stein © Humana Press, Inc., Totowa, NJ

The events caused by the injection of cytokine-transduced tumors include both the early infiltration of granulocytes and then of macrophages and lymphocytes, and the release of secondary cytokines. Tumor-cell debris derived from tumor destruction may represent the source of tumor antigens that APC process and bring to draining lymph-nodes, which appear often enlarged with expanded cortical and paracortical area and rich of tingible-body macrophages *(2)*. Although cellular debris captured by phagocytic cells contain antigens that are presented through the Class II pathway, CD8$^+$ cytotoxic T lymphocyte (CTL) are often induced in this setting because systemic immunity and generation of cytotoxic T lymphocytes generally follow tumor destruction *(2)*.The finding of GM-CSF-dependent DC Class I presentation of soluble proteins for CTL induction *(3,4)* as well as of the role of bone marrow-derived APC *(5)* in mediating in vivo cross-priming *(6)* indicate that intratumoral DC can induce protective immunity by uptaking and processing antigen for presentation within their own major histocompatibility complex (MHC) *(5)*.

The efficacy of such vaccines largely depends on their ability to provide all the repertoire of relevant antigens and the cytokines and cosignals that favor DC recruitment and function for both T-cell priming and T-T help. The perspective should consider the possibility of favoring the interaction between tumor-cell vaccine and DC, rather than genetically manipulate tumor cells to transform them into APC-like cells that, by interacting directly with T cells, may bypass the need of DC.

1.2. Inhibition of Tumor Take, Induction of Systemic Immunity, and Curative Effects Involve Different Mechanisms and Different Players

The main criterion in the assessment of cytokine-transduced tumor-cell vaccines is the therapeutic efficacy. Tumor inhibition and/or the induction of systemic immunity are not in themselves sufficient for evaluation of treatment efficacy and curative potential. In fact, tumor inhibition has been studied by injecting tumor-cell suspensions, although it is known that solid tumor fragments often grow progressively, whereas even 10-fold-higher numbers of the identical tumor-cell type injected as a suspension are rejected *(7)*. The tumor stroma, which consists of vessels, sessile and migratory cells, and extracellular matrix, plays an important role in tumor growth and progression. In addition, tumor cells modified to produce cytokines are likely to have additional regulatory signals resulting from cytokine-extracellular matrix crosstalk. Thus, the interaction of the tumor with host immune cells and the features of the effector cells mediating destruction of a tumor injected as a cell suspension differ from those required to reject an established tumor nodule, as shown in the case of C-26 colon carcinoma transduced with the G-CSF gene *(8)*. Moreover, induction of systemic immunity with activation of CTL might not be sufficient to destroy existing tumor nodules although tumor-bearing mice still retain the ability to recognize the same antigen present within the tumor when presented on a normal tissue and outside the tumor environment *(9)*. This suggests that whereas a tumor patient could be immunized against that tumor, the induced immunity is insufficient to fight an established tumor growing within its own stroma. Tumor escape from T-cell cytotoxicity may also result from loss of MHC Class-I antigens or from impaired migration of CTL at the tumor site. The latter occurs in C-26 carcinoma cells transduced with IL-12 genes, and CD4$^+$ cell depletion can replenish CD8^1 T-cell tumor infiltration *(10)*.

1.3. Tumor and Animal Models for Preclinical Studies: Working With Known Target Antigen(s)

Other crucial points underscore the differences between experiments performed in the mouse system and ongoing clinical investigations. For some human tumors, the target antigen(s) of an antitumor immune response has been identified at the molecular level *(11)*, whereas for most murine neoplasms, the target tumor antigen remains unknown. Moreover, in the case of melanomas most of the dominant antigens cloned come from specific differentiation antigens of the melanocytic lineage whereas few are from mutated gene products *(11)*. This implies that vaccines directed against antigens common to different tumors in patients sharing the relevant HLA haplotype are possible in humans, whereas similar evidence in the mouse is lacking. Exceptions are viral-tumor antigens such as Friend-Moloney and Rauscher gag/env proteins, which are common to some lymphomas and leukemias and lung tumor-associated antigen connexin 1 *(12)*. Other antigens that are frequently expressed on different tumors are those derived from mutated oncogenes, such as *ras* or from fusion proteins derived by chromosomal translocations, such as PML/RARα, or from genes overexpressed in tumors, such as HER-2/neu. The immunogenicity of peptides deriving from these gene products has been better demonstrated in humans than in mice. Several *ras* mutations that are commonly associated with carcinogen-induced tumors are reportedly immunogenic based on the use of peptides or recombinant proteins; however, their role as tumor-transplantation antigens *(13)* is not clear in the absence of experiments with tumors carrying such mutations. By contrast, tumor antigens cloned from mouse tumors appear to be unique and tumor specific.

In all mouse experiments that require a well-characterized target antigen, proteins not classifiable as tumor antigens have been used. In fact, to test whether a recombinant vaccine carrying the gene encoding an antigen recognized by CTL can treat established metastasis, Restifo and co-workers *(14)* used the β-galactosidase (β-gal) gene of *Escherichia coli*. We have also used (β-gal by to demonstrate Class I-restricted CTL priming by dendritic cells, and cytolysis and in vivo protection against a β-gal -transduced tumor *(3)*. As a model, β-gal offers many advantages; β-gal soluble protein, its peptide, as well as a retroviral vector able to transduce the gene into tumor cells are all available. In addition, β-gal, as a soluble protein, is unable to enter the cell outside the endosomal compartment and is unable to stimulate CTL in vivo. Finally, the animal model utilizing transplantable tumors are of limited preclinical value. New models employing transgenic mice carrying oncogenes under tissue-specific promoters mimic more closely the clinical setting.

2. Materials

2.1. Solutions and Materials

2.1.1. Cell Culture

1. RPMI-1640 (Life Technologies, Bethesda, MD) supplemented shortly before use with 5–10% fetal calf serum (FCS) heat inactivated 1 h at 56°C, 2 mM L-glutamine, 25 mM HEPES buffer, 1% nonessential amino acids, 1% Na piruvate, 50 mM 2-mercaptoethanol (2-ME), 100 U/mL penicillin, 100 µg/mL streptomycin sulfate.
2. ACK lysing buffer: add to 1 L distilled sterile H_2O: 8.29 g NH_4Cl (0.15M), 1 g $KHCO_3$ (1 mM), 37.2 mg Na_2EDTA (0.1 mM) and bring to pH 7.2–7.4 with HCl 1M; filter 0.2 µm, store at 4°C.
3. Low tox-M rabbit complement: Cederlane (Hornby, Ontario, Canada), cod CL3051.
4. 1 mCi/mL $Na_2{}^{51}CrO_4$ in isotonic saline solution (ICN 620152).

2.1.2. In Vivo Reduction of Metastases

1. India Ink 15% in distilled H_2O, add 2 drops ammonia water.
2. Fekete solution (to bleach white tumor nodules against blacked lung parenchima): 100 mL 70% ethanol, 100 mL formaldehyde, 5 mL CH_3COOH.

2.1.3. In situ Hybridization

1. OCT compound (Tissue Tek II, Miles cod 4583).
2. SSC (sodium chloride/sodium citrate), 20X: 3M NaCl (175 g/L), 0.3M Na_3citrate $2H_2O$ (88 g/L), adjust pH to 7.0 with 1M HCl.
3. 100x Denhardt's solution: 10 g Ficoll 400, 10 g polyvinylpyrrolidone, 10 g bovine serum albumin (Pentax Fraction V, Miles Lab. Rexdale, Ont., Canada).
4. Ammonium acetate (Sigma A-1542).
5. Dextran sulfate (Sigma D-8906).
6. Dithiothreitolo (DTT) (BRL 5527UA).
7. Formamide (Sigma F-7508).
8. Glycine (USB 16407).

9. Triethanolamine (Sigma T-1502).
10. EDTA (Sigma E-5134).
11. Salmon Sperm DNA (SSDNA) (Sigma D-9156).

2.1.4. Immunohistochemical Staining of Tissue Sections

1. Poly-L-lysine (Sigma, MW> 150,000).
2. Tris-buffered saline (TBS): 10 mM Tris Cl, pH 7.6, 1 mM EDTA.

2.2. Mice (Short Note on Animal Care and Handling)

Ethical use of experimental animals include the concepts outlined by Russel and Burch in 1959 *(15)*, replacement, refinement, and reduction of the use of laboratory animals. Besides the ethical considerations, experiments with animal models is strictly regulated by local law, submitted for approval to Institutional Committee and eventually regulated by Institutional Guidelines for Animal Experimentation. It is important to know that health conditions may affect results, because common mycoplasma and viral infection determine immunosuppression. Thus, health monitoring is recommended and a stable environment for maintenance and quarantine of newly arrived animals should be followed. Immunocompromised mice, because of irradiation or other immunosuppressive treatment or because of genetic defects, cannot survive in conventional animal facilities and should be maintained in conditions aimed to prevent adventitious infections. Handling requires knowledge of the proper methods for avoiding injury to the handler and to the animal. Pain and distress should be avoided as far as possible, anesthesia should be used for all surgical procedures, and euthanasia by acceptable methods that minimize pain should be used, following fixed GLP standards *(16–18)*.

2.3. Hybridomas

Most, if not all, the hybridomas listed below can be obtained from American Type Culture Collection (ATCC). On-line database of ATCC http://www.atcc.org gives information on monoclonal antibodies (MAbs).

2.3.1. Antibodies for Immunocytochemistry

1. hamster antimouse CD3ε (154-2C11 clone)
2. rat antimouse CD8 (53.6.72 hybridoma)
3. rat antimouse CD4 (GK1.5 hybridoma)
4. rat antimouse CD28 (37.51 hybridoma)
5. rat antimouse CD31/PECAM-1 (MEC 13.3 hybridoma)
6. rat antimouse CD34 (14.7 MEC hybridoma)
7. rat antimouse CD45 (M1/9.3.4.HL2 hybridoma)
8. rat antimouse CD51/αv integrin (H9.2B8 hybridoma)

9. rat antimouse CD54 (3C2 hybridoma)
10. rat antimouse CD61/β_3 integrin (2C9.G2 hybridoma)
11. rat antimouse CD86 (GL-1 hybridoma)
12. rat antimouse Mac-3 (M3/84,6,34 hybridoma)
13. rat antimouse MHC-II (B21-2 hybridoma)
14. rat antimouse GR-1 (RB6-8C5 hybridoma)
15. rat antimouse DEC205 (NDLC-145 hybridoma)
16. rabbit antiasialo GM1 serum (Wako, Osaka, Japan)

2.3.2. Antibodies for In Vivo Leukocyte Depletion

1. rat antimouse CD4 (GK1.5 hybridoma)
2. rat antimouse CD8 (2.43 hybridoma)
3. rat antimouse NK1.1 (PK136 hybridoma)
4. rat antimouse granulocytes (RB6.8C5 hybridoma)
5. rabbit antiasialo GM1 serum (Wako, Osaka, Japan)

2.3.3. Antibodies for TCR Vβ Usage

1. rat antimouse Vβ 2 (B20.6 hybridoma)
2. hamster antimouse Vβ 3 (KJ-25 hybridoma)
3. rat antimouse Vβ 4 (KT4 hybridoma)
4. mouse antimouse Vβ 5 (MR 9.4 hybridoma)
5. rat antimouse Vβ 6 (44.22.1 hybridoma)
6. rat antimouse Vβ 7 (TR310 hybridoma)
7. mouse antimouse Vβ 8 (F23.1 hybridoma)
8. mouse antimouse Vβ 9 (MR 10.2 hybridoma)
9. rat antimouse Vβ 10 (B21.5 hybridoma)
10. rat antimouse Vβ 11 (RR3-15 hybridoma)
11. rat antimouse Vβ 12 (MR 11-1 hybridoma)
12. rat antimouse Vβ 13 (MR 12.4 hybridoma)
13. rat antimouse Vβ 14 (14.2 hybridoma)
14. mouse antimouse Vβ 17 (KJ 23 hybridoma)

3. Methods

3.1. In Vivo Tumorigenicity and Challenge-Protection Assay (Tumor Growth Curves: Tumor Take, Onset, and Survival)

The induction of an in vivo measurable antitumor response in mice following immunization with genetically modified tumor cells has a major relevance for perspectives of clinical application. In fact, although in vitro methods have been developed to measure different specific effector cells or molecules involved in tumor regression, a correlation between in vitro detected antitumor responses and clinical response is still undetermined. In addition, there are instances in which the positive demonstration of antitumor reactivity in vitro bears no correlation with the extent of the antitumor response in vivo. Thus, although several aspects of the mechanisms at the basis of immune tumor destruction have been described, the related immunological parameters are likely to vary in the different tumor models and treatments tested.

In vivo tumorigenicity of engineered tumor cells can be primarily used to determine the mechanisms of tumor regression as far as lymphoid subpopulations involved by depletion experiments (*see* **Subheading 3.3.1.**) or by histological techniques. Challenge-protection assays are used to measure immunogenicity of cytokine-transduced tumors as their ability to induce a tumor rejection response. They are intended to measure a secondary or memory response rather then a primary response. Here, parental tumor cells are injected in mice that have been previously immunized with irradiated engineered cells, or that have rejected an injection of live engineered cells. Both assays require tumor-cell injection in mice and monitor of tumor growth and can follow this scheme:

1. Inject groups of syngeneic mice with engineered tumor cells and parental or mock-engineered parental cells at doses that have been predetermined in preliminary experiments. Generally, TD 50/100 tumor-cell inoculum-producing tumor growth in 50 and 100% of injected animals are used for the first experiments. Subcutaneous implant in the flank is used because the tumor growth is most easily observed. Use at least 5 mice per group. For protection assays, the number of parental tumor cells producing tumor growth in 100% of untreated animals is injected in immunized mice and control group.
2. Evaluate and record incidence and tumor growth twice weekly in a blinded fashion. Check tumor appearance by palpation and measure tumor nodules in the two perpendicular diameter by caliper.
3. To evaluate data by analyzing differences in:
   a. Tumor takes or incidence of tumor-free animals.
   b. Tumor growth curves constructed by calculation of tumor volume, in mm^3 or in mg, as: (minor diameter)^2 × (major diameter)/2 *(19)*, or πr^3. Tumor area can be alternatively used, calculated by the measures of the longest and shortest tumor diameters. Tumor growth curves are constructed by plotting the tumor measures, mg or mm^3 or mm^2, against time in days or weeks.
   c. Tumor onset, defining latency as the time period between challenge and growth of neoplastic mass.
   d. Survival, by observing tumor growth until mice die of tumors or until they become moribund or until tumor masses become excessively large. Use χ-square test to determine significance in the difference of tumor takes, and survivors, student's *t*- or Fisher test for differences in tumor growth.

3.2. Evaluation of the Curative Effect
of Genetically Modified Tumor Cell Vaccines

Different studies have shown that genetic modification of tumor cells with specific cytokine genes results in the acquisition of immunogenic properties that allow tumor rejection and development of systemic antitumor immunity *(2)*. Although this phenomenon has been extensively studied, the capacity of cytokine-transduced tumor cells vaccines to affect the progression of an established tumor growing at a distant site has received less attention. When the immunizing and curative potential of cytokine-modified tumor vaccines have been tested in parallel, they were shown to differ dramatically *(20,21)*.

It is clear that the assessment of the curative effect of a cytokine-gene-modified vaccine is the most relevant assay for determining the efficacy of a vaccine. Curative effect can be evaluated by different in vivo assays, depending also upon the tumor model studied. The most simple procedure is testing the effect of vaccines in mice transplanted with parental tumor sc. The difference between the vaccinated mice and untreated controls can be evaluated as defined in **Subheading 3.1.** Minimal residual disease models are represented by spontaneous metastases, occurring after removal of a primary tumor and experimental lung or liver metastases, determined by the intravenous or intrasplenic injection of tumor cells *(22)*. Other experimental models include transplantation of the tumor into its organ or tissue of origin (orthotopic injection) *(23–26)*.

3.2.1. Experimental and Spontaneous Metastases Models:
Survival vs Tumor Reduction

The in vivo efficacy of immunotherapy by engineered tumor vaccines can be evaluated on survival or reduction of tumor metastases.

1. For survival, follow-up mice should be controlled daily and euthanized when showing dyspnoea or other symptoms of tumor growth. Close the experiment when no deaths occur afterward in preliminary experiments. Analyze the rate of survivors by χ-square test, survival curves by Wilcoxon test.
2. For evaluating the reduction of metastases, treated and control mice are sacrificed after the therapeutic treatment (a good time-point is generally 1 wk after the end of treatments) and metastases quantitated. Spontaneous metastases are evaluated by the weight of the metastatic organ (for example lung or liver); the weight of the same organ of age-matched nontumor-bearing animals gives a baseline for this evaluation. Experimental metastases are numbered by counting the superficial tumoral foci of lungs or liver. Treated and control mice are sacrificed (generally 2–3 wk after tumor-cell injection) the organ fixed and metastatic foci counted in a blinded fashion under dissection microscope. For counting lung metastases,

lungs can be colored in black by intratracheal insufflation with 1 ml of a water solution of 15% India Ink followed by bleaching in Fekete solution *(27).*

3.3. Analysis of Effector Cells

Procedures to isolate, prepare, and study different populations of lymphoid cells have been widely described. However, because activation of antitumor T cells has been shown to be required for tumor regression, and because techniques have been adapted to the study of antitumor response, methods for the study of antitumor T cells will be given here. These include a protocol for assessing the role of T subpopulations by in vivo depletion with specific MAbs (*see* **Subeading 3.3.1.**), protocols for assaying antitumor T-cell functions in vitro (*see* **Subheading 3.3.2.–3.3.3.**). In addition, protocols for assaying antitumor Ab response, which can participate to the tumor regression mechanism, arc included in **Subheading 3.3.4.**

3.3.1. In Vivo Leukocyte Depletion to Obtain Selected Immunodeficient Mice by Antibody Depletion and Thymectomy

Mice can be effectively depleted of defined subsets of lymphocytes by high-dose antibody treatment. *In vivo* depletion experiments provide information of the direct involvement of the studied T-cell subset in the complex multifactorial phenomenon of tumor regression. The role in the initiation and in the effector phases or in a memory response of the different lymphoid cell subpopulations can be demonstrated by depletion experiments. MAbs that can be used for this assay are listed in **Subheading 2.2.** In addition, MAbs for TCR Vβ can also be used to demonstrate the role of a defined T subpopulation. Purified MAbs should be used for in vivo depletion, and IgG are better than IgM *(28).*

Once the MAb of interest is identified, do the following:

1. Inject mice with MAb, ip route, at the dose of 0.2–0.5 mg in 0.2 mL of PBS or saline solution. Inject isotype-matched antibodies in controls. Repeat treatment twice weekly for the duration of the experiment.
2. Sacrifice some treated and untreated mice (after > 5 d or at the time-points of interest) and preparing splenic and lymph-node lymphocytes to verify subset depletion.
3. Stain lymphocytes for the MAb used and for control markers and analyze by flow cytometry. When possible, use lymphocytes to verify depletion by functional assays. Near-complete depletion (more than 95%) must be observed. Verify depletion in pilot experiments and for new batches of MAb used.

Depletion before tumor injection allows to test whether a certain population is involved at the induction phase, whereas depletion carried out before challenge in immunized mice determines whether such populations are involved at the effector phase. Leukocyte depletion by repeated MAb injections is costly in terms of the amount of MAb, but is very flexible because it allows to revert the depleted state by MAb withdrawal.

3.3.2. In Vivo Leukocyte Depletion by Antibody Depletion After Thymectomy

A way to permanently deplete $CD4^+$, $CD8^+$, or both T-cell population is through thymectomy before a single antibody injection *(29)*.

To perform adult thymectomy:

1. After anesthesia, perform a skin incision over the suprasternal notch to expose the proximal part of thoracic cage and trachea. Insert scissors under the sternum and cut to the second-third rib that form a prominent V. Cut the ribs on the right side of sternum and using the blunt end of forceps, operate to spread the two sides of excision and expose the thymus lobes.
2. Thymus lobes can be removed by suction using a Pasteur pipet. A moderate vacuum pump is indicated for this operation. Pipet should be modified by operating a side hole that allows to control the amount of vacuum by varying the degree of occlusion with the forefinger during suction. Be sure that both lobes have been removed.
3. Hold the skin closed to seal the chest and secure the skin with a wound clip.

3.3.3. CTL Activation in Mixed Lymphocyte Tumor-Cell Culture (MLTC)

CTLs are a T-cell subpopulation generated from precursors T lymphocytes (CTLp) expressing the antigen-specific T-cell receptor (TCR) repertoire following stimulation by specific antigens carried by APC in the presence of costimulatory signals and helper T cells. Cytolysis of target cell results from the engagement of TCR/MHC antigen-peptide complex and of other accessory surface molecules. Antigen-specific CTL activity is thus MHC-restricted and distinguished from nonspecific non-MHC-restricted tumor-cell mediated response observed by lymphokine activated killer cell (LAK) *(30)*.

Antitumor CTL activation can be detected and measured after in vitro culture in MLTC conditions determining the restimulation/activation of in vivo primed CTLp. In MLTC, responder lymphocytes are cultured with stimulator cells (irradiated tumor cells or APC presenting tumor antigen in the form of synthetic peptide) at densities that have to be determined by titration experiments. After 5–10 d incubation, cells are harvested from cultures and used as effector cells to kill tumor cells, or cells expressing the tumor antigen because of gene modification, or target cells pulsed exogenously with relevant synthetic peptide in the ^{51}Cr release assay *(31)*. MHC-restricted antigen-specific reactivity can be further demonstrated by blocking cytotoxicity with MAbs for MHC Class I or against CD3/TCR. Although lymphoid cells to be tested functionally in vitro can be isolated from tumor, blood, or nonlymphoid organs such as liver, gut, and lungs *(30)*, the protocols given here deal with splenic cells (SPC) or lymph node cells (LNC). Systemic antitumor CTL induction is measured with SPC, the capacity of a vaccine to induce CTL can be detected with LNC from lymph nodes draining vaccination site. Lymphocytes should be prepared with the use of sterile equipment and manipulations because in vitro culture is required.

To measure antitumor CTLs, lymphocytes are cultured in MLTC and then are assayed for specific lytic activity against tumor cells in cell-mediated cytotoxicity assay.

Set up MLTC by coculturing:

1. Responder lymphocytes *(R)* as follows:
   - SPC 40–20 × 10^6 in 25 cm^2 upright flask in 10–15 mL total volume
   - LNC 1–0.5 × 10^6 in 24 wells plate in 2 mL
2. Stimulator cells *(S)*: irradiated (10–20 × 10^3 rad) tumor cells or syngeneic irradiated (2000 rad) SPC loaded with peptide, at $R:S$ ratio 80–10:1. Optimal concentration vary in the different experimental systems, and between LNC or SPC and should be determined in pilot experiments. Use lymphocyte medium added of 5–10 U/mL rIL-2.
3. Include positive and negative control, especially in pilot experiments. The first can be CTL clones specific for the assayed tumor antigen or tumor cells, alternatively the experimental lymphocytes activated by rIL-2 to develop LAK activity (culture lymphocytes without stimulator cells 10^6/mL with 500 U/mL rIL-2).
4. Incubate for 5 d in CO_2 incubator.

3.3.4. Cell-Mediated Cytotoxicity Assay (^{51}Cr Release Assay)

To test lymphocytes from MLTC in cytotoxicity assay:

1. Label target cells. Important: use standard safety procedures for radionuclides when labeling cells and then when using labeled cells. Add 50–100 µCi of Na$_2$^{51}CrO$_4$ (50–100 µL of a sterile, pyrogenic-free, saline solution at 1 µCi/mL) to 2 × 10^6 cells pellet discarded of the supernatant. If Na$_2$^{51}CrO$_4$ is more than 2 wk old, use double volumes. Incubate 1 h at 37°C (meanwhile, prepare effectors), resuspend by flicking after 30 min. For peptide testing, use mitogen activated lymphoblasts as targets (T blasts or B blasts obtained by culturing 2–5 × 10^6 cells/mL in 10 mL in 25 cm^2 flask for 2–4 d with ConA 2 µg/mL, or LPS 10 µg/mL, respectively), and add peptide (10–1 µg/mL) together with Na$_2$^{51}CrO$_4$. Label cells if viability is > 80%, avoid enrichment by Ficoll Hypaque gradient centrifugation.

2. Prepare effector *(E)* lymphocytes. Maintain lymphocytes at room temperature in their culture medium (reduced it by centrifugation for cell counting) until the assay plates are prepared. Then spin and prepare *E* diluted $1–5 \times 10^6$/mL.
3. Prepare target cells *(T)*. After 3–4 washes with cold medium, prepare target cells at $1–5 \times 10^4$/mL. In pilot experiments, check viability by cell count.
4. Prepare test plates. In 96 wells U or V bottomed plates:
   a. Add 100 μL of lymphocytes at 4 *E:T* dilution (in three replicates wells).
   b. Add 100 μL of lysing agent (NP40 nonidet 1% in water) to the total release *(TR)* wells; add 100 μL of medium to spontaneous release *(SR)* wells in six replicates.
   c. Add 100 μL of target cells to each well.
5. Spin the plates for 2 min to bring cells into contact.
6. Incubate plates for 4–6 h.
7. Spin plates for 5 min.
8. Remove 100 μL of supernatant from each well, place in tubes, and count CPM in γ-counter or in a β scintillator counter.
9. Calculate % specific release as (sample cpm - sr cpm/ tr cpm-sr cpm).

3.3.5. Limiting Dilution Analysis (LDA) of Antitumor CTL Activation

LDA is used to estimate the frequency of precursor CTL specific for a defined tumor antigen or antigenic repertoire of a tumor. The higher the frequency measured, the more potent the antitumor response assayed. The assay consists of multiple MLTC cultures set up in 96-well plates at different concentrations of lymphocytes. It is based on the difference between the presence of a positive or a negative response in individual cultures within groups of replicate cultures. The frequency is determined with the fraction of negative cultures at each lymphocyte dilution, being a negative culture considered as zero precursors with the tested specific function. Many protocols and several statistical methods to calculate CTLp by LDA analysis have been published after its first description *(32–36)*. The reading of some monographs introducing to the application of this method is highly recommended. LDA represent a sensitive method to detect response to antigens by pCTL present in the lymphocyte population at a low frequency. In addition, CTL activity is estimated with more precision by this method, because in bulk cultures a dominant response can result from a selection process favoring the expansion of clones, which do not predominate in vivo rather than from the presence of large number of precursors. The assay also has the advantage of requiring few cells and it is thus suitable for the analysis of cells prepared by sorting. On the other hand, LDA is more time consuming and expensive than bulk MLTC and requires experience in MLTC, a day's work by a skilled worker and another day for testing and calculations. LDA has not been widely applied to tumor systems, also because tumor-cell stimulation may not be successful. The possibility to use synthetic peptides for restimulation can bypass this problem and should be considered when dealing with known antigens.

The following protocol is used for determining tumor or peptide specific precursor T cells in SPC of tumor immunized mice in our laboratory.

1. Seed cells in 96-well U-bottomed microtiter plates in the following order (final volume of 200 µL/well):
   a. Feeder cells: 5×10^5 cells in 25 µL in every well of all test plates. Use syngeneic irradiated (2000 rad) SPC after removal of red blood cells; prepare single-cell suspension at 2×10^7 cells/mL.
   b. Tumor cells: 5×10^3 cells in 25 µL in every well. Prepare irradiated tumor cells (15,000 rad) at 2×10^5 /mL.
   c. Recombinant human IL-2: 40 U/mL in 100 µl in every well (final test concentration 20 U/mL).
   d. Responder lymphocytes: 50 µL/w in 32–48 replicates. Prepare cells diluted to 250, 500, 1000, 2000, 5000, 10,000, 20,000, 40,000, 80,000 cells/w, starting from $1,8 \times 10^6$/mL dilution and then diluting 1:2. Set up the same number of control wells that receive no responder cells (0 lymphocyte wells). The cpm measured by these control wells will be used to calculate a threshold to discriminate positive from negative cultures. Frozen lymphocytes can be used successfully.
2. Incubate plates at 37° C 5% CO_2 in humidified atmosphere.
3. Remove 100 µL/w medium and replace with fresh medium plus rIL-2 at 20 U/mL on days 3–4.
4. Check lymphocyte proliferation by microscope examination on day 6. In case massive proliferation is observed, test cytotoxicity on day 7, otherwise change medium again on day 6/7 and test on day 10.
5. Test cytotoxicity (days 7–10) in cell-mediated ^{51}Cr release assay. If two different targets are tested to verify specificity, split cultures by transfer 80 µL in 2 replica plates to be used for positive and negative targets. Use $1–2 \times 10^3$ target cell/w. Remember to include total and spontaneous control wells.
6. Calculate frequencies. Calculate the fraction of positive cultures at each lymphocyte dilution as those with cpm>mean cpm of culture with 0 lymphocytes $+3 \times SD$. The fraction of negative cultures is converted to its negative logarithm and the results plotted on ordinate in linear form with lymphocyte concentrations on abscissa. Regression analysis is used to fit this line. Using the Poisson equation which predicts that when the 37% of test cultures are negative there is an average of one precursor cell per well giving a crude estimate reciprocal frequency. Basic common programs such as EXCEL can be used to calculate the resulting number of pCTL by linear regression analysis. The resulting linear equation ($y = ax + b$) is then used to calculate pCTL frequency as (log 36.78794-b)/a.

3.3.6. Cytokines Production at Draining Nodes and Tumor Site: Th1/Th2 Deflected Responses by In Vitro Analysis of Cytokines produced

Naive CD4[+] T helper cells (Th) differentiate into one of two well-defined cell types during immune responses. Mature Th1 and Th2 cells regulate the type of response as a consequence of the unique cytokines that they secrete. The initial development and continued maintenance of Th1 or Th2-like responses in vivo play a pivotal role in determining immune effector mechanisms and clinical outcome. The ability of tumor vaccines to preferentially activate Th1 or Th2-dominated responses in vivo has been evaluated.

In vitro cytokine production by T cells isolated from lymph nodes draining vaccination site, from spleen or from other organs of mice undergoing vaccination treatment can be induced by culturing lymphocytes plates precoated with anti-CD3 MAb (145-2C11 hybridoma). Supernatants are recovered and assayed for IFNγ and IL-4 titers (or for other cytokines of interest) by specific commercial ELISA. In ELISA cytokine levels are calculated using standard curves constructed using recombinant murine cytokines. Results of ELISA for lymphocytes can be normalized to percentage of CD3[+] cells determined by immunostaining and FACS analysis. Purified CD4[+] cells can be alternatively tested.

To induce cytokine release by anti-CD3 MAb stimulation:

1. Add 50 µL of a 10 µg/mL solution of anti-CD3 (hybridoma 145-2C11) MAb in Tris Cl 0.05 M pH 9.5 to 96 flat-bottomed wells to obtain Ab coated wells.
2. Leave plates at room temperature for at least 1 h.
3. Three washes with PBS and 1 with PBS containing 5% FCS. Do the same for noncoated control wells.
4. Add lymphocytes 2×10^5/w in 200 µL to coated and noncoated wells.
5. Incubate plates overnight.
6. Spin plates for 5 min.
7. Collect supernatant, store in plates or vials, pool replicates.
8. Keep at −80°C until measuring cytokine content by commercially available ELISA.

3.3.7. Cytokines Production at Draining Nodes and Tumor Site: Analysis by In situ Hybridization Using Cryosections

In situ hybridization is the only useful method for studying the differential localization of cells that express a certain cytokine within a tissue sample. It is crucial, for example, to study the cytokines expressed by leukocytes infiltrating a tumor nodule and to identify which cell expresses a particular cytokine. Many different obstacles have to be overcome in order to obtain reliable results:

1. Achievement of suitable preparation of cryostatic section;
2. Choice of a fixative able to prevent the degradation of RNA and, at the same time, to allow the probe to penetrate;
3. Choice of the appropriate probe.

DNA, RNA, and synthetic oligonucleotides can be used as probes, taking into consideration the advantages and disadvantages of each in relation to the experimental condition and availability. cDNA probes, labeled by nick-translation or random priming are efficiently employed for *in situ* hybridization, but single-stranded RNA probes have several advantages:

1. They do not selfanneal in solution like DNA can do, giving a strong hybridization signal owing to the higher number of available-labeled molecules.
2. RNA/RNA hybrids are more stable than DNA/RNA ones allowing to use higher stringency conditions to reduce the background.
3. RNase digestion of unbound probe further eliminates the background.

Although cDNA appear to be a disadvantageous probe, excellent results have been obtained with this material that is easy to handle.

The introduction of synthetic oligonucleotides produced by DNA synthesizer brought other improvements in *in situ* hybridization. In fact, oligonucleotides do not require subcloning and can be designed to hybridize to any mRNA sequence. Moreover, they have an optimal tissue penetration. The choice of the labeling methods is a compromise between resolution and sensitivity. ^{3}H-labeled probes allow a good resolution, but they need long exposure (several weeks), whereas ^{32}P permits a quicker detection but, as its energy of emission is too penetrating, the resolution is poor. An acceptable compromise is ^{35}S or the recently introduced ^{33}P, which shows a lower energy and a longer half-life, although with a high economic cost.

1. Glass slides and glassware preparation
   - Place slides in a slide rack and immerse for 30 min in SDS 0.5%, 0.2 N HCl.
   - Wash with abundant running tap water.
   - Leave in 3% H_2O_2 (in distilled H_2O) for 3 h.
   - Wash with 95% ethanol.
   - Air dry and autoclave.
2. Specimen preparation
   Samples are quick frozen after inclusion in OCT by dipping in liquid N_2.
3. Sectioning
   - Autoclaved glass slides are dried at 80°C and then let them cool at RT.
   - Sections (5–8 μm thick) are cut at –20°C cryostat.
4. Tissue fixation
   - Use 4% paraformaldehyde (PFA) in PBS (pH 7.4) for 10–20 min at RT.
   - Rinse with PBS for 5 min.

- Dehydrate with ethanol for 5 min at each of the following concentrations: 30%, 70%, 95%, 100%.

5. Rehydration
   - 50 mM MgCl$_2$ in PBS for 15 min.
   - 200 mM tris-HCl pH 7.5, 100 mM glycine.
   - Dehydrate with ethanol as above.

6. Acetylation
   - Immerse slides in fresly prepared 2X SSC, 100 mM triethanolamine (pH 8).
   - Add Acetic Anhydride to a final concentration of 0.25% and leave for 20 min.
   - Wash the slides in 2X SSC for 5 min.
   - Dehydrate with ethanol as indicated above.

7. Prepare hybridization mix
   - 10% dextran sulphate.
   - 50% formamide (30% for oligonucleotides probes).
   - 300 mM NaCl, 20 mM tris HCl pH 8, 5 mM EDTA.
   - 5X Denhardt's solution.
   - Add H$_2$O to volume required.
   - 10 mM DTT.
   - 10^6 cpm probe/section.
   - 20 μg slide/SSDNA.

   a. Mix all freshly prepared ingredients, but DTT and leave at 70°C for at least 20 min until dextrane sulphate will melt.
   b. Prepare the probe by precipitation with 2μl carrier SSDNA, resuspend in H$_2$O as required to bring to final volume the hybridization mix. Add 20 μg slide/SSDNA to the probe so to denature them together. Denature probe at 100°C and chill in ice.
   c. Add the probe solution and DTT to the hybridization mix maintained at 70°C and use immediately to cover sections.

8. Hybridization
   - Prepare dehydrated sections in a moist chamber at 70°C.
   - Cover sections with 20–25 μl hybridization mix using the tip of a pipet.
   - Cover with parafilm to maintain the probe on the section.
   - Incubate in moist chamber at 42°C for 16 h (for DNA probes).

   When RNA probes are used, dehydrate with ethanol containing 0.6M ammonium acetate and hybridize the probes at 50°C. When oligonucleotides (25–40 bp) are used add 0.5% SDS to the hybridization mix and hybridize the probes at 37°C.

9. Wash the slides through the following regimen (DNA and RNA probes):
   - 20 min with 2X SSC at RT.
   - 30 min in mixer with 2X SSC, 50% formamide at 45°C.
   - 30 min in mixer with 1X SSC, 50% formamide at 45°C.
   - 15 min in mixer with 1X SSC at 45°C.
   - 30 min with 0.1X SSC at RT. A further wash with 0.6M ammonium acetate may be required if salt crystals are still there.

For oligonucleotide probes wash the slides as follows:
- 20 min with 2X SSC at RT.
- 30 min in mixer with 2X SSC, 50% formamide at 45°C.
- 2 washes of 30 min with 200 m*M* tris-HCl pH 7.5, EDTA 5 m*M*, 0.5% SDS at 40°C.
- 30 min with 20 m*M* tris at RT.

10. Detection of hybridized probe by emulsion autoradiography
- Prepare 1:2 diluted emulsion Kodak NBT2 or NBT3 in ammonium acetate 0.6*M* at 42°C.
- Leave at 42°C and stir for 2 min.
- Avoid creating bubbles and wait 1 min to remove any bubbles with a piece of paper towel.
- Test diluted emulsion for bubbles before use by dipping a clean unused slide and visualizing under incident red light.
- Dip slides smoothly into emulsion for 4 s. Withdraw slowly and let drain for 4 s.
- Place slides in a ligh-tight slide box in a vertical position.
- Wrap the slide box in aluminium foil and keep in a cold room for 24–48 h in case of ^{32}P-labeled probes, or for 5 d for the first develop when ^{35}S-probes (then after 10 d).
- Prepare developer D19 Kodak as for paper.

11. Develop in a ligh-tight darkroom in ice (10–12°C) as follows:
- 7 min in developer.
- 1 min in water.
- 5 min in rapid fixer prepared for paper.

3.3.8. Analysis of Tumor Infiltrate by Immunohistochemical Staining

Immunohistochemical staining offers the possibility to analyze tumor infiltrate induced by the cytokine produced by engineered tumor cells, or by tumor-cell vaccines, and interactions between reactive cells or between leukocytes and tumor cells *(37)*. By combining *in situ* hybridization with immunohistochemistry it is possible to detect both cytokine gene expression and the presence of a specific protein like a receptor or a cell-differentiation marker, present on the same cell or on different cells within a tissue. In this case, the fixation should preserve the antigenic site as well as the target RNA sequences (usually 0.5–1% paraformaldehyde treatment followed by a wash in 70% ethanol gives ecceptable results). RNAse inhibitors should be included at all stages to prevent RNA degradation during antibody treatments. Finally, the enzyme substrate for immunohistochemistry development should not be soluble in organic solvents, so that the reaction product is not lost during the hybridization procedures.

1. Sectioning frozen tissues
   • Routine sections are cut at 5 μm and picked up on a glass slide pretreated with polylysine (after sequential washing with ETOH 70% and 90% and drying, dip in 1% polylysine in distilled water, air dry and store in a slide box at 4°C for up to 1 mo).
   • Perform sections on the day before staining, and conserve slides at RT and light. This procedure maintains tissue antigens whereas it inhibits enzimatic activity such as endogenous peroxidase activity.
2. Fixation
   • Fix sections in acetone for 10 min at RT.
   • Allow sections to air dry for at least 15 min.
3. Blocking nonspecific binding
   • Incubate sections for 20 min in 1% BSA in TBS or in 6% serum in TBS, using serum from the species used to obtain secondary antibody.
   • Section can be rehidratated in this step by adding 0.02% Tween 20 to the solution. Frozen sections generally do not need this treatment even if nuclear antigens are stained.
4. Incubation with primary antibody
   • Wipe off excess blocking solution from around the specimen with absorbent paper tissue and immediately add 100 μL of the primary antibody diluted in TBS to completely cover the tissue section. Incubate for 30 min at RT. If antisera are used for staining, add 0.1% BSA or 1% serum.
   • Optimal dilutions are usually given for commercial antibodies; generally monoclonals are used at 2.5 μg/mL, antisera at 0.1 μg/mL while hybridoma supernatants diluted 2–5 times. Dilutions vary according to the staining method and shoud be predetermined with the staining method of choice.
5. Incubation with secondary antibody
   • Wash for 5 min with TBS three times
   • Wipe off TBS excess from around the specimen and add secondary antibody as follows:
   a. Direct method:
   • Add secondary antibody labeled with Horse Radish Peroxidase (HRP) or Alcaline Phosphatase (AP) and incubate for 30–40 min at RT. Optimal dilutions are indicated by the manufacturer.
   b. Indirect method (PAP):
   • Add secondary unconjugated "link" antibody (for example, rabbit antimouse if primary antibody is a mouse MAb) and incubate for 30 min at RT.
   • Wash with TBS and wipe as indicated above.
   • Add PAP Complex, comprised of the enzyme peroxidase and an antibody against peroxidase, from the species in which the primary antibody is made and incubate 30 min at RT.
   c. Avidin-biotin or streptoavidin indirect method:
   • Use secondary "link" antibody conjugated to biotin, incubate for 30 min at RT.
   • Wash as indicated above.

- Incubate with avidin-biotin-HRP or avidin-biotin-AP or streptoavidin-HRP or streptoavidin-AP Complex for 30 min at RT. Kits that need a shorter incubation (5–10 min) are commercially available, but they can be used only with primary antibodies from mouse, goat, and rabbit.
- Substrate incubation.
- After incubation, wash as above.
- For peroxidase, incubate for 1–5 min at RT with solution of 0.06% 3-3′–diaminobenzidine tetrahydrochloride (DAB) and 0.03% H_2O_2 in TBS (solution is visibly brown colored) prepared immediately before use. Attention: DAB is considered a possible carcinogen: handle with care and always wear gloves.
- For Alkaline Phosphatase (AP), use commercially available kits. Incubation required: 5–30 min (staining is visible).
- Block staining (both methods) in running tap water, rinse thoroughly, and counterstain.
7. Counterstaining
   - For brown or red staining, counterstain with hematoxylin (1 min incubation), wash well with gently running tap water for 5 min.
   - For blue–black reaction counterstain, using neutral red (incubate 5 min) and rinse under gently running tap water for at least 10 min.
8. Mount slides
   - For DAB and black staining (alcohol insoluble), dehydrate by using growing concentrations of ETOH and xilene and coverslip with xylene or toluene containing mounting media. Fast red, fast blue, or other reaction products that are soluble in alcohol and organic solvents should be coverslipped while still wet using a water-based mounting media.

3.3.9. Antitumor Antibody Responses

The elicitation of antitumor serum antibodies after immunization with tumor vaccines has been reported both in neoplastic patients and in tumor-bearing animals *(21,38–40)*. In order to determine if an antitumor serologic response is induced by the studied-tumor vaccine, reactivity of the sera from treated- and age-matched controls is tested on the relevant and irrelevant tumor cells by indirect immunofluorescence and FACS analysis. Functional characterization of the antitumor antibodies can be achieved by in vitro testing tumor lysis in the presence of complement or of Fc+ lymphoid cells (ADCC).

1. Mice are bled from retroorbital senus under anesthesia, blood is pooled and sera obtained by clotting at 30°C.
2. Stain positive and negative tumor cells with mice sera at dilutions ranging from 1:10–1:200 followed by a second incubation with FITC antimouse Ig or with FITC rat MAbs antimouse IgG1, IgG2a, IgG2b, IgG3, IgM, IgA, IgE to determine immunoglobulin isotype.
3. Analyze staining by flow cytometry.

3.3.10. Assays for Measuring Antitumor Activity of Serum Antibodies (C-dependent Cytotoxicity and ADCC)

To test complement-dependent cytotoxicity ^{51}Cr-release assay can be used.

1. Prepare target cells as indicated in **Subheading 3.3.2.**
2. Add 25 μL sera to 96-well V bottomed plates at four different 1:2 dilutions in triplicate samples. Add medium in Complement and Total Release control wells.
3. Add ^{51}Cr labeled tumor cells (2–10 × 10^3/well) in 25 μl.
4. Incubate plates for 45 min at 37°C.
5. Add 100 μL medium, spin the plate and discart supernatant with a micropipet.
6. Add 100 μL rabbit complement (optimal dilution should be predetermined in pilot assays). In control wells, add 100 μL medium to 100 μL NP40.
7. Incubate 2 h at 37°C.
8. Spin plates 5 min.
9. Harvest supernatants and determine cpm with a counter.
10. Calculate % cytotoxicity as: ([sample cpm] – [complement cpm](/ ([total cpm] – [complement cpm]) × 100.

To assay antitumor effect of sera in Cellular Dependent Cytotoxicity Assay (ADCC) appropriate effector cells should be identified in pilot experiments. Peritoneal-elicited macrophage, SPC and LAK cells have been used for this assay *(37,41)*. For ADCC assay, follow the above indications for complement-dependent cytotoxicity ^{51}Cr-release assay through points 1–6. Then add effector lymphocytes. Follow above points from 7 to 10.

4. Notes

1. Negative results in MLTC (*see* **Subheading 3.3.3.**) may result from several reasons including ineffective irradiation or Mycoplasma contamination of cell lines. It is important to check both these possibilities.
2. Blocking cytotoxicity (*see* **Subheading 3.3.4.**) by MAbs require a preincubation of 30 min of lymphocytes and blocking MAbs in test plates before adding target cells. % blocking is calculated as (% lysis + MAb – % lysis – MAb) × 100/% lysis – MAb *(41)*. Blocking MAbs should be titrated in pilot experiments. Controls include isotype-matched MAbs and unblocked effector cells like LAK cells *(42)*.
3. When pCTL frequencies (*see* **Subheading 3.3.5.**) in LDA experiments are measured to demonstrate differences in response between for example different vaccination groups, comparison is best made within the same experiment. Variables to be set include concentration of stimulating cells, of rIL-2, target cell choice, specificity of the effectors detected. The same method can be used to measure frequency of pCTL producing a specific cytokine upon coculture with the tumor target.
4. *In situ* hybridization (*see* **Subheading 3.3.7.**) requires many different controls. First, whenever possible, the specificity of the hybridization signal must be tested

on Northern blot, because a cross-hybridization with ribosomal RNA, which represents more than 90% of total RNA, is common. Moreover, positive and negative control sections must be set up by treating the specimens with DNAse or RNAse before hybridization or by using a sense RNA probe when riboprobes are utilized. Finally, hybridization with vectors containing sequences that are not expected to be expressed or without any insert should be performed.

5. Frozen sections (*see* **Subheading 3.3.8.**) can be fixed with several fixative agents. Acetone is recommended because it allows the maintenance of almost all antigens and it is very quick.
6. For immunohistochemical staining (*see* **Subheading 3.3.8.**), avoid inhibition of endogenous peroxidase with H_2O_2, since it can damage tissues.

Acknowledgments

We are indebted to Chiara Zilocchi, Barbara Cappetti, Mariella Parenza, and Ivano Arioli for their assistance in the definition of most of the present protocols. We thank Antonella Stoppacciaro for sharing her expertise and Grazia Barp for editing assistance.

References

1. Colombo, M. P., Modesti A., Parmiani G., and Forni G. (1992) Local cytokine availability elicits tumor rejection and systemic immunity through granulocyte-T-lymphocyte cross-talk. *Cancer Res.* **52,** 4853–4857.
2. Colombo, M. P. and Forni, G. (1994) Cytokine gene transfer in tumour inhibition and tentative tumour therapy: where are we now? *Immunol. Today* **15,** 48–50.
3. Paglia, P., Chiodoni, C., Rodolfo, M., and Colombo, M. P. (1996) Murine dendritic cells loaded in vitro with soluble protein prime CTL against tumor antigen in vivo. *J. Exp. Med.* **183,** 317–322.
4. Porgador, A., Snyder, D., and Gilboa, E. (1996) Induction of antitumor immunity using bone marrow-generated dendritic cells. *J. Immunol.* **156,** 2918–2926.
5. Huang, Y. C., Golumbeck, P., Ahmadzadeh, M., Jaffee, E., Pardoll, D., and Levitsky, H. (1994) Role of bone-marrow derived cells in presenting MHC class I-restricted tumor antigens. *Science (Wash., DC)* **264,** 961–965.
6. Bevan, M. J. (1976) Cross-priming for a secondary cytotoxic response to minor H antigens with H-2 congenic cells which do not cross-react in the cytotoxic assay. *J. Exp. Med.* **143,** 1283–1289.
7. Singh, S., Ross, S. R., Acena, M., Rowley, D. A., and Schreiber, H. (1992) Stroma is critical for preventing or permitting immunological destruction of antigenic cancer cells. *J. Exp. Med.* **175,** 139–146.
8. Stoppacciaro, A., Melani, C., Parenza, M., Mastracchio, A., Bassi, C., Baroni, C., et al. (1993) Regression of an established tumor genetically modified to release G-CSF requires granulocyte-T cell cooperation and T cell-produced IFNγ. *J. Exp. Med.* **178,** 151–161.

9. Pedrizet, G. A., Ross, S. R., Stauss, H. J., Singh, S., Koeppen, H., and Schreiber, H. (1990) Animals bearing malignant grafts reject normal grafts that express through gene transfer the same antigen. *J. Exp. Med.* **171,** 1205–1220.

10. Martinotti, A., Stoppacciaro, A., Vagliani, M., Melani, C., Spreafico, F., Wysocka, M., et al. (1995) CD4 T cells inhibits in vivo the CD8-mediated immune response against murine colon carcinoma cells transduced with IL-12 genes. *Eur. J. Immunol.* **25,** 137–146.

11. Boon, T., Cerottini, J. C., Van den Eynde, B., Van der Bruggen, P., and van Pel, A. (1994) Tumor antigens recognized by T lymphocytes. *Annu. Rev. Immunol.* **12,** 337–358.

12. Mandelboim, O., Bar-Haim, E., Vadai, E., Fridkin, M., and Eisenbach, L. (1997) Identification of shared tumor-associated antigen peptides between two spontaneous lung carcinomas *J. Immunol.* **159,** 6030–6036.

13. Peace, D. J., Smith, J. W., Chen, W., You, S. G., Cosand, W. L., Blake, J., and Cheever, M. A. (1994) Lysis of Ras oncogene-transformed cells by specific cytotoxic T lymphocytes elicited by primary in vitro immunization with mutated Ras peptides. *J. Exp. Med.* **179,** 473–479.

14. Bronte, V., Tsung, K., Rao, J. B., Chen, P. W., Wang, M., Rosenberg, S. A., and Restifo, N. P. (1995) IL-2 enhances the function of recombinant poxvirus-based vaccines in the treatment of established pulmonary metastases. *J. Immunol.* **154,** 5282–5289.

15. Russel, W. M. S. and Burch, R. L. (1959) *The Principles of Humane Experimental Technique.* Methuen, London.

16. van Zutphen, L. F. M., Baumans, V., and Beynen, A. C. (1993) *Principles of Laboratory Animal Science.* Amsterdam, Elsevier.

17. Tuffery, A. A. (1987) *Laboratory Animals: An Introduction for New Experimenters.* Wiley, Chichester, England.

18. Donovan, J. and Brown, P. (1995) Care and handling of the laboratory animals, in *Current Protocols in Immunology,* Wiley, England, pp. 1.0.1– 1.10.11.

19. Geran, R. I., Greenberg, N. H., Macdonald, M. M., Shumacher, A. M, and Abbot, B. J. (1972) Protocols for screening chemical agents and natural products against animal tumors and other biological systems. *Cancer Chemother. Rep.* **3,** 1–88.

20. Allione, A., Consalvo, M., Nanni, P., Lollini, P. L., Cavallo, F., Giovarelli, M., et al. (1994) Immunizing and curative potential of replicating and nonreplicating murine mammary adenocarcinoma cells engineered with interleukin (IL)-2, IL-4, IL-6, IL-10, TNFα, GM-CSF, and γ-IFN gene or admixed with conventional adjuvants. *Cancer Res.* **54,** 6022–6026.

21. Rodolfo, M., Zilocchi, C., Melani, C., Cappetti, B., Arioli, I., Parmiani, G., and Colombo, M. P. (1996) Immunotherapy of experimental metastases by vaccination with interleukin gene-transduced adenocarcinoma cells sharing tumor-associated antigens. Comparison between IL-12 and IL-2 gene-transduced tumor cell vaccines. *J. Immunol.* **157,** 5536–5542.

22. Kopper, L., Van Hanh, K., and Lapis, K. (1982) Experimental model for liver metastasis formation using Lewis Lung Tumor *J. Cancer Res. Clin. Oncol.* **103,** 31–38.
23. Saito, S., Bannerji, R., Gansbacher, B., Rosenthal, F. M., Romanenko, P., Heston, W. D., et al. (1994) Immunotherapy of bladder cancer with cytokine gene-modified tumor vaccines. *Cancer Res.* **54,** 3516–3520.
24. Vieweg, J., Heston, W. D., Gilboa, E., and Fair, W. R. (1994) An experimental model simulating local recurrence and pelvic lymph node metastasis following orthotopic induction of prostate cancer. *Prostate* **24,** 291–298.
25. Ashley, D. M., Faiola, B., Nair, S., Hale, L. P., Bigner, D. D., and Gilboa, E. (1997) Bone marrow-generated dendritic cells pulsed with tumor extracts or tumor RNA induce antitumor immunity against central nervous system tumors. *J. Exp. Med.* **186,** 1177–1182.
26. Salup, R. R., Herberman, R. B., and Wiltrout, R. H., (1985) Role of natural killer activity in development of spontaneous metastases in murine renal cancer. *J. Urology* **134,** 1236–1241.
27. Wexler, H. (1966) Accurate identification of experimental pulmonary metastase *J. Natl. Cancer Inst.* **36,** 641–643.
28. Cobbold, S. P., Jayasurija, A., Nash, A., Prospero, T. D., and Waldmann, H. (1984) Therapy with monoclonal antibodies by elimination of T cell subsets. *Nature* **312,** 548–551.
29. Herold, K. C., Montag, A. G., and Fitch, F. W. (1987) Treatment with anti-T-lymphocyte antibodies prevents induction of insulitis in mice given multiple doses of streptozocin. *Diabetes* **36,** 796–801.
30. Kruisbeek, A. D. *In vivo* assays for mouse lymphocyte function, in *Current Protocols in Immunology*, Wiley, England, pp. 4.1.1–4.1.4.
31. Brunner, K. T., Mauel, J., Cerottini, J. C., and Chapuis, B. (1968) Quantitative assay of the lytic action of immune lymphoid cells on ^{51}Cr labeled allogenic target cells in vitro: inhibition by isoantibody and by drugs. *Immunology* **14,** 181–196.
32. Langhorne, J. and Fisher Lindahl, K. (1981) Limiting dilution analysis of precursors of cytotoxic T lymphocytes, in *Immunological Methods vol. 2* (Lefkovits, I. and Pernis, B., eds.), Academic, New York, pp. 221–231.
33. Lefkovits, I. and Waldmann, H. (1979) *Limiting Dilution Analysis of Cells in the Immune System*, Cambridge University Press, England
34. Mac Donald, H. R., Cerottini, J. C., Ryser, J. E., Maryanski, J. L., Tarswell, C., Widmer, M. B., and Brunner, T. K. (1980) Quantitation and cloning of cytolytic T lymphocytes and their precursors *Immunological Rev.* **51,** 93–150.
35. Sharrock, C. E. M, Kaminski, E. M, and Man, S. (1990) Limiting dilution analysis of human T cells: a useful clinical tool. *Immunol. Today* **11,** 281–285.
36. Taswell, C. (1981) Limiting dilution assays for the detrmination of immuno-competent cell frequencies. I. Data analysis. *J. Immunol.* **126,** 1614–1619.

37. Musiani, P., Modesti, A., Giovarelli, M., Cavallo, F., Colombo, M. P., Lollini, P. L., and Forni, G. (1997). Cytokines, tumor-cell death and immunogenicity: a question of choice. *Immunol. Today* **18,** 32–36.
38. Pericle F., Giovarelli, M., Colombo, M. P., Ferrari, G., Musiani, P., Modesti, A., et al. (1994) An efficient Th2-type memory follows CD8$^+$ lymphocyte-driven and eosinophil-mediated rejection of a spontaneous mouse mammary adenocarcinoma engineered to produce IL-4. *J. Immunol.* **153,** 5659–5668.
39. Morton, D., Foshag, L. J., Hoon, D. S. B., Nizze, J. A., Wanek, L. A., Chang, C., et al. (1992) Prolongation of survival in metastatic melanoma after active specific immunotherapy with a new polyvalent melanoma vaccine. *Ann. Surg.* **216,** 463–469.
40. Jager, E., Chen, Y., Drijfhout, M., Karbach, J., Ringhoffer, M., Jager, D., et al. (1998) Simultaneous humoral and cellular immune response against Cancer-Testis antigene NY-ESO-1: definition of human Histocompatibility Leukocyte antigen (HLA)-A2-binding peptide epitopes *J. Exp. Med.* **187,** 265–270.
41. Hara, I., Takechi, Y., and Houghton, A. N. (1995) Implicating a role for immune recognition of self in tumor rejection: passive immunization against the brown locus protein. *J. Exp. Med.* **182,**1609–1614.
42. Bright, R. K., Shearer, M. H., and Kennedy R. C. (1994) Immunization of BALB/c mice with recombinant Simian Virus 40 Large Tumor antigen induces antibody-dependent cell mediated cytotoxicity against Simian virus 40-transformed cells *J. Immunol.* **153,** 2064–2071.
43. Rodolfo, M., Bassi, C., Salvi, C., and Parmiani, G. (1991) Therapeutic use of a long-term cytotoxic T cell line recognizing a common tumour-associated antigen: the pattern of in vitro reactivity predicts the in vivo effect on different tumours. *Cancer Immunol. Immunother.* **34,** 53–57.

2

Particle-Mediated Gene Transfer into Dendritic Cells

A Novel Strategy for the Induction
of Immune Responses against Tumor Antigens

Thomas Tüting and Andreas Albers

1. Introduction

The expression of a foreign protein in the skin following direct in vivo gene transfer results in the induction of potent cellular and humoral immune responses. This strategy, now known as genetic or DNA immunization, was first described by Johnston et al. in 1992. They reported that bombardment of murine skin with an expression plasmid encoding human growth hormone coated onto microscopic gold particles using a gene gun resulted not only in the systemic delivery of the molecule, but also in the induction of antigen-specific antibody responses (*1*). It is now well established that DNA immunization by particle-mediated gene transfer promotes broad-based and long-lasting antigen-specific immune responses capable of protecting against challenges with infectious agents and tumor cells in rodents [reviewed in (*2,3*)]. Importantly, gene gun immunization elicits both humoral and cellular immunity, consisting of antibody responses specific for conformational determinants, as well as, antigen-specific $CD8^+$ cytotoxic T cells and $CD4^+$ T-helper cells. For this reason, it represents an attractive novel approach for the clinical development of prophylactic and therapeutic vaccines against certain infectious diseases and tumors. We are currently investigating, like many other tumor immunologists, whether DNA-based immunization can lead to the induction of potent cellular and humoral immune responses against defined tumor antigens that are associated with tumor rejection activity in vivo.

From: *Methods in Molecular Medicine, Vol. 35: Gene Therapy: Methods and Protocols*
Edited by: W. Walther and U. Stein © Humana Press, Inc., Totowa, NJ

1.1. Dendritic Cells are Critical for the Induction of Immune Responses Following Cutaneous Gene Gun Immunization

The molecular mechanisms responsible for the antigen-specific stimulation of naive lymphocytes following transgenic expression of foreign proteins in the skin has been poorly understood until recently. Studies using bone marrow chimeric mice *(4–7)* have demonstrated that cellular responses to plasmid-encoded antigens are dependent upon bone marrow-derived cells rather than on keratinocytes, which are the predominantly transfected cell type after direct in vivo gene transfer to the skin. These observations were consistent with emerging evidence in the field of immunology, suggesting a pivotal role for the dendritic cell (DC) system of antigen presenting cells (APC) for the induction of cellular immune responses [reviewed in *(8,9)*]. DCs are bone marrow-derived leukocytes that are specialized for antigen capture, processing, and presentation. They are frequently found in the skin and mucous membranes where they function as sentinels of the immune system. Activation of DC in response to inflammatory stimuli followed by antigen capture, functional maturation, and subsequent migration appears to be a key event in initiating immunity. Activated, mature DC localize to T-cell rich areas of secondary lymphoid organs where they display high levels of processed antigen in association with MHC molecules on their cell surface. Most importantly, activated DC produce chemotactic factors for naive T cells and provide the antigen in the context of secondary immunostimulatory signals (costimulatory molecules like B7.1/CD80, B7.2/CD86, and CD40) and immunostimulatory cytokines (like TNF-α, IL-6, and IL-12), which promote the activation and expansion of antigen-specific T cells. Evidence has now accumulated that particle-mediated gene transfer to the skin leads to direct in vivo transfection of cutaneous DC associated with endogenous antigen synthesis and processing *(10)*. Particle bombardment itself appears to represent an activating stimulus for the DC system leading to DC migration to regional lymph nodes, where antigen-expressing DC can efficiently stimulate proliferation of antigen-specific CD8[+] as well as CD4[+] T lymphocytes *(11,12)*. DC migrating out of skin injected with plasmid DNA can stimulate antigen-specific cellular immune responses in vitro and in vivo when transferred to naive mice *(11–14)*. Advances in cell-culture technology now allow for the in vitro generation of immunostimulatory dendritic cells from precursors in bone marrow or peripheral blood *(15–16)*. Cultured DC, gene gun-transfected in vitro with antigen-encoding plasmid DNA, are also capable of stimulating antigen-specific immune responses in vitro and, following their adoptive transfer, in vivo *(17–19)*. The possibility to immunize with cultured DC genetically engineered to endogenously express a given antigen represents an exciting new method both for basic science and clinical applications.

1.2. The Immune Response Can Be Manipulated at the Molecular Level

The use of plasmid DNA as a source of antigen for gene gun immunization opens up a number of completely new strategies allowing researchers to investigate the regulation of adoptive immunity and try to deliberately influence the nature of immune responses. This can be achieved by simultaneous delivery of plasmids encoding immunomodulatory proteins, revealing their role in the recruitment, antigen-capture, activation, and migration of DC, as well as, in the stimulation of responding T and B cells. As an example, codelivery of plasmid DNA encoding the costimulatory molecules B7 and CD40L and the cytokines GM-CSF, IFN-α, or IL-12 have been shown to enhance the induction of cellular immune responses following DNA immunization in mice *(20–24)*. These factors are known to stimulate growth and maturation of DC and influence the expansion and phenotype of responding T cells. Another attractive idea is the possibility to selectively target antigen into the processing machinery of immunostimulatory DC for effective presentation to both CD8[+] and CD4[+] T lymphocytes. This is currently being attempted by translational targeting of antigen expression in dendritic cells in vivo using a DC-specific promoter element or by transfection and adoptive transfer of cultured DC. Furthermore, genetic reengineering of the actual antigen-encoding cDNA allows for targeting antigen into MHC Class I and II loading compartments by manipulation of signals governing intracellular protein transport *(25,26)*.

1.3. Gene Gun Immunization Can Be Applied for the Induction of Immune Responses Against Defined Tumor Antigens

With the molecular identification of tumor antigens *(27,28)*, there has been increasing interest in DNA immunization for the development of active specific tumor vaccines. It is envisioned that such strategies may be clinically applied in an adjuvant setting to cancer patients who are macroscopically tumor-free following successful surgery. It is hypothesized that the induction of a strong antigen-specific immune response can eliminate residual tumor cells resulting in a clinical benefit by reducing the risk of recurrence. We and others have shown that DNA immunization of mice with model tumor antigens such as chicken ovalbumin or β-galactosidase *(10,21–23)* induced protective immune responses leading to partial rejection of a subsequent, normally lethal challenge with tumor cells expressing the respective model antigen. More

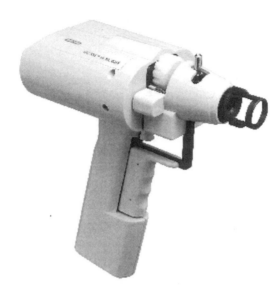

Fig. 1. Helios Gene Gun.

recently, DNA immunization has also been shown effective in murine models employing clinically relevant tumor antigens. Tumor rejection activity was observed following immunization with a mutated form of the transformation-related antigen p53 (22), with the idiotypic determinant of the immunoglobulin expressed on the surface of a B-cell lymphoma (29), with the tumor-specific "cancer-testes" antigen P815 (30), and with melanocyte differentiation antigens such as gp100, TRP-1, and TRP-2 (31–33). Studies are underway in a large number of laboratories to characterize the antitumor immune responses induced following DNA immunization in greater detail. Careful comparisons with established vaccination methods need to be performed. Furthermore, strategies for immunization need to be optimized, for example by targeting tumor antigen-expression to DC. Eventually, clinical trials will have to be conducted in cancer patients. The early results of clinical trials involving DNA immunization for the prevention and treatment of infectious diseases appear to be promising (34–37).

1.4. Particle-Mediated Gene Transfer Directly Delivers Plasmid DNA to the Nucleus

The general principles of particle-mediated gene transfer have been detailed by Rakhmilevich and Yang in Chapter 20. Briefly, plasmid DNA is precipitated onto 0.6–3 μm gold beads, which are subsequently loaded into pieces of plastic tubing as a cartridge, and placed in the gene gun (**Fig. 1**). A short helium pulse accelerates the plasmid-coated gold beads towards the target

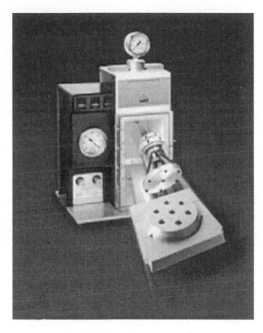

Fig. 2. Biolistic PDS/1000He with sevenfold pressure distribute.

tissue, resulting in efficient intracellular delivery of high copy numbers of DNA in vivo. Particle-mediated gene transfer has recently been technologically advanced for effective ex vivo gene delivery into cells in culture. A vacuum chamber is used for gentle acceleration of gold beads. Additionally, the ballistic approach is combined with magnetic separation of transfected cells. This system is now called ballistomagnetic vector system (BMVS) (**Fig. 2**). Gold particles are simultaneously coated with nucleic acids and superparamagnetic beads and propelled into target cells. It can be shown that plasmid DNA and magnetic beads penetrate plasma membranes and other cellular barriers and are directly delivered into the nucleus of mammalian cells. This is of particular importance for expression of transgenes because plasmid DNA can only become transcriptionally active if it reaches the nucleoplasm. Superparamagnetic beads, simultaneously delivered with the nucleic acids, allow for efficient separation of transfected and nontransfected cells in a high gradient magnetic field (Schroff et al., manuscript submitted). A new procedure of plating cells on microporous polycarbonate supports has been developed to improve gene transfer efficiency, as well as, recovery and viability of cells. In this way, subsequent enrichment of the ballistomagnetically transfected cell population via high gradient magnetic separation columns becomes much more efficient (Albers et al., manuscript in preparation).

1.5. Practical Considerations

We describe here the use of particle-mediated gene transfer for the induction of immune responses against (tumor) antigens in murine tumor models. We recommend that interested researchers begin their experiments with marker genes such as β-galactosidase and EGFP, which can be readily detected and can simultaneously serve as model tumor antigens. We have found β-galactosidase very convenient in mice, since several CTL-defined peptide epitopes have been identified for both BALB/c and C57BL/6 strains and β-galactosidase is available as a recombinant protein. Mice can be immunized by directly bombarding the skin with plasmid DNA. Here we describe the preparation of cartridges with DNA-coated gold beads and the in vivo gene transfer into skin using the Helios Gene Gun. We also describe protocols for the measurement of humoral and cellular immune responses using β-galactosidase in BALB/c mice. These protocols can subsequently be adopted to other antigens.

Alternatively to direct in vivo immunization with the Helios Gene Gun, mice can be immunized by injection of genetically modified immunostimulatory dendritic cells. Cultured DC can be transfected with the hand held gene gun. Transfected DC can subsequently be used to immunize mice and immune responses monitored. However, we believe that the ballistomagnetic transfer using the Biolistic PDS/1000He system modified by a sevenfold pressure distributor system ensuring particle distribution over the entire Petri dish will be much more suitable for efficient and reproducible gene transfer to cultured DC in vitro. This system has optimized physical parameters for in vitro particle-mediated gene delivery and allows simultaneous transfection of large numbers of cells. We are currently evaluating this system for gene transfer to cultured DC. Gold particles (usually 1.6 μm in diameter) are coated with a mixture of plasmid DNA and much smaller superparamagnetic particles (65 nm in diameter). Following ballistomagnetic gene transfer, cells are immediately washed, resuspended, and transferred onto a high gradient magnetic separation column to enrich for cells containing paramagnetic beads (and DNA). This procedure ensures that >90% of living cells contains DNA, a subset of which will express the gene (or genes) of interest. The ballistomagnetic vector system has been established for the production of genetically modified tumor cell vaccines under GMP conditions at the Centrum Somatische Gentherapie, Berlin, Germany. It has proven to be highly reproducible and can readily be quality controlled and, therefore, appears ideally suited for possible future clinical applications regarding genetic immunization with tumor antigen-transfected DC.

2. Materials

2.1. Mice, Cell Lines, Media, and Cytokines

1. Female C57BL/6 (H–2^b) and BALB/cJ (H–2^d) mice, 6–10 wks old. We have purchased from any of the large vendors (i.e., Charles Rivers, Jackson Laboratory, or Taconics).
2. EL4 is a murine thymoma available from the American Type Culture Collection (Rockville, MD). EL4-transfectants expressing β-galactosidase, EGFP or hgp100 have been generated from various laboratories. C3 is an HPV 16-transformed murine sarcoma *(38)*. C26 is a chemically induced BALB/c murine adenocarcinoma *(39)*.
3. Our cell culture medium (CM) consists of RPMI-1640 supplemented with 10% heat-inactivated FCS, 2 mM l-glutamine, 1 mM sodium pyruvate, 0.1 mM nonessential amino acids, 0.1 mM HEPES, 50 µM 2-ME, 100 IU/mL penicillin, and 100 µg/mL streptomycin. All cell culture reagents can be purchased from Life Technologies.
4. Recombinant murine IL-4, murine GM-CSF, and human IL-2. We use cytokines given to us from Schering-Plough Research Institute (New Jersey) and Chiron (Emeryville, CA). They can be bought from commercial suppliers such as Genzyme as well. Cytokines are diluted to 10^6 U/mL of complete medium and stored frozen at –80°C. Once thawed, they can be stored at 4°C and should be used within 4 wks.

2.2. Plasmid DNA, Synthetic Peptides, β-Galactosidase Detection

1. Plasmids encoding reporter genes or tumor antigens: pCI-*βgal*, pCI-*EGFP*, pCI-*E7*, pCI-*hgp100*. These plasmids were constructed by inserting fragments containing the *Escherichi coli βgal* gene, the *EGFP* gene (Clontech, Palo Alto, CA), the ORF of human papilloma virus (HPV) 16-E7, or the cDNA encoding the melanosomal protein gp100/pmel17 into the expression vector pCI (Promega, Madison, WI). We grow plasmids in *E. coli* strain DH5α, use Qiagen Endofree Plasmid Maxi Kits (Qiagen, Chatsworth, CA) for purification, resuspend in distilled water, and store plasmids at –20° (*see* **Note 1**).
2. CTL-defined synthetic peptides: We have used the H-2K^b-binding βgal-encoded peptide DAPIYTNV (βgal$_{96–103}$), the H-2L^d-binding βgal-encoded peptide TPHPARIGL (βgal$_{876–884}$), the H-2D^b-binding HPV-E7-encoded peptide RAHYNIVTF (E7$_{49–57}$), and the H-2D^b-binding hgp100-encoded peptide KVPRNQDWL (hgp100$_{25–33}$). These peptides were synthesized commercially by standard F-moc chemistry and purified by HPLC. Peptides are diluted at 10 mg/mL in PBS containing various amounts of DMSO and stored frozen at –20°C (*see* **Note 2**).
3. Reagents for detection of β-galactosidase: X-gal substrate (5-bromo-4-chloro-3-indolyl-β-D-galactopyranoside, Sigma Chemical Co., St. Louis, MO) dissolved

in dimethyl formamide at 20 mg/mL (can be stored frozen at –20°C). Mix prior to use 1:25 (40 µL/mL) with buffer solution containing 44 mM HEPES buffer, 3.1 mM K$^+$ ferricyanide, 3.1 mM K$^+$ ferrocyanide, 150 mM NaCl, 10 mM Na$_2$HPO$_4$, 10 mM Na$_2$HPO$_4$, 1 mM MgCl$_2$, pH 7.4 mL (can also be stored frozen at –20°C).

2.3. DC Culture and Phenotyping

1. 70% EtOH, scalpel, scissors, forceps, 10 cm Petri dishes, 18G and 23G needles, 10/20 mL syringes, 50 mL polypropylene tubes, 6-well plates, cell strainer (70 µm nylon, Falcon 2350) or sterile nylon mesh (*see* **Note 3**).
2. RBC lysing buffer (Sigma Chemical Co.) or self-made: Dissolve 8.29 g NH$_4$Cl in 700 ml dH$_2$O on stirrer, add 1g KHCO$_3$, and finally 0.0372 g of Na$_2$EDTA. Fill up to 1 L, filter-sterilize.
3. Hybridoma supernatants (optional): anti-mCD4 (L3T4, ATCC TIB 207); anti-mCD8 (Lyt 2.2, ATCC TIB 210); anti-B220 (ATCC TIB 146).
4. Antibodies for FACS staining: Isotype controls, anti-IA^b or -IA^d, anti-CD40, anti-B7.1 (CD80), anti-B7.2 (CD86), and anti-CD11c, anti-B220, anti-CD3, anti-GR-1, and anti-NK1.1. All antibodies are available from Pharmingen (*see* **Note 4**).

2.4. Handheld Gene Gun

1. The Helios Gene Gun System is now available from Bio-Rad (Richmond, CA) including helium regulator, tubing prep station, and tubing cutter.
2. Helium gas 4.6, personal hearing protection.
3. Gold beads: Bio-Rad sells 1.6 µm gold beads. We have also successfully used 1–3 µm beads purchased from Strem Chemicals (*see* **Note 5**).
4. Tefzel Tubing.
5. Analytical balance, microfuge, ultrasonic cleaner bath, hair clippers.
6. 15 mL and 50 mL polypropylene tubes, 1.5 mL microfuge tubes.
7. Spermidine, CaCl$_2$, 100% (dry) ethanol, polyvinylpyrrolidone PVP (Sigma Chemical Co.).

2.5. Ballistomagnetic Vector System (BMVS)

1. The Biolistic PDS 1000/He System for particle mediated gene delivery including the Hydra-Adaptor and the membrane vacuum pump Vaccubrand MZ 2C is available from Bio-Rad.
2. Gold beads/microcarrier: Bio-Rad sells good quality beads (Ø 0.6 µm, 1.0 µm, and 1.6 µm).
3. Stopping-screens.
4. Macrocarrier.
5. Rupture discs 450 psi–2200 psi.
6. Superparamagnetic beads, separation columns, and the magnet are available from Miltenyi Biotec.
7. Superparamagnetic beads: Basic MicroBeads.
8. Separation columns: Depletion Column Type AS.

9. Magnetic cell separator: VarioMACS.
10. Helium gas 4.6.
11. PBS without Ca^{2+} and Mg^{2+} (Biowhittaker).

2.6. Detection of Immune Responses

1. ELISA-Reader, dissecting microscope, gamma counter.
2. ELISA plates (we use Nunc Maxisorp).
3. Recombinant β-galacatosidase protein (Sigma).
4. Peroxidase-conjugated goat antimouse IgG Ab (Sigma), isotype-specific goat antimouse IgG_1 and IgG_{2a} Ab, peroxidase-conjugated donkey antigoat IgG Ab (Jackson Research Lab.), We use TMB peroxidase Substrate System (Kierkegaard and Perry) for detection.
5. Millipore HA ELISPOT plates.
6. Antibodies to mouse IFN-γ: purified antimouse IFN-γ (clone R4-6A2, Pharmingen) for capture and biotinylated rat antimouse IFN-γ (clone XMG1.2, Pharmingen) for detection; streptavidin-peroxidase conjugate (Boehringer Mannheim, Mannheim, Germany); peroxidase substrate kit DAB (Vector Labs., Burlingame, CA).
7. BSA fraction V, Tween 20, PBS, Thimerosal (Sigma).
8. Na_2CO_3, $NaHCO_3$, NaCl, $NaH_2PO_4 \times 2H_2O$.
9. 24-well and 96-well round-bottom plates.
10. $Na_2{}^{51}CrO_4$ (NEN-Dupont, Bedford, MA).
11. Titer tubes (Bio-Rad).

3. Methods

3.1. Gene Transfer Directly to Skin In Vivo

3.1.1. Coating DNA on Gold Particles

1. We routinely use 0.5-in cartridges containing 1 µg DNA coated onto 0.5 mg gold beads. In each preparation we aim for 50 cartridges and need 25 mg gold and 50 µg DNA.
2. Make a 0.05M Spermidine solution and a 1M $CaCl_2$ solution. Dissolve PVP at 1 mg/mL in 100% ethanol and seal with parafilm. All solutions can be stored frozen at –20°C.
3. Weigh 25 mg gold for 25 inches of tubing (= 50 bullets) in a 1.5-mL microcentrifuge tube.
4. Resuspend 25 mg gold in 100 µL 0.05M spermidine, vortex and sonicate briefly in the ultrasound cleaner bath to disrupt clumps. Add 50 µg of plasmid DNA in 50 µL water and vortex. Plasmid DNA should be at 1 µg/mL in distilled water.
5. While vortexing, slowly add 100 µL of 1M $CaCl_2$ dropwise to precipitate DNA onto gold beads. Allow gold beads to settle for 10 min (*see* **Note 6**).
6. Centrifuge beads and remove supernatant. Disrupt pellet and wash three times with 100% ethanol to remove H_2O. Resuspend gold beads in 200 µl of 100%

ethanol containing 0.075 mg/mL of PVP and transfer to a 15-mL polypropylene tube. Add 3 mL of 100% ethanol containing 0.075 mg/mL. The DNA-coated bead suspension can be stored several weeks at –20°C. Seal tubes with parafilm before freezing.

3.1.2. Loading DNA-Coated Gold Particles into Tefzel Tubing

1. Set up tubing prep station and connect to nitrogen tank. Flush tubing 15 min with nitrogen prior to loading with beads to dry completely (*see* **Note 7**).
2. Vortex and sonicate the ethanol solution containing the DNA-coated gold beads. Immediately draw the solution into the tubing using the syringe and load into the tubing prep station.
3. Allow beads to settle for 3–5 min.
4. Remove ethanol at 0.5–1.0 in/s from the Tefzel tubing, quickly turn the tubing by hand, and start to rotate the tubing to distribute the gold beads evenly.
5. After 30 s, turn on the nitrogen flow (0.4 LPM) and dry gold beads inside the tubing for about 5–10 min (*see* **Note 8**).
6. Cut tubing in bullets 0.5-m inches long. Store in 50 mL polypropylene tubes along with dessiccant pellets. Seal with parafilm and store bullets at 4°C. Bullets are stable for several months (*see* **Note 9**).

3.1.3. Gene Gun Immunization of Mice

1. Shave the abdominal skin of the mice and label the cages. Load the cartridges into the cartridge holder. Put on hearing protection.
2. Prepare the gene gun and test its function with an empty cartridge holder, setting the discharge pressure to 400 psi (*see* **Note 10**).
3. Load gene gun with full cartridge holder and immunize mice.
4. We routinely immunize by bombarding the abdomen. In this way, one can conveniently hold the mouse and shoot without anaesthesia. We usually shoot twice, resulting in the delivery of 2 μg of plasmid DNA for each immunizations.
5. You can sacrifice mice 24–36 h following particle-mediated gene transfer, depilate and harvest bombarded skin, snap freeze in liquid nitrogen, and store at –80°. Cryosections can be fixed in 0.5% glutaraldehyde, stained for β-gal expression with X-gal (5-bromo-4-chloro-3-indolyl-β-D-galactopyranoside, Sigma Chemical Co.) 1 h at room temperature, counterstained with hematoxylin, and analyzed. EGFP expression can be directly visualized under a fluorescent microscope.

3.2. Gene Transfer to DC In Vitro and Adoptive Transfer

3.2.1. Culture of DC

1. Sacrifice mouse immediately before harvest. Clean mouse with 70% EtOH. Make a transverse incision across belly and deskin mouse to expose the entire hind legs.
2. Using scalpel or fine sterile scissors, remove femur and tibia bilaterally, taking care to remove as much surrounding muscle as possible (bone does not need to be completely clean). Place bones in Petri dish on ice.

3. Put 3 Petri dishes under hood, one with 70% EtOH, two with RPMI-1640 (no serum). Place bones for 2 min in alcohol, then wash in RPMI-1640 and transfer to third dish with RPMI-1640.

4. Taking the femur, cut off the epiphyseal plates at both ends of the bone (area of thickening) until the red bone marrow is visible centrally. Using a 23G needle attached to a 10/20 mL syringe, squirt 1–2 cc RPMI-1640 through the bone marrow canal (from top to bottom) into the Petri dish. You should see the red marrow contents exit the bone. Harvest the bone marrow from the tibia similarly.

5. Disrupt cell clusters by vigorous pipeting and filter through a cell strainer (70 μm nylon, Falcon 2350) or sterile nylon mesh into a 50 mL tube to remove all debris.

6. Centrifuge at 600g for 5 min at RT. Decant supernatant.

7. Resuspend the pellet in 1 mL/per mouse of red blood cell lysing buffer, incubate at RT for 2 min. Neutralize with 10–20 mL complete medium.

8. Centrifuge cells again and resuspend pellet in 10–20 mL complete medium and count. Yield should be approximately 25×10^6 cells/mouse. Dilute and distribute cells into 6-well (we used Costar or Falcon plates) at 10^6 cells/3 mL medium containing 500 U/mL mGM-CSF + 500 U/mL IL-4/well (*see* **Notes 11** and **12**).

9. After 48 h, remove 2 mL of the medium after *gentle* swirling of the plate. This removes many of the contaminant B cells, granulocytes, and NK cells. Care must be taken not to disrupt the DC clusters that are loosely adherent. Add 2 mL of fresh cytokine-containing medium.

10. After 4 and 6 d, fresh cytokine-containing medium should be added/replaced (2 mL/well). After 7–8 d, you will have about 20×10^6 cells per mouse with approximately 60–80% of total cells exhibiting DC morphology and phenotype (MHC II$^+$, CD40$^+$, B7.1$^+$, B7.2$^+$, CD11c$^+$, B220$^-$, Gr1$^-$, CD3$^-$, NK1.1$^-$) (*see* **Note 13**).

11. This system has also been developed using 1.5% freshly harvested autologous mouse serum (MS) instead of FBS in the culture medium. If MS is used, yields are reduced significantly on day 7–8 harvests.

3.2.2. In Vitro Gene Transfer to DC Using the Hand-Held Gene Gun

1. Harvest murine bone marrow-derived DC, count, and centrifuge. Meanwhile, prewet 6-well plates with HEPES-buffered complete medium and prepare the gun.

2. Carefully resuspend DC in HEPES-buffered complete medium at 2×10^6 cells/ 25μL per transfection and place on ice. Completely remove medium from 6-well plates, leaving only a film that will allow the DC suspension to spread evenly.

3. Place 2×10^6 DC/25μl in the center of the well, shoot from optimal distance as recommended by the manufacturer, and immediately add CM. We have bombarded at a pressure range of 250–300 psi of helium with the Accell device using a "spinner," which is placed in front of the cylinder and rotates the helium flow to give an even distribution of gold beads over the target range (*see* **Note 14**).

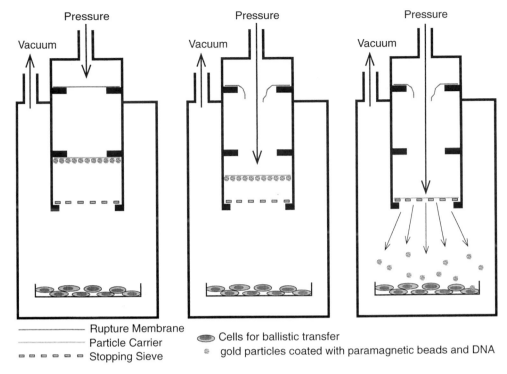

——————— Rupture Membrane
················· Particle Carrier   Cells for ballistic transfer
= = = = = Stopping Sieve   gold particles coated with paramagnetic beads and DNA

Fig. 3. Operation of the Biolistic Device for in vitro gene transfer to cell suspension.

3.2.3. In Vitro Gene Transfer Using the Ballistomagnetic Vector System (BMVS) Operation of the Biolistic Device (**Fig. 3**)

1. Pipet 15 µL of a colliodal gold suspension (60 mg Au/mL H_2O) in the center of seven macrocarrier, let the gold particles sediment, remove carefully excess supernatant water (*see* **Note 15**).
2. Resuspend the gold particles in 30 µl of a mixture of three parts of DNA (1 µg/µl) and one part superparamagnetic bead solution (*see* **Note 16**).
3. Let the gold particles sediment again, remove the supernatant, let the gold particles dry (*see* **Note 17**).
4. Load the seven macrocarrier into the launch assembly and mount the pressure distributor and the launch assembly into the Biolistic PDS/1000He system.
5. Remove all supernatant from the cells to be transfected.
6. Place the Petri dish containing the cells into transfection chamber.
7. Draw vacuum to 20 in Hg and operate the Biolistic PDS/1000He.
8. Resuspend the cells immediately after transfection in PBS containing 1% FCS and 2 m*M* EDTA.

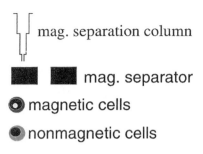

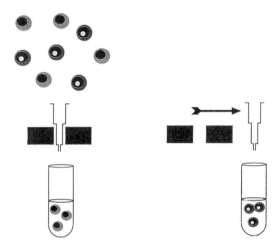

Fig. 4. Magnetic enrichment of cell populations containing plasmid DNA on paramagnetic beads.

3.2.4. Enrichment of the Transfected Cell Population (**Fig. 4**)

1. Equilibrate the separation column carefully according to the supplier's protocol (*see* **Note 18**).
2. Sediment the cells at 400*g* at 4°C for 7 min, resupend cells in 1 mL PBS containing 1% FCS and 2 m*M* EDTA.
3. Keep an aliquot of the unsorted cell fraction for reference and total cell count.
4. Place the assembled column in the magnetic separator.
5. Load the cells onto the column and wash with 3 mL PBS (*see* **Note 19**).
6. Collect the effluent as "nonmagnetic fraction."
7. Remove the column from the separator and flush back the retained cells.
8. Place the column in the magnetic separator and wash with 3 mL PBS containing 1% FCS and 2 m*M* EDTA.

9. Collect the effluent as "wash fraction."
10. Remove the column from the separator.
11. Elute the enriched cell population.
12. Wash the cells and proceed with your protocol.

3.2.5. Genetic Immunization of Mice by Adoptive Transfer of Genetically Engineered DC

1. You should let the DC recover in the incubator for 2–3 h before carefully washing and injecting them into mice. Keep them in polypropylene tubes (slightly open) because of their tendency to adhere to plastic.
2. Place the tubes on ice to detach DC before washing them two times with PBS followed by centrifugation at 600g for 5 min with PBS. Carefully resuspend the cells each time and fill into 1 mL insulin syringes with a 30G needle.
3. We recommend to immunize mice by injecting 2.5 x 105 DC suspended in 0.5 mL of PBS via the tail vein. We are currently comparing the efficacy of intraperitoneal and subcutaneous DC injections, which would be much more simple to perform.
4. You may repeat the immunization after 7 d and monitor immune responses 7 d later.

3.3. Detection of Immune Responses

3.3.1. Detection of Antigen-Specific Antibodies

1. Obtain serum samples from mice at various time-points after gene gun immunization by tail vein bleeding. Anti-βgal antibodies can be measured easily by ELISA using rβgal as a solid-phase Ag.
2. Coat ELISA microtiter plates with 5 µg/mL rβgal in 100 mM carbonate buffer (30 mM Na$_2$CO$_3$ and 70 mM NaHCO$_3$, pH 9.6) for 16 h at 4° and block with PBS containing 3% BSA and 0.05% Tween for at least 1 h.
3. Dilute serum samples serially in PBS containing 1% BSA and 0.05% Tween (assay buffer), fill into the ELISA plate and incubate 1 h at RT.
4. Detect bound antibodies using peroxidase-conjugated goat antimouse Ab (Sigma) at a 1 : 10,000 dilution for 1 h at RT.
5. Alternatively, you can detect γ_1 and γ_{2a} isotypes using isotype-specific goat antimouse Ab (Sigma) at a 1 : 10,000 dilution in assay buffer followed by peroxidase-conjugated donkey antigoat Ab (Jackson Research Lab., Bar Harbor, ME) at a 1:20,000 dilution in assay buffer.
6. Develop color using TMB (Peroxidase Substrate System, Kierkegaard and Perry, Gaithersburg, MD) according to the manufacturers instructions and read the OD450 in an ELISA plate reader (*see* **Note 20**).

3.3.2. Detection of Antigen-Specific Cytokine Release (ELISPOT)

1. Prepare ELSIPOT plates by coating sterile Millipore HA overnight at 4°C with 10 µg/mL purified anti-IFN-γ coating mAb in sterile PBS (50 µL/well). Wash plates with sterile PBS and block with 200 µL of complete medium at 37°C.

2. Harvest and pool splenocytes from two immunized mice in each group (including two nonimmunized littermates) at various time points after immunization. Mince spleens with scissors or with a stainless steel mesh, filter through 70 μm cell strainer, deplete red blood cells in lysing buffer as described for DC culture, and wash splenocytes twice in complete medium.

3. Restimulate lymphocytes in triplicates for about 22 h in ELISPOT plates at 1×10^6 and 3×10^5 cells in 200 μL of CM containing 1 μg/mL $\beta gal_{876-884}$ peptide and 25 IU/mL recombinant human IL-2 (Chiron) per well. Include control peptides and medium alone.

4. Wash ELISPOT plates three times in PBS containing 0.1% Tween 20. Add 2.5 μg/mL biotinylated anti-IFN-γ MAb (50 μL/well) and incubate for 2 h at 37°C.

5. Wash ELISPOT plates three times in PBS containing 0.1% Tween 20. Add SA-POD diluted 1 : 1000 in assay buffer (see above) for 1/2 h at RT.

6. Wash ELISPOT plates three times in PBS containing 0.1% Tween 20. Mix DAB substrate according to the manufacturer's instruction and develop color with 50 μL/well. It should take about 5 min, check under a dissecting microscope, which you can also use for quantitation.

7. Rinse the plates thoroughly under tap water and let dry overnight. You can detach the filter membranes by mounting them on an adhesive membrane normally used to seal ELISA plates.

8. Count the fuzzy spots on the filter under the dissecting microscope (*see* **Note 21**).

3.3.2. Detection of Antigen-Specific Cytotoxicity

1. Alternatively, you can restimulate lymphocytes in 24-well plates (at 37°C in 5% CO_2-humidified air) at 4×10^6 cells in 2 mL of CM containing 1 μg/mL $\beta gal_{876-884}$ peptide and 25 IU/mL recombinant human IL-2 (Chiron) per well.

2. Harvest lymphocytes after 5 d and test for their cytolytic reactivity against peptide-pulsed target cells in standard 4 h ^{51}Cr release assays using 96-well round-bottom plates. We use EL4 or C26, which grow well and are reliably loaded with chromium. You still need to be religious with the culture. The cells have to be in log phase growth and very happy. We pass them 4 and 2 d before each assay.

3. Label 2×10^6 target cells with 100 μCi $Na_2^{51}CrO_4$ for 1 h at 37°C. Wash two times. Prepare peptide-pulsed targets by addition of 1 μg/mL peptide during radiolabeling.

4. Set up the assay in triplicate using 5000–10,000 target cells and titrated numbers of effectors in 200 μL of complete medium per well (for example 50 : 1, 25 : 1, and 12.5 : 1). Set up maximum release with target cells in 5% Triton-X and spontaneous release with target cells in medium only (*see* **Note 22**).

5. Centrifuge the plates and incubate for 4 h at 37°C and 5% CO_2. Centrifuge again, harvest 100 μL of supernatant into titer tubes, and count in a gamma counter.

6. The percentage of ^{51}Cr release is determined by the following formula: mean experimental release-mean spontaneous release/mean maximum release-mean spontaneous release.

3.3.3. Assessment of Antitumor Immunity In Vivo: Resistance to Tumor Challenge

1. The prinicple goal of an effective tumor vaccine is the induction of immune protection against a tumor challenge.
2. We recommend starting tumor challenge experiments using tumor cells stably transfected with immunogenic model antigens such as β-galactosidase. You can challenge subcutaneously or intravenously (for lung metastases). Determine the minimal tumorigenic dose and the tumor growth curve. Challenge with 2–10x cells following DNA immunization. This should work reasonably well. You can then switch to your tumor antigen of choice.
3. We have successfully used genetic immunization in mice for the viral tumor antigen HPV16-E7, which is latently expressed by the HPV16-transformed murine sarcoma C3. Gene gun immunizations with a plasmid expressing HPV16-E7 or with gene gun transfected DC expressing HPV16-E7 completely protected C57BL/6 mice against a tumor challenge with C3.

4. Notes

1. A clean preparation of plasmid DNA resuspended in destilled water at 1 μg/mL should be employed. We routinely check by restriction digest and have never had any trouble with plasmid DNA purified using Quiagen columns. CsCl-purification, however, should work equally well.
2. Depending on the hydrophobicity of the respective peptide, you should try to dissolve the peptide in a smaller amount of either PBS or DMSO. If you have problems getting the peptide into solution, you can then adjust accordingly. The DMSO content should be as low as possible (usually 10–50%), because it is toxic to cells.
3. You need to use polypropylene for DC handling. Cultured DC tend to stick to the plastic and polysterene is even worse.
4. For a minimal FACS analysis of DC, you need to have antibodies to MHC Class II, CD11c, and CD86. The major contaminating cell types are granulocytes, B cells, and NK cells.
5. Gold particles can be obtained of different sizes and shapes. Each lot should be microscopically examined. One must bear in mind that the shape and size of the gold beads will determine their impulse and, consequently, their penetration into tissues and cells. For in vivo transfection, a mixture of different sizes may be beneficial since gold will penetrate the skin to various depths. For in vitro gene transfer to suspension cells in a monolayer, a homogenous sample of gold beads is paramount in order to reach exactly the same level of penetration.
6. This procedure sounds difficult, but is actually rather simple and foolproof. We have never had any trouble coating the gold with plasmid DNA.
7. Especially during humid weather conditions, it is important to dry the tubing first. The major problem preventing an even loading of the tubing with gold beads

appears to be residual water in the ethanol. For this reason you seal PVP and beads in 100% ethanol with parafilm and wait until they acquire room temperature before opening. Try to use fresh 100% ethanol whenever possible.

8. Loading rarely turns out perfect. The quality of the DNA appears to influence the fine distribution of the beads in the cartrdge. Surprisingly, even rather unevenly loaded cartridges work well for immunization. You can test the DNA precipitation onto the gold beads. Place three bullets in a 1.5 mL microfuge with 600 μL destilled water. Vortex, sonicate, rinse, and centrifuge. Measure OD_{260}. It should be close to 0.05 (= 1.5 μg/mL).

9. You can also test the cartridges by discharge onto parafilm or into agar plates (you can use plates to grow bacteria or prepare some with 3% water agar). Cut sections and observe the distribution of gold beads under the microscope.

10. We have had best results at 400 psi in mice. You should start the experiments with β-gal and EGFP as marker genes and simultaneous test antigens. Expression in the skin can be conveniently detected and immune responses analyzed.

11. Immunodepletion of contaminant cells can be performed on the bone marrow cell suspension using hybridoma supernatants (0.5–1 mL of anti-B220, ATCC TIB 146, anti-IA, anti GR-1) and either magnetic beads or rabbit complement according to standard protocols. In our hands, this has not consistently increased the purity of the DC culture. However, it can reduce the yield considerably, depending on the reagents.

12. DC can be enriched by density gradient centrifugation over metrizamide gradients (14.5 mg/mL complete medium). There is considerable debate how to obtain the best and most immunostimulatory DC population. The addition of CD40L or TNF-α during the last 2 d of culture has been reported to increase the percentage of dendritic cells expressing high levels MHC Class II and B7.2. These cultures have been more efficient in vivo.

13. For phenotyping, DC are washed in PBS supplemented with 2%FCS, 1 m*M* EDTA, 0.1% NaN_3 (FACS-staining buffer) and incubated (30 min at 4°C) with one of the following mAb: Isotype controls, anti-IA^b or -IA^d, anti-CD40, anti-B7.1 (CD80), anti-B7.2 (CD86), and anti-CD11c for the detection of dendritic cells. Contaminating cells can be visualized by using anti-B220, anti-CD3, anti-GR-1, and anti-NK1.1 (C57BL/6 only). Antibodies are either directly PE- /FITC-conjugated or a secondary antibody is used.

14. We have used the prototype Accell helium pulse gun kindly provided by Geniva (Middleton, WI). We have not extensively tested the Helios Gene Gun available from Bio-Rad for this purpose yet. Overall, transgene expression has been rather low when bombarding primary dendritic cell cultures as assessed by luciferase assays. However, gene gun transduction has been very reliable in our hands when compared to other nonviral gene delivery methods. We recommend to use one of the longterm dendritic cell lines which have been established in various labs *(18)*.

15. To avoid clumping of the gold particles, wash them two times in 70% ethanol p.a and two times in aqua ad in inectablia under sterile conditions.

16. Plasmid DNA needs to be prepared under sterile conditions. We routinely use endotoxin free plasmid preps (Qiagen, Chattsworth, CA) and dilute plasmids in aqua ad iniectabilia under sterile conditions.
17. When loading the macrocarrier with gold particles, do not let the gold dry out too much.
18. Avoid air bubbles in the column, when equilibrating the column. Do not load aggregated cells onto the column; resuspend or filter cells carefully before loading.
19. If buffer or cell suspension does not flow well tap hard onto the column to liberate air bubbles or cell clumps in the column, capillary or flow resistor. Use capillary G23 as flow resistor.
20. Any number of detection reagents can be used. Secondary reagents have to be titrated to yield optimal results and low background. In BALB/c mice, the relative amount of antibodies of the IgG1 and IgG2a isotype is indicative of a Th2 versus a Th1-type immune response, repsectively. Care must be taken to exclude cross-reactivity of isotype-specific secondary antibodies.
21. We have adopted our ELISPOT from Schneider, et al. *(40)*. When assaying splenocytes from DC-immunized mice, you need to enrich for CD8$^+$ T cells, because there is considerable background IFNγ release in whole splenocyte suspensions, presumably resulting from the FCS which is normally used for DC culture. We are currently developing protocols to replace FCS with NMS in DC culture and/or ELISPOT.
22. Anti-CD4 and anti-CD8 MAb (hybridoma supernatants or purified antibody) followed by separation with magnetic beads or complement mediated depletion can be used to remove (or enrich) effectors.

References

1. Tang, D. C., DeVit, M. J., and Johnston, S. A. (1992) Genetic immunization: a simple method for eliciting an immune response. *Nature* **356,** 152–154.
2. Donnelly, J. J., Ulmer, J. B., Shiver, J. W., and Liu, M. A. (1997) DNA vaccines. *Ann. Rev. Immunol.* **15,** 617–648.
3. Tüting, T., Storkus, W. J., Falo, L. D. (1998) DNA immunization targeting the skin: Molecular control of adaptive immunity. *J. Invest. Dermatol.* **111,** 183–188.
4. Corr, M., Lee, D. J., Carson, D. A., and Tighe, H. (1996) Gene vaccination with naked plasmid DNA: mechanism of CTL priming. *J. Exp. Med.* **184,** 1555–1560.
5. Fu, T-M., Ulmer, J. B., Caulfield, M. J., Deck, R. R., Friedman, A., Wang, S., et al. (1997) Priming of cytotoxic T lymphocytes by DNA vaccines: requirements for professional antigen presenting cells and evidence for antigen transfer from myocytes. *Mol. Med.* **3,** 362–371.
6. Iwasaki, A., Torres, C. A. T., Ohashi, P. S., Robbinson, H. L., and Barber, B. H. (1997) The dominant role of bone marrow-derived cells in CTL induction following plasmid DNA immunization at different sites. *J. Immunol.* **159,** 11–14.
7. Doe, B., Selby, M., Barnett, S., Baenziger, J., and Walker, C. M. (1996) Induction of cytotoxic T lymphocytes by intramuscular immunization with plasmid DNA

is facilitated by bone marrow-derived cells. *Proc. Natl. Acad. Sci. USA* **93**, 8578–8583.

8. Cella, M., Sallusto, F., and Lanzavecchia, A. (1997) Origin, maturation and antigen presenting function of dendritic cells. *Curr. Opin. Immunol.* **9**, *10–16*.

9. Banchereau, J. and Steinman, R. M. (1998) Dendritic cells and the control of immunity. *Nature* **392**, *245–252*.

10. Condon, C., Watkins, S. C., Celluzzi, C. M., Thompson, K., and Falo, L. D. (1996) DNA-based immunization by in vivo transfection of dendritic cells. *Nature Med.* **2**, 1122–1128.

11. Porgador, A., Irvine, K. R., Iwasaki, A., Barber, B. H., Restifo, N. P., and Germain, R. N. (1998) Predominant role for directly transfected dendritic cells in antigen presentation to CD8+ T cells after gene gun immunization. *J. Exp. Med.* **188**, 1075–1082.

12. Akbari, O., Panjwani, N., Garcia, S., Tascon, R., Lowrie, D., and Stockinger, B. (1999) DNA vaccination: Transfection and activation of dendritic cells as key events for immunity. *J. Exp. Med.* **189**, 169–177.

13. Casares, S., Inaba, K., Brumeanu, T-D., Steinman, R. M., and Bona, C. A. (1977) Antigen presentation by dendritic cells after immuniation with DNA encoding a major histocomapatibility complex class II-restricted viral epitope. *J. Exp. Med.* **186**, 1481–1486.

14. Walker, P. S., Scharton-Kersten, T., Rowton, E. D., Hengge, U., Bouloc, A., Udey, M. C., and Vogel, J. C. (1998) Genetic immunization with glycoprotein 63 cDNA results in a helper T cell type immune response and protection in a murine model of leishmaniasis. *Hum. Gene. Ther.* **9**, 1899–1907.

15. Labeur, M. S., Roters, B., Pers, B., Mehling, A., Luger, T. A., Schwarz, T., and Grabbe, S. (1999) Generation of tumor immunity by bone marrow-derived dendritic cells correlates with dendritic cell maturation stage. *J. Immunol.* **162**, 168–175.

16. Jonuleit, H., Kuhn, U., Muller, G., Steinbrink, K., Paragnik, L., Schmitt, E., Knop, J., and Enk, A. H. (1997) Pro-inflammatory cytokines and prostaglandins induce maturation of potent immunostimulatory dendritic cells under fetal calf serum-free conditions. *Eur. J. Immunol.* **27**, 3135–3142.

17. Tüting, T., DeLeo, A. B., Lotze, M. T., and Storkus, W. J. (1997) Bone marrow-derived dendritic cells genetically modified to express tumor-associated antigens induce antitumor immunity in vivo. *Eur. J. Immunol.* **27**, 2702–2707.

18. Timares, L., Takashima, A., and Johnston, S. A. (1998) Quantitative analysis of the immunopotency of genetically transfected dendritic cells. *Proc. Natl. Acad. Sci. USA* **95**, 13,147–13,152.

19. Tüting, T., Wilson, C. C., Martin, D., Kasamon, Y., Rowles, J., Ma, D. I., et al. (1998) Autologous human monocyte-derived dendritic cells genetically modified to express melanoma antigens elicit primary cytotoxic T cell responses in vitro: Enhancement by cotransfection of genes encoding the Th1-biasing cytokines IL-12 and IFN-α. *J. Immunol.* **160**, 1139–1147.

20. Conry, R. M., Widera, G., LoBuglio, A. F., Fuller, J. T., Moore, S. T., Barlow, D. L., et al. (1996) Selected strategies to augment polynucleotide immunization. *Gene Ther.* **3,** 67–74.

21. Irvine, K. R., Rao, R. B., Rosenberg, S. A., and Restifo, N. P. (1996) Cytokine enhancement of DNA immunization leads to effective treatment of established pulmonary metastases. *J. Immunol.* **156,** 238–245.

22. Tüting, T., Gambotto, A., Storkus, W. J., De Leo, A. B. (1999) Co-delivery of T helper 1-biasing cytokine genes enhances the efficacy of gene gun immunization of mice: Studies with the model tumor antigen β-galactosidase and the BALB/c Meth A p53 tumor-specific antigen. *Gene Ther.* **6,** 629–636.

23. Corr, M., Tighe, H., Lee, D., Dudler, J., Trieu, M., Brinson, D. C., and Carson, D. A. (1997) Costimulation provided by DNA Immunization enhances antitumor immunity. *J. Immunol.* **159,** 4999–5004.

24. Gurunathan, S., Irvine, K. R., Wu, C-Y., Cohen, J. I., Thomas, E., Prussin, C., et al. (1998) CD40ligand/trmer DNA enhances both humoral and cellular immune responses and induces protective immunity to infectious and tumor challenge. *J. Immunol.* **161,** 4563–4571.

25. Dyall, R., Bowne, W. B., Weber, L. W., LeMaoult, J., Szabo, P., Moroi, Y., et al. (1998) Heteroclitic immunization induces tumor immunity. *J. Exp. Med.* **15,** 553–1561.

26. Parra-Lopez, C. A., Lindner, R., Vidavsky, I., Gross, M., and Unanue, E. R. (1997) Presentation on class II MHC molecules of endogenous lysozyme targeted to the endocytic pathway. *J. Immunol.* **158,** 2670–2679.

27. Boon, T. and Van der Bruggen, P. (1996) Human tumor antigens recognized by T lymphocytes. *J. Exp. Med.* **183,** 725–729.

28. Rosenberg, S. A. (1997) Cancer vaccines based on the identification of genes encoding cancer regression antigens. *Immunol. Today* **18,** 175–182.

29. Syrengelas, A. D., Chen, T. T., and Levy, R. (1996) DNA immunization induces protective immunity against B-cell lymphoma. *Nat. Med.* **2,** 1038–1041.

30. Rosato, A., Zambon, A., Milan, G., Ciminale, V., D'Agostino, D. M., Macino, B., et al. (1997) CTL response and protection against P815 tumor challenge in mice immunized with DNA expressing the tumor-specific antigen P815. *Hum. Gene Ther.* **8,** 1451–1458.

31. Schreurs, M. W., de Boer, A. J., Figdor, C. G., and Adema, G. J. (1998) Genetic vaccination against the melanocyte lineage-specific antigen gp100 induces cytotoxic T lymphocyte-mediated tumor protection. *Cancer Res.* **58,** 2509–2514.

32. Weber, L. W., Bowne, W. B., Wolchok, J. D., Srinivasan, R., Qin, J., Moroi, Y., et al. (1998) Tumor immunity and autoimmunity induced by immunization with homologous DNA. *J. Clin. Invest.* **102,** 1258–1264.

33. Tüting, T., Gambotto, A., De Leo, A. B., Robbins, P. D., Lotze, M. T., and Storkus, W. J. (1999) Induction of tumor antigen-specific immunity using DNA immunization in mice. *Cancer Gene Ther.* **6,** 73–80.

34. Ugen, K. E., Nyland, S. B., Boyer, J. D., Vidal, C., Lera, L., Rasheid, S., et al. (1998) DNA vaccination with HIV-1 expressing constructs elicits immune responses in humans. *Vaccine* **16**, 1818–1821.
35. MacGregor, R. R., Boyer, J. D., Ugen, K. E., Lacy, K. E., Gluckman, S. J., Bagarazzi, M. L., et al. (1998) First human trial of a DNA-based vaccine for treatment of human immunodeficiency virus type 1 infection: safety and host response. *J. Infect. Dis.* **178**, 92–100.
36. Calarota, S., Bratt, G., Nordlund, S., Hinkula, J., Leandersson, A. C., Sandstrom, E., and Wahren, B. (1998) Cellular cytotoxic response induced by DNA vaccination in HIV-1-infected patients. *Lancet* **351**, 1320–1325.
37. Wang, R., Doolan, D. L., Pe, T. P., Hedstrom, R. C., Coonan, K. M., Charoenvit, Y., et al. (1998) Induction of antigen-specific cytotoxic T lymphocytes by a malaria DNA vaccine. *Science* **282**, 476–480.
38. Feltkamp, M. C. W., Smis, H. L., Vierboom, M. P. M., Minnaar, R. P., de Jongh, B. M., Drijfhout, J. W., et al. (1993) Vaccination with cytotoxic T lymphocyte epitope-containing peptide protects against a tumor induced by human papillomavirus type 16-transformed cells. *Eur. J. Immunol.* **23**, 2242.
39. Brattain, M. G. et al. (1980) Establishment of mouse colonic carcinoma cell lines with different metastatic properties. *Cancer Res.* **40**, 2142–2146.
40. Schneider, J., Gilbert, S., Blanchard, T. J., Hanke, T., Robson, K. J., Hannan, C. M., et al. (1998) Enhanced immunogenicity for CD8+ T cell induction and complete protective efficacy of malaria DNA vaccination by boosting with modified vaccinia virus Ankara. *Nature Med.* **4**, 397–402.

3

Cancer Gene Therapy With Heat Shock Protein-65 Gene

Katalin V. Lukacs and Artit Nakakes

1. Introduction

Heat shock proteins (HSPs) are highly conserved proteins present in every living cell. Many members of the HSP family are essential for cellular functions under physiologic conditions, others are induced by various forms of cellular stress (including sudden increase in temperature) to protect cells from environmental damage (1,2). Involvement in protein folding and transport led to designation of HSPs as molecular chaperones (3).

Work over the past decade has demonstrated the importance of HSPs in the immune response to many infectious agents. Mycobactrial HSPs are among the most potent antigenic stimuli for the mammalian immune system. In addition to their highly immunogenic nature, HSPs have been shown to chaperone small tumor-derived antigenic peptides to MHC molecules for more effective antigen presentation (4). As a result, weakly immunogenic tumor antigens become capable of inducing an effective antitumor immune response.

We were the first to show that tumor cells expressing the mycobacterial HSP65 gene after in vitro gene transfer lose their ability to form tumors and protect animals against the otherwise lethal challenge of nonmodified parent tumor cells (5,6). In addition, in vivo HSP65 gene transfer results in regression of existing tumors in J774 murine sarcoma (7) and malignant mesothelioma (unpublished). In this chapter we describe both ex vivo and in vivo gene therapy with the mycobacterial HSP65 gene.

From: *Methods in Molecular Medicine, Vol. 35: Gene Therapy: Methods and Protocols*
Edited by: W. Walther and U. Stein © Humana Press, Inc., Totowa, NJ

2. Materials

2.1. Ex Vivo Gene Therapy

2.1.1. Transfection and Selection of HSP65 Transfected Cells

1. Exponentially growing cells.
2. DMEM-10: Dulbecco's modified eagle's medium HEPES modification (Sigma Chemical Co., St. Louis, MO) containing 10 mM HEPES supplemented with 10% foetal calf serum and 1 mM L-glutamine (Sigma).
3. Liposome: Transfection reagent (DOTAP) (Boehringer Mannheim, Mannheim, Germany).
4. Endotoxin-free plasmid DNA (*see* **Note 1**): using EndoFree™ plasmid purification kit (Qiagen GmbH, Hilden, Germany).
5. Opti-MEM 1 reduced serum medium (Life Technologies Ltd., Paisley, UK).
6. Geneticin G418 sulphate (Life Technologies).
7. 10 cm tissue culture plate (Nunc, Life Technologies Ltd.).
8. Polystyrene tube (Falcon, Becton Dickinson, Lincoln Park, NJ).

2.1.2. Detection of HSP65 Expression (see **Note 2**)

1. 4M Guanidinium thiocyanate (BDH, Merck Ltd., Poole, UK) (*see* **Notes 3** and **4**).
2. 1M Sodium citrate (BDH) (*see* **Note 4**).
3. 10% Sarcosyl (Sigma) (*see* **Note 4**).
4. 2-mercaptoethanol (Sigma).
5. 2M Sodium acetate (BDH). Store at room temperature for 3 mo.
6. Acid phenol (Amresco Inc., Solon, OH). Store at 4°C in the dark.
7. Chloroform (May and Baker Ltd., Dagenham, UK).
8. Isopropyl alcohol (BDH).
9. 80% ethanol (Hayman Ltd., Witham, UK).
10. RNase-Free DNase 1 U/µl (Promega Corp., Madison, WI).
11. 50 mM Magnesium sulphate (BDH). Store at room temperature for 3 mo.
12. Oligo(dT) 12 to 18 mer, 1 mg/mL; (Pharmacia Biotech, Amersham Pharmacia Biotech, St. Albans, Herts, UK) stock 0.5 mg/mL. Store at –20°C.
13. DEPC water: 0.1% Diethyl Pyrocarbonate (Sigma) in double distilled water (autoclave sterilized).
14. Acetylated BSA (Life Technologies) 0.5 mg/mL.
15. 10 mM of 2'-deoxynucleoside-5'-triphosphates (dNTP) (Pharmacia).
16. Murine monkey leukemia virus reverse transcriptase (MMLVRT) 150 U/µL (Life Technologies) supplied with 5X RT buffer and DTT.
17. RNase inhibitor: RNasin® Ribonuclease Inhibitor 20–40 U/µL (Promega).
18. Sterile water (Sigma).
19. 20 µM of 5' Primer (for HSP65: 5'-TTGAGCAGGTCCTCGTACTCA-3'; for β-actin: 5'-GTGGGCCGCTCTAGGCACCAA-3').
20. 20 µM of 3' Primer (for HSP65: 5'-ATGGCCAAGACAATTGCGTAC-3'; for β-actin: 5'-CTCTTTGATGTCACGCACGATTTC-3').

21. Taq polymerase 5 U/μL (Appligene Oncor, Co., Durham, UK) supplied with 10X PCR buffer.
22. Mineral oil (Sigma).

2.1.3. Injection of Mice with HSP65 Expressing Tumor Cells

1. 6 to 12-wk-old female Balb/c and SCID (severe combined immune deficiency) mice (*see* **Note 5**).
2. Normal saline solution, 0.9% (NSS) (Sigma).

2.2. In Vivo Gene Therapy

2.2.1. Tumor Initiation

1. Balb/c and SCID mice.
2. Exponentially growing cells.

2.2.2. In Vivo Gene Transfer

1. Endotoxin-free plasmid DNA (*see* **Note 1**).
2. Liposome (DOTAP) (Boehringer Mannheim, Mannheim, Germany).
3. Normal saline solution (0.9%) (NSS) (Sigma).
4. Polystyrene tube.

3. Methods

3.1. Ex Vivo Gene Therapy

3.1.1. Transfection of Tumor Cells with HSP65 Plasmid-liposome Complexes

1. Exponentially growing cells can be obtained by plating 5×10^5 J774 mouse macrophage tumor cells in 10-cm tissue culture plate in 10 mL of 10-DMEM and incubate overnight before the day of transfection (*see* **Note 6**).
2. On the day of transfection, remove the medium from the cells and gently layer 5 mL of fresh DMEM-10 medium, prewarmed to 37°C, over the cells. Return the cells to the incubator.
3. Prepare DNA solution by diluting 5–10 μg of plasmid DNA complex into 100 μL with Opti-MEM1 medium in a polystyrene tube.
4. Prepare liposome solution for each transfection by diluting 25–50 μL of DOTAP liposome into 100 μL with Opti-MEM 1.
5. Mix the two solutions by gently pipeting up and down (do not vortex or centrifuge) and allow to stand at room temperature for 15–30 min (white precipitate may form at this stage. This does not interfere with the transfection procedure).
6. Add 4.8 mL of Opti-MEM 1 to the mixture. Mix the solution by inversion and gently layer over the cells. Gently mix the plate and return immediately to the incubator (*see* **Notes 7–9**).
7. After 24 h, remove the medium and gently wash the cells twice with 10 mL of prewarmed DMEM-10.

8. Gently add 15 mL of prewarmed fresh medium over the cells. Return the cells to the incubator and incubate for another 48 h.

3.1.2. Selection of HSP65 Transfected Cells

The cells can be selected with 15 mL of DMEM-10 plus G418 (1 mg/mL) (*see* **Note 10**) and they need to be fed with fresh medium every 5–7 d. The transfected colonies would appear after 10–14 d (*see* **Notes 11** and **12**). The selected colonies can be picked when there are at least 200 cells/colony and transferred to grow in 24-wells plates.

3.1.3. Detection of HSP65 Expression

Positive clones can be selected by RT/PCR(reverse transcription and polymerase chain reaction) technique, i.e., isolation of total RNA from the selected clones *(8)*; treatment of the RNA with DNase to eliminate any contaminating DNA; obtaining cDNA by reverse transcription of the DNase treated RNA; then using PCR to probe the cDNA for HSP65 by specific pair of primers *(9)*.

9. Prepare lysis buffer ($4M$ Guanidinium thiocyanate 5 mL; $1M$ sodium citrate 125 µL; 10% Sarcosyl 250 µL and 2-mercaptoethanol 45 µL). Store at room temperature for 1 mo.
10. Wash 2×10^6 cells or 3×3 mm of tissue once in ice-cold PBS and homogenize in 500 µL of ice-cold lysis buffer.
11. The sample can be stored at –70°C (we stored our samples for up to 6 mo).
12. For each 500 µL of the sample, sequentially add 50 µL of $2M$ sodium acetate, 500 µL of acid phenol and 100 µL of chloroform; briefly vortex the mixture after the addition of each reagent. Leave on ice for 15 min; vortex for 30 s every 5 min.
13. Centrifuge at $10,000g$ at 4°C for 20 min.
14. Transfer the upper aqueous phase to a fresh tube avoiding the interface.
15. Precipitate the RNA with equal volume of isopropyl alcohol at –20°C for at least 1 hour.
16. Centrifuge at $10,000g$ at 4°C for 30 min.
17. Wash once with 1 mL of 80% ethanol (centrifuge at $10,000g$ at 4°C for 10 min.)
18. Vacuum dry and dissolve in 85 µL of DEPC water.
19. DNase treatment: Add 5 µL of $2M$ sodium acetate, 10 µL of 50 mM magnesium sulphate, 1 µL of RNase-free DNase and incubate in a water bath at 37°C for 10 min; place the tube on ice; add 400 µL of DEPC water; then repeat **steps 12–16.**
20. Wash twice with 800 µL of 80% ethanol.
21. Vacuum dry and dissolve the pellet in 8 µL of DEPC water.
22. The amount of RNA used for the next step should be between 1–2 µg in 8 µL of DEPC water.
23. Add 2 of oligo(dT) 0.5 mg/mL.
24. Incubate at 65°C for 10 min and place the tube on ice.

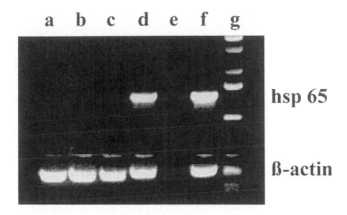

Fig. 1. PCR products of cDNA preparations using HSP-65 and β-actin primers. Lanes: **a**, untransfected J774 cells; **b**, vector transfected cells; **c**, clone 1 (negative); **d**, clone 2 (positive); **e**, negative control (contained sterile water) **f**, positive control (contained 0.1 pg of HSP 65 plasmid DNA used in transfection); **g**, 1-kb ladder size standard. Corresponding equal amount of the products from each set of primers were mixed together with DNA loading buffer and run in the same lane.

25. Prepare reverse transcription mix (for 25 µL, 5X RT buffer 10 µL; DTT 5 µL; DEPC water 2 µL; BSA 2 µL; dNTP 2 µL; MMLVRT 2 µL, and RNase inhibitor 2 µL).
26. Add 10µL of reverse transcription mix and incubate at 37°C for 1 h.
27. Incubate at 95°C for 5 min.
28. Add 80 µL of DEPC water. The sample is now ready for PCR.
29. Prepare PCR mix (for 45 µL, sterile water 33.75 µL; 10X PCR buffer 5 µL; 10 mM dNTP 1 µL; 20 µM of 5′ Primer 2.5 µL; 20 µM of 3′ Primer 2.5 µL and 200U/µL Taq polymerase 0.25 µL). Add 5 µL of cDNA to 45µL of the PCR mix.
30. Layer 50 µL of mineral oil over the mixture.
31. The sample was subjected to the following PCR conditions, i.e., 35 cycles of 96°C/45 s; 60°C/45 s; 72°C/90 s followed by the extension cycle of 72°C for 5 min.
32. The PCR product was ready to be visualized by the agarose gel electrophoresis (*see* **Fig. 1**).

3.1.4. Injection of Mice with HSP65 Expressing Tumor Cells

Subconfluent culture of J774-HSP65 tumor cells are washed twice with NSS. The cells are diluted in NSS and inoculated intraperitoneally at 2×10^6 cells/500 µL/mouse 4 times at weekly intervals. One week after the last injection, tumor-specific protection can be detected. Challange with otherwise lethal nonmodified parent tumor cells (2×10^6 J774 cells/mouse) results in no tumor formation.

3.2. In Vivo Gene Therapy

3.2.1. Tumor Initiation

Inject mice intraperitoneally with 2×10^6 cells from subconfluent culture of J774 in 500 µL of NSS per mouse.

3.2.2. In Vivo Gene Transfer (see **Note 13**)

1. Prepare DNA-liposome complexes by incubating 100 µg plasmid DNA in 100 µL NSS with 400 µg DOTAP for 15 min at room temperature for each mouse to be treated.
2. Dilute complexes to 1 mL final volume/mouse with NSS.
3. Inject the DNA-liposome complexes ip.
4. Repeat treatment twice weekly for two weeks.
5. Mice should be observed daily. Untreated controls develop terminal tumors in 21–24 d after tumor initiation. Animals showing any two of the following symptoms: 20% weight loss, permanent hunching, labored respiration or permanent pilo-errection, should be sacrificed. Tumor size can be determined and histological evaluation can be carried out. After four injections of HSP65 DNA-liposome complexes, mice have been observed for up to two years without developing terminal tumors.
6. Because of the inseparable aggregation of primary tumors and abdominal organs, tumor size can be calculated by weighing the primary tumor and abdominal organs of the test mice and subtracting the average weight of abdominal organs obtained from five age-matched normal controls.

4. Notes

1. Endotoxin can be toxic to some cells. The amount of endotoxin should be lower than 100 EU/mg of plasmid DNA.
2. In RT/PCR, all the water used to prepare every solution is DEPC water. We recommend the use of sterile disposable plastics to store solution.
3. Guanidinium thiocyanate is hazardous. We recommend ordering a small amount and dissolving in the manufacturer-supplied bottle.
4. Lysis buffer can be stored for three months at room temperature if 2-mercaptoethanol is left out, only to be added just before use.
5. The use of immunodeficient (SCID) mice is recommended to confirm in vivo HSP65 gene expression. Two days after in vivo gene transfer, HSP65 mRNA easily detectable in tumor samples of treated immunodeficient mice (SCID and nude mice) but not in immunocompetent Balb/c mice. HSP65-transfected cells express a foreign, bacterial protein, therefore they are rapidly eliminated in immunocompetent hosts.
6. For stable transfection, the cells should be plated to obtain no more than 50% confluency on the day of tranfection.

7. For different cell lines used, the ratio of plasmid DNA to liposome complex must be optimized. In general, use 1X plasmid DNA to 4-5X DOTAP.
8. The plasmid DNA/liposome complex can cause toxicity to the cells. A small-scale experiment should be done first to determine the amount of plasmid DNA to be used. We recommend using 6 wells (35 mm) multidishes (Nunc) and scaling down the experiment by the factor of 5. We prefer the concentration that give 80–90% viability after 24 hr.
9. During transfection, it is recommended to try to use reduced serum medium (no more than 5% serum) and antibiotics must be omitted.
10. For every cell line used, the optimum concentration of selectable markers, i.e., G418, must be predetermined. A small-scale standardization can be done in a 24-well-plate. For G418, we use the range between 0.3–1.0 mg/mL. We prefer to use the concentration that kills the cells after 5–7 d of selection. Each lot of G418 can have different potency, so buying in a large amount of one lot for standardization is recommended.
11. There may be difficulty in obtaining a stable transfection. We have found that supplementing the selection medium with 10–20% of the 24-hr supernatant of the exponentially growing cells (filtered through 0.2 μm filter) improves efficiency. The supernatant can be aliquoted and stored at –70°C for 3 mo.
12. During selection, the plate should be kept for at least 4 wk because the transfected cells might take a long time to form colonies. Frequent changes of the medium should also be avoided in order to maintain any soluble factors that help the colonies to grow.
13. For in vivo gene therapy, we recommend 2–4 treatments at 2–7 d intervals starting at 7 or 14 d after tumor initiation.

References

1. Goff, S. A. and Goldberg, A. L. (1985) Production of abnormal proteins in E. coli stimulates transcription of Lon and other heat shock genes. *Cell* **41,** 587–595.
2. Johnson, C., Chandrasekhar, C. N., and Georgopoulos, C. J. (1989) Echericia coli DNA K and GrpE heat shock proteins interact both in vivo and in vitro. *Bacteriol.* **171,** 1590–1596.
3. Ellis, J. (1987) Proteins as molecular chaperones. *Nature* **328,** 378–379.
4. Suto, R. and Srivastava, P. K. (1995) A mechanism for the specific immunogenicity of heat shock protein-chaperoned peptides. *Science* **269,** 1585–1588.
5. Lukacs, K. V., Lowrie, D. B., Stokes, R. W., and Colston, M. J. (1993) Tumor cells transfected with a bacterial heat-shock gene lose tumorigenicity and induce protection against tumors. *J. Exp. Med.* **178,** 343–348.
6. Lukacs, K. V., Lowrie D. B., and Colston M. J. (1996) Protection against tumours by stress protein gene transfer, in *Stress proteins in Medicine*, (Eden, W. and Young, D. B., eds.) Marcel Dekker, New York, pp. 249–265.
7. Lukacs, K. V., Nakakes, A., Atkins, C. J., Lowrie, D. B., and Colston, M. J. (1997)

In vivo gene therapy of malignant tumours with heat shock protein-65 gene. *Gene Therapy* **4,** 346–350.

8. Chomczynski, P. and Sacchi, N. (1987) Single-step method of RNA isolation by acid guanidinium thiocyanate-phenol-chloroform extraction. *Anal. Biochem.* **162,** 156–159.

9. Walker, K. B., Butler, R., and Colston, M. J. (1992) Role of Th-1 lymphocytes in the development of protective immunity against *Mycobacterium leprae.* *J. Immunol.* **148,** 1885–1889.

4

Recombinant Vaccinia Virus MVA for Generation and Analysis of T Cell Responses Against Tumor Associated Antigens

Ingo Drexler, Karl Heller, Marion Ohlmann, Volker Erfle, and Gerd Sutter

1. Introduction

Live attenuated viruses used as vaccines are known for their efficacy to elicit protective immunity against viral diseases. More recently, with an increasing number of tumor-associated antigens (TAA) being identified and molecularly cloned *(1)* the development of vaccines for cancer immunotherapy has gained considerable interest. In particular, live recombinant viral vectors seem to be appropriate delivery systems for efficient presentation of TAA to the immune system. The promise of viral vectors is likely to be founded on their capacity for high-level expression of target genes combined with their intrinsic property to activate immunological control systems mimicking an infection with a disease causing agent.

Vaccinia virus (VV), the prototype live viral vaccine, serves as a basis for well-established viral vectors [for review *see (2)*] which already have been successfully evaluated as anticancer vaccines in a variety of animal model systems *(3)*. However, VV replicates in humans and its imperfect safety record as a smallpox vaccine was a concern for its use as a vector in clinical applications. Recently, the development of highly attenuated vaccinia viral vectors was attained by the construction of recombinant viruses from modified vaccinia virus Ankara (MVA), a strain with established clinical safety *(4)*. MVA has been generated by long-term serial passage in avian cells and it is characterized by its avirulence and severe deficiency to replicate in cells of mammalian origin *(5–7)*. Importantly, recombinant MVA (rMVA) has been found

From: *Methods in Molecular Medicine, Vol. 35: Gene Therapy: Methods and Protocols*
Edited by: W. Walther and U. Stein © Humana Press, Inc., Totowa, NJ

immunogenic and protective against disease when used as candidate recombinant vaccine in animal models for viral or parasite infections *(8–11)*. Furthermore, vaccines based on rMVA producing an artificial tumor antigen have already demonstrated their protective capacity in a mouse-tumor cell-challenge model *(12)* and ongoing efforts aim at the design of rMVA for delivery of human TAA *(13)*. Apart from their appealing use as a candidate vaccine against cancer, MVA-based vectors represent an extremely valuable experimental system for the identification and evaluation of TAA as targets for CD8+ cytotoxic and CD4+ T-cell responses.

Here, we describe an up-to-date methodology for generation and characterization of rMVA expressing target antigens. As stable coexpression of reporter genes might not always be desirable, we propose the use of transient marker gene expression as a convenient screening procedure for the isolation of rMVA vector virus. Additionally, we will outline an in vitro-approach to use these rMVA for induction and analysis of TAA-specific CTL. The protocol contains an optimized procedure for MVA-infection of immunocompetent cells (e.g., dendritic cells (DC) / B cells (BC) / lymphoblastoid cells (LCL)), to be used as TAA-presenting cells (1) to induce or activate primary and secondary T-cell responses directed against TAA; (2) to clone or subclone TAA-reactive CTL; or (3) to assess the TAA-specificity of CTL in chromium release assays.

2. Materials

2.1. Generation of Recombinant MVA

2.1.1. Cloning of Target Genes

1. Plasmid pII LZdel P7.5. Plasmid DNA is prepared using plasmid purification kits (Qiagen GmbH, Hilden, Germany).
2. Restriction endonucleases.
3. DNA modifying enzymes, e.g., Klenow DNA polymerase.

2.1.2. Transfection of MVA-Infected Cells with Vector Plasmids

1. Subconfluent monolayers of primary chicken embryo fibroblasts (CEF) or baby hamster kidney cells (BHK 21) (ATCC no. CCL-10) grown on 6-well plates in RPMI 1640 medium supplemented with 2–10% heat inactivated fetal calf serum (FCS) (Seromed, Biochrome KG, Berlin, Germany), 0.03% L-glutamine (L-glu), 100 µg/mL streptomycin, 100 IU/mL penicillin, and 25 µg/mL amphothericin B (AB/AM) (Life Technologies, Grand Island, NY) at 37°C in a humidified and 5% CO_2 atmosphere.
2. Plasmid pII LZdel P7.5-TG.
3. OptiMEM medium (Life Technologies, Gaithersburg, MD) (store at 4°C).
4. Lipofectin (Life Technologies) (store at 4°C).

2.1.3. Plaque Purification of Recombinant MVA

1. Cup sonicator (Sonopuls HD 200, Bandelin, Germany).
2. X-gal-solution: X-gal (5-bromo-4-chloro-3-indolyl β-D-galactoside, Boehringer Mannheim, Mannheim, Germany) 4% in dimethylformamide (DMFA, Sigma-Aldrich, Deisenhofen, Germany) (store at –20°C, light-sensitive, toxic).
3. 2X RPMI1640 medium supplemented with 5% FCS, L-glu and AB/AM (store at 4°C).
4. LMP-agarose 2%: 2 g low-melting-point agarose (LMP-agarose) (Life Technologies)/100 mL Aqua dest. (store at RT).

2.1.4. Amplification of Recombinant MVA

1. Confluent monolayers of CEF or BHK 21 cells grown on 60 cm² dishes, T75 and T175 tissue culture flasks (for growth conditions *see* **Subheading 2.1.2.**)
2. Cell scraper.
3. Phosphate buffered saline (PBS) pH 7.5 (Life Technologies).

2.2. Characterization of Recombinant MVA

2.2.1. PCR Analysis of MVA DNA

1. 10X TEN buffer pH 7.4 (10X TEN pH 7.4): 100 mM Tris-HCl, 10 mM EDTA, 1M NaCl.
2. DNA grade proteinase K prepared as 1 mg/mL stock solution in Aqua dest. (prot K), (store at –20°C, AGS GmbH, Heidelberg, Germany).
3. 20% sodium dodecyl sulfate in Aqua dest. (SDS 20%) (DNAse free; sterile filtered).
4. Phenol-chloroform 1:1 mixture (Applied Biosystems, Foster City, CA, store at 4°C).
5. 3M sodium acetate in Aqua dest. (3M NaAc, Merck KGaA, Darmstadt, Germany).
6. Ethanol absolute (EtOH abs) (Merck KGaA).
7. 70% ethanol in Aqua dest. (EtOH 70%, Merck KGaA).
8. Primer 1 (MVA-II-5′) and primer 2 (MVA-II-3′) dissolved in sterile Aqua dest. to final concentration of 80 pmol (store at –20°C): MVA-II-5′ (Primer 1): 5′-CTC TCT AGC AAA GAT GCA TTT AAG GCG GAT GTC-3′, MVA-II-3′ (Primer 2): 5′-TGG CCA TTA TAC TAG AAC TAT AGG TGC GTT GTA-3′.
9. Template DNA:
   a. Viral genomic DNA prepared as described in **Subheading 3.2.1.**
   b. Plasmid DNA diluted to a final concentration of 100 ng/μL.
10. PCR master kit (Boehringer Mannheim) (store at 4°C).
11. Thermocycler.

2.2.2. Titration of Recombinant MVA by Immunostaining

1. Subconfluent monolayers of CEF or BHK 21 cells grown on 96-well flat-bottom tissue-culture plates (for growth conditions, *see* **Subheading 2.1.2.**).

2. Laboratory shaker (Froebel, Wasserburg, Germany).
3. Fixing solution: 1 : 1 mixture of aceton:methanol (Merck KGaA, laboratory use grade) (store at 4°C).
4. Phosphate buffered saline (PBS) pH 7.5 (Life Technologies).
5. Blocking buffer: PBS pH 7.5 + 2 % bovine serum albumine.
6. 1st antibody (1st Ab): Polyclonal rabbit antivaccinia antibody (IgG fraction, Biogenesis Ltd, Poole, England, Cat.No. 9503-2057) diluted 1 : 1000 in blocking buffer.
7. 2nd antibody (2nd Ab): horseradish peroxidase-conjugated polyclonal goat antirabbit antibody (IgG (H+L)) (Cat.No. 111-035-114; Dianova, Hamburg, Germany) diluted 1 : 500 in blocking buffer.
8. o-dianisidine (Sigma).
9. Ethanol absolute (EtOH abs) (Merck KGaA).
10. Hydrogen superoxide >30% (H_2O_2 > 30%) (Sigma).
11. Multichannel pipet (8 or 12 channels).

2.2.3. Immune-Detection of Target Protein Made by rMVA

See **Subheading 2.2.2.** with following variations:

1. Confluent monolayers of CEF or BHK 21 cells on 6-well tissue culture plates (for growth conditions, *see* **Subheading 2.1.2.**).
2. 1st antibody (1st Ab): directed against target protein and diluted in blocking buffer as appropriate (*see* **Note 4.5.**).
3. 2nd antibody (2nd Ab): horseradish peroxidase-conjugated antibody binding to 1st Ab and diluted in blocking buffer (*see* **Note 4.5.**).

2.3. Infection of Antigen-Presenting Cells with Recombinant MVA

2.3.1. Generation of Stimulator Cells for Isolation or Activation of TAA-Specific CTL

1. Conditioned tissue-culture medium (may depend on the stimulator cells used).
2. Stimulator cells at 1×10^6 cells/100 µL medium.
3. rMVA-TG (and parental MVA, if needed as a control) at 1×10^7 IU/100 µL medium.

2.3.2. Generation of Target Cells for Analysis of TAA-Specific CTL Activity in [^{51}Cr] Release Assays

1. Serum and conditioned tissue-culture medium (may depend on the target cells used).
2. Target cells prepared as described for stimulators in **Subheading 2.3.1.**
3. rMVA-TG and control parental MVA prepared as described in **Subheading 2.3.1.**
4. Stock solution of ^{51}chromium (^{51}Cr): 1–1.5 mCi/mL.

3. Method

3.1. Generation of Recombinant MVA

3.1.1. Cloning of Target Genes

Recombinant genes to be transferred into the MVA genome are subcloned into a MVA plasmid vector such as pII LZdel P7.5. This plasmid contains a moderate strength vaccinia virus early/late promoter, P7.5, with one unique restriction endonuclease site for insertion of target genes. A vaccinia virus late promoter, P11, allows expression of an *E. coli lacZ*-reporter gene. Segments of MVA-DNA flanking these expression cassettes allow an integration into the MVA genome precisely at the site of a naturally disrupted MVA gene sequence (deletion II), *(14)*. The expression cassette of the *lacZ* gene is designed to contain repetitive DNA sequences, which allow deletion by homologous recombination to inactivate reporter gene expression in the final MVA vector virus *(13)*, **Fig. 1**.

Blunt-ended DNA-fragments containing the coding sequence of the target gene (TG), including authentic start (ATG) and stop (TAA/TAG/TGA) codons, are cloned into the unique *Sma*I restriction endonuclease site of LZdel P7.5 to generate the transfer vector plasmid pII LZdel P7.5-TG (**Fig. 1**).

The correct orientation of the TG is determined by the direction of P7.5-specific transcription (as indicated by the arrowhead symbol for P7.5). It should be taken care that no other ATG sequence is accidentally introduced between the P7.5 sequence and the start codon of the TG. Amplify stock DNA of pII LZdel P7.5-TG for use in **Subheading 3.2.**

3.1.2. Transfection of MVA-Infected Cells with Vector Plasmids

Recombinant plasmids are transfected into MVA infected cells and homologous recombination between MVA and plasmid DNA generates a recombinant virus.

1. Grow CEF or BHK cell monolayers to 80% confluency in 6-well tissue-culture plates. One well is used per transfection.
2. Discard medium and overlay cells with serum-free medium containing MVA at a multiplicity of infection (MOI) of 0.01 (e.g., an inoculum 5×10^3 IU MVA in 1 mL medium for one well with 5×10^5 cells). Incubate for 1 h at 37°C in 5% CO_2-atmosphere. Remove inoculum and wash twice with 2 mL OptiMEM per well.
3. Overlay cell monolayer with Lipofectin/plasmid DNA-mix (total volume: 1 mL) prepared as described by the manufacturer (Life Technologies) using 15 μg plasmid DNA.

MVA   *Hin*dIII

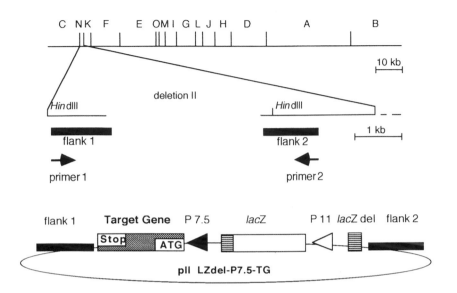

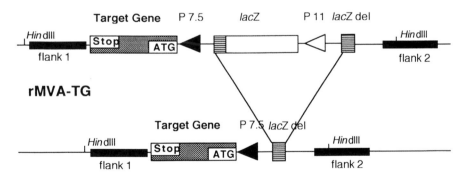

Fig. 1. Schematic representation of the MVA genome and MVA vector plasmid pII LZdel-p7.5-TG. Target gene sequences are integrated into the MVA genome by homologous recombination of MVA DNA sequences (flank 1 and flank 2) designed to target the site of deletion II. After generation of rMVA-TG/LZ by screening for *LacZ* gene expression, the reporter gene sequences are deleted during a second step of recombination resulting in the final vector virus rMVA-TG.

4. Incubate for 5–12 h at 37°C in 5% CO_2-atmosphere.
5. Remove Lipofectin/plasmid DNA-mix and overlay with 1.5 mL fresh medium supplemented with 10% FCS.

6. At 48 h after infection, detach cell monolayer with a cell scraper and transfer cells and medium into 2 mL-microcentrifuge tubes. Store transfection harvest at −20 to −80°C.

3.1.3. Plaque Purification of Recombinant MVA

rMVA expressing the target gene and transiently coexpressing β-galactosidase coding sequences (rMVA-TG/LZ) are cloned by consecutive rounds of plaque purification in CEF/BHK cell monolayers stained with X-gal *(13)*. rMVA being liberated from the reporter gene and expressing the target gene only (rMVA-TG) are isolated in an additional round of plaque purification screening for nonstained viral foci in the presence of X-gal.

1. Freeze thaw the transfection harvest three times (3x) and homogenize the material in cup sonicator (Sonopuls HD 200, Bandelin, Germany). To use cup sonicator, fill cup with ice water (50% ice), place tube containing transfection harvest in ice water, and sonicate at maximal power for 1 min. Repeat three times and take care to avoid heating of the sample by replenishing ice in cup. Make four 10-fold serial dilutions (10^{-1} to 10^{-4}) of the virus suspension in RPMI/L-glu/AM/AB medium + 2% FCS.
2. Remove growth medium from confluent cell monolayers grown in 6-well tissue culture plates and infect with 1.0 mL diluted virus suspension per well. Incubate at 37°C in CO_2-incubator for 2 h.
3. Melt 2% LMP-agarose and hold at 42°C until needed. Prewarm 2X RPMI medium and hold at 37°C until needed. Mix equal amounts of 2% LMP-agarose and 2X RPMI, and allow to temperature equilibrate at 37°C until needed.
4. After 2-h infection of cell monolayers, aspirate inoculum and overlay cell monolayer of each well with 2 mL of the medium/LMP-agarose mixture. Allow agar overlay to solidify at RT, and incubate for 48 h at 37°C in 5% CO_2-atmosphere.
5. Prepare second agarose overlay containing X-gal as described in **step 3** by mixing equal amounts of 2% LMP-agarose and 2X RPMI medium supplemented with 1/100 volume of X-gal solution (e.g., 40 µL X-gal/4 mL 2X RPMI medium). Add to each well 1 mL of the medium/LMP-agarose/X-gal mixture, allow to solidify at RT, and incubate for 4–12 h at 37°C in 5% CO_2-atmosphere.
6. Add 0.5 mL RPMI/L-glu/AM/AB medium + 2% FCS to sterile microcentrifuge tubes. Pick foci of cells infected with recombinant MVA by inserting the tip of a sterile cotton-plugged Pasteur pipet through agarose onto blue-stained viral foci. Scrape and aspirate cells together with agarose plug by squeezing a rubber bulb on Pasteur pipet, and transfer material to the tube containing 0.5 mL medium. Pick 5 to 15 foci, using separate pipet and placing each in separate tube.
7. Freeze thaw, sonicate, and replate virus material obtained from plaque picks as described in **step 1** and **step 2** or store at −80°C. Proceed as in **steps 3–6**.
8. Repeat as described in **steps 1–7** until clonally pure rMVA-TG/LZ is obtained (needs usually 5 to 10 rounds of plaque purification). Use PCR analysis of

viral DNA to monitor for absence of parental non-rMVA (*see* **Subheading 3.2.1.**).

9. Continue plaque purification in the presence of X-gal now picking nonstaining viral foci. Repeat steps as described in **steps 1–7** until all viral isolates fail to produce any blue foci in the presence of X-gal. Amplify (*see* **Subheading 3.1.4.**) and analyze (*see* **Subheading 3.2.**) the cloned rMVA-TG.

3.1.4. Amplification of Recombinant MVA

Here, we describe how to amplify rMVA-TG to generate MVA stock virus used in experiments for analysis or generation of tumor-specific CTL (*see* **Subheading 3.3.**). This protocol can equally be used to grow stocks of parental non-rMVA. If titered MVA starting material is available for amplification, use an MOI of 1 to 3 IU/cell for all infections. To allow efficient infection of cell monolayers growth medium is removed from cells before virus material is added.

1. Infect appropriate confluent cell monolayer grown in a Ø35-mm tissue culture dish with 250 µL virus suspension of isolated rMVA-TG obtained from the last passage of plaque purification, and incubate at 37°C in 5% CO_2-atmosphere for 2 d or until cytopathic effect (CPE) is obvious.
2. Discard medium, harvest cell monolayer in 1 mL RPMI/L-glu/AM/AB medium + 2% FCS, transfer into 1.5 mL microcentrifuge tube, freeze thaw, and sonicate as described in **Subheading 3.1.3., step 1**, and proceed to **step 3** or store at –20 to –80°C as 1st passage of rMVA-TG.
3. Infect cell monolayer grown in Ø60-mm tissue culture dish with 0.5 mL virus suspension obtained from 1st passage of rMVA-TG. Allow virus to adsorb for 1 h at 37°C, add 4 mL RPMI/L-glu/AM/AB medium + 2% FCS and incubate at 37°C in 5% CO_2-atmosphere for 2 d or until CPE is obvious.
4. Scrape cells, transfer to 15-mL conical centrifuge tube, centrifuge 5 min at 1800*g*, discard medium and resuspend cells in 2 mL RPMI/L-glu/AM/AB medium + 2% FCS, freeze thaw and sonicate as described in **Subheading 3.1.3., step 1**, and proceed to **step 5** or store at –20 to –80°C as 2nd passage of rMVA-TG.
5. Infect cell monolayer in 75-cm² tissue-culture flask by adding mixture of 0.5 mL of virus material from 2nd passage of rMVA-TG and 1.5 mL RPMI/L-glu/AM/AB medium + 2% FCS. Allow virus adsorbtion for 1 h at 37°C, rocking flask at 20-min intervals. Overlay with 10 mL RPMI/L-glu/AM/AB medium + 2% FCS, and incubate at 37°C in 5% CO_2-atmosphere for 2 d or until CPE is obvious.
6. Scrape cells, transfer to 15-mL conical centrifuge tube, centrifuge 5 min at 1800*g*, discard medium and resuspend cells in 5 mL RPMI/L-glu/AM/AB medium + 2% FCS, freeze thaw and sonicate as described in **Subheading 3.1.3., step 1**, and proceed to **step 7** or store at –20 to –80°C as 3rd passage of rMVA-TG.
7. Infect cell monolayer in 175-cm² tissue culture flask with 2 mL of virus material from the 3rd passage of rMVA-TG. Allow virus adsorbtion for 1 h at 37°C,

rocking flask at 20-min intervals, add 30 mL RPMI/L-glu/AM/AB medium + 2% FCS, and incubate at 37°C in 5% CO_2-atmosphere for 2 d or until CPE is obvious.

8. Scrape cells in medium, transfer to 50-mL conical centrifuge tube, centrifuge 5 min at 1800g, discard medium and resuspend cells in 15 mL RPMI/L-glu/AM/AB medium + 2% FCS, freeze thaw and sonicate as described in **Subheading 3.1.3., step 1**, and proceed to **step 9** or store at –20 to –80°C as 4th passage of rMVA-TG.

9. Infect cell monolayers of ten 175-cm² tissue-culture flasks by inoculating each flask with 1 mL virus suspension from the 4th passage of rMVA-TG. Allow virus adsorbtion for 1 h at 37°C, rocking flasks at 20 min intervals, add 30 mL RPMI/L-glu/AM/AB medium + 2% FCS per flask, and incubate at 37°C in 5% CO_2-atmosphere for 2 d or until CPE is obvious.

10. Remove about 25 mL medium from each flask, scrape cells in left-over medium, and transfer to two 50-mL centrifuge tubes. Centrifuge 5 min at 1800g, discard medium, resuspend, and combine cell pellets in 20 mL RPMI/L-glu/AM/AB medium + 2% FCS. Freeze thaw and sonicate virus material as described in **Subheading 3.1.3., step 1**, prepare 1-mL aliquots and store as rMVA-TG stock virus (5th passage) at –80°C.

3.2. Characterization of Recombinant MVA

3.2.1. PCR Analysis of MVA-DNA

MVA-DNA is analyzed by PCR using oligonucleotide primers (MVA-II-5′ and MVA-II-3′), which are designed to specifically amplify DNA fragments at insertion site of deletion II within the MVA genome. Thus, genomes of rMVA and parental non-rMVA can be easily identified and distinguished in DNA preparations from infected cell cultures. The method serves to monitor for the elimination of parental MVA during plaque purification of rMVA. Furthermore, correct insertion of foreign DNA (TG) within the MVA genome is ascertained. Primers MVA-II-5′ and MVA-II-3′ anneal to template MVA-DNA sequences adjacent to insertion site II and PCR will produce DNA fragments that are specific for parental non-rMVA (*Frag A*), rMVA-TG/LZ coexpressing the *lacZ*-marker gene (*Frag B*), or for rMVA-TG the final MVA vector virus (*Frag C*):

Fragment	Specificity	Size in kb
Frag A	non-rMVA	0.45
Frag B	rMVA-TG/LZ	4.2 + TG
Frag C	rMVA-TG	4.2 + TG – LZ

Amplification product *Frag A* has a defined size of 0.45 kb indicating that no foreign DNA has been introduced into MVA insertion site II. The expected molecular weight of PCR product *Frag B* can be calculated by adding the size of the TG insert to the 4.2 kb PCR product, which is obtained using empty plasmid vector pII LZdel P7.5 as template DNA. DNA extracted from cells infected with parental MVA and plasmid DNA from pII LZdel P7.5-TG are used as control templates amplifying *Frag* A and *Frag B*, respectively. Finally, the size of the PCR fragment specific for the final recombinant virus rMVA-TG (*Frag C*) results from the molecular weight of *Frag B* being reduced by 3.2 kb DNA corresponding to the desired loss of *lacZ* reporter gene sequences.

In the following example, sizes of PCR products are shown for a TG with given size of 1 kb:

Fragment	Specificity	Control		Size in kb
Frag A	non-rMVA	parental MVA		0.45
Frag B	rMVA-TG/LZ	pII LZdel P7.5-TG	(4.2 + 1.0)	5.2
Frag C	rMVA-TG		(5.2 – 3.2)	2.0

1. Infect cell monolayer of one well in 6-well tissue-culture plate with 2 mL of 10^{-1} dilution of the virus suspension obtained from the last round of plaque purification, and incubate for 3 d at 37°C in 5% CO_2-atmosphere.
2. Discard medium, harvest cell monolayer in 400 µL Aqua dest., transfer into 1.5 mL microcentrifuge tube, add 50 µL 10X TEN pH 7.4, and freeze thaw 3X.
3. Mix by vortexing and microcentrifuge at 450g for 5 min at RT to remove cellular debris.
4. Transfer supernatant into fresh 1.5 mL microcentrifuge tube. Add 50 µL prot K and 23 µL SDS 20 %. Mix by pipeting and incubate for 1 h at 56°C.
5. Extract suspension twice with phenol-chloroform: add equal volume of phenol-chloroform 1:1, mix and microcentrifuge at top speed for 5 min at RT, pipet supernatant into new 1.5 mL microcentrifuge tube.
6. Add 1/10 vol 3M NaAc and 2 vol of EtOH abs., mix gently, and cool for 30 min at –80°C. Centrifuge at top speed for 10 min at 4°C.
7. Aspirate supernatant, wash DNA pellet twice with EtOH 70%, air dry for 10 min, and resuspend in 50 µL Aqua dest..
8. Prepare PCR reaction mix on ice by adding in fixed order 39 µL Aqua bidest, 5 µL primer 1, 5 µL primer 2, 1 µL template DNA, and 50 µL PCR master mix to obtain total volume of 100 µL.
9. Mix and centrifuge briefly to collect sample at the bottom of the tube.
10. Put samples in thermocycler for PCR amplification. A typical PCR profile is given as an example (*see* also **Notes 4.3.**):
    Step 1: Denaturation at 94°C for 3 min
    Step 2: Cycle 1–25: Denaturation at 94°C for 1 min
    　　　　　　　　　 Annealing at 55°C for 1 min
    　　　　　　　　　 Elongation at 72°C for 3 min
    Step 3: Final elongation at 72°C for 7 min
    Step 4: Storage at 4°C

11. Use 20-μL aliquot of each PCR reaction to perform agarose gel electrophoresis, visualize amplificated DNA fragments, and determine molecular weights in comparison to double stranded DNA standards (e.g., 1-kb DNA Ladder, Life Technologies).

3.2.2. Titration of Recombinant MVA by Immunostaining

To titrate the infectivity of MVA stock preparations, foci of MVA infected cells are visualized by specific immuno-peroxidase-staining of cells containing vaccinia viral antigen.

1. After thawing, homogenize MVA stock virus preparation by sonication as described in **Subheading 3.1.3., step 1**.
2. Make 10-fold serial dilutions (ranging from 10^{-1} to 10^{-10}) of virus material in RPMI/L-glu/AM/AB medium without FCS.
3. Add 100 μL of each dilution in replicates of eight to subconfluent cell monolayers grown in 96-well plates using a multipipet and incubate at 37°C in 5% CO_2-atmosphere for 24–48 h.
4. Remove medium from infected tissue culture plates. Fix and permeabilize cells with 200 μL fixing solution per well for 10 min at RT.
5. Remove fixing solution, wash twice with 200 μL PBS per well, add 200 μL blocking buffer per well to block nonspecific binding and incubate for 30 min at RT rocking at 5 cycles per min.
6. Remove blocking buffer, add 100 μL 1st antibody solution (1st Ab) per well and incubate for 1 h at RT rocking at 5 cycles per min.
7. Remove 1st Ab and wash 3X with 200 μL PBS per well. For each washing step, allow to incubate with PBS for 10 min at RT rocking at 10 cycles per min. Add 100 μL 2nd antibody solution (2nd Ab) per well and incubate for 30–45 min as in **step 6**.
8. Remove 2nd Ab and wash 3X with 200 μL PBS per well as in **step 7**.
9. Prepare substrate solution in two steps as follows.
   First, make saturated dianisidine solution by putting a flock of dianisidine on bottom of a 1.5 ml microcentrifuge tube. Add 500 μl EtOH abs., mix by vortexing for 2 to 5 min. Centrifuge for 30 s at top speed at RT. Use supernatant only.
   Prepare final substrate solution for peroxidase-staining by adding 200 μl saturated dianisidine solution to 9.8 ml PBS in a 15-mL conical centrifuge tube. Mix by vortexing, add 15 μL H_2O_2 > 30%, gently mix again, and use immediately.
10. Add 100 μL of substrate solution per well and leave at RT for 10 to 30 min to clearly see stained viral foci.
11. Monitor 96-well plate under microscope and count all wells positive in which viral foci can be detected. Calculate titer according to the method of Kaerber *(15)*. First, determine the end-point dilution that will infect 50% of the wells inoculated calculating in the following way:
$\log_{10}$ 50% end-point dilution = $x - d/2 + (d \Sigma r/n)$

$x =$ highest dilution in which all eight wells (8/8) are counted positive

$d =$ the $\log_{10}$ of the dilution factor ($d = 1$ when serial 10-fold dilutions are used)

$r =$ number of positive wells per dilution

$n =$ total number of wells per dilution ($n = 8$ when dilutions are plated out in replicates of eight)

Given that all eight wells are counted positive in dilution 10^{-7}, x is 7. Additionally, five infected wells are found in dilution 10^{-8}, and the number of infected wells in dilution 10^{-9} (the highest dilution in which positive wells can be found) is 2. Then, the log 50% end-point dilution would be: $7 - 1/2 + (8/8 + 5/8 + 2/8) = 7 - 0.5 + (1.875) = 7 + 1.375 = 8.375$

As the end-point dilution that will infect 50% of the wells inoculated is $10^{-8.375}$ the reciprocal of this number yields the titer in terms of infectious dose per unit volume. As the inoculum added to an individual well was 0.1 mL, the titer of the virus suspension would therefore be: $10^{8.375}$ TCID$_{50}$/0.1mL = $10^{9.375}$ TCID$_{50}$/mL.

3.2.3. Immune-Detection of the Target Protein Produced by rMVA-TG

A modified protocol of the one described in **Subheading 3.2.2.** allows to conveniently confirm the synthesis of your target antigen upon infection with rMVA-TG. An antibody that reacts with your target gene product is used as 1st antibody (instead of the antivaccinia serum used in **Subheading 3.2.2.**). Therefore, the immunostaining will allow to specifically detect cells which are infected with rMVA-TG and produce the antigen of interest.

1. Homogenize rMVA-TG virus preparation by sonication as described in **Subheading 3.1.3., step 1**.
2. Infect cell monolayers grown in 6-well tissue-culture plates with rMVA-TG or parental MVA (as control) at an MOI of 0.01, 0.001, and 0.0001 IU/cell (e.g., inoculate three wells each containing 1×10^6 cells with 10^4, 10^3, or 10^2 IU rMVA-TG resuspended in 2 mL medium and incubate at 37°C in 5% CO_2-atmosphere for 48 h. Use one cell monolayer as mock-infected control.
3. After 24-h infection remove medium, fix and permeabilize cells by overlaying with 1 mL fixing solution per well for 10 min at RT.
4. Remove fixing solution, rinse twice with PBS, add 2 mL blocking buffer per well to block nonspecific binding, and incubate for 30 min at RT rocking at five cycles per min.
5. Remove blocking buffer, rinse twice with PBS, add 1 mL diluted 1st antibody (1st Ab) per well and incubate for 1 h at RT rocking at five cycles per min.
6. Remove 1st Ab and wash 3X with 2 mL PBS per well for 5 min at RT on rocking device at 10 cycles per min. Add 1 mL 2nd antibody dilution (2nd Ab) per well and incubate for 30–45 min at RT rocking at five cycles per min.
7. Remove 2nd Ab and wash as in **step 6**.

8. Prepare substrate solution as described in **Subheading 3.2.2., step 9**.
9. Add 1 mL of substrate solution per well. Incubate for up to 30 min at RT until foci of stained cell can be detected. Continue to monitor staining under microscope. When specific staining has stopped to intensify, remove substrate solution and rinse cell monolayers with PBS.

3.3. Infection of Antigen-Presenting Cells with Recombinant MVA

CTL activities to be measured in in vitro experiments will critically depend on the stimulatory or activatory capacity of stimulator or target cells. Here, we describe an optimized protocol for rMVA-TG infection of various types of antigen presenting cells, including primary cells (e.g., DC, BC, monocytes) as well as cell lines (e.g., LCL). The protocol may be applicable for infection of stimulator or target cells used in a variety of immunoassays measuring target cell lysis (e.g., chromium release assay), T-cell proliferation (e.g., [^{3}H]thymidine uptake) or T-cell activation (e.g., cytokine release). As the number of cells to be infected may vary with assays performed, we used in this protocol a given cell number of 1×10^6 cells per infection as an example.

3.3.1. Generation of Stimulator Cells
for Isolation or Activation of TAA-Specific CTL

1. After thawing, homogenize rMVA-TG preparation by sonication as described in **Subheading 3.1.3., step 1**.
2. Infect 1×10^6 stimulator cells resuspended in 100 μL medium in a 15-mL conical centrifuge tube with an MOI of 10 IU rMVA-TG/cell by adding 100 μL medium containing 1×10^7 IU of virus. Mix and incubate at 37°C in 5% CO_2-atmosphere for 1.5 h. Mix gently in 15-min intervals by snapping tube or by continuous movement with a mechanical device. Add 800 μL fresh medium and incubate for additional 1.5 h.
3. Wash cells twice with 10 mL medium (centrifuge for 5 min at 470g at RT) to remove free-virus particles.
4. Resuspend cells in appropriate volume of medium, transfer cells to tissue culture plates appropriate to the assay to be performed, and incubate for additional 10 to 12 h at 37°C in 5% CO_2-atmosphere.
5. Add responder T cells to infected stimulator cells. Perform individual assay.
6. Repeat **step 1–4** for any further stimulator cell preparation.

3.3.2. Generation of Target Cells for Analysis
of TAA-specific CTL Activity in [^{51}Cr] Release Assays

1. After thawing, homogenize rMVA-TG preparation by sonication as described in **Subheading 3.1.3., step 1**.
2. *See* **Subheading 3.3.1., step 2**.
3. Centrifuge tube for 5 min at 470g at RT. Discard medium, add the required μCi

of ^{51}Cr (e.g., 150 µCi / 150 µL / tube), add 1/10 vol serum (e.g. 15 µL) and incubate for 1 h at 37°C in 5% CO_2-atmosphere.

4. Wash labeled cells 4X with 10 mL medium (centrifuge for 5 min at 1500g at 4°C) to remove free-virus particles and free-chromium.

5. Resuspend target cells in appropriate volume of medium, transfer cells to appropriate plates for chromium release assay, and incubate for additional 7–8 h at 37°C in 5% CO_2-atmosphere. In total allow for a 12-h period of infection.

6. Add responder T cells (at varying E:T ratios) to target cells and incubate for 4–5 h. Harvest supernatants and measure ^{51}Cr activities.

4. Notes

4.1. Plaque Purification of Recombinant MVA

1. In order to pick rMVA plaques, preferably choose well-separated viral foci from wells infected with 10^{-3} or 10^{-4} dilutions. This will drastically reduce the number of plaque passages needed to isolate clonally pure rMVA.

2. As the expression cassette of the *lacZ* marker gene is designed to be efficiently deleted from the rMVA genome nonstaining MVA foci may be observed during plaque purification even after all non-rMVA has been successfully eliminated. To avoid needless plaque passages, it is important that the absence of non-rMVA is confirmed by PCR analysis. In the following, non-staining MVA foci can be picked to obtain final rMVA expressing only the target gene of interest (rMVA-TG).

4.2. Amplification of Recombinant MVA

3. When infecting cell monolayers grown in larger tissue-culture flasks (e.g., 185-cm^2 flasks), avoid drying of the cell monolayer by rocking flask by hand at 20-min intervals.

4. Having obtained the rMVA-TG stock virus, the following procedures are recommended:
   a. Titer the virus stock on infected CEF or BHK cell monolayers (*see* **Subheading 3.2.2.**).
   b. Analyze clonal purity and genomic stability of rMVA-TG by PCR (*see* **Subheading 3.2.1.**) or Southern blot analysis of viral DNA.
   c. Characterize synthesis of target protein by specific immunostaining of viral foci expressing recombinant gene(s) (*see* **Subheading 3.2.3.**), by immunoblot analysis of lysates from rMVA infected cell cultures, or by immunoprecipitation of the target antigen made during rMVA infection following labeling with radioactive amino acids.

5. It is recommended to prepare a first virus stock as primary stock which is used to amplify *working* stocks of rMVA.

4.3. PCR Analysis of MVA DNA

6. Virus material harvested from a cell monolayer grown in a 6-well/12-well tissue-culture plate and infected for 24 h with an MOI of 10 IU/cell will yield an amount

of viral DNA (*see* **Subheading 3.2.1., step 2**) adequate for PCR/Southern blot analysis. To monitor the presence of non-rMVA during plaque purification, viral DNA sufficient for PCR analysis is isolated from cell monolayers infected with the 10^{-1}-dilution of virus suspensions plated out for plaque passage.

7. Avoid sonication of infected tissue-culture material to be used for DNA extraction because unpackaged viral DNA will be destroyed and lost for analysis.

8. Alternatively, DNA precipitation may be done on dry ice for 15 min or at $-20°C$ for 2–12 h.

9. Carefully air dry the pelleted DNA material to remove all ethanol.

10. Always use DNA of non-rMVA and pII LZdel P7.5-TG as control templates for PCR analysis.

11. As DNA preparations might contain variable quantities of viral DNA, the amount of template DNA used for PCR may be optimized.

12. PCR conditions (temperatures and number of cycles) may be optimized according to the size of the expected fragment to be amplified. Conditions as stated in the protocol have been used for amplification of up to 4 kb DNA inserted into the MVA genome.

13. If template DNA is derived from mixed virus populations containing both, rMVA-TG/LZ as well as rMVA-TG, PCR may amplify preferentially *Frag C* because of its smaller size and *Frag B* may not be detectable.

4.4. Titration of Recombinant MVA by Immunostaining

14. Before titration, virus material *must* be homogenized by sonication. Sonicate aliquots of maximal 1.5 mL virus suspension as described in **Subheading 3.1.3., step 1**.

15. Alternatively, incubation with blocking buffer can be done overnight at 4°C.

16. To remove small clumps of dianisidine, filter the PBS/dianisidine mix through 0.2-μm filter into a new tube before adding the $H_2O_2 > 30\%$.

4.5. Immune-Detection of Target Protein Produced by rMVA

17. As the nature and origin of the 1st Ab may vary, an appropriate peroxidase-conjugated 2nd Ab must be chosen. Optimal dilutions of Abs should be determined for best results.

4.6. Generation of Stimulator Cells for Isolation or Activation of TAA-Specific CTL

18. Always remember to homogenize virus material by sonication, as this will ensure equal distribution of infectious particles and standardized infections.

19. For infection, cells and vector virus should be concentrated at low volume to allow most efficient virus/target interaction (e.g., 1×10^6 cells and 1×10^7 virus particles in 100 μL, respectively). Depending on the cell type used for infection appropriate medium is chosen.

4.7. Generation of Target Cells for Analysis of TAA-Specific CTL Activity in [^{51}Cr] Release Assays

20. Time for optimal chromium uptake may vary with different cell types and may be extended up to 1.5 h.
21. Time of incubation may depend on the time needed for chromium labeling, washing, and plating out targets. Usually, responder T cells are added after 12 h of infection to allow for efficient synthesis of the recombinant TAA.

Acknowledgements

This work was supported by the European Community Grant BIO4-CT96-0473 and by the Deutsche Forschungsgersinschaft Grant SFB 456–B7.

References

1. Van den Eynde, B. J. and Van der Bruggen, B. (1997) T cell defined tumor antigens. *Curr. Opin. Immunol.* **9,** 684–693.
2. Moss, B. (1996) Genetically engineered poxviruses for recombinant gene expression, vaccination and safety. *Proc. Natl. Acad. Sci. U.S.A.* **93,** 11,341–11,348.
3. Rosenberg, S. A. (1997) Cancer vaccines based on the identification of the genes encoding cancer regression antigens. *Immunol. Today* **18,** 175–182.
4. Sutter, G. and Moss, B. (1992) Nonreplicating vaccinia vector efficiently expresses recombinant genes. *Proc. Natl. Acad. Sci. USA* **89,** 10,847–10,851.
5. Meyer, H., Sutter, G., and Mayr, A. (1991) Mapping of deletions in the genome of the highly attenuated vaccinia virus MVA and their influence on virulence. *J. Gen. Virol.* **72,** 1031–1038.
6. Drexler, I., Heller, K., Wahren, B., Erfle, V., and Sutter, G. (1998) Highly attenuated modified vaccinia virus Ankara replicates in baby hamster kidney cells, a potential host for virus propagation, but not in various human transformed and primary cells. *J. Gen. Virol.* **79,** 347–352.
7. Carroll, M. W. and Moss, B. (1997) Host range and Cytopathogenicity of the highly attenuated MVA strain of vaccinia virus: Propagation and generation of recombinant viruses in a nonhuman mammalian cell line. *Virology* **238,** 198–211.
8. Sutter, G., Wyatt, L. S., Foley, P. L., Bennink, J. R., and Moss, B. (1994) A recombinant vector derived from the host range-restricted and highly attenuated MVA strain of vaccinia virus stimulates protective immunity in mice to influenza virus. *Vaccine* **12,** 1032–1040.
9. Hirsch, V. M., Fuerst, T. R., Sutter, G., Carroll, M. W., Yang, L. C., Goldstein, S., et al. (1996) Patterns of viral replication correlate with outcome in simian immunodeficiency virus (SIV)- infected macaques: Effect of prior immunization with a trivalent SIV vaccine in modified vaccinia virus Ankara. *J. Virol.* **70,** 3741–3752.
10. Durbin, A. P., Wyatt, L. S., Siew, J., Moss, B., and Murphy, B. R. (1998) The immunogenicity and efficacy of intranasally or parenterally administered replication-defiecent vaccinia-parainfluenza virus type 3 recombinants in rhesus monkeys. *Vaccine* **16,** 1324–1330.

11. Schneider, J., Gilbert, S. C., Blanchard, T. J., Hanke, T., Robson, K. J., Hannan, C. M., et al. (1998) Enhanced immunogenicity for CD8+ T cell induction and complete protective efficacy of malaria DNA vaccination by boosting with modified vaccinia virus Ankara. *Nat. Med.* **4,** 397–402.
12. Carroll, M. W., Overwijk, W. W., Chamberlain, R. S., Rosenberg, S. A., Moss, B., and Restifo, N. P. (1997) Highly attenuated modified vaccinia virus Ankara (MVA) as an effective recombinant vector: a murine tumor model. *Vaccine* **15,** 387–394.
13. Drexler, I., Antunes, E., Schmitz, M., Wölfel, T., Huber, C., Eifle, V., Rieber P., et al. (1999) Modified vaccinia virus ankara for delivery of human tyrosinase as Melanoma—associated antigen: Induction of tyrosinase—and Melanoma-specific human leukocyte antigen A*0201-restricted cytotoxic T cells in vitro and in vivo. *Cancer Res.* in press.
14. Sutter, G., Ohlmann, M., and Erfle, V. (1995) Non-replicating vaccinia vector efficiently expresses bacteriophage T7 RNA polymerase. *FEBS Lett.* **371,** 9–12.
15. Kaerber G. (1931) Beitrag zur kollektiven Behandlung pharmakologischer Reihenversuche. *Arch. exp. Pathol. Pharmakol.* **162,** 480.

I

EXPERIMENTAL APPROACHES IN CANCER GENE THERAPY

B: Suicide Gene Therapy

5

Selection of Cytochrome *P450* Genes for Use in Prodrug Activation-Based Cancer Gene Therapy

Jodi E. D. Hecht and David J. Waxman

1. Introduction

Prodrug activation-based cancer gene therapy is a molecular strategy to improve the efficacy of cancer chemotherapy by conferring upon tumor cells the capability to metabolize specific anticancer prodrugs into lethal intracellular toxins. The overall goal of this strategy is to increase the generation of cytotoxic drug metabolites locally, at their site of action within the tumor. This therapy can provide for an increase in drug efficacy and potentially also a reduction in host toxicity, which may be achieved by a lowering of the therapeutically effective drug dosage, thereby reducing the need to expose host tissues to high cytotoxic plasma drug concentrations. This chapter describes the cytochrome P450-based prodrug activation strategy for cancer gene therapy *(1–3)*, with a particular emphasis on the selection of suitable P450 gene/prodrug combinations.

Two widely studied prodrug activation-gene therapy strategies are bacterial cytosine deaminase and the herpes simplex virus thymidine kinase *(4,5)*. Transduction of target tumor cells with these genes confers upon the target tumor cell the capacity to metabolize the prodrugs 5-fluorocytosine and ganciclovir, respectively. Although these strategies have shown potential in preclinical trials and may eventually be used in clinical applications *(6)*, they both have several limitations. These include:

1. The expression of these non-mammalian genes may induce an immune response in the host that precludes repeated rounds of therapeutic gene delivery.
2. The prodrugs 5-fluorocytosine and ganciclovir have not been developed as anticancer drugs, and hence their ultimate therapeutic potential in the clinic is uncertain.

From: *Methods in Molecular Medicine, Vol. 35: Gene Therapy: Methods and Protocols*
Edited by: W. Walther and U. Stein © Humana Press, Inc., Totowa, NJ

3. The activated, phosphorylated ganciclovir metabolites do not readily cross cell membranes and require cell to cell contact for an effective bystander cytotoxic effect *(7)*.
4. Both of these drugs are active in a cell cycle-dependent manner.

An alternative prodrug-activation gene-therapy strategy involves the use of genes that encode specific drug-metabolizing cytochrome P450 enzymes *(1,2)*. This P450-based strategy uses mammalian genes, to minimize host-immune responses, in combination with well-established and clinically useful anticancer prodrugs. Cytochrome P450 enzymes are mixed-function oxidases that metabolize many therapeutic drugs and other foreign chemicals. P450 enzymes in conjunction with electron transfer from NADPH via the flavoprotein P450 reductase catalyze the monooxygenation of structurally diverse drugs and xenobiotics both in the liver and certain extrahepatic tissues. P450 metabolism of anticancer drugs most often results in detoxification, but in some cases leads to drug activation to produce DNA-alkylating, cytotoxic metabolites *(8,9)*. However, intratumoral expression of P450 enzymes is typically very low *(10,11)* and, consequently, in the absence of P450 gene transfer to tumor cells, the therapeutic activity of a P450-activated prodrug will generally be dependent on drug metabolism carried out by the liver, which expresses high levels of drug-metabolizing P450 enzymes.

Administration of anticancer agents in the form of prodrugs increases drug stability and may lead to prolonged therapeutic activity. In the case of the antineoplastic drug cyclophosphamide, multiple human P450 enzymes (CYPs) including CYP2B6, CYP3A4, and CYP2C9 activate the drug by a 4-hydroxylation reaction *(12)*. Ifosfamide, an isomer of cyclophosphamide, is primarily activated by human CYP3A4 *(12,13)*. Other examples of P450-activated anticancer prodrugs include dacarbazine, procarbazine, and thio-TEPA *(8)*. In addition, the antiestrogen prodrug Tamoxifen is metabolized to more active metabolites by CYP3A4 and CYP2D6 *(14)* and the chemotherapeutic prodrug 4-ipomeanol is specifically activated by the rabbit P450 enzyme 4B1 *(15)*.

Preclinical studies have demonstrated that P450-based anticancer gene therapy is an effective way to sensitize tumor cells to anticancer prodrugs. Introduction of the rat P450 gene CYP2B1 into rat 9L gliosarcoma or C6 glioma cells by stable transfection, adenoviral infection, or infection with replication-conditional oncolytic virus confers tumor-cell sensitivity to the anticancer prodrug cyclophosphamide *(2,16,17)*. In vivo studies, cyclophosphamide treatment of rats bearing P450-expressing 9L solid tumors grown subcutaneously *(2)* or intracranially *(1)* results in a substantial delay in tumor growth and an enhanced survival rate compared to that which can be achieved in the absence of P450 gene transfer, i.e., based on liver prodrug activation alone. Similarly, ex vivo transfection of the rat CYP2B1 gene into MCF7 human breast cancer cells confers sensitivity to cyclophosphamide in vitro, and also in vivo in the case of solid tumors grown subcutaneously in nude mice *(18)*. A further enhancement of intratumoral P450-catalyzed prodrug activation can be achieved by coexpressing the flavoprotein P450 reductase together with a prodrug-activating P450 enzyme *(16,19)*. Although CYP2B1, an active catalyst of cyclophosphamide activation *(20)*, has been used in all of these earlier studies, other P450 genes, including several human P450 catalysts of cyclophosphamide activation *(21)*, may have more useful properties in terms of their enzyme activity or kinetics of prodrug activation. Studies to examine the potential utility of several human P450 genes for cancer gene therapy have recently been carried out *(19)*.

Several factors should be considered when choosing suitable P450 gene/ prodrug combinations for anticancer gene therapy. Prodrug activation reactions that are catalyzed at a low rate or not at all by endogenous human liver P450 enzymes are ideal in terms of maximizing intratumoral prodrug activation. This situation is exemplified by the rabbit CYP4B1 gene and the chemotherapeutic drug 4-ipomeanol combination *(15)*, insofar as the corresponding human P450 enzyme does not activate 4-ipomeanol. In addition, the use of a P450 gene from a nonhuman species, e.g., a rodent P450 in place of its human P450 ortholog, may sometimes provide benefits in terms of the nonhuman P450 enzyme's specificity for related prodrug substrate. For example, rat CYP2B1 activates the isomeric anticancer prodrugs ifosfamide and cyclophosphamide *(22)* whereas its human ortholog, CYP2B6, activates cyclophosphamide with the same efficiency as CYP2B1, whereas ifosfamide is activated at a much lower rate *(23)*. Detailed enzymatic studies of closely related P450 genes from several mammalian species *(24)* including rat, mouse, dog, and rabbit should, therefore, be carried out.

A second consideration is that the P450 enzyme must have a V_{max} with the prodrug substrate that is sufficiently high to generate within the tumor an elevated level of activated drug metabolites. This is required to obtain a strong cytotoxic response in both the P450-expressing tumor cell and in adjacent tumor cells that are not transduced with the P450 gene. This bystander cytotoxic effect *(7)* is essential for achieving an enhanced chemotherapeutic response because currently available vectors for gene delivery to tumors provide for low efficiencies of gene transduction. In the case of cyclophosphamide and P450 2B1 or P450 2B6, cytotoxic metabolites that do not require cell-to-cell contact for bystander activity are generated *(2,19)*. This property is a reflection of the intrinsic diffusibility of the primary P450 metabolite, 4-hydroxycyclophosphamide, which is normally generated in the liver, but nonetheless exerts significant cytotoxicity toward distant tumor cells. By contrast, phosphorylated ganciclovir, produced by the prodrug-activating enzymes

HSV thymidine kinase, requires direct cell-to-cell contact via gap junctions for bystander cytotoxic activity *(25)*.

Finally, it is preferable if intratumoral expression of the therapeutic P450 does not stimulate a host immune response. Although many rat and human P450s have closely related amino acid sequences and similar substrate specificities, expression of some heterologous, nonhuman P450 genes may induce an immune response in the human host. In tumor model studies, immunogenic responses can lead to tumor growth rates that are not consistent, and consequently, the efficacy of drug therapy may be difficult to determine in this environment. Although cellular immune responses can enhance antitumor activity, and perhaps also increase the bystander killing effect *(26)*, this effect is difficult to control and the response may vary from one patient to another.

The specific P450 enzymes that activate cancer chemotherapeutic prodrugs can be identified in the following manner. First, a panel of tumor cell lines, each of which expresses a single, individual P450 gene can be developed using retroviral transduction methods, as described elsewhere in this volume (*see* Chapter 6). Both established and new antitumor agents can be tested or screened using these P450 cell lines by growth inhibition and cytotoxicity assays, as described in Chapter 7. Commercial lymphoblast or baculovirus P450 cDNA expression systems are widely available and, at present, represent more than a dozen different human P450 genes (e.g., 'Supersomes' from Gentest, Inc., Woburn, MA). In vitro analysis of drug metabolism can, therefore, be carried out using these expressed P450s to identify the biochemical pathways of prodrug metabolism. Finally, animal models can be employed to evaluate in vivo the therapeutic potential of specific prodrug/P450 combinations using tumor excision and tumor growth delay assays, as described in Chapter 8.

In conclusion, the use of cytochrome P450 genes for prodrug activation-based cancer therapy has the potential of becoming an effective therapy for cancer treatment, either alone or in combination with other prodrug activation genes *(27)*, such as HSV thymidine kinase/ganciclovir or cytosine deaminase/5-fluorocytosine. The efficacy of this approach requires that prodrug activation occur at a rate that is sufficiently high to kill a high proportion of the target tumor cells. Ideally, the tumor-expressed P450 enzyme will have high metabolic activity for the prodrug substrate so that a significant fraction of the prodrug can be activated intratumorally, rather than in other tissues (e.g., liver). The activated drug metabolite should have a significant bystander effect whereby diffusion of the cytotoxic species into adjacent tumor cells readily occurs, even in the absence of direct cell-to-cell contact. Finally, the increased intratumoral prodrug activation provided by this strategy must be achieved without increasing cytotoxicity to the host. The ultimate success of this prodrug-activation gene-therapy paradigm requires suitable viral or nonviral vectors with a high specificity for P450 gene transfer to tumor cells. Selective gene delivery to tumor cells may be achieved using cellular or transcriptional targeting approaches *(28,29)*, including tumor hypoxia-based strategies *(30,31)* currently under development.

Acknowledgments

Preparation of this Chapter was carried out with the support of NIH Grant CA49248 (to D. J. Waxman).

References

1. Wei, M. X., Tamiya, T., Chase, M., Boviatsis, E. J., Chang, T. K. H., Kowall, N. W., et al. (1994) Experimental tumor therapy in mice using the cyclophosphamide-activating cytochrome P450 2B1 gene. *Hum. Gene Ther.* **5,** 969–978.
2. Chen, L. and Waxman, D. J. (1995) Intratumoral activation and enhanced chemotherapeutic effect of oxazaphosphorines following cytochrome P450 gene transfer: development of a combined chemotherapy/cancer gene therapy strategy. *Cancer Res.* **55,** 581–589.
3. Waxman, D. J., Chen, L., Hecht, J. E. D., and Jounaidi, Y. (1998) Cytochrome P450-based cancer gene therapy: recent advances and future prospects. *Drug Metab. Rev.* **31,** 503–522.
4. Moolten, F. L. (1994) Drug sensitivity ("suicide") genes for selective cancer chemotherapy. *Cancer Gene Ther.* **1,** 279–287.
5. Freeman, S. M., Whartenby, K. A., Freeman, J. L., Abboud, C. N., and Marrogi, A. J. (1996) In situ use of suicide genes for cancer therapy. *Semin. Oncol.* **23,** 31–45.
6. Roth, J. A. and Cristiano, R. J. (1997) Gene therapy for cancer: what have we done and where are we going? *J. Natl. Cancer Inst.* **89,** 21–39.
7. Pope, I. M., Poston, G. J., and Kinsella, A. R. (1997) The role of the bystander effect in suicide gene therapy. *Eur. J. Cancer* **33,** 1005–1016.
8. LeBlanc, G. A. and Waxman, D. J. (1989) Interaction of anticancer drugs with hepatic monooxygenase enzymes. *Drug Metab. Rev.* **20,** 395–439.
9. Kivisto, K. T., Kroemer, H. K., and Eichelbaum, M. (1995) The role of human cytochrome P450 enzymes in the metabolism of anticancer agents: implications for drug interactions. *Br. J. Clin. Pharmacol.* **40,** 523–530.
10. Smith, G., Harrison, D. J., East, N., Rae, F., Wolf, H., and Wolf, C. R. (1993) Regulation of cytochrome P450 gene expression in human colon and breast tumour xenografts. *Br. J. Cancer* **68,** 57–63.
11. Huang, Z., Fasco, M. J., Figge, H. L., Keyomarsi, K., and Kaminsky, L. S. (1996) Expression of cytochromes P450 in human breast tissue and tumors. *Drug Metab. Dispos.* **24,** 899–905.
12. Chang, T. K. H., Weber, G. F., Crespi, C. L., and Waxman, D. J. (1993) Differential activation of cyclophosphamide and ifosphamide by cytochromes P450 2B and 3A in human liver microsomes. *Cancer Res.* **53,** 5629–5637.

13. Walker, D., Flinois, J. P., Monkman, S. C., Beloc, C., Boddy, A. V., Cholerton, S., et al. (1994) Identification of the major human hepatic cytochrome P450 involved in activation and N-dechloroethylation of ifosfamide. *Biochem. Pharmacol.* **47,** 1157–1163.

14. Dehal, S. S. and Kupfer, D. (1997) CYP2D6 catalyzes tamoxifen 4-hydroxylation in human liver. *Cancer Res.* **57,** 3402–3406.

15. Rainov, N. G., Dobberstein, K. U., Sena-Esteves, M., Herrlinger, U., Kramm, C. M., Philpot, R. M., et al. (1998) New prodrug activation gene therapy for cancer using cytochrome P450 4B1 and 2-Aminoanthracene/4-Ipomeanol. *Human Gene Ther.* **9,** 1261–1273.

16. Chen, L., Yu, L. J., and Waxman, D. J. (1997) Potentiation of cytochrome P450/ cyclophosphamide-based cancer gene therapy by coexpression of the P450 reductase gene. *Cancer Res.* **57,** 4830–4837.

17. Chase, M., Chung, R. Y., and Chiocca, E. A. (1998) An oncolytic viral mutant that delivers the CYP2B1 transgene and augments cyclophosphamide chemotherapy. *Nature Biotech.* **16,** 444–448.

18. Chen, L., Waxman, D. J., Chen, D., and Kufe, D. W. (1996) Sensitization of human breast cancer cells to cyclophosphamide and ifosfamide by transfer of a liver cytochrome P450 gene. *Cancer Res.* **56,** 1331–1340.

19. Jounaidi, Y., Hecht, J. E. D., and Waxman, D. J. (1998) Retroviral transfer of cytochrome P450 genes for oxazaphosphorine-based cancer gene therapy. *Cancer Res.* **58,** 4391–4401.

20. Clarke, L. and Waxman, D. J. (1989) Oxidative metabolism of cyclophosphamide: identification of the hepatic monooxygenase catalysts of drug activation. *Cancer Res.* **49,** 2344–2350.

21. Chang, T. K., Yu, L., Goldstein, J. A., and Waxman, D. J. (1997) Identification of the polymorphically expressed CYP2C19 and the wild- type CYP2C9-ILE359 allele as low-Km catalysts of cyclophosphamide and ifosfamide activation. *Pharmacogenetics* **7,** 211–221.

22. Weber, G. F. and Waxman, D. J. (1993) Activation of the anti-cancer drug ifosphamide by rat liver microsomal P450 enzymes. *Biochem. Pharmacol.* **45,** 1685–1694.

23. Roy, P., Yu, L. J., Crespi, C. L., and Waxman, D. J. (1999) Development of a substrate-activity based approach to identify the major human liver P450 catalysts of cyclophosphamide and ifosfamide activation based on cDNA-expressed activities and liver microsomal P450 profiles. *Drug Metab. Rev.* **27,** 655–666.

24. Nelson, D. R., Koymans, L., Kamataki, T., Stegeman, J. J., Feyereisen, R., Waxman, D. J., et al. (1996) Cytochrome P450 superfamily: Update on new sequences, gene mapping, accession numbers, and nomenclature. *Pharmacogenetics* **6,** 1–42.

25. Mesnil, M., Piccoli, C., Tiraby, G., Willecke, K., and Yamasaki, H. (1996) Bystander killing of cancer cells by herpes simplex virus thymidine kinase gene is mediated by connexins. *Proc. Natl. Acad. Sci. USA* **93,** 1831–1835.

26. Gagandeep, S., Brew, R., Green, B., Christmas, S. E., Klatzmann, D., Poston, G. J., and Kinsella, A. R. (1996) Prodrug-activated gene therapy: involvement of an immunological component in the "bystander effect." *Cancer Gene Ther.* **3,** 83–88.

27. Aghi, M., Chou, T. C., Suling, K., Breakfield, X. O., and Chiocca, E. A. (1999) Multimodal cancer treatment mediated by a replicating oncolytic virus that delivers the oxazaphosphorine/rat cytochrome P450-2B1 and ganciclovir/herpes simplex virus thymidine kinase gene therapies. *Cancer Res.* **59,** 3861–3865.

28. Dachs, G. U., Dougherty, G. J., Stratford, I. J., and Chaplin, D. J. (1997) Targeting gene therapy to cancer: a review. *Oncol. Res.* **9,** 313–325.

29. Miller, N. and Whelan, J. (1997) Progress in transcriptionally targeted and regulatable vectors for genetic therapy. *Hum. Gene Ther.* **8,** 803–815.

30. Dachs, G. U., Patterson, A. V., Firth, J. D., Ratcliffe, P. J., Townsend, K. M., Stratford, I. J., and Harris, A. L. (1997) Targeting gene expression to hypoxic tumor cells. *Nat. Med.* **3,** 515–520.

31. Brown, J. M. and Giaccia, A. J. (1998) The unique physiology of solid tumors: opportunities (and problems) for cancer therapy. *Cancer Res.* **58,** 1408–1416.

6

Construction of P450-Expressing
Tumor Cell Lines Using Retroviruses

Jodi E. D. Hecht, Youssef Jounaidi, and David J. Waxman

1. Introduction
1.1. Construction of P450-Expressing Tumor Cell Lines

Studies of tumor cell lines expressing individual cytochrome P450 genes are essential for evaluation of the utility of P450 prodrug activation-based cancer gene therapy (*1*). *P450*-expressing tumor cells may also be useful to identify novel *P450* gene /prodrug combinations (*see* Chapter 5). The evaluation of candidate *P450* genes for use in prodrug activation gene therapy is greatly facilitated by the availability of *P450*-expressing tumor cell lines, which can be prepared by the retroviral transduction methods described in this chapter. Finally, it should be noted that the methods described in this chapter are not limited to P450 gene transduction, and can readily be applied to the transduction of other genes of interest to cancer gene therapy. In vitro cytotoxicity assays using these cell lines can then be carried out as described in Chapter 7 prior to initiating more costly and labor intensive in vivo tumor studies in animal models (described in Chapter 8).

P450-expressing tumor cell lines are readily established by transduction of tumor cells with a retroviral vector that carries the *P450* gene of interest. Retroviruses are excellent vectors for laboratory studies of cancer gene therapy because they can infect dividing tumor cells with high efficiency and may contain nonviral inserts of up to 7.5 kb (cf., full-length *P450* cDNA coding sequence ~1.5 kb). These retroviral vectors are prepared in high-titer replication-deficient retrovirus packaging cell lines that express key genes required for retroviral replication (*2*). Viral titers of $\geq 10^6$ particles per mL of culture supernatant are readily generated, and can be used directly for transduction of

From: *Methods in Molecular Medicine, Vol. 35: Gene Therapy: Methods and Protocols*
Edited by: W. Walther and U. Stein © Humana Press, Inc., Totowa, NJ

tumor cells in vivo *(3)*, or more commonly, in cell-culture. For cell culture studies, selection with an appropriate drug-resistance marker enzyme encoded by the retrovirus (e.g., puromycin or hygromycin resistance) yields a pool containing thousands of independent, clonal tumor cells, each of which expresses the specific P450 gene of interest (albeit at levels that may differ from one clone to the next). The retroviral long-terminal repeat, which contains the retroviral enhancer and promoter region, ensures stable integration of the P450 gene into the host genome *(4)*.

2. Materials
2.1. Transfection

1. Bosc 23 cells: Ecotropic packaging cell line *(5)*.
2. Growth medium for Bosc 23 cells: Dulbecco's Modified Eagle Medium (DMEM) (Life Technologies, Gaithersburg, MD, cat. # 12100-046) supplemented with 3.7 g of sodium bicarbonate, 10 mL of penicillin (5000 U/mL), and streptomycin (5000 µg/mL) (Life Technologies, cat. # 15070-063) in 900 mL of deionized water. Adjust the pH of the medium to pH 7.1 with concentrated HCl. Filter-sterilize with 0.2 µm bottle-top filters. Store at 4°C for up to 6 mo. To prepare DMEM containing serum supplement 450 mL of complete DMEM with 50 mL of heat-inactivated (56°C for 30 min) fetal bovine serum (Sigma, St. Louis, MD, cat. # F-2442) (final serum concentration, 10%). Store FBS-DMEM at 4°C for up to 2 mo. Prewarm 10% FBS-DMEM to 37°C before adding to cells.
3. Freezing Medium for Bosc 23 cells: 10% dimethyl sulfoxide and 90% heat-inactivated fetal bovine serum. The medium may be stored at –20°C in 50 mL aliquots for up to 1 yr. Freeze the Bosc 23 cells at 1×10^6 cells/mL and store in liquid nitrogen.
4. 2 × HBS (42 m*M* HEPES, 274 m*M* NaCl, 10 m*M* KCl, 1.4 m*M* Na$_2$HPO$_4$, 11 m*M* glucose), adjusted to pH 6.95 (*see* **Note 1**). Filter-sterilize with 0.2 µm bottle-top filters. Store at –20°C in 10 mL aliquots. Stable for 1 yr.
5. 0.25*M* CaCl$_2$ (autoclave or filter-sterilize). Store at room temperature or at –20°C.
6. 25 m*M* Chloroquine (Sigma, cat. # C-6628). Prepare in phosphate-buffered saline or growth medium and filter- sterilize. Store at –20°C in 100 µL aliquots for up to 1 yr.
7. PBS: Phosphate Buffered Saline (without Mg^{+2} or Ca^{+2}) 0.146*M* NaCl, 0.01*M* NaHPO$_4$, 2.68 m*M* KCl, 1.76 m*M* KH$_2$PO$_4$ Filter-sterilize and store at room temperature. The pH will be about 7.4 with the mixture of these salts. Prewarm buffer to 37°C before using.
8. Syringe filters: 0.2 µm 25 mm low-protein binding filter (Gelman, Ann Arbor, MI, cat. # 4454).
9. Syringe filters: 0.45 µm 25 mm low-protein binding filter (Gelman, cat. # 4184).
10. 100 mm tissue culture dishes–Greiner, Solingen, Germany (Intermountain Scientific, Kaysville, UT, cat. # T-2881-2).

2.2. Retroviral Infection and Cell Selection

1. Tumor cell lines: 9L wild-type *(6)* and 9L/lacZ cell line (β-galactosidase) (ATCC CRL 2200).
2. Polybrene (Hexadimethrine bromide 1,5-dimethyl-1,5, diazaundecamethylene polymethobromide) (Sigma H-9268). Dissolved at 1 mg/mL in DMEM or PBS (*see* **Subheading 2.1., items 2** and **7**). Store at –20°C. Stable at 4°C at 1 mg/mL for 1 yr.
3. Retroviral supernatant, frozen aliquot stored at –80 °C (prepared as described in **Subheading 3.2.**).
4. Stock Puromycin (2 mg/mL) (Sigma P-7255) dissolved in PBS (*see* **Subheading 2.1., item 7**). Filter-sterilize the puromycin solution using a 0.2 μm syringe filter. Store at 4°C for up to 1 yr.
5. Stock Hygromycin B (50 mg/mL) (Sigma H-0654) (sterile). Store in the dark at 4°C for up to 1 yr.
6. Stock G-418 (1 mg/mL) (Geneticin) (Life Technologies, cat. # 11811-031). Prepare fresh in 10% FBS-DMEM. Geneticin solution is filter-sterilized using a 0.2 μm syringe filter. A solution of 50 mg/ml of active geneticin is stable at 4°C for up to 1 yr. The geneticin stock value is based on the drug activity for cell selection, which is reported by the manufacturer of each product lot.
7. Stock Blasticidin (3 mg/mL) (ICN Pharmaceuticals, Costa Mesa, CA, cat. # 150477). Prepare fresh in deionized, distilled water. Blasticidin solution is filter-sterilized using a 0.2 μm syringe filter. Aliquots of 100 μL can be frozen and stored at –20°C for up to 6 mo.
8. 9L Cell Freezing Medium: DMEM supplemented with 20% FBS and 10% dimethyl sulfoxide. May be stored at –20°C in 50 mL aliquots for up to 1 yr.
9. 1 × Trypsin-EDTA: 10 × Trypsin-EDTA (Life Technologies, cat. # 15400-054) diluted 10-fold in 1 × HBSS (see below). Store at 4°C for up to 6 mo. Prewarm to 37°C before adding to cells.
10. 1 × HBSS: Hank's Balanced Salt Solution (Life Technologies, cat. # 21250-014) containing 0.35 g of $NaHCO_3$/L. Filter-sterilize and store at 4°C for up to 1 yr.

2.3. Establishing Individual Clonal Cell Lines

1. 96-well tissue-culture dishes (Greiner–Intermountain Scientific T-3025-1).
2. Cyclophosphamide M.W. 279.1 g/mol (Sigma, cat. # C-0768) *potential carcinogen*. Prepare fresh for each assay. Dissolve in 10% FBS-DMEM and filter-sterilize using a 0.2 μm syringe filter.

3. Methods

3.1. Method Overview: Construction of P450-Expressing Tumor Cell Lines Using Retroviral Technology

The following is a summary of the steps required for the construction of tumor cell lines that stably express specific cytochrome P450 genes and can be used for preclinical studies of the utility of P450 genes for prodrug activation-based cancer gene therapy. Individual steps are described in greater detail in

Subheadings 3.2., 3.3., and **3.4.** Several of these steps have been modified or adapted from the protocol described in *(5)*.

1. Subclone the P450 cDNA that is to be expressed into a suitable retroviral plasmid (*see* **Note 2**). Expression of the cDNA can be controlled by the retroviral LTR promoter or by an internal promoter (e.g., SV40 or CMV), depending on the retroviral vector chosen.
2. Transform retroviral plasmid DNA into competent bacteria (*see* **Note 3**).
3. Select positive clones by growing the transformed bacteria on agar plates containing the appropriate prokaryotic drug marker, e.g., ampicillin or tetracycline.
4. Identify positive bacterial clones by either PCR or restriction enzyme digestion (*see* **Note 4**).
5. Sequence the plasmid across the cDNA cloning site to verify the identity of the retroviral plasmid construct (*see* **Note 5**).
6. Amplify the retroviral plasmid in bacteria and isolate the plasmid by a maxi preparation (*see* **Note 6**).
7. Transfect plasmid DNA into a suitable retrovirus packaging cell line to obtain infectious retroviral supernatant (*see* **Note 7**). Following transfection, harvest the supernatant, which contains retrovirus encoding the P450 gene under study (*see* **Subheading 3.2.**).
8. Infect tumor cell line with retroviral supernatant and then select a population of retrovirally infected cells with a selection drug appropriate to the retrovirus (e.g., puromycin, in the case of pBabe-puromycin retrovirus) to obtain a pool of retrovirally transduced cells (*see* **Subheading 3.3.**).
9. If required, clone out individual cell lines from the heterogeneous pool of retrovirus-infected cells to obtain one or more clonal cell lines with elevated P450 expression levels (*see* **Subheading 3.4.**).
10. Characterize pools or clonal cell lines for P450 gene expression by Northern blot, Western blot *(7)*, enzymatic assay and/or immunofluorescence using an anti-P450 antibody.
11. Evaluate the impact of P450 gene expression on the cell's chemosensitivity to P450-activated prodrugs of interest using the in vitro cytotoxicity assays described elsewhere in this volume (*see* Chapter 7).

3.2. Transfection of Retroviral Plasmid DNA and Harvesting of Retroviral Supernatant

1. Plate 2.5×10^6 Bosc 23 cells per 60-mm tissue-culture dish approx 24 h prior to transfection. Grow cells in a 37°C humidified incubator containing 5% CO_2 (*see* **Note 8**).
2. Remove the 10% FBS-DMEM medium and add 4 mL of fresh culture medium containing 25 μM chloroquine (final concentration) 3 h before transfection (*see* **Note 9**).
3. Dissolve 24 μg of retrovirus plasmid DNA in 0.5 mL of $0.25M$ $CaCl_2$ (*see* **Note 10**).
4. Add to the $CaCl_2$-DNA solution an equal volume (0.5 mL) of $2 \times$ HBS slowly and evenly, by dropwise addition, over approx 1 min (*see* **Note 11**).

5. Remove a small aliquot (about 40 µL) of the calcium phosphate-DNA solution and place on a glass microscope slide. Examine the sample by magnifying the drop with a 40 × objective under a phase-contrast microscope for the presence of small precipitated particles. Typically, a fine precipitate is observed within 1 to 2 min after adding 2 × HBS. At that point, add the remainder of the 1 mL sample of calcium phosphate-DNA solution to the 60-mm tissue-culture dish. Swirl the dish gently to distribute the calcium phosphate-DNA precipitates evenly.

6. Remove the culture medium a minimum of 5 h after DNA transfection, but no longer than 12 h (*see* **Note 12**).

7. Wash the cells twice with PBS and replace with 4 mL fresh 10% FBS-DMEM (*see* **Note 13**). Place the Bosc 23 cells back in the tissue-culture incubator.

8. Incubate the cells for 24 h to allow for cell recovery, then aspirate and discard the medium (*see* **Note 14**). Replace with 4 mL of fresh 10% FBS-DMEM. Place the cells back in the tissue-culture incubator.

9. After a second 24-h period (*see* **Note 15**), harvest the cell-culture medium by gently removing the supernatant with a sterile pipet. Transfer the supernatant to a 15 mL polypropylene centrifuge tube.

10. Spin for 5 min at ~ 200g at 4°C.

11. Filter supernatant through a 0.45 µm low protein binding syringe filter into a sterile 5 mL polypropylene centrifuge tube (*see* **Notes 16** and **17**).

12. Store the Bosc 23 cell supernatant containing retrovirus on ice only if the recipient tumor cells are to be infected within ~ 2 h (*see* **Subheading 3.3.**). For long-time storage of the retrovirus, snap-freeze the centrifuge tube containing the retroviral supernatant in liquid nitrogen and then place at –70°C (*see* **Note 18**).

3.3. Retroviral Infection and Cell Selection

1. Plate sufficient recipient tumor cells to give a confluency of about 50% 24 h later. For 9L gliosarcoma cells and NIH-3T3 cells, plate 0.5×10^6 cells/100-mm dish 12 to 18 h prior to infection.

2. For each 100-mm dish of recipient cells, replace the 10% FBS-DMEM cell-culture medium with 3 mL of retroviral supernatant (*see* **Subheading 3.2.**) containing 12 µg of filter-sterilized polybrene (final concentration 4 µg/mL) (*see* **Note 19**).

3. As a control, incubate a second plate of cells with 3 mL of culture supernatant that is devoid of virus and is prepared by mock-transfection of Bosc 23 cells. These control cells can be used to determine the efficiency of drug selection (i.e., the percentage of cell death in uninfected cells treated with the selection drug).

4. After 3 h, supplement the retroviral supernatant by adding 7 mL of fresh 10% FBS-DMEM to the culture plate. Return the cells to the incubator for an additional 45 h (*see* **Note 20**).

5. After a total of 48 h of infection, trypsin digest and divide the near-confluent infected Bosc 23 cells into 4 new 100-mm plates for drug selection. Passage the mock-infected cells at a 1:4 dilution into one new 100-mm plate.

6. After the cells have attached to the tissue-culture plate (between 4 and 16 h), add filter-sterilized antibiotic (e.g., puromycin or hygromycin) to select a population

of retrovirally infected cells that stably express the drug-resistance marker (*see* **Note 21**). Add the selection drug to the mock-infected cells as a positive control. The concentration of drug and length of selection time vary with the cell line and with the type of selection drug (*see* **Note 22**). For rat 9L gliosarcoma cells, typical conditions for drug selection are as follows:

    a. Puromycin: 2 μg/mL for 2 d.
    b. Hygromycin: 300 μg/mL for 3 d.
    c. G-418: 1.0 mg active G-418/mL for 6 d (replacing medium and G-418 every 2 d up to 6 d).
    d. Blasticidin: 3 μg/mL for 2 d.

7. After selection, prepare frozen stocks of the pool of stable cell lines at a concentration of 2×10^6 cells/mL of freezing medium and store in liquid nitrogen.
8. Characterize the cell line for P450 protein expression (*see* **Note 23**).
9. Verify that the retrovirally transduced cell line does not generate and does not contain replication-competent retrovirus (*see* **Note 24**).

3.4. Establishing Individual Clonal Cell Lines from Heterogeneous Pool of Retrovirally Transduced Cells

In some cases, biochemical analysis of a pool of drug-resistant retrovirally infected cells may reveal a lower than desired overall level of expressed-P450 protein. It may be possible to increase the level of expression of the transduced-P450 gene several-fold by dilution cloning to obtain individual clonal sublines that have a higher level of P450 protein expression than the heterogeneous cell population obtained during the original retroviral infection and drug-selection procedure. These methods are now described.

1. Dilute pool of retroviral transduced cells (*see* **Subheading 3.3.**) to calculated concentrations of 0.5, 1, and 4 cells per 200 μL of 10% FBS-DMEM. Distribute the diluted cells into at least one 96-well tissue-culture plate per concentration. Incubate the plate for about 10 d to 2 wk, until single colonies are visible under the microscope in individual wells (*see* **Note 25**).
2. Detach the cells growing as single colonies with trypsin-EDTA and divide the colony into two wells of a new 96-well culture plate (*see* **Notes 26** and **27**).
3. Allow the cells to attach overnight. When dealing with cells transduced with a prodrug-activating gene, such as a cytochrome *P450* gene that activates the prodrug cyclophosphamide, cells in one of the two wells may be treated with the prodrug to identify individual transduced cells that express a higher level of prodrug-activation P450 enzyme.
4. If cyclophosphamide is chosen as the P450 prodrug of interest, add cyclophosphamide (1 m*M*) to one of the two wells. The paired well remains drug free. Wait 2–3 d, and examine the wells to identify cells that are dying from the drug treatment. When cyclophosphamide-sensitive clones are identified, detach and replate the corresponding untreated cells derived from the same cell colonies into 60-mm dishes.

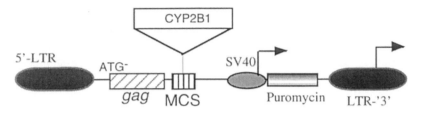

Fig. 1. Schematic map of the pBabe vector that is used for retroviral transduction to establish stable rodent cell lines expressing P450 or other genes. The retroviral vector contains the retroviral long-terminal repeat (LTR) promoter, a gag gene that lack the initiator methionine start sequence (ATG) and a multiple cloning site (MCS) with unique restriction sites for cloning a P450 cDNA. The mammalian selectable marker encoded by the puromycin resistance gene, in the example shown, is transcribed from the SV40 promoter. The pBabe vector also contains a bacterial selectable marker the ampicillin resistance gene for selection in bacteria (not shown).

5. When the cells are confluent, freeze a portion in liquid nitrogen for cell stocks. Characterize the remainder of cells for P450 protein expression and drug sensitivity.

4. Notes

1. The pH of the 2 × HBS solution is critical for obtaining fine DNA precipitates, which are necessary for efficient transfection.
2. Suitable vectors for retroviral infection include pBabe-based retroviral plasmids with puromycin or hygromycin selectable markers (*see* **Fig. 1**) *(8,9)*. Clonetech® sells two retroviral vectors, pLXSN and pLNCX, which transcribe the cDNA insert to be expressed from the viral 3′-LTR or from an internal CMV promoter, respectively. The above two retroviral vectors both confer G-418 resistance to transduced target cells.

    The availability of retrovirus plasmids that encode different drug resistance markers allows for the sequential transduction of tumor cells with several genes that can be selected for individually. In this way, cell lines that encode multiple therapeutic genes, or a *P450* gene in combination with the P450 reductase *(10)* can be obtained. Alternatively, multiple genes linked by internal ribosome entry sequence (IRES) elements can be expressed from a single retrovirus.
3. A standard bacterial transformation protocol can be found in *(11)*.
4. Specific PCR primers, complementary to the retroviral vector and the cDNA insert, respectively, can be used in PCR analysis *(12)* of bacterial extracts to identify positive clones and to directly establish the orientation of the cDNA insert. Alternatively, restriction digestion *(13)* of the isolated plasmid DNA can be carried out to identify positive clones and to establish the orientation of the cDNA insert.
5. A standard method for plasmid DNA sequencing is described in *(14)*.
6. A plasmid maxi prep method can be found in reference *(15)*.
7. For ecotropic infection of virus into rodent cells, Bosc 23 is an excellent packaging cell line *(2,5)*. Amphotropic packaging cell lines such as Bing permit viral infection of rodent cells as well as primate cells *(5)*.

8. It is important to use Bosc 23 cells that have not been passaged too frequently (i.e., less than 20 passages). Bosc 23 cells should not be plated too sparsely (≤ 25% confluent) or too densely (≥ 75% confluent). Bosc 23 cell monolayers that appear clumpy rather than uniform may have reduced DNA uptake efficiency.

9. Chloroquine enhances the efficiency of DNA transfection by inhibiting lysosomal formation, thus preventing DNA sequestration and DNA degradation.

10. It is generally not necessary to filter-sterilize the $CaCl_2$-DNA solution if the DNA is prepared using phenol/chloroform extraction methods and if the DNA is dissolved in Tris-EDTA buffer (10 m*M* Tris-HCl Ph 8.0 1 m*M* EDTA). If required, filtration of the $CaCl_2$-DNA solution through a 0.2 μm syringe filter can be carried out to ensure that bacteria from the plasmid DNA preparation do not contaminate the Bosc 23 cell culture.

11. Dropping the 2 × HBS slowly and evenly is essential for obtaining small calcium phosphate-DNA precipitates. The efficiency with which the cells take up the DNA depends on the size of the precipitate. Large clumpy DNA pellets are too large to enter the cell. Very fine pellets are too light to settle on the surface of the cell and remain suspended in the medium.

12. Chloroquine and the calcium phosphate-DNA transfection precipitates are both toxic to Bosc 23 cells. It is thus essential that they be removed between 5 h (minimum transfection time) and 12 h (maximum transfection time) after addition *(5)*.

13. Wash the Bosc 23 cells very gently. Bosc 23 cells are readily detached from the tissue-culture dish.

14. Place the retroviral supernatant to be discarded in a designated biohazard compartment. Inactivate the infectious virus with a viricidal agent, such as Conflikt (manufactured by Decon Labs and distributed by Fisher Scientific, cat. # 04-35S-52).

15. If the Bosc 23 cells are not yet confluent, it may be useful to wait an additional 24 h before harvesting the supernatant.

16. Use polypropylene rather than polystyrene tubes to avoid cracking the tube when placing it in liquid nitrogen. Store the viral supernatant in 3- to 5-mL aliquots.

17. Spinning and filtering the supernatant (**steps 10** and **11**) ensures that no Bosc 23 cells remain in the supernatant. Failure to remove all of the Bosc 23 cells could result in mixing of Bosc 23 cells with the recipient cell line and continued generation of fresh infectious virus particles.

18. Do not store viral supernatant in a liquid nitrogen tank that contains tissue-culture cells because the stored cells may become infected by the viral particles. The retroviral supernatant is stable at −70°C. The viral titer decreases if the supernatant is frozen and thawed too often (more than three times).

19. Polybrene is a polycation that facilitates efficient and stable introduction of plasmid DNA into cells *(5)*.

20. The cells are incubated during the first 3 h with a more concentrated retroviral supernatant (i.e., 3 mL of undiluted supernatant) in order to increase the efficiency of viral transduction.

21. The specific drugs that are used to select the retrovirally transduced cells are determined by the drug-resistance marker encoded by the retrovirus. pBabe-based

retroviral vectors are available with drug-resistance genes selectable with puromycin, hygromycin, geneticin (G418), and blasticidin, among others *(8,9)*.

22. The cell line under study should first be tested with the selection drug to determine the minimum drug concentration that kills ~ 99% of the uninfected cells within a defined time period (typically ~ 2 to 3 d).

23. P450-expressing cell lines may be characterized for P450 protein expression by Western blotting or specific enzyme assays *(7,16)*.

24. The replication-defective nature of the retrovirus can be verified in the following way. Passage retrovirally infected cells at least three times. Remove the supernatant from the final passage and place on wild-type uninfected cells. Proceed with the infection and drug selection protocol of **Subheading 3.3., steps 1–6**. Compare the survival of these cells following drug selection to the survival of uninfected cell controls. If replication-competent retrovirus is present, virus amplification will occur resulting in a significant number of recipient cells acquiring drug resistance.

25. Some wells will contain single colonies, whereas others may contain either no cells and or perhaps two or more colonies. Single colonies are readily identifiable by their round shape. An oblong or amorphous shape indicates more than one colony is likely to be present. Wells containing two or more colonies should be discarded. Typically, only 20–40% of the individual wells will contain colonies derived from single cells.

26. If the colonies are large, count the cells in the colony and plate the cells at a density of 1 to 2×10^3 cells/well.

27. As an alternative to the drug-sensitivity assay described in **Subheading 3.4., steps 3** and **4**, half the cells from each single colony can be used to seed two or three wells of a 6-well tissue-culture plate. Once these cells have grown to near confluency, they may be used to prepare total cell extracts for analysis by anti-P450 Western blotting to identify individual clones that express the P450 protein of interest at a high level. The remaining cells derived from the single colony may be grown in several wells of a 6-well tissue-culture dish. Once the cells have grown to near confluency, passage the cells and replate into several 100-mm dishes. Cells may then be grown and prepared for storage in liquid nitrogen.

Acknowledgments

Preparation of this chapter was carried out with the support of NIH Grant CA49248 (to D. J. Waxman).

References

1. Waxman, D. J., Chen, L., Hecht, J. E. D., and Jounaidi, Y. (1999) Cytochrome P450-base cancer gene therapy: Recent advances and future prospects. *Drug Metab Rev.* **31,** 503–522.

2. Pear, W. S., Nolan, G. P., Scott, M. L., and Baltimore, D. (1993) Production of high-titer helper-free retroviruses by transient transfection. *Proc. Natl. Acad. Sci.* **90,** 8392–8396.

3. Kondo, S., Tanaka, Y., Kondo, Y., Ishizaka, Y., Hitomi, M., Haqqi, T., et al. (1998) Retroviral transfer of CPP32beta gene into malignant gliomas in vitro and in vivo. *Cancer Res.* **58,** 962–967.

4. Verma, I. M. and Somia, N. (1997) Gene therapy–promises, problems and prospects. *Nature.* **389,** 239–242.

5. Pear, W. S., Scott, M. L., and Nolan, G. P. (1996) Generation of high-titer helper-free retroviruses by transient transfection in *Gene Therapy Protocols* (Robbins, P., ed.), Humana, Totowa, NJ. pp. 41–57.

6. Barker, M., Hoshino, T., Gurcay, O., Wilson, C. B., Nielsen, S. L., Downie, R., and Eliason, J. (1973) Development of an animal brain tumor model and its response to therapy with 1,3-bis(2-chloroethyl)-1-nitrosourea. *Cancer Res.* **33,** 976–986.

7. Waxman, D. J. (1991) Rat hepatic P450IIA and P450IIC subfamily expression using catalytic, immunochemical, and molecular probes. *Methods Enzymol.* **206,** 249–267.

8. Morgenstern, J. P. and Land, H. (1990) Advanced mammalian gene transfer: high titre retroviral vectors with multiple drug selection markers and a complementary helper-free packaging cell line. *Nucleic Acids Res.* **18,** 3587–3596.

9. Morgenstern, J. P. and Land, H. (1990) A series of mammalian expression vectors and characterisation of their expression of a reporter gene in stably and transiently transfected cells. *Nucleic Acids Res.* **18,** 1068.

10. Jounaidi, Y., Hecht, J. E. D., and Waxman, D. J. (1998) Retroviral transfer of human cytochrome P450 genes for oxazaphosphorine-based cancer gene therapy. *Cancer Res.* **58,** 4391–4401.

11. Aubusel, F. M., Brent, R., Kingston, R. E., Moore, D. D., and Seidman, J. (1994-1997) *Introduction of Plasmid DNA into Cell.* Current Protocols in Molecular Biology, (Chanda, V. B., ed.), Vol. 1, supplement 40, Wiley, New York, pp. 1.8.2–1.8.3.

12. Aubusel, F. M., Brent, R., Kingston, R. E., Moore, D. D., and Seidman, J. (1994–1997) *The Polymerase Chain Reaction.* Current Protocols in Molecular Biology, (Chanda, V. B., ed.), Vol. 2, supplement 40, Wiley, New York, pp. 15.1.1–15.1.9.

13. Aubusel, F. M., Brent, R., Kingston, R. E., Moore, D. D., and Seidman, J. (1994–1997) *Restriction Endonucleases.* Current Protocols in Molecular Biology, (Chanda, V. B., ed.), Vol. 1, supplement 40, Wiley, New York, pp. 3.1.1–3.1.4, 3.2.1–3.2.5.

14. Sambrook, J., Fritsch, E. F., and Maniatis, T. (1989) *DNA Sequencing.* 2nd ed. *Molecular Cloning–A Laboratory Manual* (Nolan, C., ed.), Vol. 2, Cold Spring Harbor Laboratory Press, New York, pp. 13.3–13.18.

15. Sambrook, J., Fritsch, E. F., and Maniatis, T. (1989) *Plasmid Vectors.* 2nd ed. *Molecular Cloning–A Laboratory Manual,* (Nolan, C., ed.), Vol. 1, Cold Spring Harbor Laboratory Press, New York, pp. 1.36–1.37.

16. Phillips, I. R. and Shephard, E. A. (1997) in *Methods in Molecular Biology: Cytochrome P450 Protocols* (Phillips, I. R. and Shephard, E. A., eds.), Vol. 107, Humana, Totowa, NJ, pp. 95–102.

7

In Vitro Methods for Evaluation
of *P450*-Based Anticancer Gene Therapy

Jodi E. D. Hecht and David J. Waxman

1. Introduction
1.1. In Vitro Methods for Evaluation
of P450-Based Anticancer Gene Therapy

Cytochrome *P450* genes encode drug-metabolizing enzymes that bioactivate a number of widely used anticancer prodrugs. These genes have recently been shown to be useful for prodrug activation-based cancer gene therapy *(1)*. Approaches to identify new *P450* gene/prodrug combinations that may potentially be useful in *P450*-based cancer gene therapy are discussed in Chapter 5 of this volume. These studies are greatly facilitated by the use of in vitro cytotoxicity and growth inhibition assays, which are described in the present chapter. These in vitro assays are very useful for studying the efficacy of *P450*-based gene therapy prior to proceeding to in vivo experimentation for the following reasons: 1) cell-culture assays are much more cost effective than in vivo tumor model studies carried out in rats or mice; 2) in vitro experiments can be performed much more readily than in vivo tumor model studies; 3) a large throughput of *P450* genes and drugs can readily be tested to identify novel prodrug activation gene and prodrug combinations. This chapter describes growth inhibition and cytotoxicity assays that can be used to rapidly characterize the drug sensitivity of tumor cell lines transduced with a prodrug activation *P450* gene (*see* Chapter 6). These assays are general in nature, and can readily be adapted for use with other prodrug activation gene/prodrug combinations currently under evaluation for cancer gene therapy *(2)*.

From: *Methods in Molecular Medicine, Vol. 35: Gene Therapy: Methods and Protocols*
Edited by: W. Walther and U. Stein © Humana Press, Inc., Totowa, NJ

2. Materials

2.1. In Vitro Growth Inhibition and Cytotoxicity Assays

1. Tumor cell lines: 9L wild-type *(3)* and 9L/lacZ cell line (β-galactosidase) (ATCC CRL 2200). 9L/*P450* cell line (e.g., 9L/2B1) [prepared by retroviral transduction (Chapter 6) or by stable transfection] *(4)*.
2. Growth medium for 9L cells: Dulbecco's Modified Eagle Medium (DMEM) (Life Technologies, Gaithersburg, MD, cat. # 12100-046) supplemented with 3.7 g of sodium bicarbonate, 10 mL of penicillin (5000 U/mL)–streptomycin (5000 μg/mL) (Life Technologies, cat. # 15070-063) in 900 mL of deionized water. Adjust the pH of the medium to pH 7.1 with 1N HCl. Filter-sterilize with 0.2 μm bottle top filters. Store at 4°C for up to 6 mo. To prepare DMEM containing serum supplement 450 mL of complete DMEM with 50 mL of heat-inactivated (56°C for 30 min) fetal bovine serum (Sigma, St. Louis, MO, cat. # F-2442) (final serum concentration, 10%). Store DMEM-containing FBS at 4°C for up to 2 mo. Prewarm 10% FBS-DMEM to 37°C.
3. PBS: Phosphate Buffered Saline 0.146M NaCl, 0.01M Na_2HPO_4, 2.68 mM KCl, 1.76 mM KH_2PO_4. Filter-sterilize and store at room temperature for up to 6 mo. The pH should be about 7.4. Prewarm buffer to 37°C before adding to cells.
4. 1 × Trypsin-EDTA: 10 × Trypsin-EDTA (Life Technologies, cat. # 15400-054) diluted 10-fold in 1 × HBSS (*see* below). Store at 4°C for up to 6 mo. Prewarm to 37°C before adding to cells.
5. 1 × HBSS: Hank's Balanced Salt Solution (HBSS) (Life Technologies, cat. # 21250-014) containing 0.35 g of NaHCO3/L. Filter-sterilize and store at 4°C for up to 1 yr.
6. Cyclophosphamide M.W. 279.1 g/mol (Sigma cat. # C-0768) *potential carcinogen*. Prepare fresh for each assay. Dissolve in 10% FBS-DMEM and filter-sterilize using a 0.2 μm syringe filter.
7. Mafosfamide, a chemically activated derivative of cyclophosphamide, M.W. 400.55 g/mol (gift from Dr. J. Pohl, ASTA Pharma, Bielefeld, Germany) *potential carcinogen*. Dissolve in 10% FBS-DMEM and filter-sterilize using a 0.2 μm syringe filter.

2.2. Crystal Violet Staining

1. Crystal Violet Stain: 1.25 g crystal violet (Sigma C-3886) mixed with 50 mL of 37% formaldehyde solution (Sigma, cat. # F-8775) and 450 mL methanol. To prepare the stain, mix the above three components and store in a tightly closed container. The stain can be stored at room temperature for up to 1 yr provided that the methanol does not evaporate.
2. ELISA microplate reader: SLT Spectra Shell (Tecan US, Research Triangle Park, NC) or any similar instrument.

2.3. SRB assay

1. 0.4% Sulforhodamine B (w/v) (Sigma, cat. # S-9012) in 1% glacial acetic acid. The SRB solution can be stored at room temperature for up to 6 mo.

2. TCA: 50% (v/w) Trichloroacetic acid (Fisher, Pittsburgh, PA, cat. # A323-508) dissolved in distilled water. Store at 4°C for up to 1 yr.
3. 1% (v/v) Glacial acetic acid in distilled water. Store at room temperature for up to 1 yr.
4. 10 mM Tris base (pH 10.5). Store at room temperature for up to 1 yr.

2.4. Cell Counting

1. 0.4% Trypan Blue Solution (Sigma, cat. # T-8154).
2. Hemacytometer (VWR Scientific Counting Chamber Levy Double, cat. # 15170-208).

2.5. XTT Assay

1. XTT (sodium 3-[1-phenylamino-carbonyl)-3,4-tetrazolium]-bis (4-methoxy-6-nitro)benzene sulfonic acid hydrate) (Sigma, cat. # X-4626). To prepare stock of XTT, dissolve 10 mg of XTT in 10 mL of warmed cell-culture medium (60°C) (*see* **Note 1**). The stock solution is stable for up to 1 mo when stored at 0–4°C.
2. Phenazine methosulfate (PMS) (N-methyldibenzopyrazine methyl sulfate) (Sigma, cat. # P-5812). To prepare stock solution of PMS, dissolve 0.383 mg of PMS into 1 mL of PBS 1.25 mM (**Subheading 2.1., item 3.**). The stock solution is stable for at least 2 wk at –20°C.

3. Methods

3.1. In Vitro Growth Inhibition and Cytotoxicity Assays

The following is a description of the general steps required for in vitro growth inhibition and cytotoxicity assays. The growth inhibition assay can be used to measure the effect of continuous (e.g., 4–5 d) drug treatment on the growth of a tumor cell population. By contrast, the cytotoxicity assay measures the viability of cells, in terms of their ability to grow and form colonies, after a short period (e.g., 1–4 h) of drug treatment. The cytotoxicity assay is particularly suitable for *P450* gene/prodrug combinations that do not require longer-term metabolite accumulation for efficient cell killing. The protocol outlined below has been optimized for *P450*-expressing 9L gliosarcoma cells treated with cyclophosphamide or mafosfamide and may need to be optimized for other tumor cell lines and other drugs. **Subheadings 3.2.–3.5.** detail four different methods for analyzing the effects of *P450* expression on anticancer drug activity leading to tumor cell growth inhibition and/or cytotoxicity in cell culture. The methods described for evaluating growth inhibition (**Subheading 3.1.1.**) are crystal violet staining, staining with the SRB dye, cell counting, and XTT assay for mitochondrial dehydrogenase activity. The crystal violet staining and SRB staining methods can also be used for evaluating drug-induced cytotoxicity as outlined in **Subheading 3.1.2.**

3.1.1. In Vitro Growth Inhibition Assay

1. Plate 9L tumor cells or 9L/*P450* tumor cells (100 μl volume containing a suspension of 1×10^3 cells) into each well of a 96-well tissue-culture microtiter plate (*see* **Note 2**). Include a sufficient number of wells so that each treatment condition (e.g., each drug concentration) is assayed in triplicate. For experiments involving cell counting, two sets of wells are required: cells without drug and cells with drug. When using a staining method to evaluate the drug's effect on cell growth, a third set of wells is required: wells containing culture medium without cells (background absorbance measurement).
2. Incubate the 9L cells for 16 to 24 h in a 5% CO_2 humidified incubator at 37°C, prior to anticancer drug treatment (*see* **Note 3**).
3. Prepare drug(s) to be tested (e.g., cyclophosphamide at 0–1 m*M*, final concentration) by dissolving in 10% FBS-DMEM, with vortexing, if necessary (*see* **Note 4**). Filter-sterilize the drug solution using a 0.2 μm syringe filter (*see* **Note 5**).
4. Aspirate the cell-culture medium and add the sterile drug solution to the attached 9L cells.
5. Observe the cells daily and record any changes in cell morphology. The experiment must be terminated if there is bacterial or fungal contamination in the cell culture.
6. After 4–5 d, evaluate the effect of drug treatment using one of the quantitative assays (e.g., crystal violet, SRB, cell counting or XTT) described in **Subheadings 3.2.–3.5.** of this chapter.

3.1.2. In Vitro Cytotoxicity Assay (5)

1. Plate 9L wild-type tumor cells or 9L/*P450* cells at a cell density of 1×10^5 cells/ 60-mm tissue-culture dish in 5 mL of 10% FBS-DMEM (*see* **Note 6**). Allow the cells to attach for 12–16 h prior to drug treatment.
2. Remove the cell culture medium and add 10% FBS-DMEM containing the drug under investigation. In this example, mafosfamide (50 μM) is added to the cells for 1 h at 37°C (*see* **Note 7**). As a control, incubate one plate of cells without drug.
3. Remove the drug-containing culture medium. Wash the cells with 5 mL of PBS.
4. Trypsin digest the washed cell monolayer with 1 mL trypsin-EDTA and then resuspend in 4 mL of 10% FBS-DMEM. Count the cells by the trypan blue dye-exclusion assay (*see* **Subheading 3.4.**).
5. Plate the cell suspensions in duplicate wells to give cell densities of 200, 1000, 10,000 cells/well in 6-well plates (*see* **Note 8**).
6. Place the cells at 37°C in a humidified incubator containing 5% CO_2. Change the medium after the cells attach (i.e., 4 to 12 h). Incubate the cells for a further 7 to 10 d (*see* **Note 9**).
7. Stain the cells with either crystal violet (*see* **Subheading 3.2.**) or SRB stain (*see* **Subheading 3.3.**) and dry the stained plate overnight (*see* **Note 10**).
8. Count colonies and calculate the survival fraction as follows (*see* **Note 11**):

Calculations *(6)*
Plating Efficiency (PE):
$$= \frac{\text{Number of colonies in the control plate} \times 100}{\text{Number of control cells originally plated}}$$
Colony Forming Efficiency (CFE):
$$= \frac{\text{PE of drug-treated group} \times 100}{\text{PE of control group}}$$
The CFE represents the surviving fraction of cells from a treated tumor.

3.2. Crystal Violet Staining

Of the four techniques described for evaluation of cytotoxicity assays (*see* **Subheading 3.1.2.**), crystal violet staining is the simplest method to carry out and is highly reproducible. This method can also be used for the evaluation of the growth inhibition assays described above (*see* **Subheading 3.1.1.**). One disadvantage of this method is that the efficiency of crystal violet staining varies from one cell line to another *(7)*. A second potential disadvantage is that crystal violet stains the nucleus of both viable and nonviable cells *(8)*.

1. Treat cells with drug for time periods from 1–2 h up to ~5 d as described in the cytotoxicity and growth inhibition assays (*see* **Subheading 3.1.**). Remove culture medium from each of the wells (including medium-only control wells) of the 96-well tissue-culture plate.
2. Gently wash the cells in each well with 100 µL of PBS (volumes based on a 96-well plate format) (*see* **Subheading 3.1.1.** and **Note 12**).
3. Remove the PBS wash by vacuum aspiration.
4. Add 100 µl of crystal violet stain (*see* **Subheading 2.2.1.**) to each well. Stain for 10 min at room temperature.
5. Remove the stain from the wells by gentle aspiration (*see* **Note 13**).
6. To remove the remaining unbound stain, gently rinse the wells by immersing the microtiter plate in a basin filled with tap water at room temperature.
7. Change the water several times until the water no longer colors purple.
8. Air dry the tissue-culture plates overnight and, if desired, photograph the plate to obtain a record of the results (*see* **Note 14**).
9. To quantitate the staining, reconstitute the dye in each well with 100 µL of 70% ethanol.
10. Shake the covered microtiter plate at room temperature on a shaker for approx 1 h or until the dye dissolves completely.
11. Determine the cell number of each well by directly placing the 96-well plate in an ELISA microplate reader and measuring the absorbance at 595 nm. Alternatively, the absorbance of the dye may be quantified in a 0.5 mL spectrophotometer cuvet after dilution of each well with 400 µL of water (*see* **Note 15**).
12. Calculations for percent cell survival
    a. Subtract the background absorbance (culture medium without cells) from the drug-free and drug-treated values.

    b. Determine percent survival by dividing the absorbance value of the treated-cell group by the absorbance value of the control-cell group (no drug) then multiply by 100.

3.3. SRB Assay

Sulforhodamine B in an aminoxanthene dye with two sulfonic groups that binds to basic amino acids of proteins. This stain is very stable and nondestructive to the cellular architecture *(7)*. This staining procedure is suitable for both the growth inhibition assay and the cytotoxicity assay.

1. Treat cells with drug for time periods from 1–2 h up to ~ 5 d as described in the cytotoxicity and growth inhibition assays *(see* **Subheading 3.1.**). Remove the culture medium from each of the wells (including medium-only control wells) of the 96-well tissue-culture plate.
2. Place 200 µL of fresh culture medium in each well of a 96-well plate containing drug-treated and control cells. Add 50 µL of 50% TCA *(see* **Subheading 2.3., item 2**) to the 200 µl of medium in each well to give a final concentration of 10% TCA *(see* **Note 16**).
3. Incubate for 1 h at 4°C *(see* **Note 17**).
4. Remove the TCA fixative and rinse the plates five times with tap water by inverting the plate into a container filled with tap water. Air dry the plate or dry by gently blowing warm air over the plate.
5. Stain the TCA-fixed cells with 0.4% SRB (w/v) in 1% acetic acid *(see* **Subheading 2.3., item 1** and **item 3**) for 30 min at room temperature.
6. Remove excess stain by inverting the plate. Quickly destain the plate with four washes of 1% acetic acid *(see* **Subheading 2.3., item 3** and **Note 18**).
7. Dry the plates overnight before proceeding to resuspend the dye *(see* **Note 19**).
8. Solubilize the bound SRB dye with 100 µl of 10-m*M* Tris base *(see* **Subheading 2.3., item 4**). Shake on a gyratory shaker for 5 min.
9. Determine the cell number of each well by directly placing the 96-well plate in an ELISA microplate reader and measuring the absorbance at 564 nm. Alternatively, the absorbance of the dye may be quantified in a 0.5 mL spectrophotometer cuvette after dilution of each well with 400 µL of the Tris buffer *(see* **Note 20**).
10. Calculations for percent cell survival
    a. Subtract the background absorbance (culture medium without cells) from the drug-free and drug-treated control absorbance values.
    b. Determine percent survival by dividing the absorbance value of the treated-cell group by the absorbance value of the control-cell group (no drug) then multiply by 100.

3.4. Cell Counting

This method is more labor-intensive than the crystal violet, SRB, and XTT staining methods described in this chapter. However, cell counting is a highly sensitive method that is preferred in cases where there is extensive cytotoxicity, as it can allow for quantitation of multilog cell killing. Moreover, the cell-counting assay can be carried out using a minimum of reagents and specialized equipment. These are limited to trypan blue (exclusion dye), a phase contrast microscope, a hemacytometer and a hand-held cell counter. Cell counting is also necessary for plating cells at the beginning of a growth inhibition or cytotoxicity assay and is suitable for determining percent cell survival in a growth inhibition assay.

1. Treat cells with drug for time periods from 1–2 h up to ~5 d as described in the cytotoxicity and growth inhibition assays (*see* **Subheading 3.1.**).
2. Remove culture medium from each of the wells (including medium-only control wells) of the 96-well tissue-culture plate (*see* **Note 21**).
3. Gently wash the cell monolayer with 100 µL of PBS (*see* **Subheading 2.1.** and **Note 22**).
4. Remove the PBS wash.
5. Add 50 µL of trypsin-EDTA solution to each well. Wait 2 to 5 min for the cells to detach, then add 150 µL of 10% FBS-DMEM.
6. Mix cell suspension with 200 µL of trypan blue. The cell suspension is now diluted by a factor of 2.
7. Place 10 µL of the trypan blue cell mixture onto each of two hemacytometer chambers. For each well, count at least 100 unstained cells in the hemacytometer (*see* **Note 23**).
8. Calculate the number of cells using the following formula (*see* **Note 24**):
   Number of cells/mL:
$$= \frac{\text{No. of unstained cells x dilution factor x } 1 \times 10^4 \text{ cells/mL}}{\text{Number of total squares counted in the hemacytometer}}$$
   The total number of cells:
$$= \text{number of cells/mL} \times \text{the total cell volume}$$
   In this example, the dilution factor is 2 and the total number of squares that can be counted in a standard hemacytometer is 9.
9. To calculate the percent survival of cells, divide the cell number of the treated cell group by the cell number of the control cell group (no drug treatment) then multiply by 100.

3.5. XTT Assay

The XTT method is widely used for determination of cell viability following anticancer drug treatment (*9*). This assay is suitable for evaluating percent cell survival in an in vitro growth inhibition assay. In our experience, this method is less sensitive than either the crystal violet staining or cell counting assays. The XTT assay measures the activity of viable cells by measuring the activity of mitochondrial dehydrogenases. Mitochondrial dehydrogenases in the presence the aid of an electron-coupling reagent like phenazine methosulfate (PMS) cleave the tetrazolium ring of XTT to yield a product with a peak absorbance at approximately 450 nm *(9)*.

1. Treat cells with drug for time periods from 1–2 h up to ~5 d as described in the cytotoxicity and growth inhibition assays (*see* **Subheading 3.1.**).
2. Prepare XTT/PMS reagent fresh prior to use by adding 0.1 mL of PMS stock (*see* **Subheading 2.5., item 2**) to 4.9 mL of XTT stock (*see* **Subheading 2.5., item 1**) in the dark. Mix well in a dark container.
3. Remove the cell-culture medium from each well of the 96-well microtiter plate containing drug-treated cells.
4. Wash each well once with 100 µL of PBS.
5. Add 100 µL of phenol red-free medium to each well. Add 50 µL of the XTT-PMS solution. The final concentration of XTT in each well is 0.3 mg/mL.
6. Incubate the cells at 37°C for a total of 8 h. Measure the absorbance of the cells at 450 nm and the background at 690 nm at 1-h intervals using an ELISA microplate reader.
7. Calculations:
   a. For each well, subtract the background absorbance measured at 690 nm from the absorbance at 450 nm.
   b. To determine the net absorbance, subtract from the corrected absorbance values, determined in **step 7a** above, the absorbance at 450 nm of wells without cells.
   c. Finally, divide the net absorbance of drug-treated wells by the net absorbance of control wells and multiply by 100. This represents the percent cell survival.

4. Notes

1. The XTT reagent does not need to be filter-sterilized. To reduce background absorbance it is preferable to use cell-culture medium not containing the pH dye indicator phenolthalein (e.g., DMEM Life Technologies, cat. # 1300021). If medium containing phenolthalein is used, each of the negative control wells must also contain medium with the pH indicator.
2. The initial cell density number is chosen to give ~ 5% confluency. The number of cells plated should be such that at the end of drug treatment the control cells (no drug treatment) are almost confluent.
3. This ensures good cell attachment and that the cells are in log phase.
4. Cyclophosphamide is readily soluble in 10% FBS-DMEM up to 100 mM. Drugs that are not soluble in 10% FBS-DMEM may be soluble in organic solvents like dimethyl sulfoxide (DMSO), methanol or ethanol. Once the drug is dissolved in solvent, dilute into 10% FBS-DMEM. An equivalent volume of solvent vehicle is added to wells corresponding to untreated cells (drug-free control wells). 9L tumor cells can tolerate up to 0.1% of methanol or ethanol or up to 1% DMSO. Higher concentrations of these solvents are toxic to the cells.
5. Filtration minimizes the possibility of microbial and fungal contamination.
6. A relatively large number of cells is used (e.g., 1×10^5 cells/60 mm tissue culture

plate) to facilitate counting and replating. If necessary, the assay may be scaled down to accommodate a lower cell number and/or limited drug availability of drug (e.g., begin with 2×10^4 cells/well of a 6-well plate and replate cells in 12-well culture dishes to give densities of 100, 500, and 1000 cells/well).

7. The concentration of drug and length of drug exposure need to be optimized for each drug and each cell line. Mafosfamide is a chemically activated analog of cyclophosphamide that decomposes to yield the cytotoxic 4-hydroxy-cyclophosphamide with high efficiency. Consequently, mafosfamide is cytotoxic to the cells at much lower concentrations than cyclophosphamide, which must undergo P450-catalyzed 4-hydroxylation to generate a cytotoxic metabolite.

8. Ensure that the cells are well disaggregated before plating. Plating of a single cell suspension is essential for distinguishing colonies from cell clusters (*see* **Note 11**). The cell densities given in **Subheading 3.1.1.** are values suggested for 9L cells. Other cell types and other drug treatments may require modifications to this protocol. For instance, lower cell densities (e.g., 50 cells/well) or higher cell densities (e.g., 50,000 and 100,000 cells/well) may be needed to determine the colony formation efficiency in other cases.

9. The cells may be stained earlier than 7 d (e.g., after only 5 d) if the number colonies from the nondrug-treated cells plated at a density 200 cells/well becomes too dense to count individual colonies. The cells may be grown longer than 7 d before staining (e.g., 10 d) if there are fewer than 50 cells in the nondrug-treated colonies.

10. The staining procedures for the cytotoxicity assay are outlined in **Subheadings 3.2.** and **3.3.** When using the crystal violet or SRB-staining protocols to stain cells for the cytotoxicity assay, the plates are stained, but, the dye is not reconstituted and absorbance measurements are not carried out.

11. The most precise method for counting colonies is to record for each dilution (e.g., at both 200 and 1000 cells/well) the number of cell colonies that contain 50 or more cells. Try to distinguish between cell clusters and cell colonies. Cell clusters are groups of cells that arise from single cells that have attached adjacent to each other on the tissue-culture plate surface. Cell colonies, but not cell clusters, represent the products of cell division from a single cell. To aid in counting, use a transparency film showing a graph paper grid. Cut out an 8 cm × 12 cm rectangle and tape it to the bottom of the tissue-culture plate that is to be counted. Alternatively, the number of cell colonies can be counted with the aid of a bacterial colony counter. By this method, the tissue-culture wells are magnified but clusters and colonies cannot be distinguished and the number of cells in a colony cannot be determined.

12. To scale up the staining procedure for the cytotoxicity assay, use 500 μL of PBS to wash the monolayer of each well of a 6-well plate and 1-mL volume per well of crystal violet stain.

13. Do not touch the surface of the well with the pasteur pipet during aspiration because this could disrupt the cell monolayer and lead to detachment of sheets of fixed cells.

14. The dried crystal violet-stained plates can be stored indefinitely at room temperature before reconstitution with ethanol.

15. If desired, the wells can be restained with crystal violet after removal of the crystal violet-ethanol solution. Four or more washes with 70% ethanol may be necessary to remove all the crystal violet from the cells.

16. This step fixes the cells to the microtiter plate. Add the TCA gently to the cell monolayer to avoid detachment of the cells by shearing forces.

17. Do not fix the cells longer than one hour, because increased crosslinking of serum proteins and cell debris to the tissue-culture wells will increase background absorbance and reduce the overall sensitivity of the assay.

18. Rinse the plates by inverting them rather than by aspirating each well (as done in the crystal violet assay). This allows for rapid removal of the reagents while minimizing desorption of SRB dye from the stained cellular proteins.

19. The plates can be stored for several weeks at room temperature before resuspending the SRB stain with the Tris solution.

20. The SRB assay is generally linear up to ~1.8 absorbance units at 564 nm, with the precise value dependent on the ELISA plate reader or the spectrophotometer. If the absorbance of the wells is outside the linear range of the instrument, the samples can be diluted with Tris solution and the absorbance values redetermined. Alternatively, results can be quantified at a submaximal wavelength chosen between 490 and 530 nm to give absorbance values within the linear absorbance range.

21. The volumes suggested for cell counting are based on a 96-well tissue-culture plate. Adjust the volumes of PBS and trypsin accordingly for larger tissue-culture wells (e.g., for a 48-well plate use 200 µL per well).

22. The PBS wash removes any excess fetal bovine serum that could react with the trypsin and inhibit proteolysis of cell attachment proteins.

23. Cells that are not viable will not exclude the trypan blue dye and will appear blue in color. It should be noted that viable cells may take up the trypan blue dye if left for > 15 min in the cell counting solution.

24. Each of the nine large squares in the standard hemacytometer has an area of 1 mm^2 and a depth of 0.1 mm *(8)*. Therefore, the volume of each square is 0.1 mm^3 and the concentration of cells is n divided by 0.1 mm^3 or 1×10^{-4} mL, which equals $n \times 10^4$ cells/mL.

Acknowledgments

Preparation of this chapter was carried out with the support of NIH Grant CA49248 (to D. J. Waxman).

References

1. Waxman, D. J., Chen, L., Hecht, J. E. D., and Jounaidi, Y. (1999) Cytochrome P450-base cancer gene therapy: Recent advances and future prospects. *Drug Metab Rev.* **31,** 503–522.

2. Rigg, A. and Sikora, K. (1997) Genetic prodrug activation therapy. *Mol. Med. Today* **3,** 359–366.

3. Barker, M., Hoshino, T., Gurcay, O., Wilson, C. B., Nielsen, S. L., Downie, R., and Eliason, J. (1973) Development of an animal brain tumor model and its response to therapy with 1,3-bis(2-chloroethyl)-1-nitrosourea. *Cancer Res.* **33,** 976–986.

4. Chen, L. and Waxman, D. (1995) Intratumoral activation and enhanced chemotherapeutic effect of oxazaphosphorines following cytochrome P-450 gene transfer: development of a combined chemotherapy/cancer gene therapy strategy. *Cancer Res.* **55,** 581–589.

5. Chen, G. and Waxman, D. J. (1995) Identification of glutathione S-transferase as a determinant of 4-hydroperoxycyclophosphamide resistance in human breast cancer cells. *Biochem Pharmacol.* **49,** 1691–1701.

6. Stephens, T. C. (1987) Measurement of tumor cell surviving fraction and absolute numbers of clonogens per tumor in excision assay, in *Rodent Tumor Models In Experimental Cancer Therapy* (Kallman, R. F., ed.), Pergamon, New York, pp. 90–94.

7. Skehan, P., Storeng, R., Scudiero, D., Monks, A., McMahon, J., Vistica, D., et al. (1990) New colorimetric cytotoxicity assay for anticancer-drug screening. *J. Natl. Cancer Inst.* **82,** 1107–1112.

8. Dawson, M. (1992) *Initiation and maintenance of cultures in cell culture.* (Butler, M. and Dawson, M., eds.), BIOS Scientific, Oxford, pp. 25–42.

9. Scudiero, D. A., Shoemaker, R. H., Paull, K. D., Monks, A., Tierney, S., Nofziger, T. H., et al. (1988) Evaluation of a soluble tetrazolium/formazan assay for cell growth and drug sensitivity in culture using human and other tumor cell lines. *Cancer Res.* **48,** 4827–4833.

8

Tumor Models for Evaluation of *P450* Gene Therapy In Vivo

Jodi E. D. Hecht, Pamela Schreiber Schwartz, and David J. Waxman

1. Introduction

1.1. Evaluation of P450 *Gene Therapy In Vivo*

P450 prodrug activation-based cancer gene therapy strategies have been developed and show striking effectiveness in both in vitro cell culture and preclinical antitumor animal models *(1,2)*. In vivo tumor models play an important role in the evaluation of the therapeutic efficacy of these strategies, and complement in vitro approaches (*see* Chapter 7) designed to evaluate and compare different *P450* genes and different *P450* gene/prodrug combinations. This chapter describes methods required for in vivo tumor models and their use in evaluating the therapeutic impact of intratumoral *P450* gene expression on a tumor's chemosensitivity to cancer chemotherapeutic agents.

Important factors to consider when choosing a suitable tumor model for such studies include the following *(3)*:

1. The stability of the tumor with respect to reproducible growth, morphology, drug sensitivity, and any effect that *P450* gene expression itself may have on tumor growth.
2. The immunogenicity of the tumor to the host animal, which may be an important determinant of the tumor's sensitivity to drug therapy.
3. Cell kinetics must be considered with regard to growth fraction, cell death and cell cycle time.
4. The extent to which tumor heterogeneity could arise with the emergence of subpopulations of hypoxic or quiescent tumor cells.

From: *Methods in Molecular Medicine, Vol. 35: Gene Therapy: Methods and Protocols*
Edited by: W. Walther and U. Stein © Humana Press, Inc., Totowa, NJ

5. The emergence of subpopulations of cells with altered (e.g., decreased) *P450* expressions in response to drug treatment.
6. The metastatic potential of the tumor model.

The potential for a human *P450* gene to elicit an immune response when expressed within a tumor growing in the animal host is an important consideration when choosing an appropriate animal model for in vivo studies. Evidence of an immune response in an in vivo tumor model includes *(4)*:

1. Poor tumor take or no tumor take.
2. Spontaneous tumor regression in animals not treated with anticancer agents.
3. Changes in drug response profile of a tumor.
4. Animals that are cured of tumors at a very low drug dose.
5. Tumors that are more drug-responsive in a late stage of the disease than at an earlier stage.

These immune responses can contribute to an antitumor effect and may thus lead to overestimation of the efficacy of *P450* gene-dependent prodrug activation-based therapeutic responses. It is, therefore, preferable to avoid these complications in the interpretation of drug responses by carrying out in vivo tumor model studies in an immunodeficient animal background, such as nude or SCID mice.

Two useful assays for determining the responsiveness of tumors expressing cytochrome *P450* genes or other prodrug-activating genes are the tumor-growth delay and the tumor-excision assay. Each assay has its own purposes and advantages, as discussed below. The methods described in this chapter utilize *P450*-expressing tumor cell lines, which may be prepared by retroviral transfection as described in Chapter 6. This method thus represents an ex vivo *P450* gene transfer model, however, the same assay methods can readily be adapted to in vivo *P450* gene transfer studies.

2. Materials

2.1. Tumor Implantation

1. Tumor cell lines: 9L wild-type *(5)* and 9L/lacZ cell line (β -galactosidase) (ATCC - CRL 2200).
2. Culture medium for 9L cells: Dulbecco's Modified Eagle Medium (DMEM) (Life Technologies, Gaithersburg, MD, cat. # 12100-046) supplemented with 3.7 g of sodium bicarbonate, 10 mL of penicillin (5000 U/mL), and streptomycin (5000 μg/mL:) (Life Technologies, cat. # 15070-063) in 900 mL of deionized water. Adjust the pH of the medium to pH 7.1 with concentrated HCl. Filter-sterilize using a 0.2 μm bottle top filter. Store at 4°C for up to 6 mo. To prepare DMEM containing serum supplement 450 mL of complete DMEM with 50 mL of heat-inactivated (56°C for 30 min) fetal bovine serum (Sigma, St. Louis, MO,

cat. # F-2442) (final serum concentration, 10%). Store FBS-DMEM at 4°C for up to 2 mo. Prewarm 10% FBS-DMEM to 37°C before adding to cells.

3. PBS: Phosphate Buffered Saline 0.146M Na$_2$Cl, 0.01M NaHPO$_4$, 2.68 mM KCl, 1.76 mM KH$_2$PO$_4$. Filter-sterilize and store at room temperature for up to 6 mo. The pH should be about 7.4. Prewarm to 37°C before adding to cells.

4. 1X Trypsin-EDTA: 10X Trypsin-EDTA (Life Technologies, cat. # 15400-054) diluted 10-fold in 1X HBSS (see below). Store at 4°C for up to 6 mo. Warm to 37°C before use.

5. 1X HBSS: Hank's Balanced Salt Solution (HBSS) (Life Technologies, cat. # 21250-014) containing 0.35 g of NaHCO$_3$/L. Filter-sterilize and store at 4°C for up to 1 yr.

6. 1 cc syringes (Becton Dickinson, Rutherford, NJ, cat. # BD309602).

7. 27 gauge, 1/2″ needles (Becton Dickinson, cat. # BD305109) or insulin syringes ICC, 29 gage, 1/2″.

8. Animals: (*see* **Notes 1** and **2**). Fischer 344 rats (*see* **Note 3**). Immunodeficient mice (*see* **Note 4**).
   a. Severe combined immuodeficiency mice (ICR Fox Chase ICRTM SCID mice; Tac:ICR:Ha(ICR)-scid) (SCID).
   b. Athymic nude mice (Tac:Cr:(NCr)-nu) (nude). Taconic Farms (Germantown, NY) is one supplier of the Fischer 344 rats, SCID, and nude mice. These animals can also be obtained from other animal suppliers.

9. Ear tags (National Band and Tag Company, Newport, KT).

10. Cyclophosphamide M.W. 279.1 g/mol (Sigma, cat. # C-0768), *potential carcinogen*. Prepare fresh in sterile saline (0.9% NaCl). For rats inject 0.9 mL (100 mg/kg) for each intraperitoneal injection (i.p.) and for mice inject 0.3 mL (150 mg/kg) for each i.p. injection.

2.2. Tumor-Growth Delay Assay

Vernier Caliper - Manostat Corporation, Switzerland (distributed in the USA by VWR).

2.3. Tumor-Excision Assay (6)

1. 95% ethanol.

2. Sterilized surgical instruments for tumor excision: scissors, forceps, long-handled scissors (Harvard Apparatus, South Natick, MA).

3. Cell strainer, 70 micron (Falcon, Los Angeles, CA, cat. # 2350).

4. 50-mL centrifuge tubes (Falcon, cat. # 2095).

5. 27 g 1/2″ needles (Becton-Dickinson, cat. # BD305109).

6 DMEM with and without fetal bovine serum (*see* **Subheading 2.1., item 2**).

7. PBS (*see* **Subheading 2.1., item 3**).

8. Alpha Minimum Essential Medium (α-MEM) (Life Technologies, cat. # 12000-022).

9. Stock Collagenase Type IV–(Sigma, cat. # C-5138) (4500 U/mg). Prepare collagenase Type IV solution in sterile α-MEM at a final concentration of 4500 U/mg (see above). Filter-sterilize through a 0.45 µm syringe filter only if the collagenase was not prepared by resuspending an unopened jar of collagenase under

aseptic conditions. The solution is highly viscous and difficult to filter. The collagenase solution can be prepared and stored at –80°C for 2 wk prior to use.

10. Stock DNase I Type IV (1 mg/mL)–(Sigma, cat. # D-5025). Prepare DNase I solution in α-MEM at a final concentration of 1 mg/mL. Filter-sterilize through a 0.2 μm syringe filter. The DNase I solution can be prepared and stored at –80°C for up to 2 wk prior to use.

11. Crystal Violet Stain (1.25 g crystal violet (Sigma, cat. # C-3886) dissolved in 50 mL of 37% formaldehyde (Sigma, cat. # F-8775) and 450 mL methanol). Mix well and store in a tightly closed container at room temperature for up to 1 yr provided that the methanol does not evaporate.

3. Methods
3.1. Tumor Implantation

1. Handle and ear tag the animals several days before injection of 9L tumor cells (*see* **Notes 5** and **6**).

2. Shave the flanks of the rats with an electric razor 1–2 d before tumor-cell injection (*see* **Note 7**). When shaving the SCID mice with an electric razor, detach, and sterilize the razor blade by autoclaving prior to use. The nude mice are hairless.

3. Tumor cells to be implanted are grown in cell culture to approximately 75% confluency. For Fischer 344 rats and 9L tumors, prepare to have on-hand a sufficient number of tumor cells to inject 2×10^6 cells per subcutaneous (sc) site on the day of injection (*see* **Note 8**). For SCID or nude mice, inject 3 to 4×10^6 tumor cells per site.

4. Prepare tumor cells for injection as follows:
   a. Remove culture medium from cells. Wash the cell monolayer with 5 mL of PBS. Detach tumor cells from the monolayer with 2 mL of 1X trypsin-EDTA per 100-mm tissue-culture dish.
   b. Resuspend the tumor cells from the tissue culture dish in ~ 5 mL of 10% FBS-DMEM/100-mm dish (i.e., for ~ 4×10^6 cells/plate). Pool cells from four dishes of the same tumor-cell line per 50-mL centrifuge tube.
   c. Rinse each 100-mm dish with an additional 2–3 mL of culture medium to harvest remaining cells from the tissue-culture plate. Add this rinse to the 5 mL of cells collected in **step b**, above.
   d. Centrifuge the cells at ~200g for 5 min.
   e. Remove the supernatant and wash the cell pellets in 5 mL of PBS. Centrifuge the cells as in **step d**, above.
   f. Remove the supernatant and resuspend the cells in serum-free DMEM in an approximate volume based on 0.5 mL per injection site for rats or from 0.3–0.5 mL per injection site for mice.
   g. Take a small aliquot of cells and count the number of viable tumor cells by trypan blue exclusion in a hemacytometer (*see* Chapter 7, Subheading 3.4.). For injection of tumor cells in rats, adjust the total volume to give a cell concentration of 4×10^6 viable cells/mL. For injection of tumor cells in mice,

adjust the cell volume to give either 10 or 13.5×10^6 cells/mL (for either 3 or 4×10^6 cells/injection site, respectively).

5. Weigh the animals prior to injection. Maintain a body-weight record over the course of the experiment.
6. Inject the tumor cells sc by lifting the skin of the shaven flank and injecting 2×10^6 tumor cells in 0.5 mL (0.3–0.5 mL for mice) in the base of the skinfold using a 27 g 1/2″ needle and 1 cc syringe or insulin syringe (*see* **Notes 9** and **10**).
7. Check the injection site of the animals the day after tumor-cell inoculation to inspect for any bleeding, bruising, or infection caused by the injection. Examine the mice 1 wk later to ascertain whether small tumors are palpable under the skin (*see* **Note 11**).

3.2. Tumor-Growth Delay Assay

The tumor-growth delay assay measures the response of tumors to drug treatment in vivo. Tumor growth is not only influenced by the specific drug treatment, but also by hormones and the immune response of the host animal. In particular, rodent tumors expressing human *P450* genes should be implanted in immunodeficient animals to eliminate host immune response effects (*see* **Subheading 1.**). The site of the tumor in the animal model and the size of the tumor when drug treatment is initiated also influence the efficacy of drug treatment *(7)*.

1. When the tumor is at least 25 mm^2, tumor area can be measured by calipers (*see* **Notes 12** and **13**).
2. Take tumor-size measurements twice a week (*see* **Note 14**).
3. Treat the animals with the chemotherapeutic drug under investigation by either intraperitoneal or intravenous injection, as required, when the tumors are approximately 80 to 100 mm^2 in size (*see* **Notes 15** and **16**).
4. Continue to monitor tumor areas and body weights of the rats or mice (*see* **Note 17**) until the drug-treated tumors regress, or the tumor burden in untreated rats reach an average area of 1000–1500 mm^2 in each flanking tumors (*see* **Note 18**), or until the animal dies (*see* **Note 19**).
5. Kill the animals by CO_2 asphyxiation or cervical dislocation at the end of the experiment (*see* **Note 20**).
6. Determine tumor-growth delay and tumor-cell kill for the *P450*-expressing tumor cells *(4)*.
   a. Tumor-Growth Delay (TGD) = [*T*(test) - *C*(control)]. TGD is the median time in days required for the treatment group (test) to reach a predetermined size compared to untreated tumors (control).
   b. Tumor-Cell Kill

$$\log 10 \text{ cell-kill total (gross)} = \frac{\text{TGD (d)}}{3.32 \times T_d}$$

T_d = tumor volume doubling time estimated from the best-fit straight line from a log linear growth plot of the control group tumors in exponential growth (unique for each cell type). 3.32 = number of cell doublings per one log of growth (a fixed factor).

Specific growth delay (SGD) values can also be calculated: SGD = $(T_2-T_1) \div T_1$, where T_1 and T_2 are the times in days for control (T_1) and drug-treated tumor (T_2) to double in area. SGD provides an estimate of the number of tumor area doublings by which growth is delayed, and facilitates comparisons of therapeutic responses between tumors that differ in their intrinsic growth rates *(8)*.

3.3. Tumor Excision Assay (see Note 21)

The tumor excision assay is designed to quantitate the fraction of tumor cells that retains proliferative potential following drug treatment in vivo, as measured in an in vitro colony formation assay. This assay is appropriate for *P450*-expressing tumor cells that can be grown as a monolayer. The tumor-excision assay allows for a determination of the effectiveness of drug treatment with greater sensitivity compared to the tumor-growth delay assay. Doses of drug that would otherwise be too toxic to the host when used in the longer-term tumor-growth delay assay (*see* **Subheading 3.2.**) may be used in the tumor-excision assay provided that overt toxicity is not manifest during the first 24 h after drug treatment. Finally, tumor excision experiments have a lower animal maintenance cost and give results more quickly than the tumor-growth delay assay (results obtained in ~ 1 mo compared to about 3 mo required for completing the tumor-growth delay assay) *(9,10)*.

The disadvantages of the tumor-excision assay include the following. First, host and microenvironmental interactions with the tumors that occur after the initial 24 h period of drug exposure are lost. Second, the tumor cell suspension obtained after enzymatic digestion of the isolated solid tumor may not be representative of the overall tumor cell population in terms of its response to drug treatment. In addition, inadequate cell-culture conditions may influence the in vitro growth of subpopulations of tumor cells. Finally, the time at which the tumor is excised may influence the apparent effectiveness of cell survival *(8)*. Typically, tumor excision is carried out 24 h after drug treatment to allow for repair of potentially lethal drug-induced DNA damage. Consequently, a significant number of tumor cells may be lost during the initial 24 h period following drug treatment and prior to tumor excision. Cells lost during this time period will not be counted, resulting in an underestimation of the number of tumor cells killed by the drug. Similarly, cells not killed by drug treatment may proliferate and a delay in the time of tumor excision may allow for repair of the lethal DNA damage resulting in an overestimation of cell survival *(10)*. In addition, the cloning efficiency of many tumors studied using the tumor excision assay is about 10%: typically, only about 20% of the disaggregated tumor cells are recovered and under the best circumstances only half of those cells that are recovered attach to the tissue-culture plates. For example, for each 1000 nondrug treated tumor cells excised from the tumor and then plated on tissue-culture plates, approximately 100 colonies will be formed and counted at the end of the experiment *(9)*.

1. When the tumors reach a size between 50 and 100 mm^2, treat the animals with the chemotherapeutic drug under investigation by either intraperitoneal or intravenous injection, as required (*see* **Notes 22** and **23**).
2. 24 h after drug delivery, kill rats or mice by CO_2 suffocation or cervical dislocation.
3. Remove and pool the two tumors (i.e., provided the tumors are the same cell type) from each rat or mouse using the following methods:
    a. Clean around the area where the tumor is to be excised with 95% ethanol.
    b. Lift the skin and cut around the tumor with sharp scissors.
    c. Remove fat, blood, and necrotic tissue from the outside of the tumor.
    d. Place the remainder of tumor in 20 mL of sterile DMEM in a sterile 50-mL centrifuge tube (*see* **Note 24**).
4. Once the tumors are excised, work with the tumors in a sterile environment using a laminar flow hood.
5. Wash the tumors twice more in separate aliquots of 20 mL DMEM in 50-mL centrifuge tubes.
6. Place the tumors in 10 mL of DMEM in 50-mL centrifuge tubes. Mince the tumors into small pieces using long handled scissors (*see* **Note 25**).
7. Spin the pieces of tumor at ~200g for 3 min at 4°C. Remove the supernatant (*see* **Note 26**).
8. Resuspend the pellet in 8 mL of DMEM. Add 1 mL of collagenase solution and 1 mL of DNase I solution.
9. Incubate the minced tumor pieces for 15 min at 37°C while shaking at high speed (*see* **Note 27**).
10. Add an additional 1 mL of collagenase solution and 1 mL of DNase I solution to each tube containing two tumor samples. Incubate for 15 min at 37°C while shaking at high speed.
11. Spin at ~200g for 5 min at 4°C. Remove the supernatant and add 10 mL of DMEM to the cell pellet.
12. Strain the cell suspension in a cell strainer and collect the cells in a 50-mL centrifuge tube. Wash the cell strainer and original tube containing the disaggregated tumors with 5 mL of DMEM (*see* **Note 28**).
13. Spin the cells at ~200g for 3 min at 4°C.
14. Remove the supernatant and resuspend in 10 mL of DMEM. Spin as in **step 11**.
15. Remove the supernatant and resuspend in 10 mL of DMEM (*see* **Note 29**).
16. Count the viable tumor cells using trypan blue and a hemacytometer (*see* **Note 30**).
17. Dilute cells over a wide range of densities to facilitate analysis. Plate cells in duplicate wells of 6-well tissue-culture dishes (*see* **Note 31**).

18. Change the medium once the cells have attached. This should be done between 4 and 12 h after plating the cells (*see* **Note 32**).
19. Incubate the tumor cells in a tissue culture incubator for 7–10 d before staining colonies with crystal violet (*see* **Note 33**).
20. Count colonies using a phase contrast microscope or a magnifying colony counter (*see* **Note 34**).
21. Data Analysis *(10)*.
    Plating Efficiency (PE):

$$\frac{\text{Number of colonies in the control plate}}{\text{Number of control cells plated}} \times 100$$

Colony Forming Efficiency (CFE):

$$\frac{\text{PE treated cells}}{\text{PE control cells}} \times 100$$

The CFE represents the surviving fraction of cells from a treated tumor.

4. Notes

1. Experiments can be carried out using either male or female animals; however, this choice may affect the results, because of sex-differences in liver *P450* enzyme profiles that can influence the extent of hepatic drug metabolism [e.g., *(11)*].
2. Typical weights and ages of animals at the time of tumor inoculations for both the tumor growth delay and tumor excision assays are listed below. Animals should be obtained from the supplier 1–2 wk younger than the ages listed below so that the animals can acclimate to the animal facility and be handled and prepared for tumor-cell injections.
   8-wk-old Fischer 344 rats: male—165–200 g; female—130–140 g.
   6-wk-old SCID mice: male—23–27 g; female—19–23 g.
   6-wk-old Nude mice: male—22–25 g; female—17–22 g.
3. Fischer 344 rats can be used for tumors that are syngeneic in this rat strain (e.g., 9L gliosarcoma), provided that a rat *P450* gene is to be expressed in the tumor cells.
4. Use immunodeficient mice for growing nonsyngeneic tumors expressing heterologous *P450* genes. These mice require special care including sterile cages and cage lids equipped with filters, sterile bedding, food, and water. Mice must be handled with sterile gloves in a laminar flow hood.
5. The number of animals required for each experiment will depend on the number of treatment groups. Four animals containing two tumors per animal for each experimental treatment is sufficient for many studies. If additional resources are available, it may be useful to inoculate five to six animals per treatment group. This allows the investigator to select at the time of drug treatment a group of four animals with a uniform tumor size for inclusion in the experiment.
6. Handling the animals for 5 min on each of two consecutive days immediately prior to tumor-cell injections will make the animals more comfortable with human

touch and more compliant during the experiment. Male Fischer 344 rats have a better disposition than female Fischer 344 rats. Handling the nude or SCID mice before tumor-cell injections improves their behavior only slightly.

7. Shaving the animals clears the skin for injection. The hair grows back quickly so the shaving should be carried out within 2 d of tumor-cell injection. The hind flank is a good site for sc injection of tumor cells because of its easy access for tumor-size measurement. Tumors grown at this site also cause less distress for the animal than tumors grown on the forelimbs or the back.

8. For 9L tumors, cells of a low cell-passage number (≤ 25) should be used to reduce the variability of growth between individual tumors. It is preferable to inject 9L cells harvested in cell culture prior to confluence, e.g., cells at a density of 4×10^6 9L cells per 100-mm culture dish. This helps to ensure that a high proportion of the injected cells will be in log phase. It is critical that the cells should be mycoplasma and bacteria-free when injecting them into the immunodeficient mice.

9. To facilitate the injections, one person may hold the animal while a second person injects the tumor cells. Lift up the skin on the hind flank and inject the needle into the base of the raised skin while keeping the needle parallel to the animal's body (longitudinal axis) or at a 30° angle from the animal's body surface. This will help avoid making an intramuscular injection. Make sure that the needle punctures completely through the base of the raised skin to avoid an intradermal injection. A 'bubble' will form under the skin with minimal redness when the injection is sc. Remove the needle slowly from the injection site to minimize tumor cell leakage caused by the release of sc pressure following the injection.

10. Each mouse or rat can tolerate the growth of two sc tumors (e.g., one on each hind flank). The two tumors may both express the same transfected gene or may be selected to express different genes (e.g., 9L/lacZ tumor on right flank and 9L/*P450* 2B1 tumor on left flank). Implantation of two of the same tumor types/ animal eliminates the possibility of intratumoral affects on tumor-growth rate or drug responsiveness.

11. Tumor-growth rates depend on the tumor cell type and on the animal model. The tumor may become palpable as early as 7 d to as late as several wk after inoculation. Lift the skin and feel for a hard bump; this may indicate that a tumor is forming. A tumor will be about 4 mm^2 in area at the earliest point of detection.

12. To determine tumor area, measure the width and length of the tumor. Measuring the tumor area rather than tumor volume generally gives a very good indication of the tumor size, provided the tumor mass is less than 6 g *(12)*.

13. The growth rate of the tumor will be markedly different if the tumor is grown intramuscularly compared to subcutaneously. Ensure that the tumors in each experiment are all growing in the same tissue compartment (i.e., sc).

14. Ideally, all tumor-area measurements in a given experimental series should be taken by a single individual to improve the consistency of the data. The measurements should also be taken double-blind, i.e., without prior knowledge of which animals received which tumors and treatments.

15. The sensitivity of the tumors to drug may be dependent on its size at the time of drug treatment. Large tumors become necrotic in their centers with little cellular material present. In immunocompetent animals, if the tumors are too small at the time of drug treatment, immunogenic factors may influence tumor growth.

16. Fischer 344 male and female rats can tolerate a single injection of cyclophosphamide (*see* **Subheading 2.1., item 10**) at 100 mg/kg body weight. Nude and SCID mice can tolerate a total injection of 450 mg of cyclophosphamide per kg body weight administered over 6 d (i.e., drug treatment every other day × 3 at 150 mg/ kg per drug treatment). Additional drug treatments are possible after a suitable drug-free recovery interval.

17. With many anticancer drugs given at therapeutic doses, weight loss during the first 1–2 wks following drug treatment is common, and provides an index of systemic drug exposure. In male and female Fischer 344 rats given cyclophosphamide, a 5 to 10% body-weight loss is a good indication that the animal received the drug. Immunodeficient mice do not show a significant weight loss after cyclophosphamide injection at 300 mg/kg.

18. In the case of 9L tumors, the maximum tumor burden that the average 30 g nude or SCID mice can tolerate is two 1000-mm^2 necrotic flanking tumors.

19. Monitoring the survival of tumor-bearing animals is done for experiments designed to assess the effects of the *P450*/prodrug combination on length of animal survival.

20. Once the animals are killed, the tumors can be excised on ice. At this point, the tumors are verified as having grown subcutaneously. The tumors are then weighed, rinsed in cold 1.15% potassium chloride to remove blood, placed in scintillation vials, and frozen quickly in liquid nitrogen and then stored at –80°C for in vitro biochemical analyses, e.g., microsomal isolation and analysis of *P450* enzyme activity.

21. This procedure is long and arduous and it is best to be carried out by two people working together. It takes approx 12 h for two people to process 12 animals that each have two tumors. It is recommended to prepare the day before the excision assay by labeling tubes and aliquoting medium.

22. Fischer 344 male and female rats can readily tolerate a single injection of cyclophosphamide (*see* **Subheading 2.1., item 10**) at 100 mg/kg body weight. Nude and SCID mice can tolerate a single injection of cyclophosphamide of 300 mg per kg body weight.

23. The size of the tumor will influence the efficacy of drug treatment.

24. Transfer the tumor from one tube to another using long forceps. Clean and sterilize the forceps and scissors with 70% ethanol then flame to vaporize the alcohol.

25. Spend about 5 to 10 min cutting each group of two tumors into small pieces. Mincing the tumors is a critical, albeit tedious step. Transferring the tumors to a 100 mm sterile tissue culture dish may facilitate mincing of the tumors. Return the tumor pieces to a centrifuge tube for the collagenase and Dnase step. The smaller the tumor pieces, the more effective the tumor disaggregation step will be.

26. The pellet is very soft and loose. Be careful not to aspirate the tumor cells.
27. For most effective disaggregation, position the centrifuge tubes at an angle in the water bath so that the tumor homogenate is well mixed. Ensure that the centrifuge tubes are immersed in the warm water during this shaking step.
28. Use a plunger from a 3-mL syringe to pass cells through the strainer. Periodically lift the strainer from the mouth of the centrifuge tube to disrupt any vacuum that may inhibit cell flow. If the cells are difficult to strain, use a 27G 1/2″ needle attached to a vacuum line to aid in straining.
29. 10 mL is a convenient volume for dilution for cell counting for an average-size tumor (e.g., 0.6–1 g, corresponding to ~ 90–110 mm^2 in area). For smaller tumors use 5 mL and for larger tumors use 20 mL. Note the exact volume used so that the total cell number recovered from the excised tumor can be calculated.
30. Count at least two aliquots from the cell homogenate. Ensure that at least 100 cells are counted in the hemacytometer. Methods for cell counting can be found in Chapter 7, Subheading 3.4.
31. Ensure that the cells are well disaggregated before plating. Plating of a single-cell suspension is essential for distinguishing colonies from cell clusters (*see* **Note 34**). Suggested dilutions are 100, 1000, 5000, 10,000, 50,000 and 100,000 cells/well of a 6-well tissue-culture plate. The drug-treated cells can be plated at higher density (10,000, 50,000, 100,000 cells/well) and the untreated cells may be plated at lower density (100, 1000, 5000 cells/well) if time or tissue-culture supplies are limiting.
32. Remove dead cells and other debris by changing the medium on the plates once the cells are attached (i.e., wait a minimum of 4 h but less than 12 h).
33. Stain the cells with crystal violet after the colonies grow for 7–10 d. To stain with crystal violet: remove medium from each well and gently wash monolayer with 1 mL of PBS. Aspirate the PBS and add 1 ml of stain for 10 min. Remove stain by gentle aspiration. Do not allow the pasteur pipet to touch the surface of the well because this will disrupt the monolayer. De-stain by gently rinsing the wells in a container filled with tap water. Change the water until the wells no longer stain the water purple (~ 4 rinses with water). Air dry overnight, then count colonies.
34. The most precise method for counting colonies is to record for each dilution (i.e., at both 200 and 1000 cells/well) the number of cell colonies that contain 50 or more cells. Try to distinguish between cell clusters and cell colonies. Cell clusters are groups of cells that arise from single cells that have attached adjacent to each other on the tissue-culture plate surface. Cell colonies, but not cell clusters, represent the products of cell division from a single cell. To aid in counting, use a transparency film showing a graph paper grid. Cut out a 8 cm × 12 cm rectangle and tape it to the bottom of the tissue culture plate that is to be counted. Alternatively, the number of cell colonies can be counted with the aid of a bacterial colony counter. By this method, the tissue culture wells are magnified, but clusters and colonies cannot be distinguished and the number of cells in a colony cannot be determined.

Acknowledgments

Preparation of this chapter was carried out with the support of NIH Grant CA49248 (to D. J. Waxman).

References

1. Chen L., Yu, L. J., and Waxman, D. J. (1997) Potentiation of cytochrome P450/cyclophosphamide-based cancer gene therapy by coexpression of the P450reductase gene. *Cancer Res.* **57,** 4830–4837.
2. Chase, M., Chung, R. Y., and Chiocca, E. A. (1998) An oncolytic viral mutant that delivers the CYP2B1 transgene and augments cyclophosphamide chemotherapy. *Nat. Biotechnol.* **16,** 444–448.
3. Corbett, T. H. and Valeriote, F. A. (1987) Rodent models in experimental chemotherapy, in *Rodent Tumor Models–In Experimental Cancer Therapy* (Kallman, R. F., ed), Pergamon, New York, pp. 233–247.
4. Corbett, T., Valeriote, F., LoRusso, P., Polin, L., Panchapor, C., Pugh, S., et al. (1997) In vivo methods for screening and preclinical testing–use of rodent solid tumors for drug discovery, in *Anticancer Drug Development Guide–Preclinical Screening, Clinical Trials, and Approval* (Teicher, B. A., ed.), Humana, Totowa, NJ, pp. 75–99.
5. Barker, M., Hoshino, T., Gurcay, O., Wilson, C. B., Nielsen, S. L., Downie, R., and Eliason, J. (1973) Development of an animal brain tumor model and its response to therapy with 1,3-bis(2-chloroethyl)-1-nitrosourea. *Cancer Res.* **33,** 976–986.
6. Teicher, B. A., Holden, S. A., and Jacobs, J. L. (1987) Approaches to defining the mechanism of enhancement by Fluosol-DA 20% with carbogen of melphalan antitumor activity. *Cancer Res.* **47,** 513–518.
7. Begg, A. C. (1987) Principles and practices of the tumor growth delay assay, in *Rodent Tumor Models In Experimental Cancer Therapy* (Kallman, R. F., ed.), Pergamon, NY, pp. 114–121.
8. Lartiqau, E. and Guichard, M. (1996) The effect of tirapazamine (SR-4233) alone or combined with chemotherapeutic agents on xenografted human tumors. *Br. J. Cancer* **73,** 1480–1485.
9. Hill, R. P. (1987) Excision assays, in *Rodent Tumor Models–In Experimental Cancer Therapy* (Kallman, R. F., ed.), Pergamon, NY, pp. 67–75.
10. Stephens, T. C. (1987) Measurement of tumor cell surviving fraction and absolute numbers of clonogens per tumor in excision assay, in *Rodent Tumor Models In Experimental Cancer Therapy* (Kallman, R. F., ed.), Pergamon, NY, pp. 90–94.
11. Yu, L. and Waxman, D. J. (1996) Role of cytochrome P450 in oxazaphosphorine metabolism. Deactivation via N-dechloroethylation and activation via 4-hydroxylation catalyzed by distinct subsets of rat liver cytochromes P450. *Drug Metab. Dispos.* **24,** 1254–1262.
12. Tomayko, M. M. and Reynolds, C. P. (1989) Determination of subcutaneous tumor size in athymic (nude) mice. *Cancer Chemother. Pharmacol.* **24,** 148–154.

I

EXPERIMENTAL APPROACHES IN CANCER GENE THERAPY

C: Anti-Oncogene and Suppressor Gene Therapy

9

Intracellular Single-Chain Antibodies for Gene Therapy

Guadalupe Bilbao, Jesus Gomez-Navarro, Keizo Kazano, Juan Luis Contreras, and David T. Curiel

1. Introduction

The delineation of the molecular basis of cancer in general, allows for the possibility of specific intervention at the molecular level for therapeutic purposes. To this end, three main approaches have been developed: mutation compensation, molecular chemotherapy, and genetic immunopotentiation. The strategy of mutation compensation aims to correct the specific genetic defects in cancer cells. Such correction is accomplished by either ablation of oncogenic products, replacement of cellular tumor suppressor genes, or interference with dysregulated signal transduction pathways. A second strategy is molecular chemotherapy, which aims to increase the specificity of drug delivery or to increase tolerance to standard chemotherapeutic regimens. A third strategy, genetic immunotherapy, aims to augment the specificity and/or the magnitude of the normal immune response to tumors. For each of these conceptual approaches, human clinical protocols have entered Phase I clinical trials to assess dose escalation, safety, and toxicity issues.

The genetic lesions etiologic of malignant transformation may be thought of as a critical compilation of two general types: aberrant expression of "dominant" oncogenes or loss of expression of "tumor suppressor" genes. Gene therapy strategies have been proposed to achieve correction of each of these lesions. For approaching the loss of function of a tumor suppressor gene, the logical intervention is replacement of the deficient function with a wild-type tumor suppressor gene counterpart. The disregulation of oncogenes by mutation, gene amplification, gene rearrangement, or overexpression

From: *Methods in Molecular Medicine, Vol. 35: Gene Therapy: Methods and Protocols*
Edited by: W. Walther and U. Stein © Humana Press, Inc., Totowa, NJ

contributes the aberrant expression of the corresponding gene product that elicits the associated neoplastic transformation. One approach to gene therapy for cancer is to "knock out" dominant oncogenes and thereby reduce the tumor's growth or invasive potential. Inhibition or ablation of oncogenic function can be attempted at three levels. First, the translation of the oncogene can be targeted. This strategy involves the use of the most universally employed methodology the "antisense" molecules to sequester oncogene mRNA *(1–4)*. However, despite the fact that antisense inhibition can be demonstrated in many contexts, targeting the uptake of oligonucleotides into cells, the stability of the antisense molecules, and pharmokinetic considerations within animals, have greatly limited translation of this approach into human clinical trials *(5–6)*. Second, the function of the gene product can be targeted. This approach uses polypeptides containing dominant interfering mutations to downregulate signal transduction in tumor cells. Third, the nascent oncogenic protein can be prevented from reaching its proper intracellular location. This approach uses intracellular single-chain Fv molecules (scFv) to preempt the cellular localization machinery and sequester proteins inside the cell. In this regard, single-chain immunoglobin (scFv) molecules retain the antigen-binding specificity of the immunoglobulin from which they were derived, however, they lack other functional domains characterizing the parent molecule. The basis of constructing scFvs has been established. Pastan et al. have developed methods to derive cDNAs which encode the variable regions of specific immunoglobins *(7–8)*. Specifically, a single-chain antibody (scFv) gene is derived which contains the coding sequences for variable regions from the heavy chain (V_H) and the light chain (V_L) of the immunoglobulin separated by a short linker of hydrophilic amino acids (*see* **Fig. 1**). The resultant recombinant molecule, when expressed in prokaryotic systems, is a single-chain antibody (scFv) which retains the antigen recognition and binding profile of the parental antibody *(9–11)*. The development of recombinant immunotoxins employing scFv moieties achieves cell-specific binding of the toxin to the exterior of the target cell, allowing receptor-mediated endocytosis to accomplish toxin internalization. A variety of strategies employing the recombinant scFv-directed immunotoxins have been developed by a number of investigators *(7,8,12–15)*. In addition, it has recently been shown that scFv molecules may be expressed intracellularly in eukaryotic cells by gene transfer of scFv cDNAs. The encoded scFv may be expressed in the target cell and localized to specific, targeted subcellular compartments by appropriate signal molecules. Importantly, these intracellular scFvs may recognize and bind antigen within the target cell. Target for the intracellular antibody knockout method have included viral antigens in the context of HIV infection (phase I clinical trial), transformed oncoprotein like erbB2 and cRas, and tumor associate antigens like CEA *(16–18)*. In this regard, our

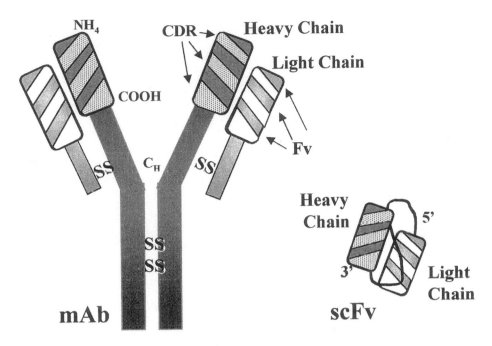

Fig. 1. Antibody structure, showing the heavy and light chain of an immunoglobulin. S-S denotes inter- or intramolecular disulfide bonds. The CDR residues, which form the antibody-binding site, are shown in dark in the variable regions. Single-chain Fv with VH and VL regions joined by a linker (black line).

group has recently exploited this technology to develop an anti-erbB-2 scFv that down-modulates the erbB-2 oncoprotein in erbB-2 overexpressing tumor cells *(19–26)*. This method of genetic intervention achieved diverse antineo plastic effects specifically in tumor cells overexpressing the targeted oncoprotein. Importantly, this approach to human carcinoma of the ovary based on the anti-erbB-2 scFv strategy is now approved for a Phase I clinical trial (htpp://www.nih.gov/od/orda/protocol.htm).

This chapter will review in detail practical procedures to generate a single-chain intracellular antibody (*see* **Fig. 2**). Most of the methods we employ in our lab utilize commercially available kits for convenience. We will emphasize in this review the different steps in our protocol that we have employed to develop scFvs to a variety of target proteins. The Recombinant Phage Antibody System (RPAS) from Pharmacia (Uppsala, Sweden), is based on a phage-display technology where fragments of antibodies are expressed as fusion with gene-3 protein and displayed on the tips of M13 phage. Once antigen-positive clones have been identified by phage rescue, they are used to infect a nonsuppressor strain of *E. coli* HB2151 for the purpose of producing soluble

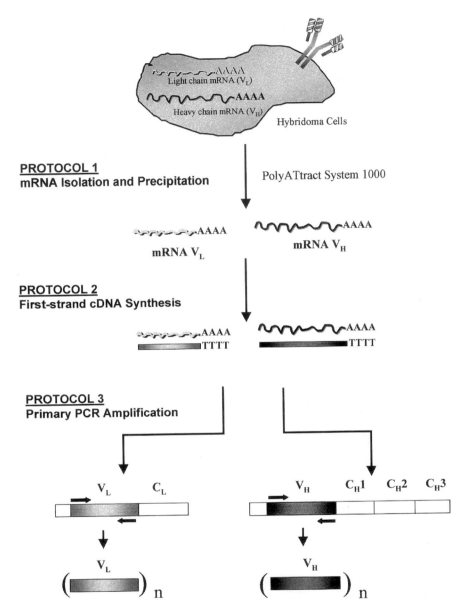

Fig. 2. Construction and screening of a single-chain antibody library.

antibodies. In our laboratory, we used a modified colony lift technology to identified antigen-positives clones directly into the nonsuppressor HB2151 *E. coli*. This modification in the expression module is a very simple way of screening your recombinant single-chain antibodies, saving time-consuming steps.

PROTOCOL 4 and 5
Gel Analysis, Purification and quantification of
Primary V_H and V_L PCR Products

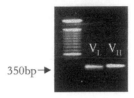

PROTOCOL 6
Assembly And Fill In Reactions

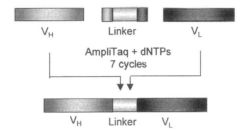

PROTOCOL 7
Second PCR Amplification and Purification

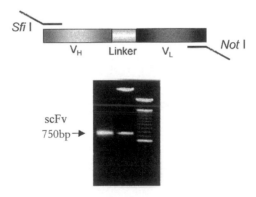

Fig. 2. *(continued)*.

PROTOCOL 8
Restriction Digestion and Purification

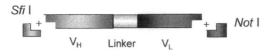

PROTOCOL 9
Ligation of the scFv cDNA into the Phagemid Plasmid pCANTAB5E

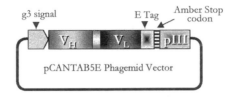

PROTOCOL 10
Transformation

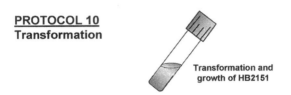

PROTOCOL 11
Modified Colony Lift Assay

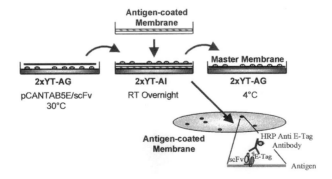

Fig. 2. *(continued).*

2. Materials

All water used in these protocols should be sterile, deionized, and distilled. All reagents, plastic-and glassware should be sterile.

PROTOCOL 12
Production of Soluble Antibodies (Periplasmic Extract)

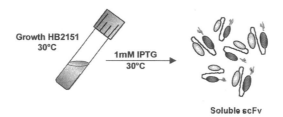

PROTOCOL 13
Detection and Binding Specificity of E-Tagged scFvs

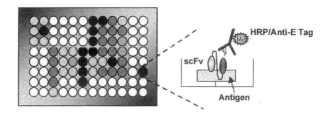

PROTOCOL 14
Western Blot Analysis of E-Tagged scFvs

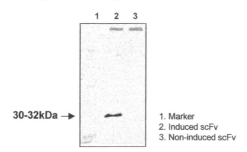

Fig. 2. *(continued)*.

2.1. Kits

1. mRNA Purification PolyATtract 1000 Kit (Promega, Madison, WI, cat. # Z5420). Store at 4°C.
2. First-Strand cDNA Synthesis Kit (Pharmacia Biotech cat. # 27-9261-01). Store at –20°C.

3. Mouse scFv Module Recombinant Phage Antibody System (Pharmacia Biotech cat. # 27-9400-01). Store at –20°C.
4. Mouse Ig-Prime Kit System (Novagen, Madison, WI, cat. # 70082-3). Store at –20°C.
5. QIAquick Gel Extraction Kit (Qiagen, Chatsworth, CA, cat. # 28704). Store at room temperature.
6. pShooter Mammalian Expression Vector collection (Invitrogen, San Diego, CA, pCMV/myc/nuc cat. # V821-20, pCMV/*myc*/mito cat. # V822-20, pCMV/*myc*/cyto cat. # V820-20). Store at –20°C

2.2. Reagents

1. β -Mercaptoethanol: is toxic, dispense in a fume hood and wear appropriate personal protective equipment. Store at 4°C.
2. RNase Zap (Ambion, Austin, TX, cat. # 9780). Store at room temperature.
3. Isopropylthio-β-D-galactopyranoside (IPTG). Store at –20°C.
4. Ethanol. Store at room temperature.
5. Mineral oil: Light Mineral Oil (Fisher, Pittsburgh, PA, cat. # 0121-1). Store at room temperature.
6. AmpliTaq® DNA Polymerase from (Perkin-Elmer, Norwalk, CT, cat. # N808-0038). Store at –20°C.
7. Ultrapure DNA grade Agarose (Bio-Rad, Richmond, CA, cat. # 162-0133). Store at room temperature.
8. 0.5X and 1X TAE Buffer: 50X TAE 121g Tris, 50 mL 0.5M EDTA pH 8.00, 28.55 mL glacial acetic acid, QS to 500 mL with ddH$_2$O. Store at room temperature.
9. RNase-Free Solutions: Add diethylpyrocarbonate [DEPC] (Sigma, St. Louis, MO, cat. # D-5758) to solution to a concentration of 0.05% (i.e., add 0.5 mL per liter of solution); shake well, incubate several hours to overnight at 37°C of 42°C; autoclave at least 45 min, or until DEPC scent is gone. Store at room temperature.
10. 0.5*M* EDTA: 186.1 g EDTA, 20 g NaOH pellets, pH to 8.00 with NaOH, QS to 1 L with ddH$_2$O. Store at room temperature.
11. 100 Base-Pair ladder (Life Technologies, Gaithersburg, MD, cat. # 15-628-019). Store at –20°C.
12. Ethidium bromide 100 mg/mL (Bio-Rad cat. # 161-0433). Store at room temperature.
13. 6X Loading Dye: 30% glycerol and 0.25% bromophenol blue in 10 m*M* TE, pH 7.6. Store at room temperature.
14. dNTP Mix (100 m*M* each of dATP, dCTP, dGTP, dTTP in sterile water). Store at –20°C.
15. 25 m*M* MgCL$_2$ sterile. Store at room temperature.
16. 10X PCR buffer (Perkin-Elmer cat. # N808-0038). Store at –20°C.
17. TE Buffer: 10 m*M* Tris-HCl (pH 8.0) and 0.1 mM EDTA. Store at room temperature.

18. *Sfi* I (Boehringer Mannheim, Mannheim, Germany, cat. # 1288-016). Store at –20°C.
19. *Not* I (Boehringer Mannheim cat. # 1014-706). Store at –20°C.
20. 3 *M* NaCl: 175.35 gr of NaCl, QS to 1 L with ddH$_2$O. Store at room temperature.
21. Phenol:chloroform:isoamyl alcohol (25:24:1), equilibrated against TE (Amresco, Solon, OH, cat. # 0883). Store at –20°(C.
22. Phosphate Buffered Saline (PBS): 0.2 g KCl, 0.24 g KH$_2$PO$_4$, 8 g NaCl, 1.44 g Na$_2$HPO$_4$, QS to 1 L with ddH$_2$O. Store at room temperature.
23. T4 DNA Ligase (Boehringer Mannheim cat. # 481-220). Store at –20°C.
24. 30% H$_2$O$_2$ (any company). Store at 4°C.
25. 2M glucose. Do not autoclave, filter sterilize. Store at room temperature.
26. HRP/Anti-E Tag Conjugate (Pharmacia cat. # 27-9412-01). Store at –20°C.
27. Chloro-1-Naphthol (4C1N) tablets (30mg) (Sigma cat. # C-6788). Store tablets at –20°C. Protect from heat, light and moisture. Allow to reach room temperature before use.
28. Triethanolamine saline pH 7.5: Add 7.5 gr of NaCl, 2.8 mL of triethanolamine (Sigma cat. # T-1377), and 17 mL of 1*M* HCl to approx 800 mL of dH$_2$O. Adjust the pH to 7.5 if necessary and QS to 1 L with dH$_2$O. Store at room temperature.
29. ABTS (2′, 2′-Azino-Bis[3-Ethylbenzthiazoline-6-Sulphonic Acid] Diammonium) add the following to a 500 mL: 450 mL of 0.05*M* citric acid pH4.0, and 100mg of ABTS. Filter sterilize the 1X ABTS stock solution and store at 4°C until needed.
30. 40% Acrylamide/Bis Solution 37.5 : 1(Bio-Rad cat. # 161-0148). Store at 4°C.
31. 10% SDS (Life Technologies, cat. # 24730-012). Store at room temperature.
32. Ammonium-Persulfate (APS) (Fisher cat. # BP179-25). Store at room temperature in the desicator.
33. TEMED (Bio-Rad cat. # 161-0800). Store at room temperature.
34. 1X Western Blot Running Buffer: 25 m*M* Tris, and 192 m*M* Glycine. Store at room temperature.
35. X Western Blot Transfer Buffer: 25 m*M* Tris, 192 m*M* Glycine, and 20% methanol. Store at room temperature.
36. 4X Western Blot Sample Buffer (100 mL): Tris-HCl/SDS, pH6.8 (20 mL ddH$_2$O, 3.03 g Tris Base, and 0.2 g SDS), 8 g SDS, 20 mL Glycerol, 0.1 g Bromophenol Blue. QS with ddH$_2$O to 100 mL. This is a nonreducing buffer. For reducing conditions, you need to add 6.2 g of dithiothreotol (DTT) per every 100 mL. Aliquots into 1 mL and store at –20°C.

2.3. Media

Store media at room temperature and all plates (and LBG medium) at 4°C. Use media and plates within 2 weeks if they contain antibiotics.

1. Luria Broth Base Media "LB" (Sigma cat. # L-3522).
2. LBG   LB Media + 20 m*M* glucose.
3. S.O.C. Media at room temperature (Life Technologies, cat. # 15544-018).

4. Minimal Medium Plates.
5. 2-YT Medium (Life Technologies, cat. # 22712-020).
6. 2X YT-AG   100 µg/mL ampicillin and 2% glucose.
7. 2X YT-AI   100 µg/ml ampicillin and 1 m*M* IPTG.
8. 2X YT-G   2% glucose.

2.4. Others

1. Cluster tubes (96 tubes in a microtiter format, Costar, Cambridge, MA, cat. # 4411).
2. Plate sealer (Costar cat. # 6524).
3. RNase-free pipets (USA American Scientific Plastics cat. # 1010-8810).
4. RNase-free user tubes (Ambion cat. # 12400).
5. Colony lift butterfly S&S nitrocellulose membrane pore size 0.45 µm, diameter 82 mm (Schleicher & Schuell cat. # 401149).
6. RNase Alert (Ambion cat. # 1960).
7. Tranblot Tranfer Medium 0.2 µm Pure Nitrocellulose Membrane (Bio-Rad cat. # 162-0146).
8. Blot absorbent filter paper. (Bio-Rad cat. # 170-3932).

3. Methods

3.1 mRNA Isolation and Precipitation

The success of antibody cloning depends on the purity of the mRNA. The source of the mRNA can be isolated from either mouse antibody produced hybridoma, established cell lines or spleen-derived B lymphocytes. Any kit that will provide high-quality mRNA is recommendable. In our laboratory, we recommend the use of the Promega PolyATtract System 1000 because it isolates messenger RNA directly from crude cell or tissue lysates and eliminate the need for total RNA Isolation.

3.1.1. mRNA Isolation from Hybridoma Cell Line ($1 \times 10^7 - 1 \times 10^8$)

Before starting this protocol make sure that rotors and centrifuges are at room temperature to avoid precipitation of salts and detergents from solutions.

1. Remove the GTC extraction buffer, Biotinylated Oligo (dT) Probe, Nuclease-free Water, and SSC 0.5X Solution from the refrigerator and warm to room temperature. Preheat the dilution buffer to 70°C.
2. In a 50-mL sterile screw cap conical tube, add 41 µL of β-Mercaptoethanol (48.7%) per milliliter of extraction buffer and named "Extraction/BME Buffer." The final concentration of β-Mercaptoethanol is 2%. Use RNase-free pipet and wear gloves to reduce the chance of contamination.
3. Collect ($1 \times 10^7 - 1 \times 10^8$) cells in a sterile 50 mL conical tube by centrifugation at 300*g* for 5 min. Wash the cell pellet with 23 mL of ice cold, sterile 1X phosphatase buffer saline (PBS) and centrifuge as above to collect the cells. Pour off the supernatant.

4. Add the "Extraction/BME Buffer" to the cells and mix by inversion the 50 mL tube 4 times. Homogenizing the cells by high speed for 15–30 s using a small homogenizer as Promega protocol recommends is optional.
5. Aliquot the preheated dilution buffer to a sterile tube and add 20.5 µL of β-Mercaptoethanol (48.7%) per milliter of dilution buffer. The final concentration of β-Mercaptoethanol is 1%. Add this to the homogenate and mix thoroughly by inversion. Add the biotinylated oligo (dT) Probe and mix well. Incubate this mixture at 70°C for 5 min.
6. Transfer the lysate to a clean, sterile 15 mL tube. Centrifuge at 12,000*g* for 10 min at room temperature to clean the homogenate of cell debris and precipitated proteins.
7. During the centrifugation, resuspend the SA-PMPs by gently rocking the bottle. The particles should appear as a homogeneous mixture and be fully suspended in the liquid. Transfer the 6 mL of SA-PMPs, to a sterile 50 mL conical screw cap tube away from the magnetic stand. Place the tube and the SA-PMPs on the magnetic stand. Slowly move the stand toward the horizontal position until the particles are collected at the tube side. Carefully pour off the storage buffer by tilting the tube so that the solution runs over the captured particles. Pouring in this manner decreases the chance of mixing the SA-PMPs into the solution again, which would decrease yields.
8. Resuspend the SA-PMPs to the original volume used (6 mL), in SSC 0.5X solution. Capture using the magnetic stand. Pour off the SSC solution as described in **step 7**. Repeat the washing a total of three times. Resuspend in the original volume (6 mL) with SSC 0.5X solution. Do not centrifuge these particles.
9. When the centrifugation of the homogenate is complete, carefully remove the supernatant with a sterile pipet, avoiding the pellet. The homogenate will be translucent.
10. Add the clear homogenate to the tube containing the washed SA-PMPs in SSC 0.5X solution and mix by inversion. It is important to add the homogenate away from the magnetic separation stand to ensure proper mixing.
11. Incubate the homogenate/SA-PMPs mixture at room temperature for 2 min. Capture the SA-PMPs moving the magnetic stand toward the horizontal position until the homogenate clears and then carefully pour off the supernatant as in **step 7**. Save the supernatant in a sterile tube on ice until certain that satisfactory binding and elution of the mRNA has occurred.
12. Resuspend the particles with 2 mL of SSC 0.5X solution by gently flicking the tube. Transfer the particle mixture to one of the 2 mL RNase-free user tubes. Capture the SA-PMPs by placing the tube in the magnetic stand. Carefully pipet off the SSC solution. Repeat this washing step twice. After the final wash, remove as much of the SSC solution as possible without disturbing the SA-PMPs cake.
13. To elute the mRNA, add 1 mL of RNase-free water and gently resuspend the particles by flicking the tube.
14. Magnetically capture the SA-PMPs by moving the magnetic stand toward the horizontal position, as before. Transfer the liquid containing the elute mRNA to a sterile RNase-free microcentrifuge tube.

15. To precipitate add 0.1 vol of 3*M* sodium acetate-DEPC treated and 1.0 vol of isopropanol to the eluate and incubate at –70°C overnight.

16. Centrifuge at 4°C at (12,000*g* for 30 min. Resuspend the RNA pellet in 1 mL of 70% ethanol fresh made with RNase-free water and centrifuge again. Be careful when decanting the supernatant to avoid losing the RNA pellet.

17. For short-term storage (>30 days) let the pellet dry at room temperature for about 20 min and resuspend in 50 µL of RNase-Free water and store at –70°C. For long-term storage (>30 days), resuspend the mRNA pellet in 70% ethanol at –70°C.

18. The concentration and the purity of the eluted mRNA can be determinated by spectophotometry. Determine the absorbance readings at 230, 260 and 280 nm (A_{230}, A_{260}, and A_{280}). Absorbance readings should be greater than 0.1 to ensure significance. To estimate the mRNA concentration, assume that a 40 µg/mL mRNA solution will have an absorbance of 1 at 260 nm. Also, determine the A_{260}/A_{230} ratio which will provide information on the purity of the sample. An A_{260}/A_{230} ratio less than 2 indicates that GTC or β-Mercaptoethanol from the extraction buffer is still present. If this is the case, precipitate the RNA again.

3.2. First-Strand cDNA Synthesis

This First-strand cDNA synthesis is catalyzed by Moloney Murine Leukemia Virus reverse transcriptase. The use of random hexamers eliminates the need for immunoglobulin-specific primers or oligo (dT) primers. Using this random haxamers, the resulting cDNAs are of sufficient length (7 kbases or more) to clone the V regions from both the heavy and the light chain genes. We used the First-Strand cDNA Synthesis Kit from Pharmacia Biotech.

1. Place the 20 µL mRNA sample.
2. Heat the mRNA solution to 65°C for 10 min, then chill on ice. Start the first-strand cDNA reaction within 2 min after placing on ice.
3. For each sample, label the tube as light chain or heavy chain in a 1.5 mL RNase-free microcentrifuge tube:

3.2.1. Reverse Transcriptase Reaction

mRNA	20 µL
Primed First-Strand Mix	11 µL
DTT Solution	1 µL
RNase-free Water	X µL
	33 µL

1. Incubate for 1 h at 37°C. The completed First-strand cDNA reaction product is now ready for immediate PCR amplification.

3.3. Primary PCR Amplification

Alignment of known gene sequence from the variable domains have demonstrated that there are regions of conservation within the variable domain, particularly at the 5′ and 3′ termini. This has led to the determination of species-specific consensus sequences, which have been used in the design of PCR primers. In 1991, Clackson et al. described primers for the PCR amplification of mouse variable regions. However, the light chain from some monoclonal antibodies are difficult to amplify and they have since been redesigned as part of the Recombinant Phage Antibody System (RPAS) from Pharmacia, Biotech, and Mouse Ig-Prime System from Novagen. In our laboratories, we use the RPAS, and when the light chain can not be amplified, we use the Mouse Ig-Prime Kit that contains primers for the μ, all γ, κ, and λ light chain. The First-strand antibody cDNA is used as a template for PCR amplification to generate suitable quantities of heavy (~340 bp) and light (~325 bp) chain DNA cloning.

1. Add to 500 μL microcentrifuge tubes label as "light chain" or "heavy chain" the following reagents.

3.3.1. Light Chain PCR

First-strand Reaction	33 μL
Light Primer Mix	2 μL
Sterile distilled water	64 μL
	99 μL

3.3.2. Heavy Chain PCR

First-strand Reaction	33 μL
Heavy Primer 1	2 μL
Heavy Primer 2	2 μL
Sterile distilled water	64 μL
	99 μL

1. Mix with a micropipettor and spin briefly.
2. Overlay each reaction with two drops of mineral oil. Place the tube in a thermocycler and heat at 95°C for 5 min.
3. Add 1 μL of AmpliTaq DNA polymerase to each reaction beneath the mineral oil, using separate pipets tips for each addition.
4. Run 30 cycles of 94°C for 1 min, 55°C for 2 min, and 72°C for 2 min.

3.4. Purification of Primary PCR Products

Before performing the assembly reaction, it is very important that the heavy- and the light-chain PCR products are isolated from the other reaction components. Purification of the DNA from an agarose gel can be done. In this context, our laboratory used the QIAquick Gel Extraction Kit from Qiagen. This QIAquick system combines the convenience of microspin technology with the selective binding properties of a specially adapted silica-gel membrane.

3.4.1. Agarose Gel Electrophoresis

1. Prepare a 1% agarose gel in 1X TAE Buffer with wells sufficient to accommodate 100 µL samples.
2. Remove ~90 µL from the PCR amplification reaction tube and transfer to a new centrifuge tube.
3. Save as a backup 20 µL of the PCR product of each amplification at –20°C. Add 11 µL of 6X Loading Dye (*see* **Note 4.1., item 7**) to the remanding 70 µL of PCR amplification reaction.
4. Load the PCR amplification reaction mix with the loading buffer in the well. Electrophoreses at 80 V until the bromophenol blue dye has migrated ~1/3 the length of the gel.

3.4.2. QIAquick Gel Extraction

1. Excise the DNA fragment (heavy chain ~340 bp and light chain ~325 bp) from the 1% agarose gel with a clean scalpel under a long wavelength ultraviolet (UV) light in the transilluminator. Try to minimize the size of the gel slice by removing extra agarose.
2. Weigh the gel slice in a tube. Add 3 vol of Buffer QG to 1 vol of gel.
3. Incubate at 50°C for 10 min. To help to dissolve the gel you can mix by flicking or use a thermomixer. Is very important to solubilize the agarose gel completely. The maximum amount of agarose per column is 400 mg. At this time it is very important, to check the pH because the adsorption of the DNA to silica depends on the pH. Binding efficiency during the adsorption step is typically 95% if the pH is <7.5, and is reduced drastically at higher pH. However if the loading mixture pH is >7.5, it can be lowered by adding 10 µL of 3*M* sodium acetate pH 5.0.
4. Place a QIAquick spin column in a 2 mL collection tube and load the sample.
5. Centrifuge for 1 min at 6000*g* (~9000 rpm) in a eppendorf centrifuge. The maximum loading volume of the column is 800 µL. For larger sample volumes, multiple loading of the column are necessary.
6. Discard flow-through and place the QIAquick column back in the same collection tube.
7. Add 0.5ml of Buffer QG to the QIAquick column and centrifuge for 1 min.
8. Centrifuge for 1 min at 6000*g* (~9000 rpm) in a eppendorf centrifuge.
9. To wash, add 0.75 mL of Buffer PE to the QIAquick column and let the column stand 5 min.

10. Centrifuge for 1 min at 6000*g* (~9000 rpm) in a eppendorf centrifuge.
11. Discard the flow-through and centrifuge the QIAquick column for an additional 1 min at 10,000*g* (~13,000 rpm).
12. Place the QIAquick column to air dry for 15–20 min.
13. To elute, add 50 µL of sterile water to the center of the column and let column stand for 5 min. DNA is an acid and will undergo autocatalytic degradation in the absence of a buffering agent and must therefore be stored at –20°C when eluted with water.
14. Centrifuge the QIAquick column for 1 min at 10,000*g* (~13,000 rpm).

3.5. Gel Quantification of Purified Heavy and Light-Chain From PCR Amplification Products

The success of assembly and fill-in reactions is dependent upon the molar concentration of both heavy- and light-chain PCR products. Agarose gel electrophoresis of aliquots of the purified heavy- and light-chain products alongside a known amount of V_H Marker (provided by the RPAS Kit) gives a visual estimate of the relative amounts of the fragments based on their band intensity in an ethidium-bromide-stained gel.

1. Prepare a small 1.5% TEA Agarose gel with 3 mm wells, and add ethidium bromide at the final concentration of 0.5 µg/mL.
2. To prepare marker, add 2.5 or 5 µL (12.5 or 25 ng) of V_H marker (provided by the RAPS kit) with 1 µL of loading dye.
3. Load in separate wells 10µL of each heavy- and light-chain with 2 µL of loading dye.
4. Load in separate well 1 µg of 100 bp ladder.
5. Electrophoreses TEA Agarose gel at 80 V for 30 min.
6. Photograph the gel under UV light. It may be necessary to overexpose the picture to visualize the marker and the heavy and light chain.
7. Compare the intensity of the heavy- and light-chain products with the V_H Marker.
8. Estimate the volume of purified heavy-chain product that corresponds to 50 ng. Estimate the volume of purified light-chain product that corresponds to 50 ng. This will be your 1:1 ratio.

3.6. Assembly and Fill in Reactions

In the assembly reaction, the heavy and light chain of the antibody are joined into a single-chain antibody with a linker DNA ([Gly$_4$Ser]$_3$). When the linkers anneal to the heavy- and light-chain DNA, they prime a fill-in reaction in the presence of AmpliTaq DNA polymerase. For this reaction to proceed efficiently, approximately 1:1, 1:2, 1:3, 1:4, and 1:5 ratios of heavy to light chain DNA must be added. If you do not have enough PCR products, you can reamplify heavy and light chain.

1. Add the following components to a 500 µL microcentrifuge tube:

Heavy Chain Product (50 ng)	X µL
Light Chain Product (50 ng,100 ng, etc.)	X µL
Linker-Primer Mix	4 µL
10X PCR Buffer I (without MgCl$_2$)	5 µL
dNTP Mix (10 mM of each)	5 µL
25 mM MgCl$_2$	5 µL
AmpliTaq DNA Polymerase (5 U)	1 µL
Sterile distilled water	to 50 µL
	50 µL

2. Mix with a micropipettor and spin briefly.
3. Overlay each reaction with two drops of mineral oil. Place the tube in a thermocycler and heat at 95°C for 5 min.
4. Add 1 µL of AmpliTaq DNA polymerase to each reaction beneath the mineral oil, using separates pipets tips for each addition.
5. Run 7 cycles of 94°C for 1 min, 63°C for 4 min. 1 cycle of 72°C for 10 min.

3.7. Second PCR Amplification and Purification

It is necessary to amplify the assembled scFv DNA for further cloning steps. In this second PCR, amplification restriction sites are added. These restriction sites are used to clone into the phagemid vector. The restriction site primers (RS primers) contain the *Sfi I* annealing with the heavy chain in the 5′ end, and the *Not I* site with the light chain in the 3′ end.

1. Add to the Assembly and fill-in reaction the following:

AmpliTaq (5 U)	1 µL
10X Buffer II (with MgCl$_2$)	5 µL
dNTP Mix (10 mM)	2 µL
RS Primers Mix	4 µL
Sterile distilled water	39 µL
	50 µL

2. Mix with a micropipettor and spin briefly.
3. Overlay each reaction with two drops of mineral oil. Place the tube in a thermocycler and heat at 95°C for 5 min.
4. Run 30 cycles of 94°C for 1 min, 55°C for 2 min, and 72°C for 2 min. 1 cycle of 72°C for 10 min.
5. Run a 1.5% TEA Agarose gel at 80 V for 30 min. A predominant band ~750 bp in size should be present. Some heavy and light chain monomers may be visible.
6. Follow the QIAquick gel extraction kit to extract the scFv DNA from the gel, and follow it by gel quantification.

3.8. Restriction Digestion and Purification

The assembly scFv contains the *Sfi I* and *Not I* sites introduce by the RS primer in the second PCR amplification. The scFv DNA have to be digested in order to be cloned into the phagemid plasmid pCANTAB 5E.

3.8.1. Sfi I *Digestion*

1. Gel purified scFv product (0.25-1 µg)   up to 70.0 µL
   10X *Sfi I* Restriction Buffer   8.5 µL
   Sfi I (20 U per reaction)   X µL
   Sterile distilled water   to 85.0 µL
   _____
                                                              85.0 µL
2. Mix gently and overlay with two drops of mineral oil. Incubate overnight at 50°C.
3. The next day equilibrate the *Sfi I* digested sample to room temperature and spin briefly.

3.8.2. Not I *Digestion*

1. Add to the scFv DNA *Sfi I* digested sample the following:
   10X *Not I* Restriction Buffer   12.7 µL
   Not I (20 U per reaction)   X µL
   Sterile distilled water   to 85.0 µL
   _____
                                                              85.0 µL
2. Mix gently and overlay with two drops of mineral oil. Incubate during the day (8 h to overnight) at 37°C.
3. Follow the QIAquick gel extraction kit to extract the scFv DNA from the gel, and follow it by gel quantification.

3.9. Ligation of the scFv cDNA into the Phagemid Plasmid pCANTAB5E

McCafferty et al. described in 1990 the fd-CAT1 original phage vector for antibody display *(27)*. These vectors contain all the genetic information encoding the phage life cycle. In this context, an alternative system has been used up to now. This system involves cloning into phagemid vectors that contain a copy of the gene 3 and phage packaging signal sequence. Thus, antibody fragments can be displayed as a fusion with the gene 3 protein and the genetic information is packaged thanks to the packaging signal. In our laboratory we have used the phagemid vector pCANTAB 5 E included in the Pharmacia RPAS kit. This vector allows cloning of antibody genes into *Sfi I* and *Not I* sites. This vector incorporates an amber codon between the C-terminus of the cloned scFv and the start of gene 3 sequence allowing the recombinant antibody to be made as a soluble protein. This vector also includes a peptide tag, allowing the detection of the single-chain antibody.

1. The assembled product should be gel-quantitated as described in **Subheading 3.5.**
2. For ligation of the scFv gene to the pCANTAB 5 E vector (provided by the RPAS Kit from Pharmacia), add the following into a 1.5 mL microcentrifuge tube:

scFv gene Fragment (100 ng)	X µL
pCANTAB 5 E vector (250 ng)	5.0 µL
0X Ligation Buffer	1.5 µL
T4 DNA Ligase (5 U)	1.0 µL
Sterile distilled water	to 15.0 µL
	15 µL

3. Incubate all reactions at 14°C overnight.
4. Next day, add 2 µL of sodium acetate and 500 µL of 95% ethanol.
5. Incubate at −70°C 4 h.
6. Spin at 14,000 rpm for 30 min at 4°C.
7. Discard supernatant carefully not to loss the pellet and wash with 500 µL of 70% ethanol.
8. Spin at 14,000 rpm for 20 min at 4°C.
9. Discard supernatant carefully and let the pellet air dry.
10. Resuspend in 10 µL of sterile water (for electroporation you need a low ionic strength).

3.10. Transformation

Two *E. coli* strains are used for preparation of single chain antibody libraries. To produce phage-displayed recombinant antibodies, competent TG1 cells are use. This host strain produces a suppressor tRNA which allows readthrough (suppression) of the amber stop codon. The switch to soluble recombinant antibody production is accomplished by using the *E. coli* strain HB2151 cells. The HB2151 cells are the nonsuppressor strain, allowing the recognition of the amber stop codon; thus, only soluble single chain antibodies can be produced. The *E. coli* TG1 and HB2151 are supplied as lyophilized cultures in the Expression Module/RPAS Kit from Pharmacia for phage rescue. These *E. coli* cells will need to be prepared for an electroporation protocol. We recommend that 1 ng of uncut supercoiled vector (pcDNA3 or other irrelevant vector) be used to determinate the efficiency of the competent cells.

3.10.1. Preparation of HB2151 for Electro-Transformation

1. Inoculate 1 L of broth with a 1/100 volume of a fresh overnight culture.
2. Grow cells at 37°C in a shaking incubator until the OD_{600}= 0.5–1.0.
3. Chill the cells on ice for 15–30 min.

4. Transfer cell culture to sterile centrifuge tubes and centrifuge in a cold rotor at 4000*g* (max) for 15 min.
5. Remove supernatant and discard. Resuspend cell pellet in 1 L of cold sterile 10% glycerol.
6. Centrifuge again as in **step 4**.
7. Remove supernatant and resuspend cell pellet in 500 mL of cold sterile 10% glycerol.
8. Centrifuge as in **step 4**.
9. Remove supernatant and resuspend cell pellet in 250 mL of cold sterile 10% glycerol.
10. Centrifuge as in **step 4**.
11. Resuspend cells in a final volume of 2 to 3 mL of cold 10% glycerol and dispense 40 µL per sterile eppendorf tube.
12. Quick freeze cells in dry ice/ethanol bath before storing at –70°C. These cells should be good for six months.

3.10.2. Electroporation

1. Thaw the HB2151 cells (–70°C) on ice.
2. Add 1 to 2 µL of DNA (solution of DNA should be low in ionic strength) ligation mix and let sit on ice about 1 min.
3. Set the electroporator at 1.8 kV.
4. Transfer the cell mixture to prechilled cuvettes (make sure the suspension is at the bottom of the cuvet).
5. Charge the pulser and then discharge (this should produce a pulse with a time constant of between 4 and 5 ms).
6. Add about 500 µL of S.O.C. media to cuvet, then transfer contents of cuvet to a snap capped tube containing 500 µL of media.
7. Incubate tube at 37°C (shaking) for one h.
8. Plate onto 2xYT-AG selective media.
9. Incubate overnight at 30°C. These colonies will be used for the modified colony lift assay. Make sure that these colonies are well isolated: ~200–300 colonies per plate.

3.11. Modified Colony Lift Assay

The following protocol describes a colony lift assay whereby scFv-expressing clones of *E. coli* can be rapidly identified. Because of the large number of colonies that can be simultaneously screened, it may be possible to recover not a single positive clone. Thus, we recommend that this step be repeated at least twice with each positive colon. After each panning, we strongly recommend a PCR amplification of each positive clone with the RS primer as indicated in **Subheading 3.7.** Make sure you make a glycerol stock as soon as possible of each positive clone *(28)*.

3.11.1. Antigen-Coated Membrane

1. Dilute 50 µg of the target protein in 1 mL of PBS.
2. Coat S&S nitrocellulose membrane adding the 1 mL of protein in the middle of the membrane and gently move it around until the entire membrane is wet. This side of the membrane is where your antigen is, make sure that you always have it face up.
3. Block filter with 5% milk in PBS for one h.
4. Rinse the membrane with PBS and let it dry for 15 min.
5. Lay the antigen-coated membrane on top of the 2xYT-AI agar plate.

3.11.2. Master Membrane

1. Put a new nitrocellulose membrane on top of the plate that has your colonies in the 2xYT-AG. Note: The colonies have to be well isolated. Invert "colony membrane" (colony-side up), and place on top of your "antigen-coated membrane" in the 2x-YT-AI.
2. Incubate at 30°C overnight.
3. Lift colony filter and place colony-side up onto a fresh 2x-YT-AG plate at 4°C until you have develop the antigen-coated membrane and be ready to select.

3.11.3. Development of Antigen-Coated Membrane

1. Place antigen-coated membrane (face-up) in a Petri dish and wash 5 min three times with PBS-0.1% Tween20.
2. Block membrane in 5% nonfat milk in PBS for 1 h.
3. Wash membrane with PBS-0.1% Tween20 10 min three times.
4. Add anti-E Tag-HRP antibody 1 : 1000 in 5% nonfat milk 1 h at room temperature.
5. Remove the antibody and wash 15 min three times with PBS-0.1% Tween20.
6. Develop with 4CN substrate (Sigma cat. # C-6788).

4CN substrate: Dissolve one tablet of 4-Choloro-1-Naphthol (4C1N) (30 mg) in 10 mL of methanol. This reagent is good for 2 wk when kept in the dark at 4°C. Immediately prior to development add 2 mL of stock 4CN/MeOH to 10 mL of triethanolamine saline pH 7.5. Add 5 µL of 30% H_2O_2. Neutralize with water (rinse).

3.12. Production of Soluble Antibodies (Periplasmic Extract)

The single chain antibody is clone into to the pCANTAB 5 E phagemid vector and it can be expressed as a soluble protein from this vector. Although the localization and concentration of the scFv will vary, most of the cases the bacterial periplasmic extract will yield the highest concentration of functional scFv antibodies *(28)*.

1. Grow up each of the positive clones in 2 mL of 2x YT-AG at 30°C to log phase (OD_{550} = 0.3–0.4).

2. At this point make a glycerol stock, and a PCR as indicated in **Subheading 3.7.** to check the presence of the scFv.
3. Spin down 1500*g* for 5 min.
4. Resuspend cells in 2 mL of 2x YT-AI at 30°C overnight.
5. Spin 1500*g* 20 min in a clinical centrifuge and aspirate media.
6. Resuspend in 400 mL of cold 1 m*M* EDTA in PBS.
7. Incubate at 4°C for 30 min with regular movement.
8. Spin at 16,000*g* for 10 min.
9. Transfer supernatant (soluble scFv) to a new tube.

3.13. Detection and Binding Specificity of E-Tagged scFvs

Enzyme-linked immunosorbent assays (ELISA) can be used to characterize the positive clones obtained from the colony lift assay. In this ELISA procedure, HRP/Anti-E Tag conjugate is used to detect E-tagged scFv from the periplasmic extract bound to the antigen-coated microtiter well. Because the ELISA is quantitative in nature, the signal will vary with the expression level and affinity of the scFv. When the positive clones are identified these single chain antibody can be cloned into eukaryotic expression vector for intracellular expression.

3.13.1. Coating

1. Coat wells of the microtiter plate for ELISA with 200 μL of target antigen in PBS (pH 8.0–8.5) yielding 100 ng to 10 μg per well.
2. Coat wells with appropriate controls (irrelevant protein).
3. Incubate overnight at 4°C, covered.
4. Shake out contents of plate and rinse once with PBS using a squirt bottle.

3.13.2. Blocking

1. Add 200 μL of 3% BSA and 1% gelatin in PBS to each well.
2. Incubate 1–2 h at room temperature.
3. Shake out contents of plate and rinse once with PBS using a squirt bottle.

3.13.3. scFv Periplasmic Extract

1. Add 100 μL of periplasmic extract to each well.
2. Incubate at room temperature for 2 h or at 4°C overnight.
3. Wash three times for 15 min with PBS.

3.13.4. Conjugated Antibody

1. Dilute HRP/Anti-E Tag Conjugated 1:1000 in 2% BSA, and add 100 μL to each well.
2. Incubate at room temperature for 1 h.
3. Wash three times for 15 min with PBS.

3.13.5. Developer

1. Develop with 1X ABTS substrate. Add 100 µL developer to all wells and allow color to develop 15–30 min or until color (green) reaction has occurred.
2. The reaction can be read in a microtiter plate reader set at 405–415 nm. If a microtiter plate reader is not available, a spectrophotometer set at an absorbency of 410 nm can be used to quantitate the results. The absorbency reading for your antigen should be at least two to three times higher than the absorbency reading for the negative control.

3.14. Western Blot Analysis of E-Tagged scFvs

The principle behind SDS-PAGE is the electrophoretic separation of proteins based on mobility in an electrical field as well as their molecular size. Bigger proteins move through the gel slower than smaller ones. You can vary the concentration of the acrylamide to separate proteins of low, midrange or high-molecular size. For instance, if you are interested in a 29-kDa protein, use a 12–15% gel.

3.14.1. Electrophoresis

1. Set up the plates by placing the spacers on either side and clamping the white side-clamps by turning the screws tightly.
2. Install the plates into the bottom mold stand and turn the screws to clamp it down into the base.
3. Fill up with water to test seal and to insure that no leaks occur.
4. Pour the separating gel and let harden 30 min to 1 h. Place a layer of saturated isopropanol over the gel.

Resolving gel: 0.375M Tris, pH8.8 (~30 min)

		7%	8%	9%	10%	12%	15%	20%
1.5M Tris (pH8.8)	mL	2.5	2.5	2.5	2.5	2.5	2.5	2.5
40% Acrylamide	mL	1.75	2.0	2.25	2.5	3.0	3.75	5.0
ddH$_2$O	mL	5.6	5.35	5.1	4.85	4.35	3.6	2.35
10% SDS	100 µL	————————————————————————————————————
10%APS (make fresh)	50 µL	————————————————————————————————————
TEMED	2.5 µL	———————————————— 1.5µL ——————— 1µL

5. Empty out the saturated isopropanol by inverting the plates and then pour in the stacker gel. You can either load the stacker gel into the plates using a 5 mL pipet with the combs in place or pour the stacker gel in and then place the comb between the glass plates. Be sure there is no bubbles in the bottom of the comb.

Stacker 4%: 0.125M Tris, pH 6.8 (~25 min)
0.5M Tris (pH6.8)	1.0 µL
40% Acrylamide	0.4 µL

ddH$_2$O	2.54 µL
10% SDS	40 µL
10% APS	20 µL
TEMED	4 µL

6. Allow to set 30–60 min.
7. Gently pull out comb.
8. Place the top chamber over the gels and remove the bottom screws. Now put these screws into the top chamber and turn to tighten.
9. Fill up top chamber with 500 mL of 1X Western Blot Running Buffer.
10. Load samples using round sequencing pipet tips and put lid on. Prior to loading, samples should be boiled in 1X reducing Western Blot Sample Buffer.
11. Run the gels at 150 V for 1 h.

3.14.2. Western Transfer

Here the principle is to transfer proteins to a solid support for Western blotting. The entire assembly is done between the paddles of the transfer apparatus. Place the paddle with the protruding nubbin down first, next the backing, then all the things below followed by more backing and then the other paddle without the nubbin.

1. Carefully remove the gel from the plates.
2. Wet two pieces of blot absorbent filter paper, 1 nitrocellulose membrane, and the sponges in 1X Western Blot Transfer Buffer.
3. Lay the gel on top of the sponge and blot absorbent filter paper.
4. On top of gel, place a pre-wet in 1X Western Blot Transfer Buffer piece of nitrocellulose membrane and one blot absorbent filter paper.
5. Place one more piece of pre-wet blot absorbent filter paper on top of the nitrocellulose, and then one sponge.
6. Snap the paddles together.
7. Load into the transfer chamber which has been filled with 1 L of 1X Western Blot Transfer Buffer.
8. Snap on power pack lid which has the back facing towards you (need to transfer from negative to positive). Make sure that the two protruding male electrodes in the bottom transfer tank are secured into the powerpack lid.
9. Run the transfer at 100 V for 1 h.

3.14.3. Developing Western

1. Block with PBS with 5% nonfat milk and 1% BSA for 30 min to overnight.
2. Add your primary antibody (HRP/Anti-E Tag) at 1 : 3000 in PBS 5% nonfat milk and 1% BSA at 4°C shaking overnight.
3. Wash with PBS for 30 min to 1 h, changing the PBS every 10 min (you will never overwash, but you can under-wash).
4. Develop with 4CN substrate as indicated in **Subheading 3.11.**

3.15. Intracelular Expression of the scFv

It has recently been shown that scFv molecules may be expressed intracellularly in eukaryotic cells by gene transfer of scFv cDNAs. The encoded scFv may be expressed in the target cell and localized to specific, targeted subcellular compartments by appropriate signal molecules. Invitrogen has mammalian expression vectors that allow targeted of your protein to different subcellular compartment. Each of the vectors in the pShooter collection incorporates a signal sequence that will direct the scFv to a specific subcellular location. These eukaryotic expression vectors contain a strong mammalian CMV promoter, and a C-terminal tag for rapid detection.

3.15.1. cDNA scFv Cloning in Eukaryotic Expression Vector

Excised the scFv cDNA from the pCANTAB 5 E phage vector utilizing the *Sfi I* and *Not I* restriction sites as indicated in **Subheading 3.8.**

Set up ligation reactions as indicated in **Subheading 3.9.**, follow up by transformation into *E. coli* competent cells of your choice (DH5α, SURE) as described in **Subheading 3.10.**

4. Notes

We have identified 5 major sources of problems throughout the recombinant single chain antibody system: 1) quality of isolated mRNA; 2) PCR amplification of V_H and V_L; 3) assembly reaction of the scFv; 4) ligation of the scFv to the phegamid plasmid pCANTAB5E; 5) Modified Colony Lift Assay. In this section, we will give a guide and how to identify this problems and troubleshoot them.

4.1. Quality of Isolated mRNA

The success of antibody cloning depends on the quality (purity) of the mRNA. Highly pure mRNA is required as staring material for generating a recombinant antibody. In our experience, the PolyATtract System 1000 isolates this high-quality mRNA. This system from Promega utilized Promega's MagneSphere technology for the purification of poly (A)+RNA, eliminating the need for oligo (dT) cellulose columns. The successful isolation of intact mRNA four important steps must be performed: 1) effective disruption of cells or tissue, 2) denaturation of nucleoprotein complex, 3) inactivation of endogenous ribonuclease (RNase) activity, and 4) purification of RNA away from contaminating DNA and proteins. The most important of this is the inactivation of RNases. This system combines the disruptive and protective properties to inactivate ribonuclease present in the cell extract, as well as high stringency method to obtain pure mRNA. The isolation of this high-quality mRNA with this kit is suitable for all molecular biology applications and the yields of poly (A)+RNA is two-fold greater than with other methods.

Special precautions must be observed to avoid degradation of mRNA by RNases.

1. Your hands are a major source of RNases so always wear gloves when working with RNA.
2. The second major of RNase contamination is bacteria o molds that may be present on airborne dust particules, thus glassware, etc., that is to be used for RNA preparations should be purchased new and only used for working with RNA.
3. Used RNase Zap (Ambion) to spray all work surfaces and equipment.
4. All glassware should be washed thoroughly and soaked in a 0.1% solution of diethyl pyrocarbonate (DEPC) (inhibits RNases) for at least 15 min, autoclaved, and then baked in an oven at 250°C for 3 h (to destroy traces of DEPC–DEPC decomposes into CO_2 and ethanol when heated).
5. Whenever possible, use sterile single-use plastic ware instead of glassware.
6. Chemicals should be reserved for working with RNA and always handled with DEPC treated spatulas.
7. All solutions should be treated with DEPC prior to use. The solutions should be adjusted to 0.1% in DEPC, shaken or stirred for at least 15 min and then autoclaved. Because DEPC decomposes in the presence of Tris, all solutions containing Tris should *not* be DEPC-treated but instead be made up with DEPC-treated and autoclaved ddH_2O. Likewise solutions that are not to be autoclaved should always be made up with DEPC-treated water or solutions. You may want to check with RNase Alert from Ambion your solution before using them.

4.2. PCR Amplification of V_H and V_L

It can be possible that following the primary PCR amplification (**Subheading 3.3.**) step you can not see the light- and heavy-chain products. Since we have used the PolyATtract System 1000 we have not had this problem, however if you are using other RNA purification methods the reason to fail this fist PCR amplification can be as follows:

1. The purity of the mRNA is not adequate: this problem may be resolve by using an RNA extraction kit followed by mRNA purification kit.
2. Ribonucleases are present in the mRNA preparation: follow RNase-free precautions.
3. The hybridoma was no longer producing antibody: check the hybridoma for the present of soluble antibody.
4. The primers are annealed nonspecifically to nucleic acids contamination the mRNA: you will see a smearing in the gel electrophoresis, better purification of the mRNA preparation is required.
5. If you only can see the heavy chain but not the light chain it is because the Pharmacia mouse scFv module kit contains only the kappa light chain primers

since few lambda light chain sequence have been determined (~5%). The Novagen Mouse Ig-Primer Set (Novagen cat. # 69831-3) will allow you to PCR the light chain, however you may have to follow their protocols to assemble the scFv, and continue in **Subheading 3.9.**

Special precautions must be observed to avoid PCR contamination:

1. Use the PCR hood when making reagents for PCR or putting together reactions. The pipetmen in the hood have never been used to pipet DNA and should never be removed from the hood. Likewise, DNA—or anything that has been near DNA (dirty gloves, tube racks, etc.)—should never be brought into the PCR hood.
2. Always make up your PCR reagents with stocks and solutions that have never been out on the lab bench. Always use disposable tubes and pipets to make up stocks. It's often a good idea to make up a large batch of buffer or dNTPs, test them to make sure they're clean, and divide them into small aliquots.
3. If you suspect that your PCR reagents (buffer, dNTPs, or water) are contaminated, try irradiating them on the short wave UV box (about 3–5 min). This will crosslink any contaminating DNA. You can also UV zap some primers without affecting their ability to prime, but this is primer specific. Do not UV zap the enzyme.
4. As long as your reagents are clean, most contamination occurs when you add the template to your tubes. Take care in opening the tubes that contain your DNA template. A little bit of DNA aerosolized onto your glove can easily be transferred to your PCR tube. Use pipet tips with filters or positive displacement pipets to add your template-aerosolized DNA in pipetman is the major source of contamination.
5. Always include a negative control. Make sure to treat it like the other samples (e.g., add 1 μL of water at the lab bench with the pipetman you are using to add DNA to the other tubes).
6. For RT for PCR you should include two negative controls. First, everything except RNA is added (H_2O control). (Be sure to actually add water to this tube at the same time you are adding RNA to the other tubes); and second, when RNA is added, but no RT is included (this ensures that there is no contamination of your RNA).

4.3. Assembly Reaction of the scFv

The assembly and fill in reaction of the scFv is with no doubt the trickiest step of all. We will give you some tips that with our experience have made this step easy.

1. Make sure a high quality of the cDNA of V_L and V_H is used as a start material. The QIAquick Gel Extraction Kit from Qiagen will give you this high-quality DNA. Two modifications we introduce to their protocol: 1) Skip the isopropanol step after the solubilization of the agarose gel. It is very difficult to completely

dry the isopropanol and it can interfere with downstream reactions and 2) let the column air dry at room temperature for 20 min before elution of the DNA, thus no ethanol will be present.

2. The Pharmacia protocol suggest for the assembly reaction of the scFv an equivalent amount of the heavy- and light-chain products, however, in our experience for this reaction to proceed efficiently we add an excess of light-chain product. We proposed that approximately 1:1, 1:2, 1:3, 1:4, and 1:5 ratios of heavy- to light-chain DNA must be used for this assembly reaction to be successful.

3. The final concentration of the dNTPs in the assembly reaction is critical in this step. We have modified the dNTPs molarity to 10 mM using 1/10 of the total volume in the assembly reaction as indicated in **Subheading 3.6.**

4.4. Ligation of the scFv to the Phagemid Plasmid pCANTAB5E

After ligation of the scFv in the phegamid vector pCANTAB 5 E we recommended that **Subheadings 3.9.** through **3.12.** be done within 48 hr. It is important that you make a glycerol stock of the positive clones as soon as possible. PCR amplification of the scFv library after this time, demonstrated different scFv cDNA sizes.

4.5. Modified Colony Lift Assay

Some antibodies produced by hybridoma cells cannot recognize their respective antigen if this is immobilized onto nitrocellulose. You need to try several times by colony lift assay if your hybridoma recognize the antigen-bound to the membrane. If this is the case, the colony lift assay cannot be used to detect the recombinant antibodies, and you may need to work with the Recombinant Phage Antibody System with the Phage Antibody Library by Pharmacia.

References

1. Krol, A.V. and Stuitje, A. R. (1988) Modulation of eukaryotic gene expression by complement RNA or DNA sequences. *Biotechniques* **6,** 958–976.
2. Helene, C. and Toulme, J-J. (1990) Specific regulation of gene expression by antisense, sense, and antigene nucleic acids. *Biochem. Biophys.* **1049,** 99–125.
3. Gibson, I. (1996) Antisense approaches to the gene therapy of cancer. *Cancer Metastasis Rev.* **15,** 287–299.
4. Milligan, J. F., Jones, R. J., Froehler, B. C., and Matteucci, M. D. (1994) Development of antisense therapeutics. Implications for cancer gene therapy. *Ann. NY Acad. Sci.* **716,** 228–241.
5. Stein, C. A. and Cheng, Y-C. (1993) Antisense oligonucleotides as therapeutic agents–is the bullet really magic? *Science* **261,** 1004–1012.
6. Stein, C. A. (1995) Does antisense exist? *Nat. Med.* **1,** 1119–1121.
7. Theuer, C. P. and Pastan, I. (1993) Immunotoxins and recombinant toxins in the treatment of solid carcinomas. *Amer. J. Surg.,* **166,** 284–288.

8. Brinkmann, U., Pai, L. H., and FitzGerald, D. J. (1991) B3-(Fv)-PE38KDEL, a single chain immunotoxin that causes complete regression of a human carcinoma in mice. *Proc. Natl. Acad. Sci. USA* **88,** 8616–8620.

9. Hoogenboom, H. R., Marks, J. D., Griffiths, A. D., and Winter, G. (1992) Building antibodies from their genes. *Immunol. Rev.* **130,** 41–68.

10. Jost, C. R., Kurucz, I., Jacobus, C. M., Titus, J. A., George, A. J., and Segal, D. M. (1994) Mammalian expression and secretion of functional single-chain Fv molecules. *J. Biol. Chem.* **269,** 26,267–26,273.

11. Richardson, J. H. and Marasco, W. A. (1995) Intracellular antibodies: development and therapeutic potential. *Trends Biotech.* **13,** 306–310.

12. Chen, S. Y., Bagley, J., and Marasco, W. A. (1994) Intracellular antibodies as a new class of therapeutic molecules for gene therapy. *Hum. Gene Ther.* **5,** 595–601.

13. Colcher, D., Bird, R., and Roselli, M. (1990) In vivo tumor targeting of a recombinant single-chain antigen-binding protein. *J. Natl. Can. Inst.* **82,** 1191–1197.

14. Wawrzynczak, E. J. (1992) Rational design of immunotoxins: current progress and future prospects. *Anti-Cancer Drug Design* **7,** 427–441.

15. Mykebust, A. T., Godal, A., and Fodstad, O. (1994) Targeted therapy with immunotoxins in a nude rat model for leptomenineal growth of human small cell cancer. *Cancer Res.* **54,** 2146–2150.

16. Marasco, W. A., Haseltine, W. A., and Chen, S-Y. (1993) Design, intracellular expression, and activity of human anti-human immunodeficiency virus type 1 gp120 single-chain antibody. *Proc. Natl. Acad. Sci. USA* **90,** 7889–7893.

17. Friedman, P. N., Chance, D. F., and Trail, P. A. (1993) Antitumor activity of the single-chain immunotoxin BR96 sFv-PE40 against established breast and lung tumor xenografts. *J. Immunol.* **150,** 3054–3061.

18. Werge, T. M., Biocca, S., and Cattaneo, A. (1990) Cloning andintracellular expression of a monoclonal antibody to the p21ras protein. *FEBS Lett.* **274,** 193–198.

19. Deshane, J., Loechel, F., Conry, R. M., Siegal, G. P., King, C. R., and Curiel, D. T. (1994) Intracellular single-chain antibody directed against erbB2 down-regulates cell surface erbB2 and exhibits a selective anti-proliferative effect in erbB2 overexpressing cancer cell lines. *Gen. Ther.* **1,** 332–337.

20. Deshane, J., Siegal, G. P., Alvarez, R. D., Wang, M. H., Feng, M., Cabrera, G., et al. (1995) Targeted tumor killing via an intracellular antibody against erbB-2. *J. Clinic. Investigat.* **96,** 2980–2989.

21. Deshane, J., Grim, J., Loechel, S., Siegal, G. P., Alvarez, R. D., and Curiel, D. T. (1996) Intracellular antibody against erbB-2 mediates targeted tumor cell eradication by apoptosis. *Cancer Gene Ther.* **3,** 89–98.

22. Grim, J., Deshane, J., Feng, M., Lieber, A., Kay, M., and Curiel, D. T. (1996) erbB-2 knockout employing an intracellular single-chain antibody (sFv) accomplishes specific toxicity in erbB-2-expressing lung cancer cells. *Amer. J. Respir. Cell Molec. Biol.* **15,** 348–354.

23. Barnes, D. M., Deshane, J., Siegal, G. P., Alvarez, R. D., and Curiel, D. T. (1996) Novel gene therapy strategy to accomplish growth factor modualtion induces enhanced tumor cell chemosensitivity. *Clinic. Cancer Res.* **2,** 1089–1095.

24. Wright, M., Grim, J., Kim, M., Strong, T. V., Siegal, G. P., and Curiel, D. T. (1997) An intracellular anti-erbB-2 single-chain antibody is specifically cytotoxic to human breast carcinoma cells overexpressing erbB-2. *Gene Ther.* **4,** 317–322.

25. Kim, M., Wright, M., Deshane, J., Accavitti, M. A., Tilden, A., Saleh, et al. (1997) A novel gene therapy strategy for elimination of prostate carcinoma cells from human bone marrow. *Human Gene Ther.* **8,** 157–170.

26. Curiel, D. T. Targeted tumor cytotoxicity mediated by intracellular single-chain antioncogene antibodies in *Gene Therapy in Advances in pharmacology* (Thomas August, J., ed.), Academic, New York, Vol. 40, pp. 51–84.

27. McCafferty, J., Griffiths, A. D., Winter, G., and Chriswell, D. J. (1990) Phage antibodies: filamentous phage displaying antibody variable domains. *Nature* **348,** 552–554.

28. Rodenburg, C., Mernaugh, R., Bilbao, G., and Khazaeli M. B. (1998) Production of a single cahin anti-CEA antibody from the hybridoma cell line T84.66 using a modified colony-lift selection procedure to detect antigen-positive scFv bacterial clones. *Hybridoma* **17,** 1–8.

10

Combined Adenoviral Transfer of Tumor Suppressor and Cell-Cycle Genes for Tumor-Cell Apoptosis

Karsten Brand, Volker Sandig, and Michael Strauss

1. Introduction

The loss of control over the cell cycle and the disruption of cascade mechanisms for programmed cell death are major factors in tumorigencsis. Defects in the *p53* gene and in the regulation of genes of the retinoblastoma pathway such as *p16* or cyclin *D*1 occur in a large percentage of tumors and have been well studied. Reintroduction or overexpression of genes suppressing proliferation or promoting apoptosis offers a potential for selective suicide of tumor cells. Transfer of tumor suppressor genes into growing tumors with mutations in the respective gene can indeed reduce tumor growth *(1)*. The reason for this effect is probably not just a reestablishement of the normal phenotype, but rather a severe disturbance of the cancer cell's regulatory balance of life and death, which can result in apoptosis. Retransfer of two or more cancer genes can have synergistic effects on apoptosis induction. The choice, which gene combination will be particularly efficient, depends on the pattern of mutated genes. We have recently reported that the cotransfer of *p53* and *p16* leads to a better induction of apoptosis and reduction of tumor growth than the transfer of either gene alone *(2)*. In addition, it seems that normal cells with an intact genotype are more resistant to the action of tumor supressor genes than tumor cells with mutations in the respective genes. Several approaches are now underway to exploit those gene combinations which are the most efficient for tumor cell-specific apoptosis on a given genetic background.

Apart from the appropriate transgenc to be transferred, a vehicle for gene transfer has to be selected. We have focused on adenoviral vectors, because of their high efficacy of gene transfer in vitro and in vivo and their potential capacity to carry several foreign expression units on the same vector.

From: *Methods in Molecular Medicine, Vol. 35: Gene Therapy: Methods and Protocols*
Edited by: W. Walther and U. Stein © Humana Press, Inc., Totowa, NJ

However, insertion of tumor suppresser genes into adenoviruses also interferes with the cell cycle of the producer cell line thereby generating an environment which is not optimal for virus growth. This renders the initial virus rescue more difficult or impossible. We have optimized a highly efficient protocol for virus generation by separating construction of the full length virus genome from rescue of the virus itself. Using this protocol, a large number of homogenous virus plaques is reliably produced.

Other factors need to be considered too: adenoviral vectors by themselves can cause growth retardation, deregulation of the cell cycle, and apoptosis *(3)*. These side effects, which are caused by either the infection itself, by residual gene expression, low-level replication, or combinatorial effects are increasingly important with increased multiplicity of infection (MOI). Experiments evaluating synergistic effects of tumor suppresser genes, which usually start with a combination of single gene vectors, are particularly sensitive to side effects of the virus because they require coinfection with several viruses. These side effects can be minimized by careful determination of virus titers, the application of the lowest MOIs possible, the construction of double or multiple gene vectors and the use of highly attenuated adenoviruses, lacking not only $E1$, but also other early regions ($E2$, $E4$) or the entire set of viral genes.

In this chapter, we describe improvements in virus construction, titering *(4)*, the choice of controls when exploiting double-gene transfer using two different adenoviruses in vitro and combined adenoviral gene transfer into established hepatic tumors in vivo. As model viruses, we use *Ad.CMV-p53*, *Ad.CMV-p16*, and *Ad.CMV-tk* as a control, but any other virus preparations, which will prove to kill cells specifically and efficiently, can be selected.

2. Materials

2.1. Construction of Recombinant Adenoviruses

1. Adenovirus genome plasmid (*HVAd1*) containing the complete adenovirus genome flanked by unique restriction sites next to both Inverted Terminal Repeat (ITR)s. *HVAd1* contains the *Ad5* genome with a complete deletion of *E3* (identical to the deletion in *BHG10*). The amp^R gene and the plasmid ori are located between the Pac I sites which flank the ITRs.

   This type of plasmid can be easily generated from DNA of a wild type or partially deleted (*E4,E2*) adenovirus and a plasmid containing the 3' and 5' terminal 300–500 bp of the virus next to unique restriction using the technique described below.

2. *E1* or *E3* shuttle vectors such as pdelE1sp1A *(5)*.

3. Chemical or electrocompetent cells of two strains: BJ 5813 (recA+ recBC– sbcB– sbcC–) and any common laboratory recA– strain (*XL1,XL2*, HB101).

2.2. Determination of Viral Titer by a Modified Cyto-pathic Effect (cpe) Assay

1. Phosphate-buffered saline (PBS): 10 m*M* sodium phosphate, pH 7.4, 150 m*M* NaCl.
2. Dulbecco's Modified Eagle's Medium (DMEM pure) supplemented with 10% fetal calf serum (FCS), glutamine (2 m*M*), and penicillin (100 IU/mL)/streptomycin (50 μg/mL) (DMEM comp).
3. Multichannel pipet (8-channel).

2.3. Determination of Viral Titer by Determination of the Amount of Intracellular Adenoviral DNA

2.3.1. DNA-Isolation and Southern Blotting

1. Lysisbuffer: 10 m*M* Tris-HCL pH 8.0, 400 m*M* NaCl, 2 m*M* EDTA, 0.5%. SDS. Use Tris-HCL ultrapure or filter Tris-HCL stock solution.
2. 20X PBS, pH 7.4, sterilize.
3. Proteinase K: 10 mg/mL, store at –20°C.
4. 3*M* NaOAc, pH 5.2.
5. Ethanol: 96%, 70%.
6. TE: 1X, pH 7.5.
7. RNAseA: 10 mg/mL, store at –20°C.
8. Restriction endonuclease *NcoI*: 10,000 U/mL (NEB, Beverly, MA).
9. TAE: 50X.
10. 5*M* NaOH.
11. 5*M* NaCl.
12. 20X SSC, 3*M* NaCl, 0.3*M* sodium citrate, pH 7.0.
13. 20X SSPE, 3*M* Na Cl, 0.2*M* NaH$_2$PO$_4$, 20 m*M* EDTA, pH 7.4.
14. 20X SDS.
15. Denhardt's: 50X, 1% Ficoll, 1% polyvinylpyrrolidone, 1% BSA.
16. Herring sperm-DNA: 10 mg/mL, store at –20°C.
17. 1*M* Na$_2$HPO$_4$, sterilize.
18. 1*M* NaH$_2$PO$_4$, sterilize, should be mixed with **step 17**) to obtain a 100 m*M* sodium phosphate buffer pH 6.8 (46.3 mL Na$_2$HPO$_4$ + 53.7 mL NaH$_2$PO$_4$ + 900 mL distilled H$_2$O).
19. Phenol, phenol/chloroform/isoamylalcohol (25:24:1), chloroform/isoamylalcohol (24:1) saturated with 1 × TE.
20. Whatman paper, 3 mm (Whatman, Maidstone, England).
21. Nuclear acid transfer membrane: Hybond-N+ (Amersham, Amersham, England).

2.3.2. Preparation of Radiolabled Probe

1. Random Primed labeling Kit (100760, Boehringer Mannheim, Mannheim, Germany).

2. 32-P-ATP (Amersham, 50 µCi).
3. Gelelution Kit: Easy Pure (Biozym, Hess. Oldendorf, Germany).
4. *Taq-Pol*: *AmpliTaq* (5 U/µL, Perkin Elmer, Norwalk, CT), dNTPs,
   Primer: Ad5Nco-1: –ACC TAC gAg ACC gTg TCT gg-; Tm: 69°C
             Ad5Nco-2: –AgA CTA CgC TgA CgA ggA CC-, Tm: 70°C.
5. NAP 5 Columns (Sephadex G-25, Pharmacia Biotech, Uppsala, Sweden,
   17-0853-01).

2.4. Determination of Infectivity In Vitro

1. PBS: 10 mM sodium phosphate, pH 7.4, 150 mM NaCl.
2. 0.05% Glutaraldehyde (in PBS).
3. X-Gal-staining solution (5 mL):
3413.5 µL H$_2$O	500 µL 30 mM K$_3$(Fe(CN)$_6$)
440 µL 0.5M HEPES, pH 7.4	500 µL 30 mM K$_4$(Fe(CN)$_6$)
15 µL 5M NaCl	125 µL X-Gal (20 mg/mL in DMF)
6.5 µL 1M MgCl$_2$	

2.5. Infection of Cells with Ad.p16 and Ad.p53

1. PBS: 10 mM sodium phosphate, pH 7.4, 150 mM NaCl.
2. DMEM comp.
3. 70% methanol (in PBS).

2.6. Analysis of Cell Cycle, Apoptosis, and the Actual Efficacy of Gene Transfer

1. PBS: 10 mM sodium phosphate, pH 7.4, 150 mM NaCl.
2. Blocking medium: DMEM comp.
3. Primary antibodies: *Anti-p53* monoclonal antibody (pAB1801, Oncogene Science
   (200 µg/mL), Uniondale, NY), *Anti-p16* monoclonal antibody (DCS-50.1/A,
   LabVision Europe, Allerod, Denmark).
4. Secondary antibody: FITC-conjugated sheep-anti-mouse IgG (H+L).
5. PI-staining solution: per 1 mL PBS: 10 µL RNAse A (10 mg/mL in 10 mM Tris-
   HCl, pH 7.5, 15 mM NaCl), 25 µL propidium iodide (PI, 1 mg/mL).
6. Flow Cytometer (EPICS XL-MCL, Coulter, Krefeld, Germany).
7. MultiCycle AV (Phoenix Flow Systems, Inc., San Diego, CA).

2.7. Determination of Cell Number

1. 0.4% Trypan blue solution (Sigma, Deisenhofen, Germany).
2. Hemocytometer.

2.8. Protein Blotting

1. Antibodies as described in **Subheading 2.6.**
2. Materials according to standard protocols.

2.9. Treatment of Liver Tumors
by Local Injection of Ad.p53 and Ad.p16

1. Scid mice (C.B-17/Icr/BlnA-scid/scid).
2. Narcotic: Ketamine, 50 mg/mL (Ketanest®, Parke-Davis, Berlin, Germany), Rompun, 2% (Bayer, Leverkusen, Germany).
3. Forceps (anatomical and surgical) and scissors.
4. 1-mL syringes (Omnifix®, Braun Melsungen, Germany).
5. Microlance needles (Becton Dickinson, Heidelberg, Germany).
6. Hemoclip (Edward Weck, Research Triangle Park, NC).
7. Woundclips.
8. Calipers.
9. Liquid nitrogen.
10. Formalin, 5%.
11. Suture: (Catgut, Traumafil, Markneukirchen).

3. Methods
3.1. Generation of Recombinant Viruses

The size of the adenovirus genome (36 kb) makes cloning procedures in *E. coli* difficult. For this reason, the gene of interest is usually cloned into a small shuttle vector and homologous recombination in mammalian cells is used to create the virus. This step together with the initial genome amplification limits the success rate. The protocol presented here is based on generation of the virus genome in *E. coli* by homologous recombination between a linear plasmid (vector) and a fragment (template) containing the gene to be inserted flanked by DNA homologous to the vector (**Fig. 1**). It is a modification of the procedure described by Chartier et al. *(6)* Recombination takes place in the strain BJ 5183 RecBC-sbcB-. The strain is not available commercially, but can be sent on request.

1. Prepare highly competent cells from strain BJ 5183.
2. Clone the gene of interest together with regulatory signals into a shuttle vector for insertion into the *E*1 or *E*3 region of the virus. For insertion into *E*1, pdelE1SP1A may be used.
3. Release a fragment from the shuttle vector containing the expression unit flanked by at least 150 bp homologous to the insertion site of the adenovirus genome plasmid (template). Suitable sites for pdelE1SP1A are *Sgr*A1 and *Bst*Z17.
4. Linearize the plasmid containing the full length or deleted adenovirus next to the insertion site (vector). For *HVAd*1 a unique ClaI (methylation sensitive) in *E*1 may be used.
5. Cotransform 50 ng of template DNA and 20 ng of vector DNA into BJ 5183.
6. Grow 3 colonies for 6–8 h in 2mL LB. (Selection against the linear vector is highly efficient and leads to success rates close to 100%.)

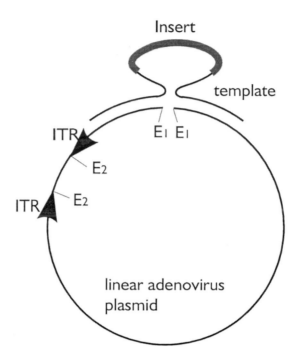

Fig. 1. Construction of recombinant adenovirus genomes by homologous recombination in *E. coli*. E1, unique restriction site used to linearize the adenovirus plasmid. E2, restriction site flanking both ITRs to release the virus genome from the plasmid.

7. Isolate plasmid DNA by alkaline lysis. An extraction with phenol/chloroform/isoamylalcohol is required before ethanol precipitation to completely remove endonucleases. The yield of plasmid DNA obtained from this strain is extremely low. Retransformation is required to generate large-scale preparations of good quality.
8. Retransform DNA into a RecA– strain (*XL1*, *XL2*, *HB*101).
9. Grow Medipreps (one of each retransformation) overnight, isolate DNA using column purification (Quiagen, Chatsworth, CA) and analyze the restriction pattern.
10. Cut 6 µg plasmid DNA with *Pac*I and transfect the digested DNA by calcium phosphate coprecipitation or Lipofection (Lipofectamin, Life Technologies) into subconfluent 293 cells. Use 3 µg DNA per 6-cm plate. Overlay cells with agarose containing media. Expect plaques between days 5 and 10. Both transfection methods work equally well and generate more than 100 virus plaques.

3.2. Determination of Viral Titer by a Modified cpe Assay

1. Seed 3×10^3 293-cells in 100 µL per well in a 96-well culture plate (plate 1) (*see* **Note 1**).

2. On the next day, mix 20 µL virus suspension with 980 µL medium to give a 1:50 dilution.
3. Place 180 µL medium into rows 1–5 of a 96-well plate (plate 2) and 108 µL into rows 6–12.
4. Add 20 µL of the initial dilution into the first row and mix. Transfer 20 µL from the first row to the second row and continue until row 5. Continue by transferring 50 µL from row 5 into row 6 and so on until row 12 (*see* **Note 2**).
5. Transfer 50 µL from plate 2 to the respective wells of plate 1.
6. After 7 d, preliminary titers can be read by detection of a cpe (**Table 1**).

Table 1.

Row	1	2	3	4	5	6	7	8	9	10	11	12
Pfu/mL	10^4	10^5	10^6	10^7	10^8	3.3×10^8	10^9	3.3×10^9	10^{10}	3.3×10^{10}	10^{11}	3.3×10^{11}

7. The three dilutions in every line following the last well with a definite cpe are subject for further propagation.
8. Place 1.5 mL medium into each well of a 24-well plate.
9. Transfer the 293-cells of each selected well of plate 1 ($n = 3 \times 8 = 24$) into the 24-well plate. 293-cells can easily be detached without trypsinizing by pipeting the respective supernatant three times up and down and transferring the whole volume.
10. Allow incubation for another 7 d.
11. Titers can be determined in 24-well plates by determination of the presence of adenoviral cpe (*see* **Note 3**).

3.3. Determination of Viral Titer by Determination of the Amount of Intracellular Adenoviral DNA

3.3.1. DNA-isolation and Southern Blotting (see **Note 4, Fig. 2**)

1. Seed 3 × 6 cm wells with 1×10^6 easily infectable cells per well for each virus preparation to be tested.
2. On the next day, transduce cells with three different MOIs for each virus preparation. The lowest MOI should lead to an efficacy of gene transfer of about 70%, the second MOI should be two times, and the third four times higher. Infection should be performed in 2 mL PBS for 1.5 h.
3. Remove virus and wash two times.
4. Add DMEM comp. and incubate for 12 h.
5. Remove medium and wash three times with DMEM pure and three times with PBS.
6. Lyse the cells with Lysis buffer (1 mL/6-cm plate; 2 mL/10-cm plate) and incubate overnight at 55°C with Proteinase K (50 µg/mL).
7. To remove protein, extract twice with phenol/chloroform/isoamylalcohol and once with chloroform/isoamylalcohol.
8. Precipitate the aqueous phase by adding 10% 3*M* sodium acetate and 2.5 vol ethanol.

Ad.p53   Ad.E2F   Ad.p21

MOI   100   200   400   100   200   400   100   200   400

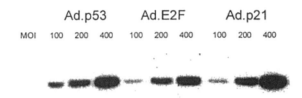

Fig. 2. Determination of viral titer by Southern blotting. AII-cells (hepatocytes derived from *p*53-knock-out mice) were transduced with *Ad.p*53, *Ad*.E2F, or *Ad.p*21 at MOIs 100 and 200 and 400 and were harvested for DNA-preparation as described in **Subheading 3.** Adenoviral DNA was probed with a 1.5-kb Nco-fragment, derived from the *Ad* 5-genome.

9. Centrifuge at 20,000*g* for 30 min. Wash DNA in 70% ethanol and resolve the pellet in an appropriate volume of TE-buffer (about 600 µL) (*see* **Note 5**).
10. Digest the DNA with *NcoI* and 100 µg/µL RNaseA at least for 3 h.
11. Purify DNA by another phenol/chloroform/isoamylalcohol extraction step (1X).
12. Precipitate, wash, and resolve DNA as described in **steps 8** and **9**. The volume of TE-buffer should not be too large considering the loading capacity of the gel-slots.
13. Measure the DNA content from each sample.
14. Load at least 3.25 µg of DNA per lane on a 1% agarose TAE gel (18 × 20 cm).
15. Run the gel at low voltage (40 V) overnight or during the day at about 80 V.
16. For DNA-denaturation, incubate the gel for 20 min in 0.5*M* NaOH/1.5*M* NaCl on a shaker at room temperature.
17. Blot the gel with a blotting device (posiblotter at 90 mmHg for 1.5–2 h). Use a solution of 0.5*M* NaOH/1.5 *M* NaCl as blotting buffer.
18. Wrap the filter in Saran Wrap (if Hybond N is used, otherwise the filter needs to be washed, dried, and UV-fixed) and mark slots by viewing the filter on a UV illuminator.
19. Wash filter twice for 10 min in 2X SSC.
20. The wrapped filter can be stored at –20°C.
21. Incubate filter in 2X SSPE, 1% SDS, 5X Denhardt's, and 50–100 µg/mL herring sperm DNA at 65°C for 3 h before adding the labeled probe. Let hybridize at 65°C overnight.
22. Wash filter:
    –2X in 2X SSC, 5 m*M* sodium phosphate buffer (pH 6.8), 0.1 % SDS, room tcmpcraturc, 10 min
    –0.5X SSC, 5 m*M* sodium phosphate buffer (pH 6.8), 0.1% SDS, room temperature, 10 min
    –2X SSC, 5 m*M* sodium phosphate buffer (pH 6.8), 0.1% SDS, 60°C, 5–10 min
    –2X SSC, 5 m*M* sodium phosphate buffer (pH 6.8), room temperature, 5–10 min (*see* **Note 6**).
23. Wrap filter in Saran Wrap and expose on imaging plate or film.

3.3.2. Preparation of Radiolabeled Probe

1. Amplify a 1.5 kb *NcoI* fragment from the adenoviral plasmid *pHVad*1 by PCR.
2. Purify the fragment by gel-elution.
3. Label 200 ng of the fragment by random priming using α-^{32}-p-ATP.
4. Boil probe for 10 min together with 50–100 µg of herring sperm DNA/mL. Add to hybridization buffer (**step 21**).

3.4. Determination of Infectivity In Vitro

1. Seed 7.5×10^4 cells into 12 wells of a 24-well plate.
2. On the next day, apply a β-gal expressing adenovirus (*AdCMV*βgal) at different MOIs (0, 10, 50, 100, 200, 500), diluted in 300 µL PBS (*see* **Notes 7** and **8**). After incubation for 1.5 h at 37°C, remove viral suspension and add 1 mL medium. Incubate at 37°C.
3. 48 h later, rinse cells two times with PBS.
4. Fix cells for 5 min with 0.05–0.5% ice cold glutaraldehyde.
5. Rinse again two times with PBS.
6. Add X-gal staining solution and incubate at 37°C.
7. Determine the percentage of blue staining cells between hour 4 and hour 24.

3.5. Infection of Cells with Ad.p16 and Ad.p53

1. Seed 1.5×10^6 cells into 10-cm plates (leading to about 50% confluence on the next day, 2 plates per group) (*see* **Note 9**).
2. On the next day, add suspensions of viruses (e.g., *p*16/*tk*, *p*53/*tk*, *p*16/*p*53) at MOIs for every single virus, which should lead to nearly 100% transduction rate (*see* **Note 10**). Incubate 1.5 h at 37°C in 4 mL PBS. Remove PBS and add 10 mL medium. Incubate at 37°C.
3. Harvest cells after 24, 48, and 72 h according to the following protocol:
4. Collect supernatant (*see* **Note 11**).
5. Rinse once with PBS and add the solution to the supernatant.
6. Trypsinize adherent cells and add the cells to the supernatant as well.
7. Centrifuge at $500 \times g^2$ and resuspend in 1 mL PBS (*see* **Note 12**).
8. Remove 50 µL for determination of cell number (trypan blue assay).
9. Divide in 450 µL and 500 µL fraction and pellet cells.
10. For determination of protein levels, freeze the pellet of the 450-µL fraction in liquid nitrogen and store at –80°C.
11. For flow cytometry, resuspend the pellet of the 500-µL fraction in 1 mL 70% methanol. Incubate for 10 min at 4°C. Centrifuge at $500 \times g^2$ and resuspend in PBS. The suspension can be stored at 4°C up to 2 wk.

3.6. Analysis of Cell Cycle, Apoptosis, and the Actual Efficacy of Gene Transfer

1. Centrifuge fixed cells at $500 \times g^2$ and resuspend in PBS. Divide cells, transduced with both viruses in two equal fractions and pellet cells again.

2. Suspend in 50 μL blocking medium, containing primary antibody against *p*53 (1:10) or *p*16 (1:10). Incubate for 1 h at room temperature.
3. Wash two times in PBS and suspend in 50 μL blocking solution, containing FITC conjugated antimouse antibody (1:25).
4. Suspend cells in 1 mL PI-staining solution. Incubate for 15 min at 37°C.
5. The cell-cycle profile, percentage of apoptosis, the efficacy of gene transfer, and the amount of expressed transgene on the single cell level can now be determined by flow cytometry (**Fig. 3**) (*see* **Note 13**). Determination of the percentage of cells in any cell-cycle phase can be determined by the "MultiCycle AV" software.

3.7. Determination of Cell Number

1. Add to the previously collected 50 μL cell suspension, 50 μL of a trypan blue solution.
2. Count viable and dead (blue) cells in a hemocytometer.

3.8. Protein Blotting

1. Determination of the content of transferred transgene products or other proteins can be performed according to conventional methods of Western blotting.
2. Concentration of antibodies used: *p*53: 1:1000, *p*16: 1:1000.

3.9. Treatment of Liver Tumors by Local Injection of Ad.p53 and Ad.p16

1. Harvest exponentially growing tumor cells and suspend in medium at a concentration of $1 \times 10^6/30$ μL.
2. Anesthesize mice with Ketanest (0.1 mg/g body weight) and Rompun (10 μL of a 0.2% solution /g body weight), given simultaneously.
3. With surgical forceps, pinch the skin, raise it, and make a small incision 5 mm below the sternum.
4. Widen the incision 5 mm towards head and tail remaining strictly medial.
5. Repeat the procedure for the peritoneum, paying attention not to damage the intestine.
6. With surgical forceps, raise the left skinflap and peritoneum.
7. With anatomical forceps, grasp the left anterior liver lobe and gently draw it out.
8. Inject 30 μL of the tumor-cell suspension close to the margin.
9. Retract the needle, and close the needle puncture by applying autoclips. This is best done by an assistant.
10. Reposition the liver.
11. Close the peritoneum with 2–4 stitches using resorbable suture.
12. Close skin with autoclips.
13. Return mice to cage.
14. After 7 d when tumors have grown, reopen the peritoneal cavity and expose the tumor bearing liver lobe.

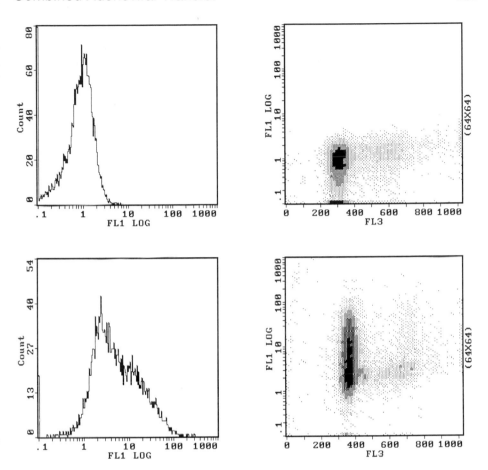

Fig. 3. Simultaneous determination of the rate of gene transfer and cell-cycle distribution using two-parameter flow cytometry. 1.5×10^6 cells (*p53* knock-out hepatocyte cell line) were plated on 10-cm culture dishes. On the next day, cells were transduced at an MOI of 100, which had previously determined to lead to a transduction rate of about 80%. Three d later, supernatant and cells were harvested, fixed and stained against *p53*, and DNA content as described in **Subheading 3.** The upper panel displays untransduced control cells, the lower panel *Ad.p53*-transduced cells. The diagrams to the left display the rate of gene transfer with the signals of *p53*-positive cells on the *x*-axis and cell count on the *y*-axis. The diagrams to the right are monitored using two-parameter flow cytometry with the DNA-content displayed on the *x*-axis and the *p53*-content displayed on the *y*-axis. Note the predominant G1-arrest of *p53*-positive cells.

15. Measure tumor size.
16. Apply 30 µL adenoviral or control solution slowly (over at least 1 min) into the tumor, carefully monitoring increases in tumor volume and eventual leakage (*see* **Notes 14** and **15**).
17. Close peritoneum and skin as described above.
18. Sacrifice animals after the observation period by cervical dislocation.
19. Excise the liver and measure the tumor size.
20. Samples can be snap frozen in liquid nitrogen for immunohistochemistry or fixed in 5% formalin for HE staining.

4. Notes

1. An accurate determination of viral titer can be expected if three independent determinations are performed. It, therefore, makes sense to first obtain large purified adenoviral preparations before titering. We have recently started to declare one virus preparation as standard, which we routinely titer with any new viruses on the same plate (4 lines each). This increases the comparability of titers obtained on different days or by different people.
2. The potency of dilution from row to row (×10 or ×3) depends on the expected titer. If extremely high titers are expected, higher initial dilutions can be made.
3. Usually not all 24 (3 × 8) terminal, which display a definite cpe at the end of the observation period are at the same level of dilution. We routinely obtain the working titer by calculating the mean of all 24 wells.
4. In our hands, the Southern blot signal of different viruses does not always fully confirm the titer as predetermined by cpe assay (*see* **Fig. 2**). Reason for this could be effects of transgenes relevant for cell cycle and apoptosis on 293 cells which could easily prevent a potent cpe. We, therefore, use the cpe only for predetermination of viral titer and determine our working titer by Southern hybridization and definition of a standard virus preparation. To define a standard, we recommend to declare one virus preparation to be the standard for any further Southern transfers. Any further blots can be standardized on the band intensity of this virus preparation.
5. It usually takes 4 d for the DNA to be resolved completely. If this is still not the case at this time, the process can be accelerated by incubation at 65°C for 3 h.
6. To further reduce the background on the filter, washing with 1X SSC, 5 mM sodium phosphate buffer (pH 6.8), 0.2% SDS, and a small amount of pyrophosphate at 65°C is recommended.
7. Most cells are transduced at 100% at MOI's between 50 and 200. In rare cases, a second round of infection at higher MOIs maybe necessary.
8. Depending on the level of accuracy required, determination of the actual cell number on the day of infection may be necessary to be able to calculate the correct MOI.
9. The number of cells required for a complete analysis of effects (determination of cell cycle, protein content, and cell number) strongly depends on the level of inhibition of proliferation and the amount of apoptosis that occurs. Two plates

are usually needed for the later time-points in cases when cell-cycle arrest is followed by apoptosis.

10. A transduction rate of nearly 100% is a compromise between the goal to transduce as many cells as possible and the side effects, which are caused by adenoviral toxicity and are seen at higher MOIs *(3)*.

11. Collection of the cellular supernatant is essential because most of the apoptotic cells will detach from the culture plate.

12. We routinely perform centrifugation of cells in swing-out rotors to prevent sticking of cells to the walls of the 1.5-mL tubes. This can be performed by placing the 1.5-mL tubes into 15-mL tubes, which than can be placed into ordinary swing-out rotors.

13. We routinely use color compensation of: FL3 (PI) = FL3 – 15% FL1 (FITC). Thereby an overestimation of the DNA content of highly transgene-positive cells because of the overlap of FITC and PI emission spectra can be prevented.

14. In principle, the therapeutic outcome is the better the more virus can be injected. We routinely obtain preparations of 5×10^{11} pfu *Ad.p*53, 4×10^{10} pfu/mL *Ad.p*16, and 1×10^{11} pfu/mL *Ad.tk*. Viral stocks can be easily concentrated by removing fluid through centrifugation in microfilter tubes. A limitation of the applicable viral dose could principally be local or systemic toxicity, which should be tested systematically for any combination of viruses.

15. The volume, which can be injected without leakage, depends on the characteristics of the tumor.

References

1. Strauss, M., Brand, K., and Sandig, V. (1997) Tumor suppressor gene therapy-growth arrest and programmed cell death, in *Concepts in Gene Therapy* (Strauss, M. and Barranger, J. A., eds.), Walter de Gruyter, Berlin, New York, pp. 521–537.

2. Sandig, V., Brand, K., Herwig, S., Lukas, J., Bartek, J., and Strauss, M. (1997) Adenovirally transferred p16[INK4/CDKN2] and p53 genes cooperate to induce apoptotic tumor cell death. *Nature Med.* **3,** 313–319.

3. Brand, K., Klocke, R., Possling, A., Paul, D., and Strauss, M. (1999) Induction of apoptosis and G2/M arrest by infection with replication-deficient adenovirus at high multiplicity of infection. *Gene Ther.* **6,** 1054–1063.

4. Sandig, V., Löser, P., Lieber, A., Kay, M. A., and Strauss, M. (1996) HBV-derived promoters direct liver-specific expression of an adenovirally transduced LDL receptor gene. *Gene Ther.* **3,** 1002–1009.

5. Bett, A. J., Haddarra, W., Prevec, L., and Graham, F. L. (1994) An efficient and flexible system for construction of adenovirus vectors with insertions or deletions in early regions 1 and 3. *Proc. Natl. Acad. Sci. USA* **91,** 8802–8806.

6. Chartier, C., Degryse, E., Ganzer, M., Dietrerle, A., Pavirani, A., and Mehtali, M. (1996) Efficient generation of recombinant adenovirus vectors by homologous recombination in Escherichia coli. *J. Virol.* **70,** 4805–4810.

I

EXPERIMENTAL APPROACHES IN CANCER GENE THERAPY

D: Antisense Gene Therapy

Inhibition of Cell Growth by Antisense Oligonucleotides Targeting the Growth-Related Protein Kinase c-raf

Doriano Fabbro, B. P. Monia, K.-H. Altmann, and Thomas Geiger

1. Introduction

1.1. Growth-related Protein Kinases in Cancer– Potential Targets for Pharmaceutical Intervention

The progress made in understanding the molecular basis of mammalian cell transformation has led to the unifying concept of growth regulation and its disorders in cancer cells. Today it is well recognized that many products of "cancer genes" encode for proteins that regulate normal mitogenesis and apoptosis. Taken together, this indicates that the carcinogenic process may be viewed as a progressive disorder of signal transduction *(1–6)*. In fact, many of the genes that are mutated or lost in cancer cells, including both the oncogenes and tumor suppressors, encode proteins that are crucial regulators for intra- as well as intercellular signal transduction *(1–6)*. This conceptual framework has provided a basis for the development of novel anticancer strategies and thera-peutic modalities with the aim to inhibit cancer growth either by blocking mitogenic signal transduction or to specifically induce apoptosis of cancer cells. Although these various approaches have not been validated clinically, these strategies are likely to identify compounds with less side effects compared to standard chemotherapeutic agents.

Specific inhibition of cancer-causing gene products can, in principle, be accomplished by appropriately designed small molecular-weight inhibitors pro-vided that the chosen targets display reasonable enzymatic functions (e.g., inhibitors for protein kinases, extracellular matrix degrading proteases,

From: *Methods in Molecular Medicine, Vol. 35: Gene Therapy: Methods and Protocols*
Edited by: W. Walther and U. Stein © Humana Press, Inc., Totowa, NJ

farnesyltransferases etc.). However, a large proportion of putative cancer-causing or cancer-associated oncoproteins either do not have intrinsic enzymatic functions like various transcription factors (e.g., Myc, Jun, Fos, etc.), cell death suppressors (*Bcl*-2 or *Bcl*-X) or their enzymatic functions are complex (multigene family of proteins like protein kinases, GTP binding proteins, etc.) and/or are not readily amenable to a conventional high throughput random screening.

1.2. General Principles of the Antisense Technology: Inhibition of Protein Expression by Antisense Oligonucleotides

The antisense approach to inhibition of gene expression at the RNA level rests on the simple basic idea that the binding of a relatively small synthetic oligonucleotide ("antisense" oligonucleotide) to a complementary base sequence on a target messenger RNA (mRNA) could lead to suppression of the expression of the corresponding protein *(7–11)*. Such an inhibitory effect on RNA translation could conceivably occur through a variety of mechanisms, including hybrid-arrested translation and RNase H-mediated cleavage of target mRNA and in its functional consequences would be equivalent to the inhibition of protein function, e.g., by small molecule-enzyme inhibitors or receptor antagonists. The first ones to demonstrate the principal feasibility of such a concept were Zamecznik and Stephenson *(12,13)* who, in 1978, showed that treatment of cultured cells infected with the Rous Sarcoma virus with a 13-mer oligodeoxyribonucleotide complementary to part of the viral RNA sequence inhibited virus replication. It has been subsequently pointed out that the antisense concept is not a manmade invention, but that many bacteria as well as eukaryotic cells make use of antisense RNA to control gene expression at the translational level *(14)*.

There are two different basic mechanisms by which the binding of an antisense oligo-deoxyribonucleotide (AS-ODN) to a target mRNA can lead to inhibition of protein expression, *physical blockage* of a variety of processes involved in the sequence of events leading from DNA to protein and/or RNAse H-mediated RNA degradation *(7–11)*. In the former case, binding of the AS-ODN, e.g., in the vicinity of the AUG start codon, may prevent binding of initiation factors or the assembly of ribosomal subunits by a steric effect. The latter mechanism, on the other hand, involves degradation of the RNA strand of the DNA/RNA duplex formed upon binding of the AS-ODN to its target RNA sequence by the endogenous RNAse H. Because of its irreversible and catalytic nature, RNA cleavage should be the most efficient mechanism of AS-ODN-mediated inhibition of protein expression. In fact, it has been demonstrated in a variety of cases that potent inhibition of translation by AS-ODN's depends on RNAse H-mediated destruction of the target RNA *(15–19)*. It should be noted, however, that specific RNA degradation can also be induced by AS-ODN's equipped with an appropriate (synthetic) chemical cleaver moiety. Attempts to design such cleaver moieties have been recently reported in the literature *(20,21)*. No cell culture or even in vivo data are yet available for such cleaver-oligonucleotide conjugates, however. The activation of RNAse L (a single-stranded ribonuclease) by 2'–5' oligoadenylate attached to an antisense oligonucleotide via an appropriate spacer group has been demonstrated to lead to RNA cleavage only in the vicinity of the bound oligonucleotide *(22,23)*. Interestingly, an antisense oligonucleotide of this type was also shown to be a potent inhibitor of the expression of the double-stranded RNA-dependent protein kinase PKR in HeLa cells *(23)*, resulting in the unresponsiveness of these cells to activation of nuclear factor-kB (NF-kB) by poly(I):poly(C).

2. Materials

2.1. Inhibition of c-raf Expression by CGP 69846A in Cancer Cells In Vitro

2.1.1. ODN Treatment of Cells

1. Opti-MEM medium (Life Technologies, Gaithersburg, MD), prewarmed to 37°C, without serum, phenol red, and antibiotics as transfection medium.
2. 1:1 (w/w) liposome fomulation of the cationic lipid N-[1-(2,3-dioleyloxy) propyl]-n,n,n-trimethylammonium chloride (DOTMA) and dioleoyl phosphotidylethanolamine (DOPE), sold as Lipofectin® by Life Technologies (Bethesda, MD).
3. ODNs dissolved in distilled water as 500- to 1000-fold concentrated solution.
4. Phosphate-buffered saline (standard PBS buffer).

2.1.2. Determination of c-raf mRNA Levels in Cells

1. $4M$ guanidinium isothiocyanate, 0.5% sodium lauryl sarcosine, 25 mM sodium citrate, pH 7.0, 0.7 mL β-mercaptoethanol/100 mL.
2. 10 mL glas Potter to homogenize the cells.
3. Chloroform:Isoamylalcohol (49:1, v/v).
4. Isopropylalcohol.
5. 1.2% agarose gel, containing 1.1% formaldehyde for separation of RNA.
6. 2.4 kb Eco R1 fragment of c-raf cDNA (ATCC) to probe Northern blots.
7. Random primer kit to label c-raf cDNA with ^{32}P-deoxycytidine (Promega, Madison, WI).
8. 20X SSPE buffer (3.6M sodium chloride, 200 mM sodium phosphate, 20 mM EDTA, pH 7.4).

9. 50X Denhardt's solution (1% Ficoll, 1% polyvinylpyrolidone, 1% bovine serum albumin, 25 mM EDTA, pH 8.0).
10. Hybridization solution: 50% formamide, 5X SSPE, 1% sodium dodecyl sulfate, 2X Denhardt's solution, 50 µ/mL salm sperm DNA. Low stingency wash buffer: 2x SSPE, 0.1% sodium dodecyl sulfate. High stingency wash buffer: 0.1X SSPE, 0.1% sodium dodecyl sulfate.

2.1.3. Determination of c-raf Protein Levels by Western Blot

1. Cell lysis buffer (20 mM Tris, pH 7.4, 1% Triton X-100, 5 mM EGTA, 2 mM EDTA, 2 mM dithiothreitol, 50 mM sodium fluoride, 10 mM sodium phosphate, 2 µg/mL leupeptin, 1 µg/mL aprotinin).
2. Protein quantification kit with bovine serum albumin as standard (Bio-Rad, Richmond, CA).
3. 2X gel loading buffer (20 mM Tris, pH 7.4, 200 mM dithiothreitol, 20% glycerol, 4% SDS, 0.02% bromphenol blue).
4. 10% SDS-polyacrylamide minigels (Bio-Rad).
5. Immobilon-P membranes (Millipore, Bedford, MA) for electrotransfer of gel-separated proteins.
6. Blocking buffer: 100 mM Tris/HCl, pH 7.4, 150 mM sodium chloride, 5% nonfat milk.
7. Monoclonal anti-c-raf antibody (IgG$_1$, Upstate Biochemicals, Lake Placid, NY). Used as a 1:1000 dilution for Western blots.
8. ^{125}I-labeled antimouse IgG$_1$ antibody (ICN Radiochemicals, High Wycombe, UK).
9. Washing buffer: TBS (Tris/HCl 100 mM, pH 7.4, 150 mM sodium chloride), containing 0.1% nonfat milk.

2.1.4. ODN Sequences (Phosphorothioates)

CGP 69846A (20-mer):	5'-TCC-CGC-CTG-TGA-CAT-GCA-TT-3'
ODN with 1 mismatch:	5'-TCC-CGC-CTG-*C*GA-CAT-GCA-TT-3'
ODN with 2 mismatches:	5'-TCC-CGC-CTG-***CT***A-CAT-GCA-TT-3'
ODN with 3 mismatches:	5'-TCC-CGC-CT***A-CT***A-CAT-GCA-TT-3'
ODN with 4 mismatches:	5-'TCC-CGC-CT***A-CTT***-CAT-GCA-TT-3'
ODN with 5 mismatches:	5'-TCC-CGC-C***CA-CTT***-CAT-GCA-TT-3'
Control ODN (7 mismatches) :	5'-TCC-CGC-***GCA-CTT-G***AT-GCA-TT-3'

2.1.5. Cell Lines

T24 human bladder carcinoma (ATCC HTB-4); A549 human lung carcinoma (ATCC CCL-185); SW480 human colon carcinoma (ATCC CCL-228); Colo 205 human colon carcinoma (ATCC CCL-222); MDA-MB-231 human breast carcinoma (ATCC HTB-26).

3. Methods

3.1. Inhibition of c-raf Expression by CGP 69846A in Cancer Cells In Vitro

3.1.1. ODN Treatment of Cells

1. Plate A549 human lung and T24 human bladder carcinoma 1 d prior to the experiment to a density that cells are 70–80% confluent at the beginning of ODN treatment. Culture medium with 10% FCS.
2. Remove FCS-containing culture medium and wash cells twice with prewarmed PBS buffer to remove serum rests. Add 0.8 mL transfection medium (Opti-MEM, without serum and phenol red) for a 6-well plate.
3. Mix ODN and Lipofectin in 200 µL transfection medium and incubate DNA and cationic lipid for 20 min at room temperature. Add ODN/Lipofectin to cells. Final concentrations: ODN: 100–500 nM, 2.5 µg Lipofectin/100 nM ODN in 1 mL Opti-Mem medium. For 300 nM ODN, use 7.5 µg Lipofectin/mL Opti-MEM medium.
4. Incubate cells for 3–4 h in the presence of ODN/Lipofectin.
5. Assays for inhibition of target gene mRNA and protein expression after 24–48 h, depending on the half-life of the target protein.
6. For the downregulation of long-lived proteins, repeated ODN/Lipofectin treatment on two consecutive days may be necessary.

3.1.2. Determination of c-raf mRNA Levels in Cells.

1. Lyse cells in 1.5 mL 4M guanidinium thiocyanate.
2. Homogenize cell extracts with 5–10 strokes in 10 mL glas potter.
3. Transfer to 2.0 mL Eppendorff cups.
4. Add 0.3 mL (0.2 vol) chloroform:isoamylalcohol and incubate for 5 min at room temperature.
5. Centrifuge for 15 min in Eppendorff microfuge.
6. Transfer water phase (above) to 1.5 mL Eppendorff cups and add 1 volume (0.75 mL) isopropanol.
7. Vortex and incubate for 10 minutes at room temperature.
8. Centrifuge for 15 minutes at 4°C in an Eppendorff microfuge.
9. Wash RNA pellet with 75% ethanol and dissolve RNA in 25–40 µL H$_2$O dest.
10. Determine RNA concentration in photometer at 260 nM.
11. Resolve 20 µg total RNA on 1.2% agarose gels, containing 1.1% formaldehyde.
12. Vacuum-transfer denatured RNA to nylon membranes (Du Pont/NEN, Wilmington, DE).
13. Hybridize Northern blot with 1–2 × 10^6 cpm/mL of ^{32}P-labeled c-raf cDNA for 8 h at 42°C (2.4 kb Eco R1 fragment of human c-raf cDNA, ATCC).
14. Wash filters twice for 20 min with low stringency wash buffer at room temperature.

15. Wash filters twice with high stringency wash buffer at 60°C.
16. Quantification of hybridization signal is done with a PhosphorImager (Molecular Dynamics, Eugene, OR).
17. Equal RNA loading is assured by reprobing the blots with a ^{32}P-labeled cDNA for glycerol-3-phosphate dehydrogenase.

3.1.3. Determination of c-raf Protein Levels by Western Blot

1. Wash cells once with prewarmed PBS buffer and lyse cells in 1 mL cell lysis buffer. Homogenize by 5–10 strokes in a glas potter.
2. Centrifuge cell lysate for 10 min at 4°C in an Eppendorff microfuge.
3. Determine protein content of cellular extract with Bio-Rad protein determination kit, bovine serum albumin as standard.
4. Denature 25–50 μg of protein by boiling for 3 min at 95°C in 1 volume gel loading buffer.
5. Separate proteins on 10% SDS-polyacrylamide gels (200 V, 30 mA for 2 h).
6. Electrotransfer separated protein to Immobilon-P membranes (Millipore).
7. Block membrane for 30 min in blocking buffer at room temperature.
8. Incubate membrane with anti-c-raf monoclonal AB for 1 h at room temperature (1 : 1000 dilution in blocking buffer).
9. Wash membrane 3 times for 30 min at room temperature with TBS buffer, containing 0.1% nonfat milk.
10. Incubate membrane with 5 μCi of ^{125}I-labeled antimouse IgG (ICN Radiochemicals) for 1 h at room temperature.
11. Wash membrane 3 times for 30 min at room temperature with TBS buffer and visualize and quantify c-raf protein levels using a PhosphorImager (Molecular Dynamics).

3.1.4. Measurement of Cellular Proliferation

1. Seed A549 cells in 6-well tissue-culture dishes at a density of 2×10^5 cells per well and allow cells to attach to the plates overnight.
2. Perform each experimental condition in triplicate and determine standard deviations for each group.
3. Treat cells with 50 or 500 nM CGP 69846A or a mismatched control ODN as described above for 4 h.
4. Remove ODNs and add culture medium containing 10% FCS.
5. Determine cell numbers by direct counting using a hemacytometer at day 1, 2, and 3 after ODN treatment and determine cell viability by Trypan blue staining.

4. Results

4.1 Identification of Antisense Inhibitors Targeting Human c-raf Kinase

The protein kinase c-raf which is believed to be deregulated in cancer cells has been selected for an antisense approach. The raf family of serine/

threonine-specific protein kinases comprises three members, A-raf, B-raf, and C-raf, which are expressed in a tissue-specific manner and are important mediators of signal transduction involving cell growth, transformation, and differentiation *(24–26)*. Experimental evidence supports a direct role for C-raf kinase in the development and maintenance of human malignancies. The raf kinases are the direct downstream mediators of the ras proteins, whose oncogenic version is associated with >30% of human solid tumor types including lung, colon, and pancreas cancers *(27,28)*.

Despite the highly important function of c-raf in signal transduction in cancer, specific low molecular-weight inhibitors of the Raf kinase have not been described yet. In order to address the functions of each protein kinase and in particular of the subtypes within one protein kinase family, the antisense approach was used, which offers an opportunity to knock out specifically an individual isoform.

Therefore, c-raf has been targeted by an antisense approach to identify highly potent and sequence-specific inhibitors. The identification of inhibitors and the optimization of their location on the target mRNA was done by a so called "gene walk." The "gene walk" for c-raf is shown as an example in **Fig. 1**. In this gene walk, 20-mer phosphorothioate ODNs were designed, covering the c-raf cDNA from the 5′-untranslated region, the AUG start codon, the coding region, and the 3′-untranslated region. The activity of these ODNs was measured by determining inhibition of c-raf mRNA expression in a suitable cell. The activity of the respective ODNs on c-raf mRNA is highly dependent on the localization on the target mRNA, as shown in **Fig. 1**. An ODN that potently inhibits expression of c-raf mRNA was identified (CGP 69846A). This ODN inhibited c-raf expression by more than 95% at a concentration of 200 n*M* in the presence of cationic lipids.

CGP 69846A is a 20-mer phosphorothioate ODN. No further optimization of the activity of CGP 69846A could be achieved by targeting the c-raf mRNA either at the 5′- or the 3′-end of the CGP 69846A site. Shortening of the ODN length was also investigated. Any attempts to shorten the ODN resulted in a considerable loss of its activity. A dose-response experiment was performed to get an idea on the IC_{50} value for inhibition of c-raf expression. CGP 69846A-inhibited c-raf expression in a dose-dependent manner with an apparent IC_{50} of 70 n*M*, as shown in **Fig. 2**. A control ODN with seven mismatches was completely inactive, indicating that CGP 69846A inhibits c-raf expression by a sequence-dependent mechanism of action (*see* **Subheadings 2.1.4.** for ODN sequences).

Inhibition of c-raf protein expression by CGP 69846A was investigated in the following experiment. Because c-raf is a protein with a long half-life, treatment of T24 cells with CGP 69846A for up to 75 h had to be performed to

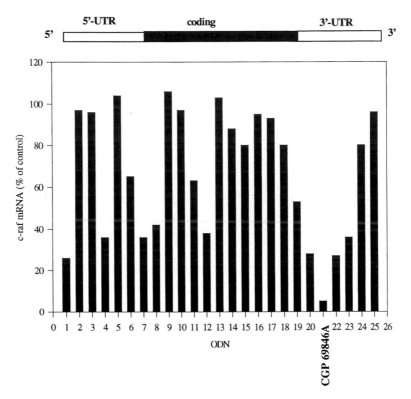

Fig, 1. Inhibition of c-raf kinase mRNA expression in cultured T24 cells by CGP 69846A. T24 human bladder carcinoma cells were exposed to phosphorothioate ODNs at a concentration of 200 n*M* in the presence of cationic lipid for 4 h. c-raf mRNA levels were analyzed by Northern blotting 24 h following ODN administration. The c-raf mRNA levels were quantitated by PhosphorImager analysis and normalized to glycerol-3-phosphate dehydrogenase mRNA levels.

allow downregulation of c-raf protein. **Figure 3** shows that c-raf protein levels start to decrease 24 h after treatment with CGP 69846A, but full reduction of c-raf protein levels by 95% is seen after 75 h only, however. This kinetics of c-raf protein downregulation is consistent with the long half-life of c-raf protein. Again, the mismatched control ODN (seven mismatches) was completely inactive.

The inhibition of c-raf expression by CGP 69846A correlated with an inhibition of proliferation of T24 cells at doses that were consistent with the IC_{50} for the inhibition of c-raf expression. CGP 69846A inhibited cell growth in culture with an IC_{50} below 100 n*M*. At doses of 500 n*M* and higher induction of apoptosis was demonstrated (data not shown). The induction of apoptosis in

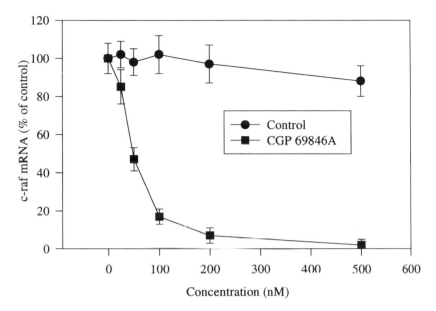

Fig. 2. Dose-dependent inhibition of c-raf mRNA expression by CGP 69846A. T24 human bladder carcinoma cells were treated with increasing concentrations of CGP 69846A and a mismatched control ODN (7 mismatches) in the presence of cationic lipid for 4 h. The c-raf mRNA levels were determined 24 hours after incubation with ODN by Northern blotting as described in **Subheading 3.1.2.** Closed squares: CGP 69846A. Closed circles: control ODN. Error bars represent standard deviation of triplicate experiments.

T24 cells by inhibition of c-raf expression is consistent with the antiapoptotic activity of c-raf. c-raf has been shown recently to prevent apoptosis in cancer cells by interaction with the antiapoptotic protein bcl-2 and phosphorylation of the proapoptotic protein Bad *(31,32)*.

4.2. Mechanism of Action of CGP 69846A: Concept Validation In Vitro

Determination of a sequence-dependent mechanism of action of antisense ODNs is crucial. To unequivocally prove a sequence-dependent effect of CGP 69846A on c-raf mRNA and protein downregulation, a series of mismatched ODNs was designed and used in in vitro experiments. *See* **Subheading 2.1.4.** for ODN sequences. As shown in **Fig. 4**, already the introduction of a single mismatch resulted in a marked inhibition of the biological effect of the ODN. ODNs with 4 or 5 mismatches were completely inactive in downregulating the expression of c-raf mRNA (**Fig. 4**). This gradual decrease of the biological effect of ODNs with the introduction of increasing numbers of mismatches is

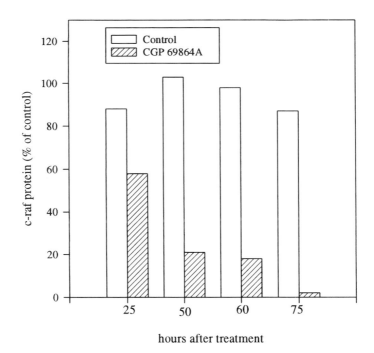

hours after treatment

Fig. 3. Inhibition of c-raf protein expression by CGP 69846A. T24 human bladder carcinoma cells were treated with CGP 69846A (hatched bars) or a control ODN (open bars) at a concentration of 200 nM for a 4-h period on two consecutive days and c-raf protein levels were analyzed by Western blot at 25, 50, 60, or 75 h following the initial ODN treatment. Protein levels were quantified by phosphorImager analysis and normalized to glycerol-3-phosphate dehydrogenase protein levels.

in perfect accordance with the decrease in the Tm values for the ODNs with mismatches (data not shown). Taken together, the experiment with the mismatched ODNs clearly indicates that CGP 69846A exerts its effects on c-raf expression by a sequence-dependent mechanism of action, most presumably an antisense mechanism of action, as it can be concluded from the sequence-dependent downregulation of c-raf mRNA in cancer cells.

4.3. Antiproliferative Effects of CGP 69846A on T24 Bladder Carcinoma Cells

T24 human bladder carcinoma cells were treated with 50 and 500 nM of CGP 69846A or a mismatched control ODN on day zero. Cellular proliferation was determined on days 1, 2, and 3 after ODN treatment by direct cell counting. **Figure 5** shows that the control ODN did not influence cellular proliferation of T24 cells. CGP 69846A, however, clearly inhibited the proliferation of T24 cells at days 1, 2, and 3 at a concentration of 50 nM and even more

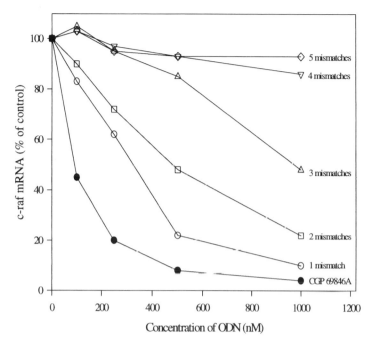

Fig. 4. Effect of increasing numbers of mismatches in CGP 69846A on c-raf mRNA expression in T24 human bladder carcinoma cells. T24 human bladder carcinoma cells were treated with increasing concentrations of CGP 69846A and a series of mismatched ODNs in the presence of cationic lipids for 4 h. c-raf mRNA levels were determined 24 h later by Northern blotting (*see* **Subheadings 2.1.4.** for ODN sequences).

pronounced at a concentration of 500 n*M*. Experimental evidence indicated that CGP 69846A inhibited cellular proliferation at a concentration of 50 n*M*, but induced apoptosis at concentrations of 500 n*M* and higher (data not shown). The antiproliferative activity of CGP 69846A is in perfect accordance with the central role of c-raf in various signal transduction cascades, resulting in the activation of the transcriptional machinery of the cell with the consequence of increased cellular proliferation. The induction of apoptosis at higher concentrations of CGP 69846A appears plausible, taking into account the antiapoptotic activity of c-raf by interaction with the antiapoptotic protein bcl-2 and phosphorylation of the proapoptotic protein Bad *(39)*.

4.4. Inhibition of c-raf mRNA Expression by CGP 69846A in Different Cell Lines

The inhibition of c-raf mRNA expression by CGP 69846A was studied in various human cell lines, including T24 bladder, A549 lung, SW480 and

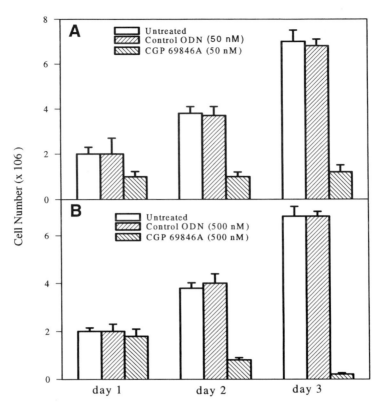

Fig. 5. Inhibition of human T24 cell proliferation by CGP 69846A. The ODNs (CGP 69846A or control ODN) were administered at a concentration of either 50 n*M* (panel A) or 500 n*M* (panel B) in the presence of cationic lipids for 4 h at day zero followed by removal of ODN and replacement with normal medium. Following ODN treatment, cell number was determined at days 1, 2, or 3 by direct counting. Effects of vehicle treatment (control), control ODN or CGP 69846A are indicated. Error bars represent standard deviation of triplicate plates.

Colo 205 colon, MDA-MB-231 breast carcinomas, and in human dermal fibroblasts. **Figure 6** shows that the inhibition of c-raf mRNA expression by CGP 69846A was highly variable even in the presence of cationic lipids in the different cell lines tested. CGP 69846A inhibited c-raf mRNA expression in T24, SW480, and A549 cells at 0.25 μ*M* and 1.0 μ*M* by 80 to 90% and 90 to 98%, respectively. In contrast, in Colo205 cells, CGP 69846A had no effect while in MDA-MB-231 cells c-raf mRNA expression was only inhibited by about 30% at a concentration of 1.0 μ*M*. This variable effect of CGP 69846A on c-raf mRNA expression in various cell lines is most probably caused by differences in the cellular uptake of phosphorothioate ODNs.

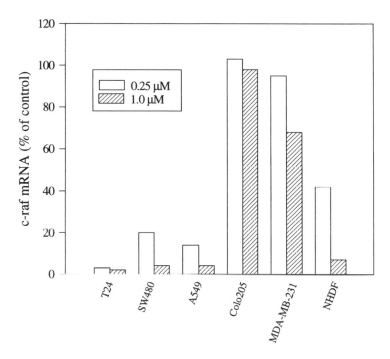

Fig. 6. Inhibition of c-raf mRNA expression by CGP 69846A in different cell lines. CGP 69846A was added to cultured T24, SW480, A549, Colo205, MDA-MB-231, and human dermal fibroblast (NHDF) cells at a concentration of 250 n*M* and 1 μ*M*. c-raf mRNA levels were analyzed by Northern blotting 24 h following ODN administration. c-raf mRNA levels were quantified by PhosphorImager analysis and normalized to glycerol-3-phosphate dehydrogenase mRNA levels.

4.5. Biological Activity of CGP 69846A and the Second Generation ODNs CGP 69845A and CGP 71849A.

Various second-generation ODNs were synthesized and their biological activities were investigated in cell culture experiments (2'-methoxy, 2'-propoxy, 2'-methoxy ethoxy). The 2'O-methoxy ethoxy modifications turned out to be the most interesting modification in our hands, in terms of hybridization efficiency and nuclease resistance, resulting in the most potent biological activity. CGP 69845A is a chimeric 2'-O-MoE ODN with MoE modifications and a phosphodiester backbone in the "wings" and a central phosphorothioate backbone in the "gap," resulting in RNase H-dependent degradation of the target mRNA. CGP 71849A is an ODN with 2'-MoE modifications in the "wings" and a full phosphorothioate backbone. This ODN is intended to be even more nuclease-resistant than CGP 69845A and is still supporting RNase H activity (*see* **Fig. 7** for structure and modifications of ODNs).

CGP 69845A (20-mer):   5'-TCC-CGC^{S}C^{S}T^{S}G^{S}T^{S}G^{S}A^{S}C^{S}A^{S}TGC-ATT-3'

                             "wing"   *"gap"*   *"wing"*

CGP 69846A (20mer):   5'-T^{S}C^{S}C^S-C^{S}G^{S}C^S-C^{S}T^{S}G^S-T^{S}G^{S}A^S-C^{S}A^{S}T^S-G^{S}C^{S}A^S-T^{S}T-3'

CGP 71849A (20-mer):   5'-T^{S}C^{S}C^S-C^{S}G^{S}C^S-C^{S}T^{S}G^S-T^{S}G^{S}A^S-C^{S}A^{S}T^S-G^{S}C^{S}A^S-T^{S}T-3'

CGP 69845A   CGP 71849A   CGP 69846A

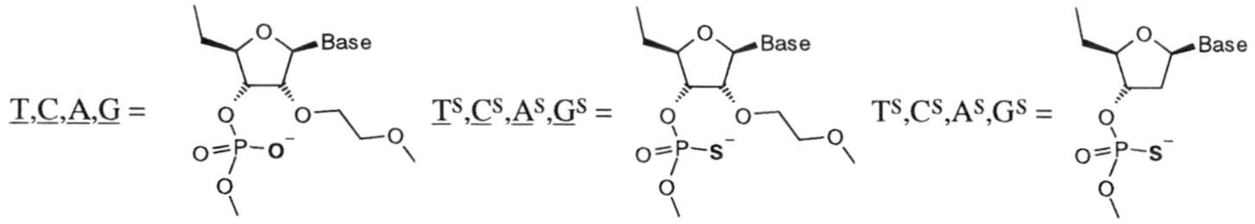

T,C,A,G =   T^S,C^S,A^S,G^S =   T^S,C^S,A^S,G^S =

Fig. 7. Structure and sequence of CGP 69845A and CGP 71849A, 2'-O methoxy ethoxy modifications of CGP 69846A. The sequence and structure of CGP 69845A, a second-generation modification of CGP 69846A, is shown. CGP 69845A is a chimeric 2'-methoxyethoxy ODN with 2'-MoE modifications in the "wings" and a phosphodiester backbone and a central 2'-unmodified phosphothioate "gap" to support RNAse H activity.

The effect of CGP 69846A on c-raf mRNA expression in A549 lung carcinoma cells was compared to the effect of CGP 69846A and CGP 71849A. A549 cells were treated for 4 h with ODNs in the presence of cationic lipids and c-raf mRNA levels were investigated 24 h later. **Figure 8** shows that CGP 69845A and CGP 71849A are equally effective in inhibiting c-raf mRNA expression with an apparent IC$_{50}$ of 70 nM. In contrast, CGP 69846A was less active in inhibiting c-raf mRNA expression with an IC$_{50}$ of 100 nM under identical experimental conditions.

When A549 cells were treated twice with the ODNs on two consecutive days, and c-raf mRNA levels were investigated 75 h following the initial ODN treatment, CGP 71849A was more active than CGP 69845A and inhibited c-raf mRNA expression with an IC$_{50}$ of approx 100 nM (**Fig. 9**). The higher activity

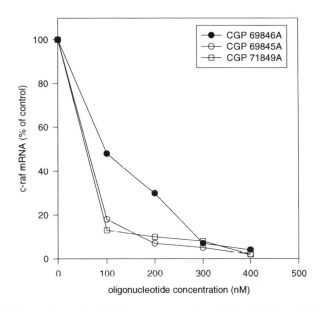

Fig. 8. Inhibition of c-raf mRNA expression by CGP 69845A, CGP 69846A, and CGP 71849A 24 h after treatment. A 549 lung carcinoma cells were treated for 4 h with CGP 69845A, CGP 69846A, and CGP 71849A in different concentrations in the presence of cationic lipids. 24 h later, mRNA was isolated and c-raf mRNA expression was measured by Northern blotting. c-raf mRNA levels were quantified using a PhosphorImager. The results are expressed as the % of control (no ODN addition).

of CGP 71849A 75 hours after ODN treatment is most presumably the result on the higher nuclease resistance and the longer half-life of CGP 71849A, compared to CGP 69845A.

4.6. Biological Activity of Various Chimeric ODNs with 2′ Sugar Modifications

Various chimeric ODNs with 2′ sugar modifications (2′-methoxy, -propoxy, 2′-methoxyethoxy) were synthesized and their activity on c-raf mRNA expression was studied in T24 bladder carcinoma cells. ODNs with 2′ methoxyethoxy modifications were most potent in inhibiting c-raf mRNA expression, followed by CGP 69846A and 2′ propoxy-modified ODNs. The 2 methoxy-modified ODN was least potent and inhibited c-raf mRNA expression only weakly in concentrations up to 300 n*M* (**Fig. 10**). From these results it was again concluded that 2′ methoxyethoxy modifications are most promising in terms of nuclease resistance, mRNA affinity and overall biological activity.

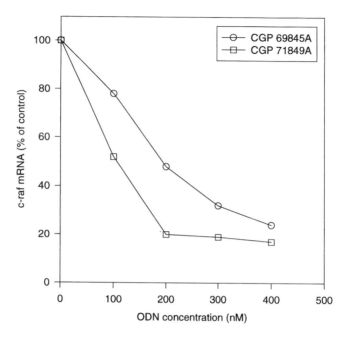

Fig. 9. Inhibition of c-raf mRNA expression by CGP 69845A and CGP 71849A 75 h after treatment. A 549 lung carcinoma cells were treated twice for 4 h with CGP 69845A and CGP 71849A in different concentrations in the presence of cationic lipids at day 0 and day 1. 75 h later mRNA was isolated and c-raf mRNA expression was measured by Northern blotting. c-raf mRNA levels were quantified using a Phosphor-Imager. The results are expressed as the % of control (no ODN addition).

5. Concluding Remarks

c-raf, one of the most important signal transducing molecules involved in growth regulation of cancer cells, has been selected for an antisense approach. A potent and sequence-specific inhibitor of c-raf expression (CGP 69846A) has been identified. It was demonstrated that this antisense ODN exerts its effects by a sequence-dependent mechanism of action, most presumably by an antisense mechanism of action. This is very important especially for phosphorothioates that have been demonstrated to often exert their activities by unspecific effects *(33–36)*. In this study, it was clearly demonstrated that the cellular activities of CGP 69846A are the result of an antisense mechanism of action. The most compelling evidence for this statement is the experiment with CGP 69846A and the series of mismatched ODNs where it could be demonstrated in vitro that the activity of the ODNs is lost by the introduction of increasing numbers of mismatches.

$$T_oC_oC_oC_oG_oC_sC_sT_sG_sT_sG_sA_sC_sA_sT_oG_oC_oA_oT_oT$$

2′ sugar modified RNase H gap 2′ sugar modified

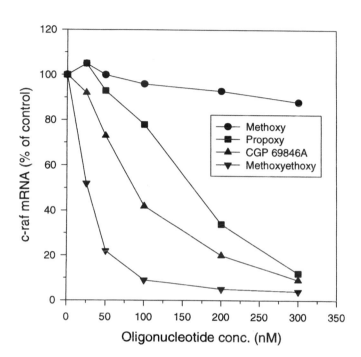

Fig. 10. Inhibition of c-raf mRNA levels by 2′ sugar modified chimeric antisense oligonucleotides. T24 bladder carcinoma cells were treated for 4 h with antisense oligonucleotides at the indicated concentrations. 2′ sugar modifications that were tested were 2′ methoxy, 2′ propoxy, and 2′ methoxyethoxy, and each was compared with the activity of the parent phosphorothioate oligodeoxynucleotide CGP 69846A. c-raf mRNA levels were determined 24 h after initial ODN treatment by Northern blot.

CGP 69846A is currently in clinical development for the indication cancer. The compound successfully completed Phase I trials where no prohibitive side effects have been seen. Our results have considerably contributed to establish the antisense technology as a promising and novel technology for the identification of therapeutic agents with a mechanism of action that is completely different from the mechanism of established anticancer drugs. We look forward very much to clinical trials with more antisense drugs and to clinical concept validation using this innovative and novel technology.

6. Notes

6.1. ODN Treatment of Cells Inhibition
of Gene Expression by Antisense ODNs

1. The cationic lipid formulation to facilitate uptake of ODNs into cultured cells has to be carefully selected for every specific cell line. Comprehensive data collections on the preferred lipid formulation for certain cell lines are available from commercial suppliers of cationic lipids.

2. The conditions for the transfection of the cells, i.e., the ODN concentration and the concentration of the cationic lipid, have to be optimized for every specific cell system. The uptake of ODNs in the presence of cationic lipids varies dramatically between different cell types. T24 bladder and A549 lung carcinoma cells took up the ODNs easily in our cell culture experiments in the presence of cationic lipids, whereas Colo 205 colon carcinoma cells were highly resistant, even in the presence of cationic lipids (**Fig. 9**).

3. Some formulation of cationic lipids are rather toxic to cells. The combination of ODN and cationic lipid results in a cumulative toxicity and therefore the adequate concentrations for maximal ODN uptake have to be determined experimentally. Usually, transfection has to be performed under serum-free conditions which increases the toxicity of the treatment. Some newer formulations of cationic lipids may be used in the presence of serum which may reduce the toxicity of the treatment.

4. The half-life of the protein to be downregulated by treatment with antisense ODNs has to be taken into account. For downregulation of long-lived proteins, multiple treatments with ODN on consecutive days may be necessary, as it was performed in this study to downregulate expression of c-raf protein. This may results in cumulative toxicity, however.

5. Northern and Western blots are widely used to monitor inhibition of mRNA and protein expression in antisense experiments. Under some circumstances, however, more refined methods, such as *in situ* hybridization and immunohistochemistry may be necessary to unequivocally demonstrate downregulation of target gene expression.

6. Cationic lipids are absolutely necessary to facilitate ODN uptake in cell-culture experiments. In animal experiments, however, the ODNs can be injected as a simple saline solution and are still taken up by the target cells. The exact mechanisms involved in ODN uptake in vivo are not yet totally clear, however.

7. For a high potency of antisense drugs, it is mandatory that the ODNs support activation of RNase H, leading to degradation of the target mRNA. This mechanism of action has been shown in the past to be most crucial for the potency of antisense compounds. A special strategy is therefore necessary for the design of second generation ODN modifications in order to preserve the activation of RNase H.

6.2. Adequate Controls for Antisense Experiments

8. Various types of control ODNs are used widely for antisense experiments both in vitro and in vivo, i.e., sense, scrambled, or mismatched ODNs.
9. The lack of biological effect of a sense or scrambled ODN does not prove a sequence-dependent effect of an active antisense ODN.
10. A sequence-dependent effect of an antisense ODN can only be proven by the introduction of single or multiple mismatches into the sequence of the ODN. Only mismatched ODNs guarantee the conservation of the overall physicochemical properties of the ODN and are, therefore, adequate controls.
11. A gradual loss of the biological effect of an antisense ODN with increasing numbers of mismatches strongly indicates a sequence-dependent effect. Experiments with a series of mismatched ODNs are described both in cell culture and in vivo in **Subheading 4.2.** and **Fig. 4**.
12. Evidence for a sequence-dependent effect of an antisense ODN can be provided by the selection of adequate control ODNs both in cell-culture experiments and in vivo. Final proof of an antisense mechanism of action in vivo is hard to achieve, however.
13. The demonstration of unchanged expression of a control protein is mandatory as a further control in antisense experiments in which the target protein is downregulated. This control protein should be related to the antisense target protein and should have a comparable half-life. If the antisense target protein belongs to a multigene family, another member of this family may be the ideal control to demonstrate a sequence-dependent effect of an antisense ODN.

6.3. First- and Second-Generation ODN Chemistries

14. Phosphorothioate ODNs are widely used for antisense experiments both in cell-culture experiments and in vivo. They have a reasonable nuclease resistance that ensures a sufficiently long half-life to exert biological effects.
15. The large-scale synthesis of phosphorothioate ODNs at affordable prices has been improved dramatically during the last few years. Phosphorothioate ODNs have entered clinical trials and the results obtained look promising.
16. It should be kept in mind, however, that especially phosphorothioate ODNs have been shown to often exert their effects by unspecific nonsequence-dependent mechanisms. Strong protein binding of phosphorothioate antisense ODNs is responsible for the major side effects in clinical trials in vivo, i.e., inhibition of clotting factors and complement activation.
17. Second-generation chemical modifications that result in higher potency of antisense ODNs and a reduced toxicity are therefore urgently needed.
18. Various chemical ODN modifications have been used both in cell culture and in antitumor experiments in vivo. The 2'-methoxyethoxy ODN modification turned out to be the best choice in our hands in terms of potency and tolerability in vivo.

19. RNase H-dependent degradation of the target mRNA turned out to be the most important activity in terms of potency of antisense ODNs. Uniformly modified 2′-modified ODNs would not support RNase H activity, however. Therefore, an alternative strategy was pursued, i.e., the design of "chimeric" ODNs with 2′-MoE modifications in the "wings" and a central unmodified "RNase H gap." These ODNs were both designed with a chimeric phosphodiester/ phosphorothioate backbone and with a full phosphorothioate backbone. CGP 71849A, the 2′-MoE ODN with a full phosphorothioate backbone, turned out to be most potent in inhibiting the expression of c-raf in cancer cells, consistent with the hypothesis that this ODN combined in an optimal manner high nuclease resistance with the ability to support RNase H-dependent degradation of c-raf mRNA.

20. The toxicology of this ODN modification has to be investigated carefully in various species, however, before this modification can be suggested as a suitable follow-up chemistry for future antisense compounds. Experiments are underway to investigate the toxicology and tolerability of 2′-MoE modifications both in rodent and primate animal studies.

References

1. Croce, C. M. (1987) Role of chromosome translocations in human neoplasia. *Cell* **49,** 155–160.
2. Alitalo, K. and Schwab, M. (1988) Oncogene amplification in tumor cells. *Adv. Cancer Res.* **46,** 235–240.
3. Bos, J. L. (1989) Ras oncogene in human cancer: a review. *Cancer Res.* **49,** 4682–4689.
4. Rabbitts, T. H. (1994) Chromosomal translocations in human cancer. *Nature* **372,** 143–148.
5. Bishop, J. M.(1991) Molecular themes in oncogenesis. *Cell* **64,** 235–248.
6. Weinberg, R. A. (1994) Oncogenes and tumor suppressor genes. *CA Cancer J. Clin.* **44,** 160–179.
7. Uhlmann, E. and Peyman, A. (1991) Antisense oligonucleotides: a new therapeutic principle. *Chem. Rev.* **90,** 543–551.
8. Milligan, J. F., Matteucci, M. D., and Martin, J. C. (1993) Current concepts in antisense drug design. *J. Med. Chem.* **36,** 1923–1931.
9. Crooke, S. T. (1992) Therapeutic applications of oligonucleotides. *Annu. Rev. Pharmacol. Toxicol.* **32,** 329–339.
10. Hélène, C. and Toulmé, J.-J. (1990) Specific regulation of gene expression by antisense, sense, and antigene oligonucleotides. *Biochimica et Biphysica Acta.* **1049,** 99–125.
11. Cohen, J. S. (1994) Gene-mimetic substances. *Adv. Pharmacol.* **25,** 319–325.
12. Zamecnik, P. C. and Stephenson, M. L. (1978) Inhibition of rous sarcoma virus replication and cell transformation by a specific oligodeoxynucleotide. *Proc. Natl. Acad. Sci. USA* **75,** 280–286.

13. Stephenson, M. L. and Zamecnik, P. C. (1978) Inhibition of rous sarcoma viral RNA translation by a specific oligodeoxyribonucleotide. *Proc. Natl. Acad. Sci. USA* **75,** 285–292.

14. Takayama, K. M. and Inouye, M. (1990) Antisense RNA. *Crit. Rev. Biochemistry.* **25,** 155–184.

15. Chiang, M-Y., Chan, H., Zounes, M. A., Freier, S. M., Lima, W. F., and Bennett, C. F. (1991) Antisense oligonuleotides inhibit intercellular adhesion molecule 1 expression by two distinct mechanisms. *J. Biol. Chem.* **266,** 18162–18171.

16. Dean, N. M. and McKay, R. (1994) Inhibition of protein kinase C-a expression in mice after systemic administration of phosphorothioate antisense oligonucleotides. *Proc. Natl. Acad. Sci. USA* **91,** 11762–11766.

17. Monia, B. P., Johnston, J. F., Ecker, D. J., Zounes, M. A., Lima, W. F., and Freier, S. M. (1992) Selective inhibition of mutant Ha-ras mRNA expression by antisense oligonucleotides. *J. Biol. Chem.* **267,** 19954–19962.

18. Monia, B. P., Lesnik, E. A., Gonzalez, C., Lima, W. F., McGee, D., Guinosso, C. J., et al. (1993) Evaluation of 2'-modified oligonucleotides containing 2'-deoxy gaps as antisense inhibitors of gene expression. *J. Biol. Chem.* **268,** 14514–14522.

19. Wagner, R. W., Matteucci, M. D., Lewis, J. G., Gutierrez, A. J., Moulds, C., and Froehler, B. C. (1993) Antisense gene inhibition by oligonucleotides containing C-5 propyne pyrimidines. *Science* **260,** 1510–1513.

20. Hall, J., Hüsken, D., Pieles, U., Moser, H. E., and Häner, R. (1994) Efficient sequence-specific cleavage of RNA using novel europium complexes conjugated to oligonucleotides. *Chem. Biol.* **1,** 185–191.

21. Magda, D., Miller, R. A., Sessler, J. L., and Iverson, B. I. (1994) Site-specific hydrolysis of RNA by europium(III) texaphyrin complexes conjugated to a synthetic oligodeoxyribonucleotide. *J. Am. Chem. Soc.* **116,** 7439–7445.

22. Torrence, P. F., Maitra, R. K., Lesiak, K., Khamnei, S., Zhou, A., and Silverman, R. H. (1993) Targeting RNA for degradation with (2'-5')oligoadenylate-antisense chimera. *Proc. Natl. Acad. Sci. USA* **90,** 1300–1305.

23. Maran, A., Maitra, R. K., Kumar, A., Dong, B., Xiao, W. X., Li, G., et al. (1994) Blockage of NF-kB signaling by selective ablation of an mRNA target by 2-5A antisense chimera. *Science* **265,** 789–792.

24. Magnuson, N.S., Beck, T., Vahidi, H., Hahn, H., Smola, U., and Rapp, U. (1994) The raf-1 serine/threonine protein kinase. *Sem. Cancer Biol.* **5,** 247–253.

25. Beck, T.W., Huleihel, M., Gunnell, M., Bonner, T.I., and Rapp, U.R. (1987) The complete coding sequence of the human A-raf-1 oncogene and transforming activity of a human A-raf carrying retrovirus. *Nucl. Acids Res.* **15,** 595–609.

26. Sithanandam, G., Kolch, W., Duh, F.M., and Rapp, U.R. (1990) Complete coding sequence of a human B-raf cDNA and detection of B-raf protein kinase with isozyme specific antibodies. *Oncogene* **5,** 1775–1780.

27. Boulikas, T. (1995) The phosphorylation connection to cancer. *Int. J. Oncol.* **6,** 271–278.

28. Powis, G. and Alberts, D.S. (1994) Inhibiting intracellular signalling as a strategy for cancer chemoprevention. *Eur. J. Cancer* **30,** 1138–1144.

29. Nishizuka, Y. (1995) Protein kinase C and lipid for sustained cellular response. *Faseb J.* **9,** 484–492.

30. Basu, A. (1993) A potential of protein kinase C as a target for anticancer treatment. *Pharmaceut. Ther.* **59,** 257–280.

31. Blagosklonny, M. V., Giannakakou, P. El- Deiry, W. S., Kingston, D. G. I., Higgs, P. I., Neckers, L., and Fojo, T. (1997) Raf-1/bcl-2 phosphorylation: A step from microtubule damage to cell death. *Cancer Res.* **57,** 130–135.

32. Wang, H. G., Rapp, U. R., and Reed, J. C. (1996) Bcl-2 targets the protein kinase Raf-1 to mitochondria. *Cell* **87,** 629–638.

33. O'Brien, S. G., Kirkland, M. A., Melo, J. V., Rao, M. H., Davidson, R., McDonald, C., and Goldman, J.M. (1994) Antisense BCR-ABL oligomers cause non-specific inhibition of chronic myeloid leukemia cell lines. *Leukemia* **8,** 2156–2162.

34. Perez, J. R., Li, Y., Stein, C. A., Majumder, S., van Oorschot, A., and Narayanan, R. (1994) Sequence-independent induction of Sp1 transcription factor activity by phosphorothioate oligonucleotides. *Proc. Natl. Acad. Sci. USA* **91,** 5957–5961.

35. Wyatt, J. R., Vickers, T. A., Roberson, J. L., Buckheit, R. W., Klimkait, T., DeBaets, E., et al. (1994) Combinatorially selected guanosine-quartet structure is a protein inhibitor of human immunodeficiency virus envelope-mediated cell fusion. *Proc. Natl. Acad. Sci. USA* **91,** 1356–1360.

36. Yaswen, P., Stampfer, M. R., Ghosh, K., and Cohen, J. S. (1993) Effects of sequence of thioated oligonucleotides on cultured human mammary epithelial cells. *Antisense Res. Dev.* **3,** 67–77.

37. Chirgwin, J. M., Przybyla, A. E., MacDonald, R. J., and Rutter, W. J. (1979) Isolation of biologically active ribonucleic acid from sources enriched in ribonuclease. *Biochem. USA* **18,** 5294–5299.

38. Maniatis, T., Fritsch, E. F., and Sambrock, J. (1992) *Molecular Cloning,* Cold Spring Harbor, New York.

39. Blagosklonny, M. V., Giannakakou, P., El-Deiry, W. S., Kingston, D. G., Higgs, P. I., Neckers, L., and Fojo, T. (1997) Raf-1/bcl-2 phosphorylation: a step form microtubule damage to cell death. *Cancer Res.* **57,** 130–135.

12

IGF-1 Antisense Strategies for Cancer Treatment

Yue Xin Pan and Donald D. Anthony

1. Introduction

The technical approaches to gene therapy for cancer utilize ex vivo and in vivo gene-transfer methodology. This chapter focuses on applicability and use of an ex vivo approach using an IGF-1 antisense RNA strategy of treatment. Insulin-like growth factor 1 (IGF-1) and IGF-2 have pivotal roles in cell proliferation and development (for review, see *1–6*). The preponderance of peptide synthesis and activity occur during fetal development, and protein synthesis is downregulated in most mature tissues except for adult liver. Further modulating the activities of these proteins are the levels of their respective cell-surface receptors and ligand-receptor interactions *(3,5,6)*.

Many different cancers and cancer cell lines produce and secrete IGF-1 and/ or IGF-2 and also express IGF-1 receptor. These include astrocytomas, glioblastoma multiforme, sarcomas, thyroid adenomas, hepatocellular cancer, teratocarcinoma, small-cell cancer of the lung, and carcinomas of breast, colon, and prostate gland *(7)*. The initiation and/or early growth of such tumors may be dependent upon changes in these mitogenic peptides or their receptors. Work in tissue culture *(8)* and animal model systyems *(7,9–11)* support a role for these growth factors in the modulation of aberrant cell growth. Downregulation in expression of IGF-1 and/or its receptor prevents tumor formation and causes regression and cure of tumor in rodents *(9,10)*. The insertion of growth factor antisense genes into tumor cells as a means to investigate, treat, and/or modify tumor growth patterns is reviewed in this chapter. The following subsections describe the various procedures involved in the process.

From: *Methods in Molecular Medicine, Vol. 35: Gene Therapy: Methods and Protocols*
Edited by: W. Walther and U. Stein © Humana Press, Inc., Totowa, NJ

1.1. Outline of Methods and Time Line for Development of Vaccine

The time from acquisition of tumor cells to successful in vitro transfection and amplification of transfected cell populations is a critical factor in determining practicality for the treatment of human cancer; particularly for those cancers with rapid and aggressive growth patterns. The procedures involved can vary requiring, in some cases, up to 3–6 mo in time. It is important to utilize strategies that can minimize time requirements (*see* **Note 1**).

1.2. Human Glioblastoma Primary Cell Culture

Characteristics of primary cell cultures with respect to cell morphology and doubling times and factors such as sensitivity to antibiotics used to selectively derive transfected cell clones can be used to obtain more time-efficient processes (*see* **Notes 2** and **3**).

1.3. Cell Transfection with pAnti-IGF-1 Vector

The episomal vector pAnti-IGF-1 (described in **Subheading 3.**) produces RNA that is Anti-sense to IGF-1 mRNA. The construct includes elements of the Epstein-Barr Virus DNA (<5 % of the EBV genome) which drive extra-chromosomal replication. The multiple copies of vector produced inside of the cell during early cell passages following transfection serve to express IGF-1 antisense RNA in quantities that strongly suppress IGF-1 synthesis (*see* **Notes 5** and **6**).

1.4. Identification of pAnti-IGF-1 Transfected Cells and Their Properties

The expression of IGF-1 antisense cDNA and RNA in transfected cells is determined by conventional Southern and Northern blot and by RT-PCR technology. Immunofluorescent flow cytometry and immunocytochemistry are used to demonstrate the range of downregulation of IGF-1 in transfected cell populations (*see* **Notes 4–6**). The procedures require adequate permeabilization of cells in order to detect the intracellular protein (*see* **Note 4**).

1.5. Preparation of Vaccine

Preliminary to preparation of vaccine, amplified populations of transfected cells are compared to the corresponding nontransfected, parental cells for downregulation in intracellular IGF-1. Following $ZnSO_4$ induction of the metallothionein-I promoter and expression of IGF-1 antisense RNA, the range of downregulation in IGF-1 of transfected, human glioblastoma cells varies between 60% and 90% as determined by immunofluorescent flow cytometry (*see* **Notes 4–6**). Appropriate sterility testing is done prior to vaccination.

2. Materials

2.1. Laboratory Facility

Human tissues are obtained in the operating room using standard surgical techniques. Tissue is transported at 25°C to a dedicated gene therapy facility in closed, sterile containers containing serum-free medium. Work with tissue and cells is performed in Category II environmental hoods or the equivalent. Laboratory personnel are clothed in sterile gowns, shoe and head covers, surgical gloves, and facial masks. All buffers and reagents for cell culture, cell transfection, and preparation of final solutions for injection into recipients are FDA approved pharmaceutical grade.

2.2. Cell Culture and Transfection

Sources of materials used are indicated in parentheses

1. Dulbecco's Modified Eagle Medium (DMEM)** 4.5 g/L glucose, 4 m*M* L-glutamine (Biowhittaker, Walkersville, MD).
2. Supplemented DMEM: DMEM supplemented with 1XMEM nonessential amino acids solution, 1 m*M* sodium pyruvate, 5 µg/mL human transferrin, 3.46 ng/mL sodium selenite, 500 ng/mL insulin (prepared as required).
3. MEM nonessential amino acids solution 10 m*M*(100X) (Life Technologies, Gaithersburg, MD).
4. Sodium pyruvate, cell culture tested (Life Technologies).
5. Transferrin, human, lyophilized, 4 mg/mL when supplemented with 10 mL sterile, distilled water (Life Technologies).
6. Sodium selenite, lyophilized 2×10^{-6} *M*, 0.346 µg/mL when supplemented with 10 mL sterile, distilled water (100X) (Life Technologies).
7. Insulin, porcine, crystal (Sigma, St. Louis, MO), stock solution (10,000X) in 0.01N HCL.
8. Fetal bovine serum (FBS) (BioWhittaker) 56°C inactivated, store at –5 to –20°C.
9. Opti-MEM I reduced-serum medium (Life Technologies).
10. F-12 nutrient mixture(Ham)1X, liquid contains L-glutamine (Life Technologies).
11. Minimum essential medium, contains Earle's salts, but no L-glutamine modified for suspension culture (S-MEM) (Life Technologies).
12. Dulbecco's Phosphate-buffered Saline (DPBS) (Life Technologies) store at 25°C.
13. Hygromycin B, MW 527.5 (CalBiochem, La Jolla, CA) stock solution 100 mg/mL in DPBS.
14. Lipofectin reagent (Life Technologies).
15. 0.05% trypsin, 0.53 m*M* EDTA (Life Technologies) store at –20°C in 10-mL aliquots.
16. Cell culture freezing medium (Life Technologies) store at –20°C in 10-mL aliquots.
17. EndoFree Plasmid Maxi Kit (Qiagen, Chatsworth, CA) store at 25°C.
18. Collagenase CSL-1 (Worthington Biochemical Corp., Freehold, NJ), DNase I DPFF (Worthington Biochemical Corp.), Pronase (CalBiochem) lyophilized; rehydrate with DPBS prior to use.

** Unless otherwise indicated, all of the items are stored at 4°C.

2.3. Characterization of Transfected and Nontransfected Cells

1. Mouse antihuman IGF-1 monoclonal antibody (Upstate Biotechnology Inc.)
2. Mouse antihuman HLA Class 1 monoclonal antibody (Serotec Inc., Oxford, UK).
3. Mouse antihuman CD80 (B7-1) monoclonal antibody, R-PE conjugate (Ancell Corp.), store in absence of light.
4. Goat antimouse IgG antibody, FITC conjugate (Kirkegaard & Perry Lab.), store in absence of light.
5. Mouse antihuman glial fibrillary acidic protein (GFAP), polyclonal antibody (Boehringer Mannheim).
6. Vectastain Elite ABC Cell staining kit (Vector Laboratories, Burlingame, CA).
7. Qiagen RNA/DNA Midi Kit (Qiagen).
8. PCR primers, specific for human IGF-1 antisense cDNA (424 bp region, forward primer 5′-GAAGATGCACACCATGTCCT-3′; reverse primer 5′-TCACTCTT CACTCCTCAGGAG-3′) (Molecular Biology Core Laboratory, Case Western Reserve University, Cleveland, OH) and PCR primers, specific for human β-actin Exon 3 DNA (289 bp region) (Research Genetics, Inc.).

3. Methods

3.1. Outline of Methods and Algorithm for Development of Vaccine

An approximate time line for preparation of vaccine from the isolation of human tissue to delivery into patient is as follows:

1. Transport of tumor tissue to gene therapy center, and separation of glioblastoma cells for tissue culture (1 d).
2. Establish and characterize primary culture of glioblastoma cells (1–2 passages, 1–3 wk).
3. Propagation and expansion of cells in culture (1–3 passages, 2–3 wk).
4. Transfection and selection of cell foci which both survive and proliferate under pressure of hygromycin B (4–8 wk).
5. Characterization of transfected cell foci (4 d).
6. Amplification of the transfected cell populations (3–6 passages, 4–8 wk, occasionally as long as 12 wk).
7. Preparation of vaccine for injection (3 d). Time required to prepare vaccine varies between 12 and 22 wk, depending upon characteristics of cell lines derived from individual patients. This procedure is described in the flow diagram below.

3.2. Human Glioma Primary Cell Culture

3.2.1. Primary Cultures

1. Primary cultures are derived according to modification of technique as described by Westphal (12). At the time of surgery, 0.5 to 5 g of tumor tissue is immediately placed into sterile serum-free DMEM at 25°C and transferred to the gene therapy facility in sterile 50-mL conical Falcon tubes.

Algorithm for Development of Vaccine

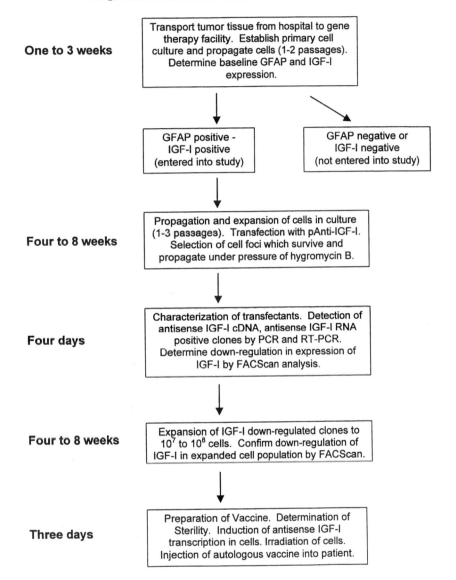

One to 3 weeks — Transport tumor tissue from hospital to gene therapy facility. Establish primary cell culture and propagate cells (1-2 passages). Determine baseline GFAP and IGF-I expression.

GFAP positive - IGF-I positive (entered into study)

GFAP negative or IGF-I negative (not entered into study)

Four to 8 weeks — Propagation and expansion of cells in culture (1-3 passages). Transfection with pAnti-IGF-I. Selection of cell foci which survive and propagate under pressure of hygromycin B.

Four days — Characterization of transfectants. Detection of antisense IGF-I cDNA, antisense IGF-I RNA positive clones by PCR and RT-PCR. Determine down-regulation in expression of IGF-I by FACScan analysis.

Four to 8 weeks — Expansion of IGF-I down-regulated clones to 10^7 to 10^8 cells. Confirm down-regulation of IGF-I in expanded cell population by FACScan.

Three days — Preparation of Vaccine. Determination of Sterility. Induction of antisense IGF-I transcription in cells. Irradiation of cells. Injection of autologous vaccine into patient.

2. Tissue is transferred in 0.5–1.0 g pieces to sterile 100-mm culture dishes and washed two times with 5 mL of DPBS to remove free blood. Washes are aspirated with sterile Pastuer pipet/electronic pipet aid.

3. Tissues are then minced into fragments 1 mm³ or smaller in size and 10 mL of DPBS containing 0.05% pronase, 0.03% collagenase, and 0.01% DNase I is added.

4. The suspension is mixed by pipet trituration, incubated at 37°C for 20–30 min with orbital shaking, and transferred to a sterile tube. Contents are allowed to settle for 2 min. At this time, the enzyme-digested mixture consists of single cells, small cell aggregates, and larger fibrous fragments.

5. The supernatant containing single cells and small cell aggregates is transferred to a separate tube and centrifuged at 100g for 5 min.

6. The cellular pellet is resuspended in 10 mL DMEM containing 4.5 g/mL glucose, 4 mM L-glutamine, 1X MEM nonessential amino acids, 1 mM sodium pyruvate, 3.46 ng/mL sodium selenite, 500 ng/mL porcine insulin, and 5 µg/mL human transferrin (supplemented DMEM) to which is added 10% FBS.

7. Cell concentration is determined by hemocytometer and adjusted with supplemented DMEM, 10% FBS to a final concentration of 1×10^5 cells/mL. 2-mL aliquots are then distributed into each well of a six-well plate. The larger fibrous fragments are resuspended separately in 10 to 15 mL supplemented DMEM, 10% FBS. 2–3 mL are distributed into each well of a six-well plate.

8. The culture media is changed at 48 h and every 4–5 d thereafter.

9. When cell growth nears confluence, medium is replaced with a 1:1 mixture of serum-free supplemented DMEM and serum-free Ham's F12 medium. Cells are maintained in this medium for a minimum of 1 wk.

10. The medium is then changed to supplemented DMEM, 10% FBS, and maintained an additional week before passage.

11. Cells are trypsinized, transferred to 60-mm dishes, and fed every 4 d. Cultures are maintained in a humidified atmosphere of 5% CO_2 and 95% air at 37°C. *See* **Note 2** for description of cell morphology, changes, and implications in respect to the time line for transfection.

3.2.2. Immunocytochemical Characterization of Human Glioblastoma Cells

Glial Fibrillary Acidic Protein (GFAP) and IGF-1 protein are localized immunocytochemically in cell populations using the Vectastain *Elite* kit according to manufacturers instructions (avidin-biotin system, Vector Laboratories).

1. Cells propagated in a 24-well plate or slide chamber are fixed with 2% paraformaldehyde for 5 min at 25°C.

2. Cells are then permeabilized with 0.1% Triton X-100 for 1 min, and incubated with 500 µL (for 24-well plates) or 300 µL (for slide chambers) of primary antibody (either antihuman GFAP or antihuman IGF-1 monoclonal antibody) at a concentration of 2–4 µg/mL × 2–4 h at 4°C.

3. Following washes three times with 0.5 mL PBS for 5 min each at 25°C, secondary antibody labeling is performed at a 1:200 to 1:1000 dilution in PBS as determined for each subset of cells (see manufacturer's instructions). Incubation at optimal dilution is carried out for 0.5 h at 25°C.

4. After washing cells three times in 0.5 mL PBS, premixed avidin and biotinylated peroxidase is added and the incubation continued 20 min at 25°C.

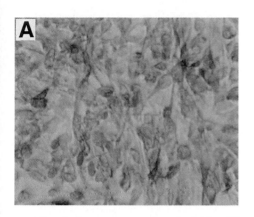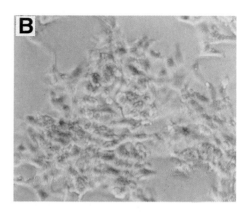

Fig. 1. Immunocytochemical identification of IGF-1 in nontransfected and trans-fected human glioblastoma cells. Cytochemical immunostaining was carried out with mouse antihuman IGF-1 monoclonal antibody as primary antibody and goat antimouse IgG as secondary label. Labeled cells were stained using Vectastain Elite ABC stain-ing kit. Both nontransfected and transfected cells were preincubated in the presence of 50 μM $ZnSO_4$ × 20 h at 37°C to optimally activate the MT-I promoter of the pAnti-IGF-1 vector. (**A**). Positive IGF-1 staining in nontransfected HG-2 human glioblas-toma cells. (**B**). Negative IGF-1 staining in transfected HG-2 cells.

5. After washing cells three times in 0.5 mL PBS, GFAP or IGF-1 antigen is visualized by addition of hydrogen peroxide and 3′, 3′- diaminobenzidene tetrahydrochloride (DAB).
6. Controls for each experiment include preincubation with normal horse serum (5% in PBS) in place of primary antibody, incubation with the primary antibody only, and incubation of the human cell line HEK 293 with both primary and secondary antibodies as described. Positively stained cells exhibit a characteris-tic brown stain over both nuclei and cytoplasm (**Fig. 1**).

3.3. Cell Transfection with pAnti-IGF-1 Vector

3.3.1. The Structure of the pAnti-IGF-1 Vector

The bacterial strain *E. coli* DH5α bearing the plasmid expression vector pAnti-IGF-1 was kindly provided by Dr. J. Ilan. This antisense expression vec-tor is episomal and includes the EBV virus origin of replication and the gene encoding nuclear antigen I, which together drive extrachromosomal replica-tion. The vector replicates readily within human cells providing a copy number of up to 100/cell *(13)*. This allows a high level of expression of IGF-1 antisense RNA within cells. The IGF-1 antisense cDNA is linked to the highly inducible mouse metallothionein promoter. Downstream of the IGF-1 antisense cDNA is a polyadenylation termination signal. The construct also contains genes for

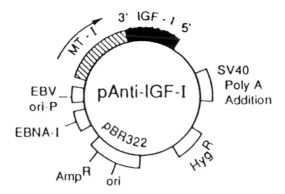

Fig. 2. Structure of pAnti-IGF-1 Episomal Vector. MT-I, metallothionein I promoter; EBNA-I, EBV-encoded nucler antigen I; SV40, Simian Virus 40; Amp®, ampicillin resistance gene; Hyg®, hygromycin resistance gene.

both hygromycin and ampicillin resistance. The physical structure is shown in **Fig. 2**.

3.3.2. Preparation of pAnti-IGF-1 Vector DNA

The vector is isolated and purified using an EndoFree Plasmid Maxi Kit (Qiagen) according to manufacturer's instructions in the vector production area of a Gene Core Facility. In this institution, the facility for experiments with vectors in human cells consists of an FDA-approved and certified Class 10,000 clean room. All air supplied to this room is HEPA filtered and ionized and the room is maintained under positive air pressure.

1. A single, large lot of DNA (400–800 µg) is prepared using the Qiagen kit.
2. The preparation of vector is suspended in sterile T_{10} E_1 buffer, adjusted to 0.5–1 µg/µL by spectrophotometry, and then filtered through a 0.2 µm sterile Acrodisc syringe filter at 25°C.
3. Lots are tested for purity and sterility as outlined under quality testing in the FDA Guidance for Human Somatic Cell Therapy and Gene Therapy *(14,15)*. Sterility testing is done in a routine hospital bacteriology laboratory.
4. Quality testing includes the determination of DNA, RNA, and protein content.
5. Lots are tested for identity using gel electrophoresis and extensive restriction endonuclease mapping to demonstrate correct sizes and orientation of the DNA fragments.
6. Efficacies for lots are standardized according to assays for two established human glioblastoma cell lines.
7. The vector capacity to downregulate IGF-1 expression in glioblastoma cells of each patient is determined individually prior to injection.
8. Each lot is divided and stored in multiple 0.1-mL aliquots in sterile $T_{10}E_1$ buffer

at a concentration of 0.5–1.0 µg/µL in sterile Eppendorf conical tubes at –80°C. Our experience is that vector stored under such conditions retains complete potency for at least 2 yr.

3.3.3. Transfection of Human Glioblastoma Cells

Human glioblastoma cells are transfected either in primary culture or during very early cell passages (i.e., passage 1–3).

1. Cells are seeded in each well of a six-well plate (1×10^5 cells in 2 mL supplemented DMEM, 10% FBS).
2. When 40–50% confluency is achieved, cells are washed two times with 2-mL aliquots of Opti-MEM I and then transfected according to manufacturer's instructions using the lipofectin reagent kit available from Life Technologies.
3. 2 µg pAnti-IGF-1 DNA in 100 µL Opti-MEM I (solution A) is added to 10 µL Lipofectin (Life Technologies) diluted in 100 µL Opti-MEM I (solution B). Solution B is maintained at 25°C × 45 min prior to addition of solution A.
4. The DNA-Lipofectin mixture is maintained at 25°C × 15 min, diluted with 1.8 mL Opti-MEM I overlaid on each well of cells and then incubated 10–12 h under routine tissue culture conditions. The medium containing DNA-lipofectin is then aspirated and replaced with supplemented DMEM, 10% FBS for 48–72 h.
5. Cells are trypsinized, transferred to cell culture dishes at a ratio of 1:5 or 1:8 in supplemented DMEM, 10% FBS containing hygromycin B at a concentration previously determined for each cell line (*see* **Note 3**).
6. Cultures are monitored daily for 2 wk for growth of cell foci developing among dying cells. Isolated foci (clones) of transfected cells are obtained using cloning cylinders.
7. Separated clones are transferred to wells of six-well plates and the population is expanded and transferred to 60-mm tissue-culture dishes or larger culture dishes, as appropriate.
8. The population of cells is then further expanded under growth conditions, which include the selective pressure of hygromycin B. To expand a single foci of transfected cells to the number needed for vaccination requires 3–5 wk, depending on the doubling time of individual cell lines. It is critical that this process take place under conditions in which cells continue to proliferate. Most expedient results are obtained when cell transfection is begun in primary culture or in early passages (*see* **Notes 2, 3**).

3.4. Identification of pAnti-IGF-1 Transfected Cells and Their Properties

3.4.1. Immunofluorescent Flow Cytometry

Immunofluorescent staining for IGF-1, HLA Class I, and CD80 antigens is performed at 4°C in a 96-well microtiter plate by modification of standard techniques (*16*).

1. Human glioblastoma cells are trypsinized and washed three times with PBS as previously described. $2.5–5.0 \times 10^5$ cells in 150 μL PBS are loaded into each well of a 96-well plate and centrifuged $800g$ for 3 min at 4°C.
2. Supernatant is aspirated and one of the following primary antibodies is added at an antibody concentration of 1:50 at 4°C for 30 min. The primary antibodies are mouse antihuman IGF-1 (Upstate Biotechnology), and mouse antihuman HLA Class I (Serotec).
3. Cells are then washed three times with 150 μL of PBS as previously described. Secondary antibody labeling is performed using fluorescein isothiocyanate (FITC) conjugated goat antimouse IgG (Kirkegaard & Perry Lab, KPL) at a dilution of 1:200 in the absence of light.
4. Surface antigen CD80 is detected using mouse antihuman CD80 (B7-1) monoclonal antibody conjugated with R-phycoerythrin (R-PE)(Ancell) by direct staining technique in the absence of light.
5. To detect intracellular IGF-1, the trypsinized and PBS washed cells are pretreated with 2% paraformaldehyde at 25°C for 5 min and permeabilized with 0.1% Triton X-100 at 25°C for 1 min (*see* **Note 4**).
6. Cells are stained as described and analyzed on a FACScan flow cytometer (Becton Dickinson, Rutherford, NJ) equipped with LYSYS II software on the day of staining and histogram analysis is performed using LYSYS II software.

For immuncytochemistry and flow cytometry studies, nontransfected or transfected cells are preincubated for 18–20 h in supplemented DMEM (no added FBS) in the presence and absence of 50 μM ZnSO$_4$. The incubation is carried out for 18–20 h in order to complete the induction and expression of IGF-1 antisense RNA prior to cell staining procedures (*see* **Note 5**).

3.4.2. Southern and Northern Blot Analysis

Southern blot analysis is done according to standard procedure (Maniatis). For Northern blot, ZnSO$_4$ induction of IGF-1 antisense RNA is done prior to the extraction of total cellular RNA from both nontransfected and transfected cells as described in **Subheading 3.4.1.** and **Note 5**. Cellular RNA is extracted using the Qiagen RNA/DNA Mini Kit following manufacturer instructions. Northern blot analysis is performed according to standard procedures (Maniatis) using ^{32}P-dCTP labeled IGF-1 cDNA fragment as probe.

3.4.3. PCR and RT-PCR

1. Cell lysates for PCR are prepared from cells by addition, to each well of a 48-well plate, of 100 μL of PCR buffer (50 mM KCl, 10 mM Tri-HCl pH 8.3, 2.5 mM MgCl$_2$) containing the nonionic detergents 0.45% NP40 and 0.45% Tween-20 plus 100 μg/mL proteinase K.
2. Following incubation for 1 h at 55°C, temperature is increased to 95°C × 10 min to inactivate proteinase K.

3. The detection of IGF-1 antisense cDNA by PCR is carried out in a Thermal Cycler 480 (Perkin Elmer, Norwalk, CT) programmed with 30 cycles of 60/45/90 s at 94/56/72°C respectively, using *Taq* polymerase.
4. RT-PCR for detection of IGF-1 antisense RNA is performed using RNA isolated with RNeasy Total RNA Kit *(20)* (Qiagen) and digested by DNase I in the presence of RNase inhibitor.
5. RT reactions are performed according to standard procedure (Maniatis), and ethanol precipitated cDNA is resuspended in PCR buffer, and PCR reactions are performed as described. The forward primer used in these experiments is the 20 base oligonucleotide 5'-GAAGATGCACACCATGTCCT-3', and the reverse primer, the 21 base oligonucleotide 5'-TCACTCTTCACTCCTCAGGAG-3'.

3.5. Preparation of Vaccine

3.5.1. Sterility Testing

Before clinical use, sterility of transfected cell cultures is tested for bacteria, fungi, virus, and mycoplasma by the Bacteriology and Virology Laboratories in a routine hospital facility.

3.5.2. ZnSO$_4$ Induction in Preparation of Vaccine

One day before vaccination of patient with autologous glioblastoma cells, cells are placed in supplemented DMEM, serum-free medium for 2–6 h. Medium is then changed to supplemented DMEM, serum-free medium containing 50 μ*M* ZnSO$_4$ for 18–20 h as described in **Subheading 3.4.1.** and **Note 5**.

3.5.3. Irradiation of Cells for Vaccine

Transfected cells in 100-mm^2 culture dishes are washed once with 10 mL DPBS, trypsinized with 1 mL of 0.05% trypsin, 0.53 m*M* EDTA at 37°C for 2–5 min and then washed again twice with 10-mL aliquots of DPBS at 4°C. The cell pellets are recovered by centrifugation at 800*g* for 5 min and the combined preparation of cells from 15–20 100-mm^2 culture dishes is then suspended in 15 mL S-MEM in a 75-mm^2 sterile flask. An aliquot of the cells is stained with Tryphan blue and viable cell count is determined with a hemocytometer. The preparation is adjusted to a concentration of 660,000 cells/mL S-MEM and irradiated with 5000 cGy delivered by cobalt source.

3.5.4. Preparation of Vaccine and Injection of Patient

Following irradiation, the cells are returned to the human gene therapy facility clean room, transferred to a sterile 50-mL conical tube, centrifuged at 800*g* at 4°C for 5 min and washed twice with 10 mL sterile saline (0.9% sodium chloride Inj., USP, preservative free, Abbott Laboratories, North Chicago, IL). The washed cells are then suspended in 1–2 mL of sterile saline and placed in a 3 cc syringe for injection.

The first injection is given between 14–18 wk after the surgical intervention. The autologous, transfected, and irradiated cells are administered subcutaneously into the forearm. Booster injections are administered into alternate forearms at 4 and 12 wk following the initial vaccination using the same predetermined dose of cells. Note, it is important to confirm downregulation of IGF-1 expression in transfected glioblastoma cells for each preparation of vaccine prior to vaccination (*see* **Note 6**).

4. Notes

1. The in vitro approaches to gene therapy have a level of precision that can be measured in control of the quantity and quality of transfected cell populations. The major handicap, in addition to monetary cost, has been the time needed to produce adequate numbers of transfected cells as immunogene vaccine or for other forms of treatment. In the case of glioblastoma multiforme, the 3–5 mo time from surgery to acquisition of vaccine frequently out-reaches the palliation produced by surgery. Vaccine becomes available after surgery, when tumor burden has again accumulated and when the patient frequently requires massive doses of steroids to help suppress the edema associated with tumor. Under similar circumstances, even bacterial infections to which the host's immune system normally reacts strongly become overwhelming if the infection is massive and in combination with an immune system suppressed by either steroids or chemotherapy. It is critical, therefore, to decrease the time for preparation(s) to a time frame in which such factors are less likely to be operative (in the case of gene therapy for glioblastoma from the 5-mo range to 3 mo or less).

2. The cell morphology in primary culture of human glioblastoma is multiplicate. The mixed appearance is composed of flat large fibrous cells, small compact apolar cells, and very differentiated bipolar or extensively branched cells. After several passages any of these cell types may predominate. After long-term culture (beyond eight passages, and usually more than 2 mo), a dominant cell type may develop with the uniform appearance of a stable cell line. Despite the multiplicate morphology, greater than 90% of cells are strongly positive for glial fibrillary acidic protein (GFAP) and more than 70% express IGF-1. Cells that rapidly develop a uniform culture appearance are predictably more stable to manipulation and can be more rapidly transfected ex vivo.

3. The selection process for foci of cells transfected with the pAnti-IGF-1 vector is based on the gene for resistance to the antibiotic hygromycin B. Studies concerning the relative sensitivity of nontransfected and transfected cells to hygromycin B show that the viability of glioblastoma cells cultured in the presence of the antibiotic varies greatly from patient to patient (**Fig. 3**). Moreover, for both the nontransfected cells lines and the corresponding transfected cell lines from each of several patients, the relative order of sensitivities to hygromycin B correlates well (**Fig. 3A,B**). Therefore, hygromycin B sensitivity curves need to be determined early in order to find the optimal concentration to use for each patient's

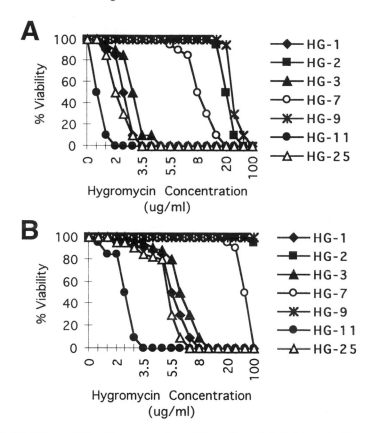

Fig. 3. Viability of Non-Transfected and Transfected Cell Lines in Hygromycin B (**A**) *Non-Transfected Cell Lines.* Three categories of cell sensitivity to Hygromycin B are shown: highly sensitive (HG-11), sensitive (HG-1, HG-3 and HG-25) and least sensitive (HG-2, HG-7 and HG-9). (**B**) *Transfected Cell Lines.* This graph demonstrates the relative changes in sensitivity to Hygromycin B after transfection with the pAnti-IGF vector. The three categories of cellular sensitivity are similar to those represented for the corresponding nontransfected cell lines. (Taken from **ref. *17***)

glioblastoma cell line. The concentration of hygromycin B used to drive the selection process for transfected cell foci is twice the concentration at which the corresponding nontransfected cells can survive, but do not proliferate well. The doubling time (defined as the time required for doubling the cell population during logarithmic cell growth) can also be correlated with the ability to survive and multiply in hygromycin B. For human glioblastoma cells in tissue culture, the range of doubling times in our experience has been between 12 and 48 h. Those cell lines exhibiting shorter doubling times survive and propagate in higher concentrations of the antibiotics *(17)*. Comparison between the doubling times of

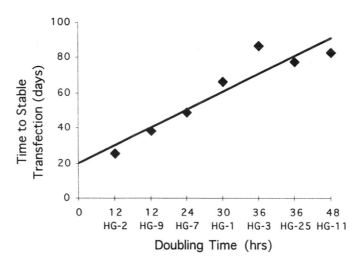

Fig. 4. Relationship Between Doubling Time and Time to Stable Transfection. Time to stable transfection is defined as the time in days required to achieve foci of cells which survive and proliferate in a Hygromycin B concentration > 2X that in which the corresponding non-transfected cells will survive and proliferate, and which maintain this property through 2 cell passages. Cell doubling time is the time required for doubling the cell population during logarithmic cell growth. (Taken from **ref. 17**)

individual cell lines and the time required to achieve stable transfection shows that those cell lines with shorter doubling times are able to be transfected more expediently (**Fig. 4**). Thus, for human glioblastoma both doubling times and relative sensitivities to hygromycin B can be used to select cell lines and cell clones that can be more expediently transfected. A critical first step is, therefore, to begin the transfection procedure early and, when the option is available, to select those cells or cell lines that have shorter doubling times and survive and replicate in higher hygromycin B concentrations. Beginning the process with ample tissue from surgery helps to provide greater numbers of cells and hygromycin B resistant cell foci from which to select for these options. Aliquots of tissue should be obtained from more peripheral and non-necrotic areas of tumor. In our experience the procedure should generally be reserved for patients with untreated cancer, particularly for those who have not received radiation therapy.

4. In order to detect intracellular IGF-1, it is important that the cells be made adequately permeable prior to staining. In the absence of this step, nonspecific binding of antibodies on cell surfaces is strong. In addition, autofluorescence of the cells contributes strongly to a high background, especially when FITC conjugates are used (most cellular fluoresence is emitted in the FITC fluorochome wavelength range of 500–550 nm). The permeablization step also alters light scattering characteristics of the cells. Fixation with paraformaldehyde before permeablization reduces the light scattering effect. The procedure as outlined in

Subheading 3.4.1. of **Methods** gives essentially the same light scattering for both untreated and permeablized cells and an optimal specific antibody staining to background ratio.

5. The vector used in this IGF-1 antisense RNA strategy of treatment contains the metallothionein promoter. Prior to vaccination, cells are incubated in the presence of $ZnSO_4$ to optimally activate the promoter in cell culture. The time required to effect the changes which occur with downregulation of cellular IGF-1 and which may be necessary for the immunogenic mechanism has not been studied. The transfected cells are, therefore, incubated in $ZnSO_4$ at 37°C for as protracted a time as the cell viability in $ZnSO_4$ allows. Human glioblastoma cells maintain viability for 16–20 h. Different tissues may have different sensitivities to $ZnSO_4$. Therefore, cell viability as function of $ZnSO_4$ concentration and duration of incubation should be determined for transfected cell lines of different tissues in order to optimize the treatment with $ZnSO_4$.

6. Molecular analysis demonstrates that the recombinant pAnti-IGF-1 vector is present predominantly in episomal form in early passages of transfected human glioblastoma cells. With late passages, the cells gradually lose the ability to express IGF-1 antisense RNA and to downregulate the expression of IGF-1. Analysis by Southern blot has demonstrated the pAnti-IGF-1 vector to be in extra chromosomal form in transfected cells until the 7–8th cell passages. Analysis, by Northern blot has demonstrated the expression of IGF-1 antisense RNA until the 9–10th cell passages. Immunocytochemical and Flow Cytometry studies have shown significant downregulation in the cellular IGF-1 until at least the 10th cell passage. It is, therefore, important to determine the persistence of desired transfection effects as a function of cell passages. The preparation of vaccines from early passages of transfected cells would seem to be advantageous. For human glioblatoma, vaccines are prepared from cells with fewer than six cell passages from the time of transfection.

Acknowledgments

We are indebted to Drs. Robert Ratcheson, Judith and Joseph Ilan, Jerzy Trojan, and Yajun Guo for their contributions to this chapter.

References

1. LeRoith, D. and Roberts, C. T., Jr. (1993) Insulin-like growth factors. *Ann. N.Y. Acad. Sci.* **692,** 1–9.
2. Roberts, C. T., Jr. (1996) Control of insulin-like growth factor (IGF) action by regulation of IGF- I receptor expression. *Endoc. J.* **43 (Suppl.),** S49–S55.
3. D'Ercole, A. J. (1996) Insulin-like growth factors and their receptors in growth. *Endocrinol. Metab. Clinics North Amer.* **25,** 573–590.
4. Rubin, R. and Baserga, R. (1995) Insulin-like growth factor-I receptor. Its role in cell proliferation, apoptosis, and tumorigenicity. *Lab. Investigat.* **73,** 311–331.
5. Ranke, M. B. and Elmlingger, M. (1997) Functional role of insulin-like growth factor binding proteins. *Hormone Res.* **48 (Suppl. 4.),** 9–15.

6. McInnes, C. and Sykes, B. D. (1997) Growth factor receptors: structure, mechanism, and drug discovery. *Biopolymers* **43,** 339–366.

7. Trojan, J., Johnson, T. R., Rudin, S. D., Ilan, J., Tykocinski, M. L., and Ilan, J. (1993) Treatment and prevention of rat glioblastoma by immunogenic C6 cells expressing antisense insulin-like growth factor I RNA. *Science* **259,** 94–97.

8. Kaleko, M., Ruther, W. J., and Miller A. D. (1990) Overexpression of the human insulin-like growth factor I receptor promotes ligand-dependent neoplastic transformation. *Mol. Cell Biol.* **10,** 464–473.

9. Trojan, J., Blossey, B. K., Johnson, T. R., Rudin, D. S., Tykocinski, M., Ilan, J., and Ilan, J. (1992) Loss of tumorigenicity of rat glioblastoma directed by episome-based antisense cDNA transcription of insulin-like growth factor I. *Proc. Natl. Acad. Sci. USA* **89,** 4874–4878.

10. Resnicoff, M., Christian, S., Rubini, M., Coppola, D., Ambrose, D., Baserga, R., and Rubin, R. (1994) Rat glioblastoma cells expressing an antisense RNA to the insulin-like growth factor-I (IGF-1) receptor are nontumorigenic and induce regression of wild-type tumors. *Cancer Research* **54,** 2218–2222.

11. Trojan, J., Johnson, T., Rudin, S., Blossey, B., Kelley, K., Shevelev, A., et al. (1994) Gene therapy of murine teratocarcinoma: separate functions for insulin-like growth factors I and II in immunogenicity and differentiation. *Proc. Natl. Acad. Sci. USA* **91,** 6088–6092.

12. Westphal, M., Hansel, M., Nausch, H., Rohde, E., and Harrmann, H. D. (1989) Culture of human brain tumors on an extracellular matrix drived from bovine corneal endothelial cells and cultured human glioma cells, in *Methods in Molecular Biology* (Walker, J. M., ed.), pp. 113–132.

13. Yates, J. L., Warren, N., and Sugden, B. (1985) Stable replication of plasmids derived from Epstein-Barr virus in virious mammalian cells. *Nature* **313,** 812–815.

14. Food and Drug Administ., Center for Biologics Eval. & Res. and National Institutes of Health, National Cancer Institute (1996) The points to consider in human somatic cell and gene therapy (1991) in *Gene Therapy Resource Book.*

15. US Dep. Health and Human Services, Food and Drug Adminis., Center for Biologics Eval. Res. (1998) Guidance for human somatic cell therapy and gene therapy.

16. Schroff, R. W., Bucana, C. D., Klein, R. A., Farrell, M. M., and Morgan, A. C. (1984) Detection of intracytoplasmic antigens by flow cytometry. *J. Immunol. Meth.* **70,** 167–177.

17. Anthony, D. D., Pan, Y. X., Wu, S. G., Shen, F., and Gou, Y. J. (1998) Ex Vivo and in Vivo IGF-1 antisense RNA strategies for treatment of cancer in humans. *Adv. in Exper. Med. Bio.* **451,** 27–34.

I

EXPERIMENTAL APPROACHES IN CANCER GENE THERAPY

E: Ribozyme Gene Therapy

13

Anti-*MDR*1 Ribozyme Gene Therapy

Takao Ohnuma, Hiroyuki Kobayashi, and Fu-Sheng Wang

1. Introduction
1.1. MDR

Multidrug resistance (MDR) in human cancer seriously limits the efficacy of anticancer agents. Circumvention of MDR is, thus, one of the urgent goals for successful cancer chemotherapy.

MDR in cancer therapeutics may be defined as the phenomenon of simultaneous resistance to drugs of different chemical structures and mechanisms of action.

The molecular basis of MDR has been demonstrated to be multifactorial. Based on the mechanisms involved, MDR can be classified as 1) P-glycoprotein (P-gp)-mediated MDR (Classical MDR); 2) MRP (Multidrug-resistance associated protein)-mediated MDR; 3) LRP (lung resistance-related protein)-mediated MDR; 4) Topoisomerase II-mediated MDR; 5) mutant p53-mediated MDR; 6) MDR associated with altered expression and/or mutations in tubulin isoforms; 7) MDR associated with altered drug-metabolism; and 8) MDR associated with increased activities of DNA repair-related proteins (modified from **ref. *1***).

Among these multiple factors, P-gp-mediated MDR is a well-characterized mechanism of MDR (*see 2–4*). P-gp is a 170-kd transmembrane glycoprotein which serves as a drug efflux pump. P-gp is a member of the ATP-binding cassette (ABC) transmembrane transporter superfamily. It is encoded by a small group of closely related genes termed *MDR* (*PGY*); only *MDR*1 is known to confer drug resistance. In humans, *MDR*1 gene is mapped to chromosome 7q21.1.

From: *Methods in Molecular Medicine, Vol. 35: Gene Therapy: Methods and Protocols*
Edited by: W. Walther and U. Stein © Humana Press, Inc., Totowa, NJ

A variety of human tumor samples was examined for *MDR*1 gene expression *(5–8)*. Generally high levels of expression were seen in tumors arisen from colon, kidney, liver, adrenal gland, in chronic myelocytic leukemia, and in carcinoid tumors. P-gp is normally present in gastrointestinal tract mucosal cells, bile duct cells, hepatocytes, renal cells, and adrenal cells. Physiological function of P-gp is postulated to be involved in protection against xenobiotics and in secretory functions in such cells as adrenal cells. The presence of P-gp in these organs explains why tumors, arisen from these organs, express high levels of P-gp and are resistant to P-gp substrate anticancer agents. In acute leukemias, neuroblastoma, pheochromocytoma, ovarian cancers, and breast cancers *MDR*1 RNA levels are increased following recurrence after chemotherapy and these tumors are more resistant to chemotherapy. High *MDR*1 expression is correlated with poor prognosis in cancer patients. P-gp up-regulation occurs in tumor cells early during treatment with P-gp substrate drugs.

P-gp substrate drugs are lipophilic heterocyclic compounds, which include vincristine, taxol, taxotere, daunorubicin, doxorubicin, mitoxantrone, mitomycin-C, etoposide, and teniposide. Various attempts have been made to block *MDR*1 overexpression *(1,9)*. Theoretically, P-gp activity can be blocked at three levels: DNA, RNA, or protein. Because amplification of *MDR*1 gene is not prerequisite to P-gp-related resistance in human tumor cells *(10–12)*, the potential loci of inhibition can be narrowed to mRNA or protein. One means to intercept a target mRNA is to use a catalytic RNA, or a ribozyme *(13,14)*.

We designed anti-*MDR*1 ribozymes targeted against MDR1 mRNA and were able to show that they could reverse MDR phenotype *(15–18)*.

1.2. Design of Anti-MDR1 Ribozymes

Ribozymes are catalytically active subsets of small RNA molecules that possess the dual properties of RNA sequence-specific recognition, analogous to conventional antisense molecules, and site-specific cleavage of RNA substrates, thereby intercepting gene expression and forestalling subsequent translation. Whereas cleavage is mediated by the ribozyme's catalytic core, substrate recognition occurs through complementary flanking sequences. Among several naturally occurring ribozymes that have been identified, the hammerhead and hairpin types are the best characterized.

In contrast to antisense RNA, ribozymes are known to be reutilized within the cell. Being an RNA, however, ribozymes are unstable molecules and are easily digested by intracellular nucleases. Therefore, after the initial report of the original structure of a hammerhead ribozyme *(13,14)*, attempts have been made to improve the ribozyme structure in terms of stability and thus efficiency of cleavage activity *(19–21)*.

1.3. Vectors

In order to transfer anti-*MDR*1 ribozyme into target cells, vectors are needed: nonviral, retrovirus, and adenovirus vectors are commonly used. Our experience with a nonviral vector, pHβAPr-1-neo, a β-actin driven vector developed by Dr. L. Kedes of the University of Southern California *(22)*, and a retroviral vector, N2A+tRNA$_i^{met}$ *(23)* will be detailed. Moloney murine leukemia virus-based double copy retroviral vector N2A was developed by Dr. Ira Gilboa of Duke University Medical Center *(24)*. A 500-bp DNA fragment containing the Δ3′-5 mutant human tRNA$_i^{met}$ gene was excised from plasmid phH2DΔ3′-5 (provided by Dr. Michael Zasloff at Magainin Research Institute, Plymouth Meeting, PA) with the restriction enzymes *Bam*HI and *Stu*I, and cloned into the *Sna*BI site present in the 3′LTR of the N2A vector. This vector, designated as N2A+tRNA$_i^{met}$, contains human met$_i$ tRNA-driven polymerase III promoter. After ligation of the Δ3′-5 mutant tRNA$_i^{met}$ gene we confirmed the sequence and orientation of the gene in the vector by DNA sequencing using Sequenase version 2.0 kit (U.S. Biochemical, Cleveland, OH).

2. Materials
2.1. Cell Lines

Human tumor cell lines used are: MOLT-3 acute lymphoblastic leukemia cell line *(25)* and it's MDR subline, MOLT-3/TMQ$_{800}$ cells *(15)*; Daudi Burkitt lymphoma cell line *(26)*; MCF-7 breast carcinoma cell line and its MDR subline MCF-7/R *(27)*. Originally, we used MOLT-3 cells for the ribozyme study, but we found that this cell line had a very poor tumor take rate when transplanted to nude or SCID mice. In contrast, Daudi cells had an acceptable take rate. If animal experiments are contemplated it is advised that Daudi or other cell lines with an acceptable take rate be used. NIH/3T3 cells were established from NIH Swiss mouse embryo cultures *(28)*. The NIH/3T3 cells are highly sensitive to sarcoma virus focus formation. GP+*env*AM 12 is a viral packaging cell line originated from the NIH/3T3 cell line *(29)*. MOLT-3, Daudi, and MCF-7 cell lines, as well as NIH/3T3 cell line, are available from American Type Culture Collection (ATCC, Rockville, MD). MOLT-3/TMQ$_{800}$ cells are available from the authors' laboratory. MCF-7/R cells are available in Dr. Kenneth Cowan's Laboratory in the NCI, Bethesda, MD. GP+*env*AM 12 cells may be obtained from Dr. Arthur Bank of Columbia University. All human tumor cell lines except MCF-7 and MCF-7/R are maintained in RPMI-1640 medium (Life Technologies, Life Technologies, Gaithersburg, MD or Bio-Whittiker, Walkersville, MD) containing 10% heat inactivated fetal bovine serum (FBS; Sigma, St. Louis, MO; or Life Technologies, or HyClone, Logan,

UT) (Daudi in 20% of FBS). The MCF-7, MCF-7/R, NIH/3T3 and GP+*env*AM 12 cells are maintained in Dulbecco's Modified Eagle Medium (D-MEM, Life Technologies) containing 10% heat inactivated FBS (*see* **Note 1**).

2.2. Reagents

1. DEPC-treated water: Add 0.5 mL of diethyl pyrocarbonate (DEPC, a RNase inhibitor) to 500 mL of dd-H_2O (a final concentration 0.1%), incubate at 37°C overnight and then autoclave.
2. Low TE buffer (10 mM Tris -HCl pH 7.4 and 0.1 mM EDTA): Mix 1 mL of 1M Tris-HCl (pH 7.4), 0.02 mL of 0.5 M EDTA (pH 8.0) and 98.98 mL of DEPC-treated water. Store at 4°C.
3. 1M Tris: Dissolve 121.1 g of Tris base in 800 mL of dd-H_2O. Adjust the pH to the desired value by adding concentrated HCl. Add 70 mL of concentrated HCl for pH 7.4, 60 mL for pH 7.6, 42 mL for pH 8.0. Allow the solution to cool to room temperature and make additional adjustments of the pH. Adjust the volume to 1 L. Sterilize by autoclaving.
4. 0.5 M EDTA (pH 8.0): Add 186.1 g of disodium ethylenediaminetetra-acetate·2H_2O to 800 mL of dd-H_2O. Stir vigorously using a magnetic stirrer. Adjust the pH to 8.0 with NaOH (~20 g of NaOH pellets). Sterilize by autoclaving.
5. 70% ethanol: Mix 70 mL of absolute ethanol and DEPC-treated water up to 100 mL. Store at –20°C.
6. 10X reaction buffer (for restriction endonuclease of DNA/RNA modifying enzymes): Use the reaction buffer supplied with each enzyme provided by suppliers.
7. TE buffer (10 mM Tris -HCl pH 7.4 and 0.1 mM EDTA): Mix 1 mL of 1M Tris-HCl (pH 8.0), 0.2 mL of 0.5M EDTA (pH 8.0) and 98.8 mL of DEPC-treated water. Store at 4°C.
8. Acid-equilibrated phenol:chloroform:isoamylalcohol: Sigma Product number P1944 (for the purification of RNA from mixture of DNA, RNA, and protein).
9. 7.5M ammonium acetate: Dissolve 57.81 g of ammonium acetate in 80 mL of DEPC-treated water. Adjust the final volume to 100 mL with DEPC-treated water.
10. 1M $MgCl_2$: dissolve 20.33 g of $MgCl_2$·6H_2O (new batch) in 80 mL of DEPC-treated water. Adjust the final volume to 100 mL with DEPC-treated water. Sterilize by autoclaving. Store as a sterile solution at room temperature.
11. Stop buffer (for in vitro cleavage reaction; 95% deionized formamide, 20 mM EDTA, 0.05% bromophenol blue, 0.05% xylene cyanol): Mix 950 µL of formamide (molecular biology grade), 20 µL of 0.5 M EDTA (pH 8.0), 15 µL of 3.3% bromophenol blue, and 15 µL of 3.3% xylene cyanol. Store at 4°C for several weeks.
12. 10X TBE Buffer (electrophoresis buffer): Dissolve 108 g of Tris base, 55 g of boric acid and 8.3 g of EDTA (disodium salt, dihydrate) in 900 mL of DEPC-treated water. Adjust the final volume to 1 L and then pass through a 0.22 or 0.45 µm filter. Store at room temperature. *Caution:* A precipitate may form when

stored for long periods. To avoid this store the 5X solution in glass bottles at room temperature.

13. 30% Acrylamide/*bis*-acrylamide (19:1) stock solution: Add 240.6 mL of dd-H$_2$O to a bottle containing 100 g acrylamide/methylene *bis*-acrylamide (19:1) (Boehringer Mannheim, Indianapolis, IN) and stir for complete dissolution of acrylamide/*bis*-acrylamide. Filter through 0.45 μm filterware (Nalgene, Fisher Scientific) and store at 4°C.

14. 10% methanol/10% acetate: Add 200 mL of methanol and 200 mL of glacial acetic acid to 2 L of H$_2$O. Store at room temperature.

15. G418 stock solution (50 mg/mL): Dissolve 1 g active Geneticin (Life Technologies) in 20 mL of 0.1M HEPES solution (Life Technologies), filter sterilize and store the aliquots at –20°C.

16. 2X (or 0.2X) SSC/0.1% SDS: dilute 50 mL (or 5 mL) of 20x SSC and 5 mL of 10% SDS in 445 mL (or 490 mL) dd-H$_2$O.

17. 20X SSC: dissolve 175.3 g of NaCl and 88.2 g of sodium citrate in 800 mL of dd-H$_2$O. Adjust the pH to 7.0 with a 10 N NaOH. Adjust the volume to 1 L with dd-H$_2$O. Dispense into aliquots. Sterilize by autoclaving.

18. 10% SDS (sodium dodecylsulfate): Dissolve 100 g of SDS (electrophoresis grade) in 900 mL of dd-H$_2$O. Heat to 68°C to aid dissolution. Adjust the pH to 7.2 by adding a few drops of concentrated HCl. Add dd-H$_2$O to the final volume of 1 L. *Caution:* Wear a mask when weighing SDS and wipe the weighing area and balance after use.

19. Hypotonic Lysis Buffer (10 mM Tris pH 7.4, 10 mM KCl, 1.5 mM MgCl$_2$, 2 mM PMSF) for the preparation of membrane fraction: dilute 100 μL of 1M Tris pH 7.4, 100 μL of 1M KCl, 15 μl of 1M MgCl$_2$, and 2 mL of 10 mM PMSF in 7.785 mL dd-H$_2$O just before use.

20. 10 mM PMSF: dissolve PMSF (phenylmethylsulfonyl fluoride) in isopropanol at a concentration of 1.74 mg/mL. Store at –20°C in aliquots. PMSF is not stable in aqueous solutions, prepare daily, and keep cold. *Caution:* PMSF is corrosive and causes severe burns on the skin. Wear gloves, protective clothing, and safety glasses. Handle PMSF in a chemical hood.

21. MRK16 (antibody which reacts with a cellular surface epitope of P-gp): available from Kamiya Biochemical, Seattle, WA in a size of 150 μg/300 μL of PBS, 0.1% NaN$_3$ and 1% bovine serum albumin. *Caution:* MRK16 has good reactivity in flow-cytometric analysis and in immunoprecipitation reaction; however, the antibody does not react in Western blotting because the antibody loses its structure in the presence of protein denaturing agents such as SDS. For Western blotting use C494 from Signet, Dedham, MA (*see* **Subheading 3.1.3.2.**)

22. Mouse IgG2a pure stock solution: use either mouse monoclonal antihuman β-2 microglobulin subtype IgG2a from BioSource International, Camarillo, CA or mouse IgG2a Pure solution containing pure mouse IgG2a from Becton Dickinson, San Jose, CA. We prefer the IgG2a from Becton Dickinson.

23. 6X (or 1X) SSPC/1% SDS: dilute 150 mL (or 25 mL) of 20X SSPE and 50 mL of 10% SDS in 300 mL (or 425 mL) dd-H$_2$O.

24. 20X SSPC: dissolve 175.3 g of NaCl, 27.6 g of $NaH_2PO_4 \cdot H_2O$, and 7.4 g of EDTA in 800 mL of dd-H_2O. Adjust the pH to 7.4 with NaOH (~6.5 mL of a 10 N solution). Adjust the volume to 1 L with dd-H_2O. Sterilize by autoclaving.

25. LB medium: add 10 g of Bacto-Tryptone (Difco Laboratories, Detroit, MI), 5 g of Bacto-Yeast Extract (Difco or Becton Dickinson, Cockeysville, MD) and 10 g of NaCl in 950 mL of dd-H_2O. Stir the solution until complete dissolution of the powders. Adjust the pH to 7.0 with 5 N NaOH (~0.2 mL). Adjust the final volume of the solution to 1 L with dd-H_2O. Sterilize by autoclaving. Store at 4°C.

26. 1X PBS (Dulbecco's Phosphate Buffered Saline solution 1x, Cellgro™): purchased from Mediatech, Herndon, VA. We used this solution for transfection experiments (*see* **Subheading 3.3.2.1.**) In these experiments we have not tested PBS solutions from Life Technologies.

27. Polybrene stock solution (8 mg/mL): dissolve 0.8 g of hexadimethrine bromide (Sigma) in 100 mL of dd-H_2O supplied by Cellgro, and filter sterilize through 0.2 μm filterware (Nalgene, Rochester, NY) and store at –20°C in aliquots.

28. 0.8% (or 1.8%) Agarose (for DNA size determination, e.g., *see* **Subheading 3.3.1.2., step 2**; **3.3.1.3., step 4**; **3.3.6.1., step 4**): add 0.8 g (or 1.8 g) of agarose (Bio-Rad, Hercules, CA) in 1X TBE buffer to 100 mL volume. Warm the solution in a microwave oven for 2–3 min for complete dissolution of agarose. Add 10 μL of ethidium bromide stock solution (5 mg/mL, see below) into 0.8% (or 1.8%) agarose solution. *Caution:* Ethidium bromide is considered to be carcinogenic. Wear disposable gloves.

29. Ethidium bromide stock solution (5 mg/mL): Add 500 mg of ethidium bromide to 100 mL of dd-H_2O. Stir on a magnetic stirrer until the dye has completely dissolved. Transfer the solution to a dark bottle and wrap it in aluminum foil and store at 4°C. *Caution:* Ethidium bromide is considered to be carcinogenic and gloves should be worn when working with solutions that contain the dye.

30. 10% ammonium persulfate stock solution: to 1 g of ammonium persulfate (Sigma), add DEPC-treated water to 10 mL. Stir at room temperature until ammonium persulfate is dissolved. Dispense the solution into small aliquots and store at –20°C.

31. FTIC-conjugated monoclonal sheep antimouse IgG2a: Sigma Product number F2883, Sigma (used as a secondary antibody, *see* **Subheading 3.3.5.**).

32. Phenol:choloroform:isoamylalcohol (25:24:1): Sigma Product number P2069, Sigma (for DNA extraction, *see* **Subheading 3.3.6.1.**).

Practically all chemicals described above are available from Sigma or Aldrich, Milwaukee, WI.

In recent years, a number of new kits have become commercially available, which has made molecular biological work much easier. We started this work in 1993. The methods described in the initial portions of this chapter were used some time ago. For the convenience of readers, similar work done in more recent years is also described in later sections of the text.

Table 1.
Template cDNA sequences of anti-*MDR*1 ribozymes (1)
(*see* Subheading 3.1.1.1.)

Ribozyme	Template cDNA sequence
RibTop	5′-CATG<u>TAATACGACTCACTATAGGG</u>-3′
179*MDR*1	5′-GATGATGTTTCGTCCTCACGGACTCATCAGTCCAAGAT
	<u>CCCTATAGTGAGTCGTATTA</u>CATG-3′
196*MDR*1	5′-CTTTCAGTTTCGTCCTCACGGACTCATCAGAATGGCAA
	<u>CCCTATAGTGAGTCGTATTA</u>CATG-3′
Mut-196*MDR*1	5′-CTTTCAGTgTCGTCCTCACGGACTCATaAGAATGGCAA
	<u>CCCTATAGTGAGTCGTATTA</u>CATG-3′

T7 promoter sequence is underlined. Small letters are mutated bases. From **ref. *15*.**

3. Methods

3.1. Anti-MDR1 Ribozyme Gene Transfer to Human Leukemic Cells In Vitro with the Aid of a Human β-Actin Expression Vector System (15)

In this section, we describe actual methods for nine experiments. 1) construction of anti-*MDR*1 ribozymes; 2) creation of a substrate for the cleavage reaction; 3) cleavage reaction in a cell-free system; 4) transduction of *MDR*1 ribozymes in human leukemic cells; and 5) five different procedures to determine the biological effects of ribozymes on multidrug resistant cells.

3.1.1. Anti-MDR1 Ribozyme Synthesis, the Creation of Substrate RNA and Determination of Cleavage Activity in a Cell-Free System

3.1.1.1. Production of Hammerhead Ribozyme

Initially, we developed two hammerhead ribozymes; one, targeted against a GUC sequence at codon 179, six amino acids upstream from amino acid codon 185, and another at codon 196, 11 amino acids downstream from the same site. The codon 185 is known to be one of the important sites for substrate preference *(15)* (**Table 1, Fig. 1**).

The ribozyme RNA structure was modeled after that of Haseloff and Gerlach *(14)*, and was made by the method described by Milligan et al. *(30)*. In this method, hammerhead ribozymes are produced by in vitro transcription from template cDNAs of ribozyme, which are synthesized by a DNA synthesizer. (We ordered them from Genset, La Jolla, CA. We received approximately 2.0 m*M* concentrations of DNAs in approximately 100 μL volume, or approximately 2 nmols/μL). The template cDNAs are composed of top strand and

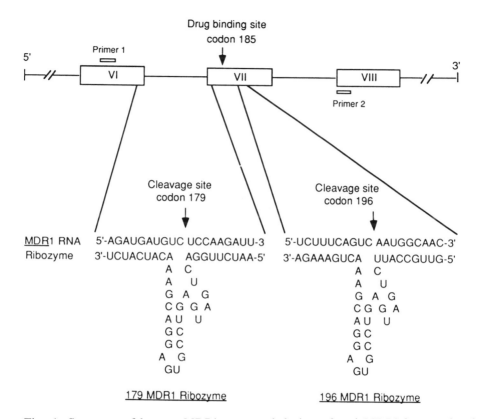

Fig. 1. Structure of human *MDR1* gene and design of anti-*MDR1* hammerhead ribozymes (modified from **ref. 15**, reprinted with permission). *See* **Subheading 3.1.1.2.1.** for the explanation of Primer 1 and Primer 2.

bottom strand. The top strand contains the bacteriophage T7 RNA polymerase promoter sequence (5′-CATGTAATACGACTCACTATAGGG-3′) (RibTop). The bottom strand contains both the T7 RNA polymerase promoter region and the complementary sequence of each hammerhead ribozyme (*see* **Note 2**). These are used to produce ribozymes by forming hemiduplex as template cDNA (*see* **Subheading 3.3.6.3.**)

1. Resuspend the oligodeoxynucleotides to a final concentration of 10 pmols/μL in DEPC-treated water and in aliquots (*see* **Note 2**).
2. Mix 2.5 μL of template cDNA (25 pmols), the same amount of RibTop, and 58 μL of low TE buffer in 1.5-mL microcentrifuge tube.
3. Place the tube at 80°C for 2 min.
4. Cool the tube slowly to room temperature to form hemiduplex with template cDNA and RibTop.

5. Add 6 μL of 100 m*M* MgCl$_2$, 2 μL of 100 m*M* ATP, 2 μL of 100 m*M* GTP, 2 μL of 100 m*M* CTP, 2 μL of 100 m*M* UTP, 3 μL of rRNasin (120 U) (Promega, Madison, WI), 10 μL of NEBuffer for RNA polymerase and 10 μL of T7 RNA polymerase (500 U) (New England Biolabs, Beverly, MA) (total volume 100 μL) (NEBuffer is supplied with T7 RNA polymerase).
6. Place the tube at 37°C for 4 h.
7. Add 10 μL (10 U) of RQI RNase-free DNase (Promega).
8. Place the tube at 37°C for 15 min.
9. Add 100 μL of acid phenol-chloroform-isoamylalcohol (phenol:chloroform: isoamylalcohol = 125:24:1, Sigma), wrap the cap of the tube with Parafilm® (Fisher Scientific, Pittsburgh, PA) and shake vigorously until an emulsion forms.
10. Centrifuge the tube at 12,000*g* for 2 min (e.g., Eppendorf centrifuge Model 5411, Brinkman Instruments, Westbury, NY).
11. Remove the lower phenol-chloroform phase.
12. Add 100 μL of chloroform and shake vigorously until an emulsion forms.
13. Centrifuge the tube at 12,000*g* for 2 min.
14. Transfer the upper aqueous phase to a new tube.
15. Add 50 μL of 7.5*M* ammonium acetate and 375 μL of 100% ethanol (–20°C), and shake the tube gently.
16. Place the tube at –80°C for 30 minutes.
17. Centrifuge the tube at 12,000*g* for 30 min at 4°C.
18. Remove the supernatant.
19. Add 800 μL of ice-cold 70% ethanol.
20. Place the tube at room temperature for 3 min.
21. Centrifuge the tube at 12,000*g* for 20 min.
22. Remove the supernatant.
23. Keep tube open on the bench (at room temperature) to air-dry for a few minutes.
24. Resuspend in 51 μL of DEPC-treated water.
25. Transfer 1 μL of the solution to a new tube and dilute it with 199 μL of DEPC-treated water.
26. Check the absorbance of the diluted solution at 260 nm with a spectrophotometer. (1.0 OD$_{260}$ = 40 μg RNA/mL).
27. Store the solution at –80°C in aliquots.

The biological activities of anti-*MDR*1 ribozymes created in **Subheading 3.1.1.1.** can be examined by their substrate cleavage efficiency. For the examination of cleavage activity, we also created a disabled 196*MDR*1 ribozyme by mutating two bases (G3→U3, A22→C22) in the sequence of ribozyme catalytic core structure, which destroyed the catalytic activity of the ribozyme (**Fig. 2**).

3.1.1.2. CREATION OF SUBSTRATE RNA

We constructed the plasmid containing a fragment of human *MDR*1 gene. With the plasmid, we produced substrates for cleavage reaction in a cell-free

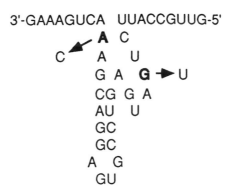

Fig. 2. Mutated 196 *MDR*1 ribozyme. Functionally indispensable residues are indicated by bold letters. These residues are mutated in order to make a disabled ribozyme that has no cleavage activity (from **ref. 15**, reprinted with permission).

system by in vitro transcription. First, we extracted total cellular RNA from MOLT-3/TMQ$_{800}$ cells and amplified the fragments of human *MDR*1 gene by RT-PCR. cDNA was synthesized by using Moloney murine leukemia virus reverse transcriptase (Life Technologies) with random hexamer (Pharmacia, Piscataway, NJ) as a primer. The reverse transcription reaction was carried out at 42°C for 1 h. Exons 6 through 8 were then amplified from this cDNA by using GeneAmp PCR Core Reagent Kit (Perkin-Elmer Cetus, Norwalk, CT) with oligonucleotide primers from exon 6 (5′-TTCATGCTATAATGCGACA GGAGATA) and exon 8 (5′-TTCTTTATCAGTAAATGAAGATAGTA). The clear and distinct 266-bp product was identified in 1.8% agarose gel and 1 × Tris-acetate EDTA buffer. PCR reaction was performed with Taq DNA polymerase (AmpliTaq™, Perkin-Elmer, Branchburg, NJ). After an initial denaturation step at 98°C for 3 min, 30 cycles of amplification were performed. Each step was as follows; denaturation at 95°C for 30 s, annealing at 60°C for 1 min and extension at 72°C for 1 min. One other cycle, in which annealing at 60°C for 2 min and extension at 72°C for 10 min, was performed after the 30 cycles. The PCR products were ligated directly to pT7Blue T-vector (Novagen, Madison, WI). After transformation of *Escherichia coli*, white colonies were selected and screened. Plasmid DNAs were prepared with Qiagen Plasmid Midi Kit (Qiagen, Valencia, CA), and the sequences and the directions were confirmed using ABI sequencer 373S (Perkin-Elmer Applied Biosystems).

To linearize plasmid DNA template by digesting with *Bam*HI:

1. Mix 5 μL of template plasmid with 5 μL of 10X Reaction buffer (supplied with enzyme purchased from company), 2 μL of *Bam*HI and add dd-H$_2$O to a volume of 50 μL.

2. Place the tube at 37°C for 3 h.
3. Add 50 µL of dd-H$_2$O.
4. Add 100 µL of refrigerated phenol-chloroform (phenol:chloroform = 1:1) and shake the tube vigorously until an emulsion forms.
5. Centrifuge the tube at 12,000g for 2 min.
6. Remove the lower phenol-chloroform phase.
7. Repeat **steps 4–6** three times.
8. Add 100 µL of chloroform and shake the tube until an emulsion forms.
9. Centrifuge the tube at 12,000g for 2 min.
10. Remove the lower chloroform phase.
11. Repeat **steps 8–10** three times.
12. Add 10 µL of 5M NaCl and 400 µL of ethanol (–20°C), and mix well.
13. Place the tube at 20°C for more than 1 h.
14. Centrifuge the tube at 12,000g for 15 min at 4°C.
15. Remove the supernatant.
16. Add 800 µL of ice-cold 70% ethanol.
17. Centrifuge the tube at 12,000g for 5 min at 4°C.
18. Remove the supernatant.
19. Keep the tube open on the bench for a few minutes to air-dry.
20. Dissolve the pellet with 19.5 µL of DEPC-treated dd-H$_2$O. Store the tube at –20°C or use immediately.

Radiolabeling of the substrate:

For the handling of [^{32}P]rCTP, proper care generally applicable to the handling of isotope-labeled substrates must be followed.

1. Mix 2.5 mg linearized plasmid in 19.5 µL of DEPC-treated water with 1.25 µL (25 U) of T7 RNA polymerase (Promega), 10 µL of Transcription Optimized 5X Buffer (Promega), 5 µL of 100 mM DTT, 1.25 µL (50 U) of RNasin (Promega), 2.5 µL of 10 mM ATP, 2.5 µL of 10 mM GTP, 0.5 µL of 10 mM CTP, 2.5 µL of 10 mM UTP and 5 µL of [^{32}P]rCTP (specific activity 800 Ci/mmol, DuPont, Boston, MA) in 1.5-mL microcentrifuge tube.
2. Place the tube at 30°C for 3 h.
3. Add 5 µL (5 U) of RQI RNase-free DNase (Promega).
4. Place the tube at 37°C for 15 minutes.
5. Add 45 µL of TE buffer (10 mM Tris-HCl pH 8.0 and 1 mM EDTA).
6. Add 100 µL of acid phenol-chloroform-isoamylalcohol (phenol:chloroform:isoamylalcohol = 125:24:1, Sigma) and shake vigorously until an emulsion forms.
7. Centrifuge the tube at 12,000g for 2 min.
8. Remove the lower phenol-chloroform phase.
9. Add 100 µl of chloroform and shake the tube until an emulsion forms.
10. Centrifuge the tube at 12,000g for 2 min.
11. Remove the lower phenol-chloroform phase.
12. Transfer the upper aqueous phase to a new tube.

13. Add 50 µl of 7.5 M ammonium acetate and 375 µl of ice-cold absolute (100%) ethanol.
14. Place the tube at −70°C for 30 min.
15. Centrifuge the tube at 12,000g for 30 min at 4°C.
16. Remove the supernatant.
17. Add 800 µl of ice-cold 70% ethanol (to rinse the pellet).
18. Centrifuge the tube at 12,000g for 20 min at 4°C.
19. Remove the supernatant.
20. Keep the tube open on the bench for a few min to air-dry.
21. Dissolve the pellet with 100 µl of DEPC-treated water.
22. Check the RNA concentration in the solution with a spectrophotometer. (1.0 OD$_{260}$ = 40 µg/ml RNA) (*see* **Subheading 3.1.1.1., steps 25** and **26**).
23. Store at −80°C in aliquots (*see* **Note 3**).

3.1.1.3. CLEAVAGE ACTIVITY OF ANTI-*MDR*1 RIBOZYMES IN A CELL-FREE SYSTEM (*SEE* **SUBHEADING 3.3.6.4.**)

Concentrations of substrate RNAs and ribozymes should be adjusted when you carry out the cleavage reaction. If you would like to carry out the cleavage reaction in various concentration of Mg^{2+}, you should change the concentration of MgCl$_2$ added to different tubes.

1. Mix substrate RNA and ribozyme in various concentrations in a total volume of 6 µL and then add 2 µL of 5 mM EDTA and 2 µL of 250 mM Tris-HCl buffer pH 7.4.
2. Heat the tube at 95°C for 2 min.
3. Place the tube on ice to be cooled quickly.
4. Add 1.1 µL of 100 mM MgCl$_2$ (final concentration 10 mM).
5. Place the tube at 37°C for more than 3 h.
6. Add 8 µL of Stop Buffer (95% formamide, 20 mM EDTA, 0.05% bromophenol blue, 0.05% xylene cyanol).
7. Transfer 8 µL of the solution to a new tube.
8. Heat the new tube at 80°C for 8 min.
9. Place the tube on ice.

3.1.1.4. ELECTROPHORESIS AND AUTORADIOGRAPHY

Electrophoresis is performed using sequencing gel apparatus. You should make sequencing gel between a set of glass plates while cleavage reactions are in progress. The gel contains 6% polyacrylamide (acrylamide : N,N′-methylene-*bis*-acrylamide = 19 : 1, Bio-Rad, Hercules, CA) and 7M urea in 1X TBE. Use DEPC-treated dd-H$_2$O in making the gel and buffer solution.

1. Assemble the glass-plate sandwich of the electrophoresis apparatus and lock the sandwich to the casing stand.

2. Prepare the solution of 6% acrylamide/7M urea gel
   25.2 g Urea (Boehringer Mannheim)
   6.0 ml 10X TBE buffer stock solution
   12 mL 30% acrylamide/*bis*-acrylamide (19:1) (Boehringer Mannheim)
   17 mL DEPC-treated dd-H_2O to a total volume of 60 mL
   Stir at room temperature until urea is dissolved. Add 480 µL of 10% ammonium persulfate in dd-H_2O and 64 µL of TEMED (Sigma) (both of which catalyze polymerization).
3. Mix briefly after adding the last two ingredients and pour gel immediately.
4. Allow the gel to polymerize for 30 min at room temperature.
5. Fix the sandwich to the electrophoresis apparatus and fill the upper and lower tanks with the 1x TBE electrophoresis buffer, which is diluted from 10X TBE stock solution with DEPC-treated water.
6. Rinse the wells with the 1X TBE electrophoresis buffer and load the RNA sample from the cleavage reactions in cell-free system.
7. Warm up the gel by running at ~1750 V for 30 min (pre-run, optional).
8. After warming up, load 2 µL of the heated solution in each well.
9. Run the gel at 1500 to 2500 V.
10. When bromophenol blue migrates to the end of gel, turn off the power pack switch.
11. Dispose of the electrophoresis buffer, and then remove the gel mold from the apparatus.
12. Remove one side of glass plates and leave the gel on the other side of the glass plate. Immerse the gel in the solution of 10% methanol/10% acetate (10% methanol (v/v) and 10% acetic acid (v/v) in dd-H_2O) for 10 min (to wash urea out of the gel).
13. Place a piece of Whatman 3MM paper (Whatman, Hillsboro, OR) on the gel. Then, place sheets of Kimwipes on the Whatman 3MM paper and press the Kimwipes to make a tight contact between the Whatman 3MM paper and the gel.
14. Dispose of Kimwipes.
15. Remove the Whatman 3MM paper with the gel from a glass plate.
16. Cover the gel with Saran Wrap.
17. Dry the Whatman 3MM paper and the gel at 80°C for 30–60 min using a gel dryer.
18. Expose the gel to X-ray film (XAR-5, Eastman Kodak, Rochester, NY, or Fuji Medical X-ray Film, Fuji Medical Systems USA, Stanford, CT) for 10 min to 2 h at –70°C.
19. Develop the films.

3.1.2. Expression of Anti-MDR1 Ribozymes in Human Leukemic Cells with the Aid of a Human β-actin Expression Vector

The 196 *MDR*1 ribozyme was found to be more active than the 179 one in a cell-free system. Because of this, we performed subsequent transfection studies with the 196*MDR*1 ribozyme. We used MOLT-3/TMQ$_{800}$ cells.

The 196 *MDR*1 ribozyme used for transfection study was designed differently from that used in the cell-free system. Two single-stranded oligodeoxynucleotides were synthesized such that the 45-base pair ribozyme contained flanking *Sal*I and *Hind*III restriction sites on each end (Genset) and were 5′ phosphorylated by T4 polynucleotide kinase (New England Biolabs, Beverly, MA), 5′-pTCGACGTTGCCATTCTGATGAGTCCGTGAGGACG AAACTGAAAGA-3′, and 5′-pAGCTTCTTTCAGTTTCGTCCTCACGGA CTCATCAGAATGGCAACG-3′ (*see* **Subheading 3.3.1.1., step 3.**). This ribozyme was cloned into the pHβAPr-1-neo *(22)*. The sequence and orientation of the ribozyme in the vector was confirmed by DNA sequencing. The disabled 196 *MDR*1 ribozyme for transfection experiments was also synthesized in the same manner, and cloned into the same vector.

1. Mix 2 μL (0.2 nmols) of each 5′-unphosphorylated oligodeoxynucleotide (*see* **Note 4**) with 2 μL (20 U) of T4 polynucleotide kinase (New England Biolabs), 3 μL of 10X Reaction Buffer (supplied with enzyme), 3 μL of 10 m*M* ATP and 20 μL of dd-H$_2$O in each microcentrifuge tube.
2. Place the tube at 37°C for 1 h.
3. Combine these two reaction mixtures into a single tube.
4. Place the tube at 95°C for 5 min.
5. Cool down the tube slowly to room temperature to form hemiduplex.
6. Dilute the **step 5** reaction mixture with dd-H$_2$O by 50-fold, and use 1 μL for the following ligation reaction.
7. Mix 0.2 μg of pHβAPr-1-neo plasmid DNA previously cut (*see* **step 7a** *below*) with *Sal*I and *Hind*III with 1 μL of diluted **step 6** reaction mixture (approx two-fold molar of the vector), 1 μL (400 U) of T4 DNA ligase (New England Biolabs), 1 μL of 10X Reaction buffer, and dd-H$_2$O up to 10 μL.
7a. Cutting of pHβAPr-1-neo plasmid DNA with *Sal*I and *Hind*III.
   a. Digest 15 μg of pHβAPr-1-neo plasmid DNA with 400 U of *Hind*III in 400 μL volume at 37°C for 1–2 h.
   b. Heat inactivate *Hind*III at 65°C for 20 min.
   c. Adjust NaCl concentration to 150 m*M*, then add 200 U of *Sal*I. Digest it at 37°C for 2 h.
   d. Electrophorese the digested product and cut the larger band.
   e. Purify the band with GeneClean® (Bio 101, Vista, CA). Measure the absorbance at 260 nm with a spectrophotometer (1.0 OD$_{260}$ = 50 μg double stranded DNA/mL).
8. Place the tube at 12°C for 4 h to overnight to complete ligation.

After transformation of DH5α competent cells (Life Technologies) (*see* **Subheading 3.3.1.2.**), the colonies are screened by PCR to check the existence of the insert. The primers used for this screening were: 5′-AGCACAG AGCCTCGCCTTT (from β-actin 5′-untranslated region) and 5′-TGGA

TCCCTCGAAGCTT (from plasmid polylinker). Plasmid DNAs were prepared with Qiagen Plasmid Midi Kit (Qiagen), and the sequences and the directions were confirmed using ABI sequencer 373S.

Transfection of plasmid DNA by electroporation:

1. Wash logarithmically growing cells twice with RPMI-1640 medium (no FBS) and resuspend the cells at a final concentration of 5×10^6 cells/500 μL in RPMI-1640 medium (no FBS) in a electroporation cuvette.
2. Add 20 μg of plasmid DNA (sterile) to the cell suspension and mix gently.
3. Incubate the cuvet on ice for 10 min.
4. Tap the cuvette gently 3–4 times.
5. Subject the cell-DNA mixture to electroporation at 330 V with a capacitance of 1000 μF using Electroporator II (Invitrogen, Carlsbad, CA).
6. After a further 10 min incubation at room temperature, dilute the cells with 10 mL of RPMI-1640 medium containing 10% FBS.
7. Plate the cells into 24-well culture dishes (Corning Glass Works, Corning, NY), and incubate them at 37°C in a humidified 5% CO_2/95% air atmosphere.
8. Change the medium 24 h later (without disturbing the cells sitting at the bottom of the wells).
9. Three days after electroporation, add G418 at a concentration of 1 mg/mL as an active moiety.
10. Change one half of the medium (plus G418 at a concentration of 1 mg/mL as an active moiety) twice a week.
11. Three to four wk later, select the well in which G418-resistant cells are growing, and subclone them by the limiting dilution method (*see below* **step 11a**).
11a. Limiting dilution method. Briefly, cells are serially diluted from 5×10^5 to 0.5 cells per 100 μL in RPMI-1640 medium supplemented with 10% FBS plus G418. Then, 24–48 aliquots of each diluted sample are placed in flat-bottomed microculture plates. Cells are fed every 4 d and incubated at 37°C for 12–24 d. Growth at each serial dilution is assessed in an "all-or-nothing" (positive or negative) fashion under an inverted phase-contrast microscope.

3.1.3. Evaluation of the Effect of MDR1 Ribozymes on Multidrug-Resistant Human Leukemic Cells

3.1.3.1. NORTHERN BLOT ANALYSIS OF MDR1 EXPRESSION

For Northern blot analysis of *MDR1* expression, the cDNA for *MDR1*, pMDR 2000XS *(31)* (kindly provided by Dr. M. Gottesman of the National Cancer Institute, Bethesda, MD) is used. The *Bst*UI-*Pme*I fragment is excised, radiolabeled, and used as the probe. The cDNA for human glyceraldehyde-3-phosphate dehydrogenase (GAPDH) (pHcGAP) is obtained from the ATCC and the *Pst*I-*Xba*I fragment is used for the probe as an internal control.

1. Harvest $5-10 \times 10^6$ cells (do not wash) and make a pellet. Add 1 mL of TRIzol® Reagent (Life Technologies) and follow steps provided in the accompanying instruction sheet to isolate total cellular RNA.
2. Size-fractionate 10 μg total RNA per lane by electrophoresis in $0.41M$ formaldehyde/1% agarose gels.
3. Transfer the size-fractionated RNA onto Maximum Strength Nytran nylon membrane using TurboBlotter™ Rapid Downward Transfer Systems (Schleicher and Schuell, Keene, NH).
4. Expose the membranes to ultraviolet light (254 nm) for fixation of RNA (for a total dose of 120 mJ/cm²).
5. Hybridize the membranes with [³²P] labeled cDNA probes at 42°C for 12–18 h using a rotator (with swirling) (For radiolabeling of cDNA probe, kits are available, e.g., NEBlot™ Kit, New England Biolabs).
6. Pour off hybridization solution and add an equal volume of 2X SSC/0.1% SDS. Incubate with gentle swirling motion for 10 min at room temperature, then wash solution and repeat once. (Dispose of the waste as if radioactive waste)
7a. (For low-stringency wash) Replace with equal volume of 0.2X SSC/0.1% SDS and incubate for 10 min with a swirling motion at room temperature.
7b. (For moderate-stringency wash) Prewarm 0.2X SSC/0.1% SDS to 42°. Replace with equal volume of 0.2X SSC/0.1% SDS and incubate for 15 min at 42°C with a swirling motion.
7c. (For high-stringency wash) Prewarm 0.2X SSC/0.1% SDS to 68°. Replace with equal volume of 0.2X SSC/0.1% SDS and incubate for 15 min at 68°C with a swirling motion.
8. After adequate washing of the membranes, expose the membranes to X-ray film (*see* **Subheading 3.1.1.4., step 18**) between two intensifying screens at –80°C for 4–24 h.
9. Develop the autoradiograph.
10. Measure the intensities of specific signals by a scanning densitometer and normalize to GAPDH signal as an internal standard.

3.1.3.2. WESTERN BLOT ANALYSIS OF P-GP EXPRESSION

For Western blot analysis of P-gp, the monoclonal antibody C494 (Signet, Dedham, MA) is used.

Plasma membranes are prepared and purified according to the method of Riordan and Ling *(32)*.

1. Wash cells twice with cold Dulbecco's phosphate buffered saline (PBS) (Life Technologies), place them in Hypotonic Lysis Buffer (10 mM Tris pH 7.4, 10 mM KCl, 1.5 mM MgCl$_2$, 2 mM PMSF), and incubate them for 30 min at room temperature.
2. Centrifuge the swollen cells at 400g for 10 min, and resuspend the pellet in 0.5 mL of Hypotonic Lysis Buffer.

3. Rupture the cells with a 2-mL Ten Broeck homogenizer (Corning Glass Works, Corning, NY). Monitor disruption by phase contrast microscopy until ≥95% of cells are broken.
4. Pool the homogenate and centrifuge them at 4,000g for 10 min (to remove cell debris).
5. Centrifuge the supernatant at 40,000g for 60 min (e.g., Beckman ultracentrifuge L5-75 or Sorval RC-5B centrifuge) (to collect the membrane pellets).
6. Resuspend the membrane pellet in a small volume of 5 mM Tris pH 7.4 and layer on the gradients. Centrifuge the gradients at 100,000g for 18 h. A discontinuous sucrose gradient consisted of 60%, 45%, 31%, and 16% sucrose (w/v).
7. Collect the membrane fraction at 16/31% interface.
8. Dilute the membrane fraction with 10-times the volume of 5 mM Tris pH 7.4 and mix well.
9. Centrifuge them at 35,000g for 60 min.
10. Dissolve the pellet in 200 μL of 8.6% sucrose in 5 mM Tris pH 7.4.
11. Measure the protein concentration by using BCA protein assay reagent (Pierce, Rockford, IL).
12. Freeze in liquid nitrogen and store at −20°C or lower.

SDS-polyacrylamide gel electrophoresis is performed according to the method of Fairbanks, et al. *(33)*.

1. Mix 50 μg of the plasma membrane preparation from **step 10** above and the one-third volume of 4X Laemmli buffer (250 mM Tris pH 6.8, 8% SDS [w/v], 40% glycerol [v/v], 20% 2-mercaptoethanol, 0.004% bromophenol blue [w/v]).
2. Incubate at 37°C for 30 min.
3. Load onto 2%SDS-5%polyacrylamide gels for electrophoresis.
4. Transfer the size-fractionated plasma membrane onto BA-S 85 nitrocellulose membranes (pore size 0.45 μm, Schleicher & Schuell) using Trans-Blot Cell (Bio-Rad, Hercules, CA).
5. Incubate the membrane with the monoclonal antibody C494 (1 : 800 dilution) for 1 h at room temperature.
6. Wash the membrane three times with 250 mL of PBS containing 0.1% Tween 20 and 0.02% NaN$_3$.
7. Incubate the membrane with the [^{125}I]-labeled Protein A (Amersham M144, Amersham, Arlington Heights, IL) in a hybridization bag with 10 mL of 2% nonfat dry milk, 0.1% Tween 20, 0.02% NaN$_3$ and PBS for 1 h at room temperature with gentle swirling.
8. Wash the membranes six or more times with 200 mL of PBS containing 0.1% Tween 20 and 0.02% NaN$_3$, dry them and subject to autoradiography (*see* **Subheading 3.1.1.4., step 18**).

3.1.3.3. FLOW-CYTOMETRIC ANALYSIS OF P-GP ON THE CELL SURFACE (SEE SUBHEADING 3.3.5.)

Cell surface expression of P-gp was analyzed with anti-human-P-gp mouse monoclonal antibody MRK16 *(34)* (Kamiya Biochemical, Seattle, WA; Kyowa Medicus, Tokyo, Japan), using a standard indirect immunofluorescence assay.

1. Wash logarithmically growing 10^6 cells and resuspend in 0.1~0.5 mL of PBS containing 1 m*M* EDTA.
2. Incubate the cell suspension with heat-inactivated human gamma-globulin (Sigma) at the final concentration of 50 μg/mL at 4°C for 30 min (in order to block nonspecific binding of the antibody to Fc receptors).
3. Incubate the cell suspension with 10 μL (5 μg) of MRK16 at 4°C for 1 h. For negative control, add isotype antibody, mouse IgG_{2a}, instead of MRK16. (To insure that the proper amount of antibody is added, titrate by adding increasing amounts of antibody. When analyzed by FACS, the mean fluorescence and the percent of cells staining positive will reach a plateau when you have reached antibody excess.)
4. After washing twice with PBS, incubate the cells with 10 μL phycoerythrin-conjugated rat anti-mouse IgG_{2a+b} (Becton Dickinson, San Jose, CA) at 4°C for another 1 h in darkness.
5. Wash again with PBS.
6. Add 0.6 mL of 1% paraformaldehyde in PBS to suspend the cells. Transfer the sample to 12 × 75-mm tube for FACS analysis.

3.1.3.4. DETECTION OF RIBOZYME EXPRESSION IN TRANSFECTED CELLS

To detect ribozyme expression in transfected cells, 200 ng of total RNA from each transfectant is subjected to RT-PCR using 2 primers: 5′-AGCA CAGAGCCTCGCCTTT (from β-actin 5′-untranslated region) and 5′-TGGA TCCCTCGAAGCTT (from plasmid polylinker). The cycling conditions are as follows: 94°C for 30 s, 47°C for 3 min, and 72°C for 2 min for 25 cycles. After RT-PCR, a filter containing an amplified 116-base pair RT-PCR product was hybridized using a probe, complementary to normal conserved catalytic sequences, 5′-CCTCACGGACTCATCAG. A high-stringency condition is used to detect normal ribozyme only, in which filters were hybridized with the oligonucleotide probe at 50°C for 4 h and then washed three times in 6X SSPE/1% SDS for 15 min at room temperature and in 1X SSPE/1% SDS for 15 min at 50°C. A low-stringency condition is used to detect not only normal ribozyme, but also disabled ribozyme containing a mismatch with the probe, where 37°C was used for hybridization and filters were washed three times in 6X SSPE/1% SDS for 10 min at room temperature and in 1X SSPE/1% SDS for 3 min at 37°C.

3.1.3.5 Cytotoxicity Assay

For the determination of vincristine sensitivity, we used the 3-(4,5-dimethylthiazol-2-yl)-2, 5-diphenyltetrazolium bromide (MTT, Sigma) assay with minor modifications *(15)*.

1. Place 4×10^3 viable cells in 100 µL of RPMI-1640 medium containing 10% FBS and 100 µL of graded concentrations of vincristine sulfate (Pharmacia, Columbus, OH) in the same medium into 0.2-mL 96-well flat-bottomed culture dishes (Falcon, Becton Dickinson, Lincoln Park, NJ).
2. Incubate the culture dishes for 72 h at 37°C in a humidified 5% CO_2/95% air atmosphere.
3. At the end of the incubation, add 10 µL 0.4% MTT (Sigma) solution (4 mg/mL in PBS) and 10 µL of 0.1M sodium succinate (Sigma) to each well, and incubate the plate for another 4 h at 37°C.
4. Following incubation, centrifuge the plate at 650g for 5 min and remove the supernatants.
5. (To solubilize the Formosan crystals produced) Add 150 µL of dimethylsulfoxide (DMSO, Sigma). Then, thoroughly mix the contents of the wells on a plate shaker for 5 min.
6. Immediately measure the absorbance of each well at 540 nm wavelength using a plate reader (e.g., MRX Automated Plate Reader, Dynex Technologies, Chantilly, VA).
7. Draw dose-response curves by plotting the absorbance, expressed as a percentage of the control value without drug treatment, against drug concentrations.

3.2. Cationic Liposome-Mediated Anti-MDR1 Ribozyme RNA Transfer to Tumor Cells In Vitro (16)

3.2.1. Ribozyme Synthesis

The method of ribozyme synthesis by in vitro transcription is described in **Subheading 3.1.1.1.** (*see* **Note 5.1.**).

3.2.2. Liposome-Mediated Anti-MDR1 Ribozyme Transfection in Human Leukemic and Solid Tumor Cells

For these experiments we used two human tumor cell lines, MOLT-3 and MCF-7, and their MDR sublines, MOLT-3/TMQ$_{800}$ and MCF-7/R, respectively. MOLT-3 and MCF-7 cells were cultured in the RPMI-1640 medium (Life Technologies) supplemented with 10% FBS and in D-MEM medium supplemented with 10% FBS and 3×10^{-3} U/mL human insulin, respectively, at 37°C under humid condition with 5% CO_2. The cells were fed twice a week with the medium at the final cell density of approximately 2×10^5/mL. We adjusted the cell density of MOLT-3 cells to $2–3 \times 10^5$/mL 24 h before transfection.

3.2.2.1. ON DAY 0.

1. Centrifuge the cells at $170g$ for 5 min.
2. Remove the supernatant.
3. Resuspend the cells in 10 mL of OPTI-MEM I Reduced Serum Medium (Life Technologies).
4. Centrifuge the cells at $170g$ for 5 min.
5. Remove the supernatant.
6. Resuspend the cells in OPTI-MEM I Reduced Serum Medium and adjust the cell density to 1.5×10^4 cells/mL.
7. Plate the 200-µL cell suspension in each well of 96-well flat-bottomed plate (3×10^3/well).
8. Mix 350 µg of ribozyme and 70 µg of liposome (DOTAP, Boehringer Mannheim) in 1 mL of 20 mM HEPES buffer and incubate for 15 min at room temperature, then add 100 µg of RNase inhibitor (rRNasin, Promega). Add 10 µL aliquot of DOTAP-ribozyme complex to each well. Prepare control wells and treat with medium only, DOTAP only or ribozyme only (*see* **Note 5.2.**).
9. Incubate the plate at 37°C under humid condition with 5% CO_2.

3.2.2.2. FROM DAY 1 TO DAY 4.

Exchange 100 µL of medium in each well and add a 100 µl aliquot of DOTAP-ribozyme complex to each well daily for 4 d. (Considering cytotoxic effects of liposome and RNase inhibitor, we exchanged only one half of the medium.)

3.2.2.3. FROM DAY 2 TO DAY 4.

With exchange of medium and addition of DOTAP-ribozyme complex, add one-tenth volume of various concentrations of vincristine to each well for three consecutive days.

3.2.2.4. ON DAY 5, PERFORM CYTOTOXICITY ASSAY

(*See* protocol described in **Subheading 3.1.3.5.**)

3.2.3. Detection of Endocytotic Activity of Target Cells

In our study, endocytotic activity of target cells was shown to correlate with the success of cationic liposome-mediated transfer of ribozymes. Determination of endocytotic activity of target tumor cells may be predictive of efficacy of liposome-mediated gene transfer.

We describe two assay methods for endocytotic activity, phase-contrast microscopy for the uptake of latex beads and confocal microscopy with the use of dextran.

3.2.3.1. PHASE-CONTRAST MICROSCOPY

1. (For MCF-7/R cells) Seed 3×10^3 cells in 200 µL of OPTI-MEM Reduced Serum Medium per well of eight-well chamber slides (Nunc, Naperville, IL). (For MOLT-3/TMQ$_{800}$ cells) Seed 3×10^4 cells in 2 mL of OPTI-MEM Reduced Serum Medium in culture tubes.
2. Prepare three groups of samples.
   a. No treatment group: Incubate for 24 h, then replace one half volume of medium by fresh medium containing 20% FBS only. Then, culture for another 24 h.
   b. DOTAP group: Incubate for 24 h in the presence of 0.7 µg of DOTAP (per 200 µL of cell culture. For MOLT-3/TMQ$_{800}$ cells the amount of DOTAP should be proportionately larger). Then, one-half volume of medium is replaced by fresh medium containing 20% FBS and 0.35 µg of DOTAP (per 100 µL of cell culture). Then, culture for another 24 h.
   c. Latex beads group: Incubate for 24 h in the presence of 2 µL of suspension of latex beads (10%, v/v) with a diameter of 0.24 µm (Sigma) (per 200 µL of cell culture). Then, one-half of medium is replaced by fresh medium containing 20% FBS and 1 µl of suspension of latex beads (per 100 µl of cell culture). Then, culture for another 24 h.
3. After a total of 48 h incubation, wash the cells (and for MOLT-3/TMQ$_{800}$ cells, attach cells on glass slides using Cytospin 2, Shandon, Pittsburgh, PA) and examine immediately with a phase-contrast microscope (Olympus BX-60, Olympus, Tokyo, Japan).

3.2.3.2. CONFOCAL MICROSCOPY

1. (For MCF-7/R cells) Seed 3×10^3 cells in 200 µl of OPTI-MEM Reduced Serum Medium per well of eight-well chamber slides (Nunc, Naperville, IL). (For MOLT-3/TMQ$_{800}$ cells) Seed 3×10^4 cells in 2 mL of OPTI-MEM Reduced Serum Medium in culture tubes.
2. Prepare four groups of samples.
   a. No treatment group: Incubate for 24 h. Then, replace one-half volume of medium by fresh medium containing 20% FBS only and culture for another 24 h.
   b. FITC-dextran group. Incubate for 24 h with 3.5 µg of FITC-dextran (MW 10,000, Sigma) per well (per 200 µL of cell culture. For MOLT-3/TMQ$_{800}$ cells the amount of FITC-dextran should be proportionately larger). Then, replace one half volume of medium with fresh medium containing 20% FBS plus 3.5 µg of FITC-dextran (per 100 µL of cell culture) and culture for another 24 h.
   c. DOTAP-FITC-dextran complex group. Incubate for 24 h with DOTAP-FITC-dextran complex, which consists of 3.5 µg of FITC-dextran (MW 10,000 Da, Sigma) and 0.7 µg of DOTAP in 10 µL per well (per 200 µL of cell culture). (Before adding to the cell culture, mix FITC-dextran and DOTAP in a total

volume of 10 μL, and incubate them at room temperature for 15 min in order to form a DOTAP-FITC-dextran complex.) Then, replace one half volume of medium with fresh medium containing 20% FBS plus DOTAP-FITC-dextran complex, and culture for another 24 h (*see* **Note 5.3.**).

d. FITC-conjugated latex beads group: Incubate for 24 h in the presence of 8 μL of a suspension of FITC-conjugated latex beads (2.55% v/v, 0.213 μm diameter, Fluoresbrite YG microspheres, Polysciences, Warrington, PA).

3. Wash cells (and for MOLT-3/TMQ$_{800}$ cells, attach cells on glass slides using Cytospin 2, Shandon), fix them with methanol at $-20°C$ for 15 min.

4. Subject to confocal imaging (Leica True Confocal Scanner 4D system; Leica, Deerfield, IL, equipped with an argon krypton laser coupled to a Leica Leitz DMR fluorescence microscope and a 40X Plan Fluotar oil objective).

3.3. Retrovirus-Mediated Anti-MDR1 Ribozyme Gene Transfer into Human Leukemic and Lymphoma Cells In Vitro (17,18)

3.3.1. Chimeric tRNA/Ribozyme Molecular Design, Anti-MDR1 Ribozyme Synthesis and Cloning of Anti-MDR1 Ribozyme DNA into a Retroviral Vector

In this section, three aspects of experiments including, first, synthesis of anti-*MDR*1 ribozyme oligonucleotides; second, transformation of *E. coli* and preparation of retroviral plasmid vector; and third, cloning of anti-*MDR*1 ribozyme gene into retroviral vector, will be described.

3.3.1.1. SYNTHESES OF ANTI-*MDR*1 RIBOZYME OLIGONUCLEOTIDES

In this section we describe synthesis of four anti-*MDR*1 ribozymes: one, 196*MDR*1-Rz, which cleaves the GUC site at codon 196 of *MDR*1 mRNA; second, 196 *MDR*1-sRz, a stem-II base modified (stabilized) (U9→G9, U13→A13, G14→A14, A18→C18) ribozyme (*see* **ref. *19,20***) against codon 196; third, i*MDR*1-sRz, a stem-II base modified ribozyme directed against the $-6~-4$ GUC sequence of the translation initiation site; and fourth, mutated i*MDR*1-sRz, by mutating two bases (G3→U3, A22→C22) in the sequence of ribozyme catalytic core structure, which destroys the catalytic activity of anti-*MDR*1 ribozyme (**Fig. 2**).

1. Four anti-*MDR*1 ribozyme complimentary oligonucleotides carrying the *Mlu*I and *Sac*II sites on 5′ and 3′ ends are synthesized (**Table 2**) and purified by means of high performance liquid chromatography. (These are custom-ordered from Genset. Original solution had oligonucleotide concentrations in a range of 200 nmols in a volume of 100 μL or 2.0 m*M*).

2. Place 10 μL of the synthesized anti-*MDR*1 ribozyme oligonucleotides (if original concentration was 2.0 m*M*) in a microcentrifuge tube and add 990 μL of sterile dd-H$_2$O (to make a 20 μ*M* solution). Store at $-20°C$ in aliquots. Mix 10 μL each of corresponding anti-*MDR*1 ribozyme oligonucleotides (196*MDR*1-Rz+ and

Table 2.
Template cDNA sequences of anti-*MDR*1 ribozymes *(2)*
(*see* Subheading 3.3.1.1.)

Ribozyme	Template cDNA sequence
196*MDR*1-Rz+	5'-GGTTGCCATTCTGATGAGTCCGTGAGGACGAAACTG AAAGCGTTTTTGGA-3'
196*MDR*1-Rz-	5'-CGCGTC<u>CCAAAAACG</u>TCTTTCAGTTTCGTCCTCACG GACTCATCAGAATGGCAACCCGC-3'
196*MDR*1-sRz+	5'-GGTTGCCATTCTGATGAGGCCGAAAGGCCGAAACT GAAAGACGTTTTTGGA-3'
196*MDR*1-sRz-	5'-CGCGTC<u>CAAAAACG</u>TCTTTCAGTTTCGGCCTTTCGG CCTCATCAGAATGGCAACCCGC-3'
i*MDR*1-sRz+	5'-GGATCCATCCCCTGATGAGGCCGAAAGGCCGAAAC CTCGCGCCGTTTTTGGA-3'
i*MDR*1-sRz-	5'-CGCGT<u>CCAAAAACG</u>GCGCGAGGTTTCGGCCTTTCGG CCTCATCAGGGGATGGATCCCGC-3'
Mut-i*MDR*1-sRz+	5'-GGATCCATCCCCTtATGAGGCCGAAAGGCCGAcACCT CGCGCCGTTTTTGGA-3'
Mut-i*MDR*1-sRz-	5'-CGCGT<u>CCAAAAACG</u>GCGCGAGGTgTCGGCCTTTCGG CCTCAT aAGGGGATGGATCCCGC-3'

Rz, ribozyme; sRz, stem II stabilized ribozyme. Poly III promoter termination sequence is underlined. Small letters are mutated bases. From **ref. *18*.**

196*MDR*1-Rz- strands, 196*MDR*1-sRz+ and 196*MDR*1-sRz- strands, i*MDR*1-sRz+ and i*MDR*1-sRz- strands, Mut-i*MDR*1-sRz+ and Mut-i*MDR*1-sRz- strand), heat the mixture to 94°C for 5 min, then cool down to room temperature (for hemiduplex formation). (The final concentration of double strand anti-*MDR*1 ribozymes becomes 10 μ*M* in 20 μL volume.)

3. (To phosphorylate the 5' end of anti-*MDR*1 ribozyme double strand DNA fragments) aspirate 20 μL (0.2 nmoles) anti-*MDR*1 ribozyme double strand DNA fragments into a separate 1.5 mL Eppendorf tube which contains 10 μL 10X Reaction Buffer for T4 polynucleotide kinase (supplied with enzyme), 10 μL ATP (final concentration: 1 m*M*), 0.4 μL T4 polynucleotide kinase (4 U) (New England Biolabs) and add sterile dd-H$_2$O to 100 μL. Incubate the reaction tube at 37°C for 30 min (*see* **Note 6.1.**).

4. After 30 min incubation, add 200 μL of 100% cold ethanol (–20°C) into the reaction tubes, hold at –20°C for 30 min, centrifuge at 12,000*g* for 10 min and pellet the DNA fragments (*see* **Note 6.2.**).

5. Resuspend the pellets into sterile 100 μL dd-H$_2$O, transfer 5 μL of the solution to a new tube and dilute it with 495 μL of dd-H$_2$O. Measure the absorbance at 260 nm with a spectrophotometer.

6. The final concentration of each ribozyme DNA fragment is adjusted to 3.0 ng/μL for ligation into retroviral vector. Store them at –70°C in aliquots.

3.3.1.2 PREPARATION OF A LARGE AMOUNT OF RETROVIRAL PLASMID DNA (VECTOR)

1. Transform the retroviral vector, N2A+tRNA$_i^{met}$ (9.678 kb) into DH5α *E. coli* competent cells following the protocol provided in MAX Efficiency DH5α™ Competent Cells Kit (Life Technologies).

2. On the following day, pick up *E. coli* colonies formed and miniculture in 3 mL of liquid LB medium containing 50 μg/mL of ampicillin at 37°C for 10–12 h and purify the plasmid DNA from 1.5 mL of *E. coli* suspension and subject to electrophoresis on 0.8% agarose gel (which contains ethidium bromide, to ascertain the size of DNAs based on the band location).

3. After confirmation of appropriate size of retroviral plasmid (9.678 kb) culture the remaining 1.5 mL *E. coli* suspension further in a large volume (e.g., 250 mL ~ 500 mL) of LB medium with 50 μg/mL of ampicillin for 14–16 h. Purify the retroviral plasmid following the protocol provided in the Qiagen Plasmid Midi (or Maxi) Kit (Qiagen).

4. Resuspend the purified retroviral plasmid DNA in 50 μL sterile dd-H$_2$O. Transfer 2 μL of the solution into a new 1.5-mL tube and dilute it with 498 μL dd-H$_2$O and measure the absorbance value of retroviral plasmid DNA at 260 nm. Store the purified retroviral vector at –70°C in aliquots.

5. Cutting the retroviral vector with *Sac*II enzyme: Transfer 4.0 μg retroviral vector DNA into a new 1.5-mL tube and add the following components: 10 μL LOX NEBuffer 4 (New England Biolabs), 0.5 μL (10 U) *Sac*II enzyme (New England Biolabs) and DNase-free water to final volume of 100 μL. Incubate the reaction mixture at 37°C for 60 min.

6. After *Sac*II digestion, add 200 μL of 100% cold ethanol and hold at –20°C for 1–2 h (for precipitation of linear retroviral vector DNA) (*see* **Note 6.2.**).

7. Centrifuge the solution at 12,000*g* for 10 min and pellet the DNA. Discard the supernatant and dry the DNA at room temperature for 5 min.

8. Cutting of retroviral vector with *Mlu*I enzyme: resuspend the retroviral vector DNA sample in 10 μL dd-H$_2$O and mix it with 10 μL H buffer (New England Biolabs, supplied with the enzyme), 1.0 μL (10 U) *Mlu*I (Boehringer Mannheim) and 79 μL dd-H$_2$O for a final volume of 100 μL. Place the reaction tube in 37°C water bath for 60 min.

9. Add 200 μL of 100% cold ethanol and hold at –20°C for 30 min. Pellet the linear retroviral vector DNA by centrifuging it at 12,000*g* for 10–15 min. Decant the supernatant carefully and dry the pellet at room temperature for 5 min (*see* **Note 6.2.**).

10. Resuspend the double enzyme digested linear retroviral vector DNA into 100 μL of sterile dd-H$_2$O. Check the absorbance value at 260 nm with a spectrophotometer. Adjust the concentration of vector DNA to 35 ng/μL by adding sterile dd-H$_2$O, which is ready for ligation reaction.

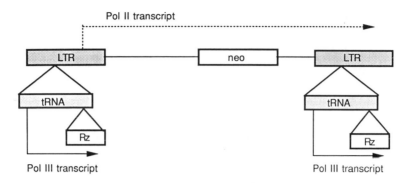

Fig. 3. Schematic presentation of integrated version of the double copy tRNA retroviral vector. By design, the expressed anti-*MDR*1 ribozymes are the chimeric tRNA-ribozymes. (From **ref.** *18*, reprinted with permission)

3.3.1.3. CLONING OF ANTI-*MDR*1 RIBOZYME GENE INTO RETROVIRAL VECTOR AND TRANSFORMATION OF *E. COLI*

When the double-stranded synthetic DNA sequences encoding 196 *MDR*1-Rz, 196 *MDR*1-sRz, and i*MDR*1-sRz are inserted into the vector N2A+ tRNA$_i^{met}$ downstream of Polymerase III promoter, three different constructs are formed: N2A+tRNA$_i^{met}$-196*MDR*1-Rz, N2A+tRNA$_i^{met}$-196*MDR*1-sRz and N2A+tRNA$_i^{met}$-i*MDR*1-sRz (**Fig. 3**). The expressed ribozymes are the chimeric tRNA-196*MDR*1-Rz, tRNA-196*MDR*1-sRz, and tRNA-i *MDR*1-sRz.

1. Mix linear retroviral vector DNA predigested by both *Sac*II and *Mlu*I enzymes (*see* **Subheading 3.3.1.2., steps 5–10**) and one of the double strand anti-*MDR*1 ribozyme DNA fragments (*see* **Subheading 3.3.1.1.**) into ligation reaction tube, respectively:
   5.7 μL retroviral vector DNA (35 ng/μL, or a total of 200 ng)
   1.0 μL anti-*MDR*1 ribozyme DNA (3.0 ng)
   2.0 μL Ligation buffer (10X) (supplied with T4 ligase)
   0.5 μL (4 U) T4 ligase
   10.8 μL sterile dd-H$_2$O
   Incubate at 16°C 12–14 h. Reserve the entire product for **step 2**.
2. Transform recombinant retroviral vectors into *E. coli* competent cells following the protocol provided in the MAX Efficiency DH5α™ Competent Cells Kit (Life Technologies) (*see* **Subheading 3.3.1.2.**).

3. On the following day, pick up colonies formed on LB agarose plate and miniculture in 3 mL of liquid LB medium containing 50 μg/mL of penicillin at 37°C for 10–12 h.
4. On the following day, transfer 1.5 mL of bacteria suspension into a new sterile microcentrifuge tube and purify the recombinant retrovirus vectors with the aid of QIAprep Spin Miniprep Kit (Qiagen). Digest the purified vectors by two restriction enzymes *Sal*II and *Mlu*I and subject to analyses with 1.8% agarose (which contains ethidium bromide) electrophoresis. After miniprep in **step 4**, verify the sequences and orientations of anti-*MDR*1 ribozymes in the constructs by DNA sequencing.
5. Culture the positive colonies containing the correct ribozyme sequences in large volume (250 ~ 500 mL) of LB medium which contains 50 μg/mL of ampicillin.
6. Purify the retroviral vector preparations using Qiagen Plasmid Midi (or Maxi) Kit. (Now ready for transfection of GP+*env*AM 12 cells for virion package.)

3.3.2. Packaging of Ribozyme-Containing Retrovirus Constructs and Viral Titration

In order to produce infectious retroviruses the recombinant retrovirus plasmid DNA purified from *E. coli* needs to be introduced into a packaging cell line. We describe the method using the amphotropic GP+*env*AM 12. In this section medium is referred to as D-MEM with high glucose (Life Technologies) with 10% heated-inactivated FBS, if not specifically addressed.

3.3.2.1. TRANSFECTION OF RECOMBINANT RETROVIRUS PLASMID CARRYING THE ANTI-*MDR*1 RIBOZYME GENE INTO GP+*ENV*AM 12 CELL LINE

Day 1. Prepare the GP+*env*AM 12 cells in 10-cm cell-culture dishes (Falcon) by 1 : 5 split of confluent cells. Incubate the dishes overnight at 37°C in a humidified 5% CO_2 incubator.
Day 2. Perform transfection.

1. Prepare the transfection mixture with Calcium Phosphate Transfection Kit (Invitrogen, San Diego, CA): Tube A: Add 36 μL of $2M$ $CaCl_2$ (supplied in the Kit) and 20 μg of retrovirus plasmid DNA (N2A+tRNA$_i^{met}$-196*MDR*1-Rz, N2A+tRNA$_i^{met}$-196*MDR*1-sRz, N2A+tRNA$_i^{met}$-i*MDR*1-sRz, N2A+tRNA$_i^{met}$-mut-*MDR*1-sRz, and empty N2A+tRNA$_i^{met}$ plasmids), adjust the volume to 300 μL with dd-H_2O supplied in the Kit. Tube B: Add 300 μL 2x HEPES Buffered Saline (HBS) in the Kit.
2. Using a Pasteur pipet, slowly add solution A dropwise over 1–2 min to solution B while bubbling air through solution B with another pipette connected to a rubber bulb. Continue until solution A is depleted.
3. Incubate the mixture at room temperature for 30 min and see if fine precipitates form.
4. Remove medium from GP+*env*AM 12 cells (approx 8×10^4 cells per culture dish) and gently pipet HBS-DNA precipitate onto the center of the dish. Expose

cells to the precipitate for 20 min under a laminar-flow hood while gently rock-ing the dish to distribute the precipitate over the entire surface of the dish (*see* **Note 6.3**).

5. After the exposure, add 10 mL medium and incubate the dishes overnight at 37°C in a humidified 5% CO_2 incubator.

Day 3: Change the medium and subject cells to glycerol shock.

1. Remove the medium from the cells.
2. Wash the cells twice with 1X PBS.
3. A glycerol shock is carried out as follows:
   a. Prepare a fresh 15% glycerol solution in 1X PBS.
   b. Add 3 mL of glycerol solution per 10-cm dish (which contains GP+*env*AM 12 cells).
   c. Incubate the dish at room temperature for 30 s.
   d. Quickly remove the glycerol solution by aspiration and gently wash cells once with 1X PBS and proceed to **step 4**.
4. Gently add fresh medium and incubate 36–48 hr at 37°C in a humidified 5% CO_2 incubator.

Day 5: Selection of the transfected cells

1. Split the transfected cells 1:10 and suspend them in medium which contains 800 µg/mL of G418. (The recombinant retroviral vector contains the neo gene and the transfected packaging cells should survive in G418-containing medium). Incubate 3–4 d.
2. Replace the medium with the fresh selection medium, incubate the cells further and exchange the selection medium every 3 d until colonies become visible.

3.3.2.2. CULTIVATION OF RETROVIRUS-PRODUCER CLONES AND HARVEST OF VIRAL STOCKS

1. After brief digestion with 0.25% trypsin-EDTA solution, pick well-isolated colo-nies carefully and transfer each clone into individual well containing 1.5 mL of fresh D-MEM with 10% FBS in 24-well tissue culture dishes (Falcon). Generally more than 50 transfected packaging cell clones can be transferred. Grow them until confluence.
2. Transfer the confluent clones into new T-25 flasks (one clone per flask) for fur-ther culture using the same medium.

3.3.2.3. TITRATION OF RETROVIRAL STOCKS USING NIH/3T3 CELLS

The viral titers of the supernatant harvested from the stable transfectants are determined using NIH/3T3 cells. (The viral titers should be in the range of 1.1–2.5 × 10^5 cfu/mL.)

Day 0: Preparation of NIH/3T3 cells:

Place aliquots of 5×10^4 logarithmically growing NIH/3T3 cells in 10 mL of the medium into the 10-cm dishes. Incubate the dishes at 37°C in a humidified CO_2 incubator overnight.

Day 1: Infection of retrovirus into target cells:

1. Remove medium from the dishes and add 2 mL of medium containing 8 µg/mL Polybrene and viral stock supernatants in a serial dilution (1:10, 1:25, 1:50, 1:100, 1:500, 1:1000). Incubate NIH/3T3 cells at 37°C for 2 h.
2. Add 8 mL of medium into the individual dishes. (Polybrene is diluted to 1.6 µg/mL final concentration). Continue to incubate retrovirus-infected cells for 2 d.

Day 3: Selection of the infectant NIH/3T3 cells:

1. Because the retroviral vectors contain the drug resistance gene neo, split the above infected NIH/3T3 cells 1:10, 1:15, 1:20 into three 10-cm dishes containing 800 µg/mL G418 in 10 mL of medium. Incubate another 3 or 4 d.
2. Exchange G418-containing D-MEM for the retrovirus-infected NIH/3T3 cells every 3–4 d and continue to incubate them at 37°C for 8–12 d. At this time cell colonies should be visible.
3. At days 8–12, count all the colonies formed in the 10-cm dishes before colonies become confluent. Calculate the retroviral titer using the following formula:

$$\text{CFU/mL} = \frac{(\text{No. of colonies/dish}) \times \text{Dilution factors of NIH/3T3 cells}}{\text{Virus volume (in mL) added per dish} \times \text{Replication factor}}$$

Use Replication factor of 2 (*see* **Note 6.4.**).

3.3.3. Development of Human Lymphoma Cells with MDR Phenotype (see **Note 6.5.**)

3.3.3.1. TRANSFECTION OF PHA*MDR*1/A EXPRESSING *MDR*1 GENE INTO GP+*ENV*AM 12 CELL LINE FOR RETROVIRAL PACKAGING

Prepare large amount of the plasmid using **Subheading 3.3.1.2., steps 1–4**. Then, proceed to **Subheading 3.3.2.1.**

The experimental protocol for transfection of pHa*MDR*1/A (provided by Dr. Michael Gottesman) *(31)* is the same as in **Subheading 3.3.2.1.** except for the steps on day 5 as follows:

Day 5: Selection of the pHa*MDR*1/A transduced cells.

1. Split the pHa*MDR*1/A-transfected GP+*env*AM 12 cells 1:10 and suspend them in the medium that contains 3×10^{-8} *M* of vincristine sulfate (VCR, Pharmacia, Columbus, Ohio) for 3–4 d (*see* **Note 6.6**).
2. Exchange the fresh VCR-containing medium every 3–4 d until colonies become visible.

3.3.3.2. Cultivation of Retrovirus-Producer Clones and Harvest of Viral Stocks

The experiment protocol is the same as in **Subheading 3.3.2.2.**

3.3.3.3 Titration of Retroviral pHaMDR1/A Stocks

The experimental protocol is the same as in **Subheading 3.3.2.3.** except for the steps on day 3.

Day 3: Selection of the infectant NIH/3T3 cells:

1. Because the retroviral pHaMDR1/A contains the drug resistance gene (*MDR1*), VCR is used in a selection medium. Split the above infected NIH/3T3 cells in 1:10, 1:15, 1:20 dilution into three 10-cm dishes containing 3×10^{-8} M of VCR in 10 mL of D-MEM medium. Incubate the dishes for another 3–4 d (*see* **Note 6.6**).
2. Exchange VCR containing D-MEM for the retrovirus-infected NIH/3T3 cells every 3–4 d and continue to incubate them at 37°C for 10–12 d. By this time cell colonies should become visible.
3. Calculate the retroviral titer as described for day 3 in **Subheading 3.3.2.3., step 3**. (In our experiments the viral titers of the supernatant harvested from the stable transfectants were $1.5–2.0 \times 10^5$ cfu/mL.)

3.3.3.4. Development of Resistant Human Lymphoma Daudi/MDR_{20} Cells Mediated by P-gp Overproduction

1. Place 2×10^6 human Burkitt lymphoma parent cells (Daudi/wt) in exponential stage in 10 ml of RPMI-1640 medium containing 20% FBS and 8 µg/mL of Polybrene (Sigma) in T-75 flask (Falcon) and add 5.0 mL of cell-free viral stock supernatant (2.0×10^5 cfu/mL) harvested from GP+*env*AM 12 packaging cells for infection of pHaMDR1/A virion (from **Subheading 3.3.3.3.**) into the flask. Incubate cells at 37°C in a 5% CO_2/humidified air atmosphere for 5 h.
2. Centrifuge the cells at 500g for 5 min, remove medium and resuspend the pellet in 10 ml of RPMI-1640 medium containing 20% FBS.
3. Repeat **steps 1** and **2** twice.
4. After the third round of infection, resuspend the infectants in 20 mL of RPMI-1640 medium containing 20% FBS; then incubate the cells at 37°C in a 5% CO_2/humidified air for 2 d, centrifuge the cells at 500g for 5 min and resuspend the cells in 20 mL RPMI-1640 medium containing 20% of FBS and $1 \times 10^{-8}M$ of vincristine sulfate (selection medium) for the next 12 d of culture. Exchange the selection medium every 3 or 4 d.
5. On day 13, start to maintain the infectants in fresh RPMI-1640 medium supplemented with 20% FBS without vincristine at 37°C in a 5% CO_2/humidified air atmosphere.
6. One week later, measure the degree of resistance of infectants by the MTT assay (*see* **Subheading 3.1.3.5.**). (In our hands, the ID_{50} of the Daudi/wt cells was $1.3 \times 10^{-9}M$ and that of pHaMDR1/A-infected Daudi cells was $2.8 \times 10^{-8}M$. On

ID_{50} basis, the infectant had approximately 20-fold resistance to VCR. We designated this resistant cell line as Daudi/MDR_{20}. The uninfected Daudi/wt cells were unable to survive in the vincristine selection medium.)

7. Expand the culture of Daudi/MDR_{20} cells in fresh RPMI-1640 medium supplemented with 20% FBS. Freeze some of them in aliquots and store in liquid nitrogen. The remainder of Daudi/MDR_{20} cells are ready for the next experiment, as described in the next section.

3.3.4. Retrovirus-Mediated Anti-MDR1 Ribozyme Transfer into Human Lymphoma Cells with MDR Phenotype

1. Suspend 1×10^6 Daudi/MDR_{20} cells grown in exponential phase in 10 mL of RPMI-1640 medium containing 20% FBS and 8 µg/mL of Polybrene (*see* **Note 6.7.**) in T-75 flask; then add 10 mL cell-free viral supernatants (viral titer: 2.5×10^5 cfu/mL). Incubate cells at 37°C in a 5% humidified atmosphere for 5 h.
2. After incubation, harvest the Daudi/MDR_{20} cells by centrifugation.
3. Repeat **steps 1** and **2** three more times in 2 d.
4. After the fourth round of infection of the cells with packaged retrovirus, remove the medium by pelleting the cells and resuspend the cells in selection medium (RPMI-1640 medium containing 20% FBS and 800 µg/mL G418) at 37°C in 5% CO_2/humidified air atmosphere. Change the selection medium every 3–4 d. (We designated the G418-resistant Daudi/MDR_{20} cells as Daudi/MDR_{20}-iMDR1-sRz, Daudi/MDR_{20}-196MDR1-sRz, Daudi/MDR_{20}-196MDR1-Rz, Daudi/MDR_{20}-mut-iMDR1-sRz sublines, respectively.) After 12 d in the selection medium, maintain the cells in fresh RPMI-1640 medium supplemented with 20% of heat-inactivated FBS.
5. Determine the levels of drug resistance with the MTT assay (*see* **Subheading 3.1.3.5.**) and characterize the infectants by carrying out such procedures as Northern blotting (**Subheading 3.1.3.2.**), Western blotting (**Subheading 3.1.3.2.**) and flow-cytometric analysis (*see next* **Subheading**).

3.3.5. Flow-Cytometric Analysis of P-gp of Infectant Cells

In **Subheading 3.1.3.3.** we described flow-cytometric analysis using phycoerythrin-conjugated rat antimouse antibody. In this section the use of fluorescein isothiocyanate (FITC) will be briefly described.

1. Harvest Daudi cells cultured in the RPMI-1640 medium with 20% FBS by centrifugation at 400g for 10 min.
2. Resuspend cells at 2×10^7 cells/mL in media or in PBS without Ca^{2+} and Mg^{2+} containing 1–2% human AB+ serum. Aliquot 50 µL volume (1×10^6 cells) of cell suspension in each Eppendorf tube.
3. Incubate the cell suspension with 10 µL (5 µg) of MRK16 at 4°C for 1 h. For unstained controls, use PBS. For nonspecific binding control, use 10 µL of mouse monoclonal anti-human β-2 microglobulin subtype IgG2a (BioSource International, Camarillo, CA) or 10 µL (0.5 µg) of Mouse IgG2a Pure stock solution containing pure mouse IgG2a (Becton Dickinson, San Jose, CA) per 1×10^6 cells.

4. (1st wash) Using 1 mL of cold PBS, wash the first antibody-binding cells and harvest the cells by centrifuging at 400g for 10 min. Repeat the procedure once. Resuspend cells in 50 µL of PBS.
5. Add 1.5–2 µL of secondary antibody, FTIC-conjugated sheep monoclonal antimouse IgG2a (Sigma). Incubate for 1 h at 4°C in the dark.
6. (2nd wash) Wash with 5 mL of cold PBS and harvest the cells by centrifugation at 400g for 10 min. Repeat the procedure once.
7. Add 0.6 mL of 1% paraformaldehyde in PBS to suspend the cells. Transfer the sample to 12 × 75-mm tube for FACS analysis.

3.3.6. Determination of Cleavage Activity of Anti-MDR1 Ribozymes in In Vitro Cell-Free System

In this section we describe methods to determine the cleavage activity of stem II-modified ribozymes and chimeric tRNA-ribozyme complex in a cell-free system (*see* **Subheadings 3.1.1.2.–3.1.1.4.**)

3.3.6.1. THE PREPARATIONS OF CDNA TEMPLATES OF RIBOZYMES (i*MDR*1-sRz, 196*MDR*1-sRz, AND 196*MDR*1-Rz)

1. The cDNA fragments of the i*MDR*1-sRz, 196*MDR*1-sRz, and 196*MDR*1-Rz are amplified from the corresponding retroviral constructs (N2A+tRNA$_i^{met}$-196*MDR*1-Rz, N2A+tRNA$_i^{met}$-196*MDR*1-sRz and N2A+tRNA$_i^{met}$-i*MDR*1-sRz) with PCR by using the following consensus primers: RzPr1: 5'-<u>TAAT ACGACTCACTATAGGGCGA</u>AGCAGAGTGGCGCAGCGGAA-3' (43-mer, the underlined sequence is T7 promoter); and RzPr2: 5'-TACTTAAGCT AGCAGCGTCCA-3' (22-mer), which are synthesized by Genset. The PCR-amplified sequence included the T7 promoter (23 bp) and the chimeric tRNA and anti-*MDR*1 ribozyme sequence. The expected products of tRNA-i*MDR*1-sRz, tRNA-196*MDR*1-sRz, and tRNA-196*MDR*1-Rz are 169 bp, 168 bp, and 168 bp, respectively.
2. PCR reaction mixture

Component		Final concentration
Sterile dd-H$_2$O	34.5 µL	
10X PCR Reaction buffer	5.0 µL	1X
10 mM dATP	1.0 µL	200 µM
10 mM dGTP	1.0 µL	200 µM
10 mM dCTP	1.0 µL	200 µM
10 mM dTTP	1.0 µL	200 µM
25 mM RzPr-1	1.0 µL	0.5 µM
25 mM RzPr-2	1.0 µL	0.5 µM
25 mM MgCl$_2$ solution	4.0 µL	2.0 µM
Taq DNA polymerase	0.25 µL	1.25 U/50 µL
Amplified DNA template	0.25 µL	0.5 µg/50 µL
Total volume	50 µL	

All PCR reagents are provided in *GeneAmp* PCR Reagents (Perkin Elmer) and for the reaction we followed the protocol supplied in the Kit.

3. Perform PCR at 95°C for 60 s; 55°C for 30 s and 72°C for 2 min for 30 cycles and extended at 72°C for 10 min and store at 4°C (*see* **Note 6.8**).
4. Add to the PCR-amplified products an equal volume of phenol:choloroform: isoamyl alcohol (25:24:1), vortex, transfer the aqueous phase solution to a new sterile 1.5-mL tube, add two volumes of 100% ethanol (to precipitate DNA) and then dissolved in 50 µL of dd-H_2O. Quantitate the products by reading the absorbance at 260 nm with a spectrophotometer and identify the expected sizes of ribozyme templates by an electrophoresis in 1.8% agarose gel (containing ethidium bromide).

3.3.6.2. THE PREPARATIONS OF cDNA TEMPLATES OF SUBSTRATES

Substrate A (185bp) and substrate B (191bp) are designed to correspond to nucleotides −72 to 113 in the translation initiation site and nucleotides 520 to 710 in the codon 196 region of the full-length *MDR*1 cDNA, respectively (*35*).

Amplify both substrate templates (A and B) by PCR from the p*MDR*2000XS plasmid (provided by Dr. Michael Gottesman) using the primers: SaPr-1, 5′-<u>TA ATACGACTCACTATAGGGCGA</u>CCACTAAAGTCGGAGTATCTTC-3′ (45-mer, the initial underlined 23 nucleotides consist of the T7 promoter sequence and the following are the nucleotides −72 to −50 in the region containing translation initiation site of the *MDR*1 gene); and SaPr-2, 5′-GAAAATACACTGACAGTTGGT-3′ (21-mer, complementary to the nucleotides 113 to 93 of *MDR*1 gene); and SbPr-1, 5′-<u>TAATACGACTCACT ATAGGGCGA</u>CGACTTACAGATGATGTCTCT-3′ (44-mer, the nonunderlined 21 nucleotides are the sense nucleotides 520 to 540 of the *MDR*1 gene); and SbPr-2, 5′-AGATAGTATCTTTGCCCAGACA-3′ (22-mer, complementary to the region from 710 to 689 of *MDR*1 gene) with the procedure described in **Subheading 3.3.6.1.**

3.3.6.3. SYNTHESES OF ANTI-*MDR*1 RIBOZYME AND SUBSTRATES A AND B BY IN VITRO TRANSCRIPTION REACTIONS

Ribozyme and substrate RNA molecules are transcribed by using the above ribozyme and substrate DNA templates that contain T7 RNA polymerase promoter.

1. The transcription reaction mixture is prepared as described in the protocol of T7-MEGAshortscript™ In Vitro Transcription Kit (Ambion, Austin, TX); for example:

Volume of RNase-free dd-H$_2$O to make final volume of 20 µL after all components are added:

    2 µl 10X Transcription Buffer
    2 µl ATP solution (75 mmol/L T7)
    2 µl GTP solution (75 mmol/L T7)
    2 µl CTP solution (75 mmol/L T7)
    2 µl TTP solution (75 mmol/L T7)
    1 µl [α-^{32}P]CTP (10 µl of 250 µCi/25 µl)
    2–3 µl template DNA (225–250 ng in total)
    2 µl T7 MEGAshortscript enzyme mix

Add dd-H$_2$O (supplied in the Kit) to a total volume of 20 µl.

2. Mix contents thoroughly by gentle flicking or brief gentle vortex and then centrifuge briefly at 12,000g for a few seconds to collect all the reaction mixture at the bottom of the tube. Incubate the reaction tube at 37°C water bath for 2 h.

3. (To remove template DNA) Add 1 µL of RNase free DNase 1 (2 U/µl) to the reaction tube, mix thoroughly by flicking tube, centrifuge briefly and then incubate at 37°C 15 min.

4. The reaction is terminated by adding 115 µL of DEPC-treated dd-H$_2$O and 15 µL of Ammonium Acetate Precipitation Solution (supplied in the Kit).

5. Precipitate the transcribed RNA with two volumes of ethanol. After addition of the alcohol, mix thoroughly, chill 30 min at –20°C, centrifuge 10 min at 12,000g and carefully remove the supernatant.

6. Resuspend the RNA pellet in RNase-free DEPC-treated dd-H$_2$O. Transfer 2 µl of RNA suspension solution into a new 1.5-mL tube and dilute it by adding 498 µL of RNase-free DEPC- treated dd-H$_2$O, and then check the absorbance at 260 nm by a spectrophotometer.

7. Transfer 1 µL of each transcribed anti-*MDR*1 ribozyme and substrates A or B RNA into the new individual tubes and dilute them with 9 µL of DEPC-treated dd-H$_2$O; add 10 µL of Formamide Gel Loading Buffer (from the Kit), centrifuge briefly at 12,000g and load them on 8% acrylamide/8M urea gel (*see* electrophoresis **Subheading 3.3.6.5.**). Run the sample at 200 V for 5–6 h and expose the gel to X-ray film (*see* **Subheading 3.1.1.4., step 18**) overnight and develop the film. Check the sizes of transcribed anti-*MDR*1 ribozymes and substrates A and B RNAs. The RNA molecule of chimeric tRNA-i*MDR*1-sRz should be 146nt in size and that of tRNA-196*MDR*1-sRz and tRNA-196*MDR*1-Rz should be 145nt in size. The sizes of substrates A and B are 185nt and 191nt, respectively.

8. Store the transcribed RNA (anti-*MDR*1 ribozymes, substrates A and B) at –70°C in aliquots. (*see* **Note 3.2**).

3.3.6.4. CLEAVAGE ACTIVITY OF ANTI-*MDR*1 RIBOZYMES IN IN VITRO CELL-FREE SYSTEM (*SEE ALSO* SUBHEADING 3.1.1.3.)

1. The ribozyme and substrate RNA quantitated spectrophotometrically at 260 nm are mixed in 2:1 ratio as follows:

Components	Final concentration
—μL anti-*MDR*1 ribozyme	10 pmol/20 μL
—μL substrate	5 pmol/ 20 μL
10 μL 100-m*M* Tris-HCl (pH 7.5) containing 10 m*M* EDTA	50 m*M* with 5 m*M* EDTA

Heat the mixture to 95°C for 2 min, quick-chill on ice, add 2 μL of 50 m*M* MgCl$_2$ (final concentration 5 m*M*), add RNase-free H$_2$O (supplied in the T7-MEGA-shortscript™ In Vitro Transcription Kit) to a final volume of 20 μl.

2. Incubate the reaction mixture at 37°C for a series of time intervals.
3. (to terminate the reaction) Add an equal volume of Formamide Gel Loading Buffer (supplied in the Kit), vortex and then heat the tube at 95°C for 3 min.

3.3.6.5. ELECTROPHORESIS AND AUTORADIOGRAPHY (*SEE* SUBHEADING 3.1.1.4.)

The cleavage activity of ribozymes is analyzed by electrophoresis in 8% polyacrylamide/8*M* urea gel in 1X TBE buffer.

1. Assemble the glass-plate sandwich of the electrophoresis apparatus and lock the sandwich to the cashing stand.
2. Prepare the solution of 8% acrylamide/8*M* urea gel
    28.8 g Urea (Boehringer Mannheim)
    6.0 mL 10X TBE buffer stock solution
    16 mL 30% acrylamide/bis-acrylamide (19 : 1) (Boehringer Mannheim)
    17 mL DEPC treated dd-H$_2$O to a total volume of 60 mL
   Stir at room temperature until urea has dissolved. Add 480 μL of 10% of ammonium persulfate in dd-H$_2$O and 64 μL of TEMED (Sigma) (both of which catalyze polymerization).
3. Mix briefly after adding the last two ingredients and pour gel immediately.
4. Allow the gel to polymerize for 30 min at room temperature.
5. Fix the sandwich to the electrophoresis apparatus and fill the upper and lower tanks with the 1X TBE electrophoresis buffer which is diluted from 10X TBE stock solution with DEPC-treated water.
6. Rinse the wells with the 1X TBE electrophoresis buffer and load the RNA sample from the cleavage reactions in cell-free system.
7. Run the samples at 200 V for 5–6 h.
8. Follow steps from **step 11** in **Subheading 3.1.1.4.**

4. Notes

1. For the maintenance of NIH/3T3 and GP+*env*AM 12 cell lines 10% newborn calf serum is usually used. We used 10% FBS and found no disadvantages.
2. Design of anti-*MDR*1 ribozymes. The PCR primer should contain several additional bases upstream of the core T7 promoter sequence. These are necessary for maximal transcription efficiency (*36*). Because the sequence of these bases is not critical, they can be used for the generation of a restriction site if desired for subsequent cloning. *Caution:* The DEPC-treated dd-H$_2$O, tubes and tips to be

used in the experiments are all autoclaved for 30 min. *Caution:* In every procedure, wear gloves to avoid the contamination of RNase enzyme.

3. Preparation of ribozymes and RNA substrate.
    1. RNAs are easily degraded during freezing and thawing procedures. We, therefore, freeze-stored the ribozyme and substrate solutions in aliquots. In this way, only necessary amounts of the solution can be thawed for each experiment.
    2. The ^{32}P-labeled ribozyme and substrate RNAs stored at –70°C must be used within a 2–3-wk period because of the short half-life (2 wk) of the isotope and prevention of radiolysis. Alternatively, ^{33}P can be used instead of ^{32}P. The lower amount of radioactivity ^{33}P contains, the safer it is.
4. Transfection with a human β-actin expression vector.
    Genset provides a data sheet with the material that includes molecular weight. The oligonucleotides are dissolved to a final concentration of 0.1 nmols/μL.
5. Liposome-mediated transfection
    1. Ribozymes to be used in liposome-mediated transfection should be sterile. Perform **Subheading 3.1.1.1., steps 21–24** at a clean bench.
    2. Do not mix DOTAP and rRNasin directly. If you mix DOTAP and rRNasin directly transfection efficiency will decrease.
    3. Cytochalasin B is known to inhibit endocytosis *(37,38)*. In order to confirm that the fluorescence uptake is due to endocytosis, cells can be pretreated with 10 μg/mL of cytochalasin B (Sigma) for 30 min at 37°C. After the pretreatment the cell samples are washed with PBS and further incubated with DOTAP-FITC-dextran complex for 24 h or FITC-conjugated latex beads for 30 min at 37°C in the continued presence of cytochalasin B.
6. Infection with N2A viral vector
    1. Phosphorylation of 5′ end (**Subheading 3.3.1.1., step 3**). In general, phosphorylation of 5′ end of a double stranded DNA is not efficient when the 5′ end is recessed. Therefore, phosphorylation procedure is performed using a single stranded DNA first and then annealed to double stranded DNA (*see* **Subheading 3.1.2.**). Here, we phosphorylated the 5′ end of double stranded DNA with sufficient amount of T4 polynucleotide kinase (4 U in 100 μL reaction volume) and it was successful.
    2. For the ethanol precipitation of DNA, salt is needed. We were able to precipitate DNA because of the presence of salt in the buffers used, NEBuffers and H Buffer.
    3. For calcium phosphate-mediated transfection, DNA precipitate is usually added to the target cells in the presence of medium. We found the transfection was more successful when the precipitate was added directly on the monolayer cells after the removal of medium.
    4. Replication factor: Calculation of viral titer is determined differently in different laboratories, partly because it is difficult to account for the number of cell divisions that occur after viral integration and before plating the cells into selection medium. Another reason is that because the titration assay involves

several steps, perfect reproducibility is unrealistic. In our titration assay, the viral titers varied within two-fold differences and approximately two cell divisions occurred prior to selection; we, therefore, chose the replication factor as two.

5. Tumor cells that are made resistant by repeated or pulse exposure to P-gp substrate drugs may contain drug resistance mechanisms other than P-gp-mediated MDR. For this reason, we developed MDR cells purely related to P-gp overexpression by infection of *MDR1* gene containing plasmid.

6. Polybrene is likely to promote retrovirus binding to the Daudi/MDR_{20} cell surface by reducing electrostatic repulsion between the negatively charged surfaces of the cell and retroviral virion.

7. PCR primers. Whereas the RzPr1 and RzPr2 have different lengths and their annealing temperatures are different, the lower annealing temperature (55°C) we chose was found to be proper for both of the primers for binding to their respective sites.

8. Selection medium for pHa*MDR*1/A transfected or infected cells: Because the retrovirus pHa*MDR*1/A contains the full length of *MDR1* gene and overexpresses the P-gp in its transfected or infected target cells, P-gp-associated anticancer agents such as VCR may be used in a selection medium. In our experiment, we used ID80 concentrations of VCR for uninfected/untransfected wide type cells as determined by MTT assay (72-h incubation of tumor cells in a series of VCR concentrations in a 96-well plate). In this condition, only the pHa*MDR*1/A-transfected or infected cells were able to grow in the VCR-containing selection medium. The wt cells which were sensitive to VCR all died in VCR-containing selection medium within 10 days of incubation. VCR sensitivity of cells we used were:

Cell lines	ID_{50} (M)	ID_{80} (M)
GP+*env*AM 12 cells (**Subheding 3.3.3.1., step 1**)	1.7×10^{-8}	3×10^{-8}
NIH/3T3 cells (**Subheading 3.3.3.3., step 1**)	9×10^{-9}	3×10^{-8}
Daudi/wt cells (**Subheading 3.3.3.4., step 4**)	1.3×10^{-9}	1×10^{-8}

Acknowledgments

This work was supported in part by the T. J. Martell Foundation for Leukemia, Cancer and AIDS Research, New York, NY, and by the United Leukemia Fund, New York, NY. We thank the following investigators for providing us with cell lines and plasmid vectors: Dr. Steven Averbuch of Zeneca Pharmaceuticals, Wilmington, DE, with MCF-7/R multidrug resistant human breast cancer cell line; Dr. Arthur Bank of Columbia University, New York, NY, with GP+*env*AM 12 packaging cell line; Dr. Laurence Kedes of University of Southern California, Los Angeles, CA, with a β-actin driven plasmid vector pHβAPr-1-neo; Dr. Ira Gilboa of Duke University Medical Center, Durham, NC, with Moloney leukemia-based N2A retroviral vector; Dr. Michael Zasloff of Magainin Research Institute, Plymouth Meeting, PA, with tRNA$_i^{met}$ gene-containing plasmid phH2DΔ3'-5; Dr. Michael M. Gottesman of National Cancer Institute, Bethesda, MD, with pHa*MDR*1/A retroviral vector as well as p*MDR*2000XS plasmid vector both of which contain full length cDNA of *MDR*1 gene.

References

1. Germann, U. A. and Harding, M. W. (1995) Chemosensitizers to overcome and prevent multidrug resistance? *J. Natl. Cancer Inst.* **87,** 1573–1575.
2. Gottesman, M. M., Pastan, I., and Ambudkar, S. V. (1996) P-glycoprotein and multidrug resistance. *Current. Opin. Genet. Dev.* **6,** 610–617.
3. Ling, V. (1997) Multidrug resistance: molecular mechanisms and clinical relevance. *Cancer Chemother. Pharmacol.* **40 (Suppl. 1),** S3–S6.
4. Bellamy, W. T. (1996) P-glycoproteins and multidrug resistance. *Ann. Rev. Pharmacol. Toxicol.* **36,** 161–183
5. Goldstein, L. J., Galski, H., Fojo, A., Willingham, M., Lai, S-L., Gazdar, A., et al. (1989) Expression of a multidrug resistance gene in human cancers. *J. Natl. Cancer Inst.* **81,** 116–124.
6. Trock, B. J., Leonessa, F., and Clark, R. (1997) Multidrug resistance in breast cancer: a meta analysis. *J. Nat. Cancer Inst.* **89,** 917–931.
7. Bradley, G. and Ling. V. (1994) P-glycoprotein multidrug resistance and tumor progression. *Cancer Metastasis Rev.* **132,** 223–233.
8. Marie, J-P. (1995) P-glycoprotein in adult hematologic malignancies. *Hematol. Oncol. Clin. North Am.* **9,** 239–249.
9. Georges, E., Sharom, F. J., and Ling, V. (1990) Multidrug resistance and chemosensitization: therapeutic implications for cancer chemotherapy. *Adv. Pharmacol.* **21,** 185–220.
10. Fuqua, S. A. W., Moretti-Rojas, I. M., Schneider, S. L., and McGuire, W. L. (1987) P-glycoprotein expression in human breast cancer cells. *Cancer Res.* **47,** 2103–2106.
11. Lemontt, J. F., Azzaria, M., and Gros, P. (1988) Increased mdr gene expression and decreased drug accumulation in multidrug-resistant human melanoma cells. *Cancer Res.* **48,** 6348–6353,.
12. Li, X. K., Kobayashi, H., Holland, J. F., and Ohnuma, T. (1993) Expression of dihydrofolate reductase and multidrug resistance genes in trimetrexate-resistant human leukemia cell lines. *Leukemia Res.* **17,** 483–490.
13. Cech, T. R. (1988) Ribozymes and their medical implications. *J. A. M. A.* **260,** 3030–3034.
14. Haseloff, J. and Gerlach, W. J. (1988) Simple RNA enzymes with new and highly specific endoribonuclease activities. *Nature* **334,** 585–591.
15. Kobayashi, H., Dorai, T., Holland, J. F., and Ohnuma T. (1994) Reversal of drug sensitivity in multidrug-resistant tumor cells by *MDR*1 (PGY1) ribozyme. *Cancer Res.* **54,** 1271–1275.

16. Masuda, Y., Kobayashi, H., Holland, J. F., and Ohnuma, T. (1998) Reversal of multidrug resistance by a liposome-*MDR*1 ribozyme complex. *Cancer Chemother. Pharmacol.* **42,** 9–16.

17. Kobayashi, H., Takemura, Y., Wang, F-S., Oka, T., and Ohnuma, T. (1999) Retrovirus-mediated transfer of anti-*MDR*1 hammerhead ribozymes into multidrug-resistant human leukemia cells: Screening for effective target sites. *Int. J. Cancer* **81,** 944–950.

18. Wang, F-S., Kobayashi, H., Liang, K-W., Holland, J. F., and Ohnuma, T. (1999) Retrovirus-mediated anti-*MDR*1 ribozymes fully restores chemosensitivity of P-glycoprotein-expressing human lymphoma cells. *Human Gene Therapy* **10,** 1185–1195.

19. Kiehntopf, M., Brach, M. A., Licht, T., Petschauer, S., Karawajew, L., Kirschning, C., and Herrmann, F. (1994) Ribozyme-mediated cleavage of the *MDR*-1 transcript restores chemosensitivity in previously resistant cancer cells. *EMBO J.* **13,** 4645–4652.

20. Sullivan, S. M. (1994) Development of ribozymes for gene therapy. *J. Invest. Dermatol.* **103,** 85S–89S.

21. Paolella, G., Sproat, B. S., and Lamond, A. I. (1992) Nuclease resistant ribozymes with high catalytic activity. *EMBO J.* **11,** 1913–1919.

22. Gunning, P., Leavitt, J., Muscat, G., Ng, S-Y., and Kedes, L. (1987) A human β-actin expression vector system directs high-level accumulation of antisense transcript. *Proc. Natl. Acad. Sci. USA* **84,** 4831–4835.

23. Adeniyi-Jones, S., Romeo, P. H., and Zasloff, M. (1984) Generation of long readthrough transcripts in vivo and in vitro by deletion of 3′ termination and processing sequences in the human tRNA$_i^{met}$ gene. *Nucleic Acids Res.* **12,** 1101–1115.

24. Hantzopoulos, P. A., Sullenger, B. A., Ungers, G., and Gilboa, E, (1989) Improved gene expression upon transfer of the adenosine deaminase minigene outside of the transcriptional unit of a retroviral vector. *Proc. Natl. Acad. Sci.* **86,** 3519–3523.

25. Minowada, J., Ohnuma, T., and Moore, G. E. (1972) Rosette-forming human lymphoid cell lines. I. Establishment and evidence for origin of thymus-derived lymphocytes. *J. Natl. Cancer Inst.* **49,** 891–895.

26. Klein, E., Klein, G., Nadkarni, J. S., Nadkarni, J. J., Wigzell, H., and Clifford, P. (1968) Surface IgM-kappa specificity on a Burkitt lymphoma cell in vivo and in derived culture lines. *Cancer Res.* **28,** 1300–1310.

27 Cowan, K. H., Batist, G., Tulpule, A., Sinha, B., and Myers, C. E. (1986) Similar biochemical changes associated with multidrug resistance in human breast cancer cells and carcinogen-induced resistance to xenobiotics in rats. *Proc. Natl. Acad. Sci. USA* **83,** 9328–9332.

28. Jainchill, J. L., Aaronson, S. A., and Todaro, G. J. (1969) Murine sarcoma and leukemia viruses: assay using clonal line of contact-inhibited mouse cells. *J. Virol.* **4,** 549–553.

29. Markowitz, D., Goff, S., and Bank, A. (1988) Construction and use of a safe and efficient amphotropic packaging cell line. *Virology* **167,** 400–406.

30. Milligan, J. F., Groebe, D., R., Witherell, G. W., and Uhlenbeck, O. C. (1987) Oligoribonucleotide synthesis using T7 RNA polymerase and synthetic DNA templates. *Nucl. Acids Res.* **15,** 8783–8798.

31. Pastan, I., Gottesman, M. M., Ueda, K., Lovelace, E., Rutherford, A. V., and Willingham, M. C. (1988) A retrovirus carrying an *MDR*1 cDNA confers multidrug resistance and polarized expression of P-glycoprotein in MDCK cells. *Proc. Natl. Acad. USA* **85,** 4486–4490.

32. Riordan, J. R. and Ling, V. (1974) Purification of p-glycoprotein from plasma membrane vesicles of Chinese hamster ovary cell mutants with reduced permeability. *J. Biol. Chem.* **254,** 12701–12705.

33. Fairbanks, G., Steck, T. C., and Wallach, D. F. H. (1971) Electrophoretic analysis of the major polypeptides of the human erythrocyte membrane. *Biochemistry* **10,** 2602–2617.

34. Hamada, H. and Tsuruo, T. (1986) Functional role for the 170- and 180-kDa glycoprotein specific to drug resistant tumor cells as revealed by monoclonal antibodies. *Proc. Natl. Acad. Sci. USA* **83,** 7785–7789.

35. Chen, C. J., Chin, J. E., Ueda, K., Clark, D., Ueda, K., Pastan, I., et al.(1986) Internal duplication and homology with bacterial transport proteins in the mdr1 (P-glycoprotein) gene from multidrug-resistant human cells. *Cell* **47,** 381–389.

36. Kain, K. C., Orlandi, P. A., and Lanar, D. E. (1991) Universal promoter for gene expression without cloning: expression-PCR. *Biotechniques* **10,** 366–373.

37. Takigawa, N., Danno, K., and Furukawa, F. (1987) Effects of colchicine and cytochalasin B on distribution of concanavalin A receptors in isolated and cultured guinea pig epidermal cells. *Arch. Dermatol. Res.* **279,** 392–397.

38. Finbloom, D. S., Martin, J., and Gordon, R. K. (1987) Endocytosis of particulate and soluble IgG immune complexes: differential effects of cytoskeletal modulating agents. *Clin. Exp. Immunol.* **67,** 205–210.

14

Anti-c-*erb*B2 Ribozyme for Gene Therapy of Breast Cancer

Toshiya Suzuki, Masami Bessho, and Kevin J. Scanlon

1. Introduction

The application of antioncogene ribozyme in the gene therapy of breast cancer by means of recombinant adenoviral vector is dicussed in this chapter. We have shown that recombinant adenovirus encoding anti-c*erb*B2 ribozyme inhibited the breast cancer cell growth in vivo efficiently *(1,2)*. We will talk about the detailed protocol here.

The c-*erb*B2 protooncogene (also called *HER-2/neu*) encodes a 185 kDa transmembrane receptor that is homologous with the epidermal growth factor receptor (EGFR) *(3,4)*. c-*erb*B2 overexpression can transform *NIH*3T3 cells in a ligand-independent manner *(5,6)* and c-*erb*B2 protein is constitutively phosphorylated and demonstrates tyrosine kinase activity without the presence of ligand when overexpressed in NIH3T3 cells *(7)*. A possible role of c-*erb*B2 in human breast cancer has been postulated through its amplification and overexpression *(8)*. c-*erb*B2 overexpression occurs in approximately 20–30% of examined tumors *(9,10)*. Moreover, there appears to be a correlation between high levels of c-*erb*B2 expression and poor clinical outcome, particularly in patients with positive axillary lymph nodes *(11–13)*. c-*erb*B2 has been implicated in the metastatic phenotype *(14)*. Because c-erbB2 protein is not expressed in most normal human tissues *(15,16)*, downregulating c-*erb*B2 expression may be an important strategy for breast cancer gene therapy to inhibit aberrant growth of the tumor. Previous studies regarding breast cancer and other c-*erb*B2 overexpressed cancers such as ovarian cancer have shown that monoclonal antibodies *(17–21)*, single-chain antibodies engineered for intracellular expression *(22–25)*, and triplex *(26,27)* or antisense oligonucle-

From: *Methods in Molecular Medicine, Vol. 35: Gene Therapy: Methods and Protocols*
Edited by: W. Walther and U. Stein © Humana Press, Inc., Totowa, NJ

otides designed against c-*erb*B2 *(28,29)* are capable of downregulating its expression, however, the effects seemed not sufficient enough to inhibit aberrant breast cancer growth.

The utility of catalytic RNAs such as hammerhead ribozymes to attenuate mRNA expression have been well demonstrated and its application to cancer gene therapy has been suggested *(30,31)*. The effectiveness of antioncogene ribozymes in reversing the malignant phenotype of cancer cells has been demonstrated in human bladder carcinoma cells *(31–34)*, malignant melanoma cells *(35–37)*, and *ras*-transformed NIH3T3 cells. These studies have targeted the mutated *H-ras* gene at codon 12 given its transforming potential *(38,39)*.

We designed anti-c-*erb*B2 ribozyme to downregulate c-*erb*B2 expression effeciently in human breast cancer cells. Because specific c-*erb*B2 mutations have not been found in human breast cancer *(40)*, we made anti-c-*erb*B2 ribozyme that cleaves normal c-*erb*B2 mRNA. We found anti-c-*erb*B2 ribozyme downregulate c-*erb*B2 mRNA expression effectively in vitro in human breast cancer BT-474 cells that overexpress c-*erb*B2 *(2)*. We were urgent to apply anti c-*erb*B2 ribozyme in vivo. In order to achieve efficient gene delivery in vivo, we engineered a recombinant adenovirus encoding the same anti-c-*erb*B2 ribozyme driven by the cytomegalovirus (CMV) promoter and designated rAdEB2Rz. In vitro studies revealed that the recombinant adenovirus had a high transduction efficacy and downregulated c-erbB2 mRNA expression in breast cancer cells *(1)*. When human breast cancer BT-474 cells were transduced with 500 PFU (plaque forming units)/cell of rAdEB2Rz, tumorigenicity of the cells was suppressed in comparison with the control recombinant adenovirus. Weekly treatments of subcutaneously established BT-474 tumors with 10 PFU/cell of rAdEB2Rz inhibited tumor growth markedly. Tumor size diminished as small as one fifth of the control. The growth inhibitory effect of rAdEB2Rz has been observed to be greater than that of a recombinant adenovirus encoding anti-c-*erb*B2 antisense.

Adenovirus-mediated anti-c-*erb*B2 ribozyme gene delivery represents a rational strategy for breast cancer gene therapy in view of its efficacy.

2. Materials

Materials and Methods have been partly described elsewhere *(2)*.

2.1. Cells

Human E1A transcomplementary 293 cells were obtained from Dr. F. Graham (McMaster University, Hamilton, Ontario, Canada) (*see* **Note 1**). BT-474 cells, established from human breast adenocarcinoma, were obtained from American Type Culture Collection (ATCC, Rockville, MD).

2.2. Culture Medium

293 cells are cultured in RPMI 1640 medium (Life Technologies, Gaithersburg, MD) supplemented with 10% fetal bovine serum (FBS, Life Technologies) with 5% CO_2 in air under humidified conditions at 37°C. BT-474 cells are cultured in RPMI 1640 medium supplemented with 10% fetal bovine serum (FBS) (Life Technologies), 300 mg/L of L-glutamine (Life Technologies), and 10 mg/mL of bovine serum insulin (Life Technologies). Cells are usually subcultured every week using Trypsin/EDTA (Life Technologies). Mycoplasm contamination is ruled out every 3 mo using Genprobe (Life Technologies) according to the manufacturer's protocol.

2.3. Infection Medium

RPMI supplemented with 2% FBS, 2 mM L-glutamine, and 0.8 mM L-arginine is used for infection experiment.

2.4. Oligonucleotides

Designing ribozyme is critical element for sufficient catalytic activity. Selecting appropriate GUC sequence in the target mRNA is the critical step for successful study. We make three different anti-c-*erb*B2 ribozymes (*see* **Note 2**). When we express the three ribozyme sequences under the control of β-actin promoter in vitro, we find the anti-c-*erb*B2 ribozyme targeting codon 71 and 72 inhibited the tumor growth most effectively *(1)*. To make the recombinant adenovirus encoding anti-c-*erb*B2 hammerhead ribozyme (**Fig. 1**), we synthesize R1 and R2 complementary oligo-deoxynucleotides targeting codon 71/72 of the c-*erb*B2 cDNA sequence *(4)* by adding linker sequence for *Sal*I -*Hind* III. The sequences for R1 and R2 are as follows.

R1: 5′-TCG ACA GGA AGC TGA TGA GTC CGT GAG GAC GAA ACA GGC TA-3′

R2: 5′-AGC TTA GCC TGT TTC GTC CTC ACG GAC TCA TCA GCT TCC TG-3′

We also synthesize oligonucleotides to construct recombinant adenoviruses encoding a corresponding anti-c-*erb*B2 mutant ribozyme (mR1/mR2) and anti-c-*erb*B2 antisense (A1/A2) targeting the same mRNA sequences (*see* **Note 3**). The mutant ribozyme has a one-base mutation, resulting in loss of cleavage activity. The structures of these inserts are shown in **Fig. 1**. The sequences of the oligos are as follows and one-point mutation of the ribozyme sequence is indicated by an asterisk.

mR1: 5′-TCG ACA GGA AGC TC*A TGA GTC CGT GAG GAC GAA ACA GGC TA-3′

mR2: 5′-AGC TTA GCC TGT TTC GTC CTC ACG GAC TCA TG*A GCT TCC TG-3′

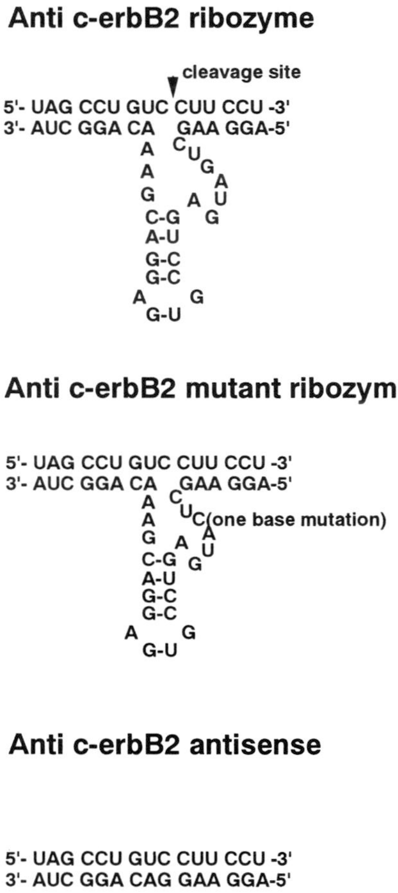

Anti c-erbB2 ribozyme

```
                       ▼ cleavage site
        5'- UAG CCU GUC CUU CCU -3'
        3'- AUC GGA CA   GAA GGA-5'
                      A  C U
                      A     G
                      G    A  A
                      C-G  A  U
                      A-U     G
                      G-C
                      G-C
                    A     G
                      G-U
```

Anti c-erbB2 mutant ribozyme

```
        5'- UAG CCU GUC CUU CCU -3'
        3'- AUC GGA CA  GAA GGA-5'
                     A  C
                     A   U C (one base mutation)
                     G     A
                     C-G A  U
                     A-U G
                     G-C
                     G-C
                   A     G
                     G-U
```

Anti c-erbB2 antisense

```
        5'- UAG CCU GUC CUU CCU -3'
        3'- AUC GGA CAG GAA GGA-5'
```

Fig. 1. Structure of anti-*c-erb*B2 hammerhead ribozyme. Target GUC is located between codon 71 and 72. The mutant ribozyme that has one base mutation in the catalytic core region of the hammerhead ribozyme shows no cleavage activity. The antisense that target the same sequence is illustrated.

A1: 5'-TCG ACA GGA AGG ACA GGC TA-3'
A2: 5'-AGC TTA GCC TGT CCT TCC TG-3'
Oligonucleotides for detecting ribozyme are synthesized (Rz stem probe).
Rz stem: 5'-CTC ACG GAC TCA TCA GC-3'
Oligonucleotides used for detecting c-erbB2 expression (P1 and P2) by RT-PCR-Southern have the following sequences.
P1: 5'-GCG TGT ACG GTG GGA GGT CT-3'
P2: 5'-GTT TCG TCC TCA CGG ACT CAT-3'

We use the *Sq*1 primer to confirm the ribozyme sequence in the PACCMVpLpARS(+) shuttle plasmid and thereafter in the recombinant adenovirus.

Sq1: 5'-GAC CAG TGT TTG CCT TTT A-3'

To rule out wild type adenovirus contamination, viral DNA is amplified with P3 and P4 primers. P3 and P4 primers are designed to amplify *E1A* gene.

P3: 5'-ATT ACC GAA GAA ATG GCC GC-3'

P4: 5'-CCCATTTAACAC GCC ATG CA-3'

2.5. Buffers

1. Calcium-free phosphate-buffered saline (PBS).
2. 50 X TAE.
   1 L of 50X Tris-acetate (TAE) stock is prepared according to the following formula: 242 g Tris base, 57.1 mL glacial acetic acid, 100 mL 0.5*M* EDTA (pH 8.0), and add dH$_2$O to a final volume of 1 L.
3. 5 X TBE.
   1 L of 5X Tris-borate (TBE) stock is prepared according to the following formula: 54 g Tris base, 27.5 g boric acid, 20 mL 0.5*M* EDTA pH 8.0, and add dH$_2$O to a final volume of 1 L.
4. QuickHyb (Stratagene, La Jolla, CA).
5. 1.33 CsCl; 454.2 g cesium chloride in 1 L of 5 m*M* HEPES, pH 7.8.
6. 1.45 CsCl; 609.0 g cesium chloride in 1 L of 5 m*M* HEPES, pH 7.8.
7. Dialysis buffer: 10 m*M* HEPES, pH 7.8, 1 m*M* KCl, and 10% glycerol.
8. Viral preservation buffer: 10 m*M* Tris HCl, pH 8.0, 100 m*M* NaCl, and 1 mg/mL BSA and 50% glycerol.

2.6. Liquid Media

1. LB medium: 10 g bacto-tryptone, 5 g bacto-yeast extract, 10 g NaCl, and add dH2O to a final volume of 1 L and autoclave. Usually, ampicillin is added to LB medium just before use at a final concentration of 50 mg/mL.
2. LA plate: 10 g bacto-tryptone, 5 g bacto-yeast extract, 10 g NaCl, 15 g bactoagar, and add dH$_2$O to a final volume of 1 L and autoclave. When the medium has cooled, add ampicillin to a final concentration of 50 µg/mL, pour into dishes, and store at 4°C.

2.7. Reagens

2.7.1. Enzymes and Reaction Buffers

1. T4 DNA kinase (Life Technologies).
2. T4 DNA kinase buffer (Life Technologies).
3. T4 DNA ligase (Life Technologies).
4. T4 DNA ligase buffer (Life Technologies).

5. Reverse transcriptase (Stratagene).
6. *Taq* DNA polymerase (Stratagene).
7. *Taq* DNA polymerase reaction buffer.
8. Deoxynucleotide mix (Stratagene).
9. Proteinase K (Boehlinger Manheim, Germany).

2.7.2. Reagens

1. DOTAP (Boehlinger Manheim).
2. $[\gamma^{-32}P]ATP$ (Dupont NEN, Boston, MA).
3. $[\alpha^{-32}P]dCTP$ (Dupont NEN).
4. Ammonium persulfate (Sigma).
5. N, N, N', N'-tetramethylethylenediamine (TEMED) (Sigma, St. Louis, MO).
6. Diethyl pyrocarbonate (Sigma).
7. abSolve (Dupont).
8. c-*erb*B2 cDNA probe (Oncogene Science, Cambridge, MA).
9. 17β-estradiol pellet (0.72 mg, 60-d release type, Innovative Research of America, Toledo, OH).
10. Matrigel (Collaborative Biomedical, Bedford, MA).

2.7.3. Miscellaneous

1. Nylon filter (Hybond-N+, Amersham, Buckinghamshire, UK).
2. G-50 column (pZ523™) (5 prime-3 prime Inc., Boulder, CO).
3. Kodak Scientific Imaging Film (Eastman Kodak, Rochester, NY).
4. 18 and 28 gage needles.
5. 1-mL insulin syringe and 10-mL syringe.

2.7.4. Kits

1. QIAquick Gel Extraction Kit (Qiagen, Chatsworth, CA).
2. QIAprep Spin Plasmid Miniprep Kit (Qiagen).
3. Endofree QIAfilter Plasmid Maxi Kit (Qiagen).
4. FastTrack mRNA isolation kit (Invitrogen, San Diego, CA).
5. Random-primed labeling kit (Life Technologies).

2.8. Animals

1. Female nu/nu mice (6-month-old, Charles River, Portage, MI).

3. Methods

3.1. Preparation of Recombinant Adenovirus Encoding anti-c-erbB2 Ribozyme

1. The R1 and R2 oligodeoxynucleotides for the anti-c-*erb*B2 ribozyme are annealed, phosphorylated by T4 DNA kinase (Life Technologies) at 37°C for 1 h. pACCMVpLpARS(+) shuttle plasmid, is prepared by digestion with *Sal*I and

*Hind*III. The plasmid is then electrophoresed on a 1% agarose gel in 1X TAE buffer. The DNA is cut from the gel and purified by using QIA quick Gel Extraction Kit according to the manufacturer's protocol (Qiagen) and then ligated with the phosphotylated ribozyme insert using T4 DNA ligase (Life Technologies) at 14°C for 16 h. The plasmid is ampicillin resistant in this experiment *(33)*.

2. After ligation, the insert is confirmed by Southern blot analysis using the 5′ end labeled Rz stem probe. DNA is electrophoresed on the 1% TAE agarose gel. The DNA is transferred to the nylon membrane filter (Hybond N⁺, Amersham, Arlinton Heights, IL) with 0.4 N NaOH using transblot apparatus. Time for blotting is usually 1 h. After blotting, DNA is fixed on the filter by Stratalinker (Stratagene).

3. Single-strand DNA probe (Rz stem) is used for the labeling by 5′ end labeling. $[\gamma^{-32}P]$ATP is purchased from Dupont NEN. Denaturing DNA is not required.

dH₂O	13 µl
10X T4 Kinase Buffer	1 µl
DNA probe (20 pmol/µl)	2 µl
$[\gamma^{-32}P]$ATP	2 µl
T4 Kinase (10 U/µl)	1 µl

    After mixing, the sample is incubated at 37°C for 1 h and gel-filtrated using G-50 column.

4. We use QuickHyb as prehybridization buffer. Prehybridization is performed at 65°C for more than 30 min and the hybridization is achieved with the 5′ end labeled hot probe at 65°C for 1 h using a rotating oven (VWR, Berlin, Germany).

5. The hybridized filter is washed in 2X SSC, 0.1% SDS at 37°C for 60 min and in 0.1X SSC, 0.5% SDS at 68°C for 60 min.

6. To visualize clear and intense ribozyme expression bands, the autoradiograph is performed using Kodak Scientific Imaging Film (Eastman Kodak) and intensifing screen (Dupont NEN) at –80°C.

7. After Southern blotting, the insert sequence is confirmed by sequencing using the Sq1 primer and the dsDNA cycle sequencing system according to the manufacturer's recommendation (Life Technologies). $[\alpha^{-32}P]$dCTP is purchased from Dupont NEN. The DNA samples are electrophoresed on a 6% polyacrylamide gel using 1X TBE. After running, the gel is dried and autoradiographed. Once the sequence is confirmed, the plasmid can be used in subsequent steps.

3.2. Large-Scale Preparation of the Plasmid

pJM17 and the sequence-confirmed shuttle plasmid are cultured in 500 mL of LB with ampicillin at a final concentration of 50 µg/mL for 37°C overnight, respectively. The cultured medium is then centrifuged at 10,000g for 20 min at 4°C and the pellet is used for DNA isolation. The DNA is isolated using Endofree QIAfilter Plasmid Maxi Kit (Qiagen) according to the manufacturer's protocol (*see* **Note 4**).

3.3. Cotransfection

The pJM17 rescue plasmid (*see* **Note 5**) and the shuttle plasmid are cotransfected with 293 cells using DOTAP (Boehlinger Manheim, Germany) according to the manufacturer's recommendation *(33)*. When first lysis appeared, the plaque is selected and purified three times.

3.4. Virus Purification

After purification, recombinant adenovirus is infected with 293 cells. Cells were cultured and harvested 48 h later. Recombinant adenovirus is isolated after three freeze-thaw cycles followed by cesium chloride density gradient ultracentrifugation. Briefly, freeze-thawed cell suspension is overlaid onto 1.33 CsCl on 1.45 CsCl cushion. Ultracentrifuge the sample at 18,000g using a swing rotor for 1.5 h at 20°C. The white viral band can be easily recognized after ultracentrifugation. Draw the band with an 18G needle and overlay again onto 1.33 CsCl on 1.45 CsCl cushion. Ultracentrifuge at 25,000g using a swing rotor for 18 h at 20°C and draw the viral band again. Viral solution is dialyzed against dialysis buffer and stocked with viral preservation buffer in small aliquots at –80°C. The resultant adenoviruses encoding anti c-*erb*B2 ribozyme, anti-c-*erb*B2 mutant ribozyme, anti-c-*erb*B2 antisense, and empty casettes are designated as rAdEB2Rz, rAdEB2mRz, rAdEB2As, and rAd-vector, respectively. rAdCMVLacZ was a kind gift from Dr. R. Gerald (University of Texas) and rAdHrasRz that encodes anti-H-*ras* ribozyme was previously reported as rAdGT6 *(33)*.

3.5. Virus Titration

Dialyzed recombinant adenovirus is infected with 1×10^6 of 293 cells at various dilutions with infection medium. Experiments should be carried out in duplicate. After 1.5 h of viral infection, the infection medium is removed and 0.65% bactoagar in infection medium is added onto the infected 293 cells. The infected cells are incubated with 5% CO_2 in air under humidified condition. The plaque forming unit (PFU) is determined using an inverted microscope on day 14.

3.6. Virus Verification

Viral DNA is isolated from the recombinant adenovirus with 100 µg/mL proteinase K, 0.6% SDS, and 10 mM EDTA at 55°C for 1 h followed by twice phenol/chlorform extraction and ethanol precipitation. To rule out E1A positive wild type adenovirus contamination, DNA is amplifed with the P3 and P4 primers and *Taq* polymerase (Perkin Elmer, Norwalk, CT) by polymerase chain reaction (PCR) using 30 thermal cycles of 94°C for 1 min, 56°C for

1 min, and 72°C for 2 min *(33)*. To confirm the presence of the expected insert, DNA is amplified by PCR similarly with the P1 and P2 primers. The PCR product is electrophoresed on 1% TAE agarose gel.

3.7. Northern Blots

1. The FastTrack mRNA isolation kit (Invitrogen, San Diego, CA) is used for the isolation of poly (A)$^+$ RNA according to the manufacture's protocol to isolate mRNA from the breast cancer cells in vitro and in vivo.
2. One µg of poly (A)$^+$ RNA species is loaded onto the formaldehyde gel and transferred to the Hybond N$^+$ nylon membrane (Amersham). In the Northern blot performed to detect cleaved c-*erb*B2 mRNA, we apply 10 µg of the poly (A)$^+$ RNA onto the gel. The blotted filter is crosslinked by Stratalinker (Stratagene), prehybridized and hybridized with labeled c-*erb*B2 cDNA (Oncogene Science), anti-c-*erb*B2 ribozyme insert (R1/R2 primers), anti-c-*erb*B2 antisense insert (A1/A2 primers), phosphoglycerate kinase (PGK) cDNA, and glyceraldehyde-3-phosphate dehydrogenase (GAPDH) primer (Oncogene Science) at 68°C with QuickHyb (Stratagene) for 1 h. c-*erb*B2 and PGK are labeled by the random-primed labeling kit (Life Technologies) with [α-^{32}P]dCTP (NEN). Ribozyme, antisense, and GAPDH primers are labeled by 5' end labeling kit (Life Technologies) with [γ-^{32}P]ATP (Dupont NEN). The hybridized filter is washed in 2X SSC, 0.1% SDS at 37°C for 60 min and in 0.1X SSC, 0.5% SDS at 68°C for 60 min. The filter is autoradiographed with an intensifying screen (Dupont) at –80°C. After hybridization using the appropriate probe, the filter was dehybridized with boiled 0.5% SDS and rehybridized with PGK cDNA or GAPDH primer to confirm equal loading on the gel.
3. Double-stranded DNA probe is labeled by the random-primed labelling kit (Life Technologies) according to the manufacturer's recommendation.
4. 1 µg of poly (A)$^+$RNA is used for reverse transcriptase-polymerase chain reaction (RT-PCR)-Southern blot to detect ribozyme expression. Poly (A)$^+$ RNA is incubated with reverse transcriptase (Stratagene) at 37°C for 1 h and the resultant cDNA is used for PCR using P1 and P2 primers, dNTP mix, and *Taq* DNA plymerase (Stratagene). The PCR cycle is 55°C for 1 min, 72°C for 2 min, and 94°C for 1 min and the cycle is repeated 30 times using the GenAmp PCR System 9600 (Perkin Elmer, Norwalk, CT). The electrophoresed PCR product is transferred to a nylon membrane (Hybond N$^+$) with 0.4 *N* NaOH using a transblot apparatus, UV crosslinked, and thereafter hybridized with 5' end-labeled Rz stem probe as previously described in Southern blot. The hybridized filter is washed in 2X SSC, 0.1% SDS at 37°C for 60 min, thereafter in 0.1X SSC, 0.5% SDS at 68°C for 60 min, and autoradiographed with an intensifying screen at –80°C.

3.8. In Vitro Effect of the Recombinant Adenovirus

2×10^4 BT-474 cells are cultured in a 35-mm dish. The cells are infected with 5 MOI (multiplicity of infection), 50 MOI, or 500 MOI of rAdEB2Rz, or

500 MOI of rAdEB2mRz, rAdEB2As, rAdCMVLacZ, rAd-vector, or rAd-HrasRz. We incubate the cells with the recombinant adenovirus for 1.5 h and exchanged the medium. Cells are trypsinized and the number of cells in each dish is determined 72 h later using a Coulter counter. Cells treated with rAdCMVLacZ are fixed with glutaraldehyde (Sigma) and stained with X-gal (Stratagene) to determine infection efficacy.

3.9. Tumor Implantation into Nude Mice

Six-wk-old female nu/nu mice are purchased from Charles River Breeding Laboratories (Portage, MI) and maintained under standard pathogen-free conditions. One day before tumor cell injection, mice are implanted with a 17β-estradiol pellet (0.72 mg, 60-d release type, Innovative Research of America). We trypsinize and harvest log-phase growing BT-474 cells. We resuspend them in PBS and inject 1×10^7 BT-474 cells in a volume of 0.1 mL subcutaneously into bilateral mice flanks with 0.1 mL of matrigel (Collaborative Biomedical, Bedford, MA) using 28-gauge needles (*see* **Note 6**). Tumor size is measured every other day and the tumor volume is calculated by the formula: (length $\times$ width^2)/2.

3.10. Intratumoral Injection of the Recombinant Adenovirus

On day 14 post implantation, we inject 10 MOI of the recombinant adenovirus into the tumors locating on both flanks of the nude mice. The amount of virus required is calculated by the assumption that 1 cm^3 of tumor contains 1×10^9 cells. The virus is resuspended in 0.1 mL of PBS and injected directly into the tumor (**Fig. 2**). PBS is always injected into the contralateral tumor. Five weekly treatments are performed. Tumor size is measured every other day (*see* **Note 7**). On day 50, mice are sacrificed and used for pathological analysis.

4. Notes

1. The passages of 293 cells should be lower than 50.
2. We recommend to design several different ribozymes. After subcloning them into some expression casette and introducing them into cultured cells, we can anticipate the cleavage activity of the specific ribozyme by the doubling time of the transformed cells *(1,2)*.
3. Ribozyme studies should be performed using ribozyme controls, a mutant ribozyme containing a point mutation that shows no in vitro cleavage activity, a nonsense ribozyme that targets an independent mRNA sequence, and an antisense control that targets the same sequence as the experimental ribozyme.
4. We recommend to use Qiagen Endofree Maxi Kit to prepare shuttle plasmid and rescue plasmid to avoid endotoxin contamination in the cotransfection experiment. Endotoxin interferes the efficacy of cotransfection significantly.

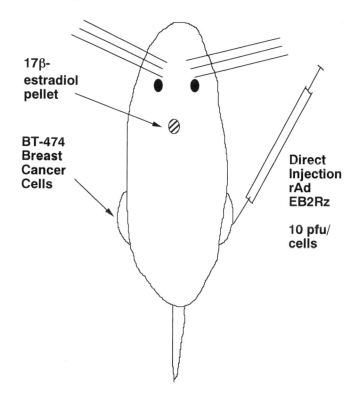

nude mouse

Fig. 2. Direct injection of the recombinant adenovirus into the breast cancer cells in the nude mouse. Six-week-old female nu/nu mouse is used. One day before tumor cell injection, mice are implanted with a 17β-estradiol pellet. 1×10^7 BT-474 cells in a volume of 0.1 mL of PBS are injected subcutaneously into bilateral mice flanks with 0.1 mL of matrigel using 28-gauge needles. Tumor size is measured every other day and the tumor volume was calculated by the formula; (length × width^2)/2. On day 14 post-implantation, 10 MOI of the recombinant adenovirus was injected into the tumors. The amount of virus required is calculated by the assumption that 1 cm3 of tumor contains 1×10^9 cells. The virus is resuspended in 0.1-mL of PBS and injected directly into the tumor. PBS was always injected into the contralateral tumor. Five weekly treatments were performed. The mouse was sacrificed for pathological examination on day five.

5. The good quality of pJM17 is critical for the successful cotransfection. Check pJM 17 with *Hind*III digestion to confirm appropriate DNA ladder formation.
6. Matrigels should be kept on ice during the injection experiment.

7. In a minority of cases, the bilateral tumors regressed spontaneously after the second injection. These cases were supposed to be caused by an immunological reaction against the adenovirus.

Acknowledgments

The work of T. Suzuki was supported by a grant from Chugai Pharmaceutical Company, Japan.

References

1. Suzuki, T., Anderegg, B., Ohkawa, T., Irie, A., Halks-Miller, M., Holm, P. S., et al. (1998) A recombinant adenovirus encoding a ribozyme targeting c-*erb*B2 inhibits tumorigenicity and growth of human breast cancer cells in vivo. Submitted.
2. Suzuki, T., Curcio, L., Tsai, J., and Kashani-Sabet, M. (1998) Anti-c-*erb*-B-2 ribozyme for breast cancer, in *Therapeutic application of ribozymes* (Scanlon, K. J., ed.), Humana, Totowa, NJ, pp. 223–239.
3. Bargmann, C. I., Hung, M-C., and Weinberg, R. A. (1986) The *neu* oncogene encodes an epidermal growth factor receptor-related protein. *Nature* (Lond.) **319,** 226–230.
4. Yamamoto, T., Ikawa, S., Akiyama, T., Semba, K., Nomura, N., Miyajima, N., et al. (1986) Similarity of protein encoded by the human c-*erb*B-2 gene to epidermal growth factor receptor. *Nature (Lond.)* **319,** 230–234.
5. Hudziak, R. M., Schlessinger, J., and Ullrich, A. (1987) Increased expression of the putative growth factor receptor p185^{HER2} causes transformation and tumorigenesis of NIH3T3 cells. *Proc. Natl. Acad. Sci. USA* **84,** 7159–7163.
6. Di Fiore, P. P., Pierce, J. H., Kraus, M. H., Segatto, O., King, C. R., and Aaronson, S. A. (1987) *erb*B-2 is a potent oncogene when overexpressed in NIH/3T3 cells. *Science* (Wash. DC) **237,** 178–182.
7. Lonardo, F., Di Marco, E., King, C. R., Pierce, J. H., Segatto, O., Aaronson, S. A., and Di Fiore, P. P. (1990) The normal *erb*B-2 product is an atypical receptor-like tyrosine kinase with constitutive activity in the absence of ligand. *New Biol.* **2,** 992–1003.
8. Gusterson, B. A. (1992) Identification and interpretation of epidermal growth factor and c-*erb*B-2 overexpression. *Eur. J. Cancer* **28,** 263–267.
9. Slamon, D. J., Godolphin, W., Jones, L. A., Holt, J. A., Wong, S. G., Keith, D. E., et al. (1989) Studies of the *HER*-2/*neu* proto-oncogene in human breast and ovarian cancer. *Science* (Wash. DC) **244,** 707–712.
10. Slamon, D. J., Clark, G. M., Wong, S. G., Levin, W. J., Ullrich, A., and McGuire, W. L. (1987) Human breast cancer: correlation of relapse and survival with amplification of the *HER*-2/neu oncogene. *Science* (Wash. DC) **235,** 177–182.
11. Perren, T. J. (1991) cv-*erb*B-2 oncogene as a prognostic marker in breast cancer (editorial). *Br. J. Cancer* **63,** 328–332.

12. Gullick, W. J., Love, S. B., Wright, C., Barnes, D. M., Guesterson, B., Harris, A. L., and Altman, D. G. (1991) c-*erb*B-2 protein overexpression in breast cancer is a risk factor in patients with involved and uninvolved lymph nodes. *Br. J. Cancer* **63,** 434–438.
13. Muss, H. B., Thor, A. D., Berry, D. A., Kute, T., Liu, E. T., Koerner, F., et al. (1994) C-*erb*B-2 expression and response to adjuvant therapy in women with node-positive early breast cancer. *N. Eng. J. Med.* **330,** 1260–1266.
14. Tan, M. and Yu, D. (1997) Overexpression of the c-*erb*B-2 gene enhanced intrinsic metastasis potential in human breast cancer cells without increasing their transformation abilities. *Cancer Res.* **57,** 1199–1205.
15. Pier, G. N., Nicortra, M. R., Bigotti, A., Venturo, I., Slamon, D. J., Fendly, B. M., and Ullrich, A. (1990) Expression of the p185 encoded by *HER*2 oncogene in normal and transformed human tissues. *Int. J. Cancer* **45,** 457–461.
16. Press, M. F., Cordon-Cardo, C., and Slamon, D. (1990) Expression of the *HER*-2/*neu* proto-oncogene in normal human adult and fetal tissues. *Oncogene* **5,** 953–962.
17. Hudziak, R. M., Lewis, G. D., Winget, M., Fendly, B. M., Shepard, H. M., and Ullrich, A. (1989) p185^{HER-2} monoclonal antibody has antiproliferative effects in vitro and sensitized human breast cancer cells to tumor necrosis factor. *Mol. Cell. Biol.* **9,** 1165–1172.
18. Fendly, B. M., Winget, M., Hudziak, R. M., Lipari, M. T., Mapier, M. A. and Ullrich, A. (1990) The extracellular domain of *HER*2/*neu* is a potential immunogen for active specific immunotherapy of breast cancer. *Cancer Res.* **50,** 1550–1558.
19. Shepard, H. M., Lewis, G. D., Sarup, J. C., Fendly, B. M., Maneval, D., Mordenti, J., et al. (1991) Monoclonal antibody therapy of human cancer: taking the *HER*2 proto-oncogene to the clinic. *J. Clin. Immunol.* **11,** 117–127.
20. Lewis, G. D., Figari, I., Fendly, B., Wong W. L., Carter, P., Gorman, C., and Shepard, H. M. (1993) Differential responses of human tumor cell line to anti-p185^{HER2} monoclonal antibodies. *Cancer Immunol. Immunother.* **37,** 255–263.
21. Vaughm, J. P., Igelehart, J. D., Demirdji, S., Davis, P., Babiss, L. E., Caruthers, M. H., and Marks, J. R. (1995) Antisense DNA downregulation of the *ERB*B2 oncogene measured by a flow cytometric assay. *Proc. Natl. Acad. Sci. USA* **92,** 8338–8342.
22. Beerli, R. R., Wels, W., and Hynes, N. E. (1994) Intracellular expression of single chain antibodies reverts *erb*-B2 transformation. *J. Biol. Chem.* **269,** 23,931–23,936.
23. Deshane, J., Loechel, F., Conry, R. M., Siegel, G. P., King, C. R., and Curiel, D. T. (1994) Intracellular single-chain antibody directed against *erb*B2 down-regulated cell surface *erb*B2 and exhibits a selective anti-proliferative effect in *erb*B2 overexpressing cancer cell lines. *Gene Therapy* **1,** 332–337.
24. Deshane, J., Grim, J., Loechel, L., Siegel, G.P., Alvarez, R. D., and Curiel, D. T. (1996) Intracellular antibody against *erb*B-2 mediates targeted tumor cell eradication by apoptosis. *Cancer Gene Ther.* **3,** 89–98.
25. Deshane, J., Siegel, G. P., Alvarez, R. D., Wang, M., Feng, M., Cabrera, G., et al. (1995) Targeted tumor killing via an intracellular antibody against *erb*B-2. *J. Clin. Invest.* **96,** 2980–2989.

26. Ebbinghaus, S. W., Gee, J. E., Roudu, B., Mayfield, C. A., Sanders, G., and Miller, D. M. (1993) Triplex formation inhibits *HER*-2/*neu* transcription in vitro. *J. Clin. Invest.* **92**, 2433–2439.

27. Noonberb, S. B., Scott, G. K., Hunt, C. A., Hogan, M. E., and Benz, C. C. (1994) Inhibition of transcription factor binding to the *HER*2 promoter by triplex-forming oligodeoxyribonucleotides. *Gene* **149**, 123–126.

28. Wiechen, K. and Dietel, M. (1995) c-*erb*B-2 anti-sense phosphorothioate oligodeoxynucleotides inhibit growth and serum-induced cell spreading of p185$^{c-erbB-2}$ overexpressing ovarian carcinoma cells. *Int. J. Cancer* **63**, 604–608.

29. Liu, X. and Pogo, B. (1996) Inhibition of *erb*B-2-positive breast cancer cell growth by *erb*B-2 antisense oligonucleotides. *Antisense Res. Dev.* **6**, 9–16.

30. Irie, A., Kijima, H., Ohkawa, T., Bouffard, D. Y., Suzuki, T., Curcio, L. D., et al. (1997) Anti-oncogene ribozyme for cancer gene therapy, in *Gene Therapy* (August, J. T., ed.), Academic, San Diego, CA, pp. 207–257.

31. Scanlon, K. J., Ohta, Y., Ishida, H., Kijima, H., Ohkawa, T., Kaminski, A., et al. (1995) Oligonucleotide-mediated modulation of mammalian gene expression. *FASEB J.* **9**, 1288–1296.

32. Kashani-Sabet, M., Funato, T., Tone, T., Jiao, L., Wang, W., Yoshida, E., et al. (1992) Reversal of the malignant phenotype by an anti-*ras* ribozyme. *Antisense Res. Dev.* **2**, 3–15.

33. Feng, M., Cabrera, G., Deshane, J., Scanlon, K. J., and Curiel, D. T. (1995) Neoplastic reversion accomplished by high efficiency adenoviral-mediated delivery of an anti-*ras* ribozyme. *Cancer Res.* **55**, 2024–2028.

34. Tone, T., Kashani-Sabet, M., Funato, T., Shitara, T., Yoshida, E., Kashfian, B. I., et al. (1993) Suppression of EJ cells tumorigenicity. *In Vivo* **7**, 471–476.

35. Ohta, Y., Tone, T., Shitara, T., Funato, T., Jiao, L. Kashfian, B. I., et al. (1994) H-*ras* ribozyme-mediated alterlation of the human melanoma phenotype. *Ann. N.Y. Acad. Sci. USA* **716**, 242–253.

36. Ohta, Y., Kijima, H., Kashani-Sabet, M., and Scanlon, K. J. (1996) Suppression of the malignant phenotype of melanoma cells by anti-oncogene ribozymes. *J. Invest. Dermatol.* **106**, 275–280.

37. Ohta, Y., Kijima, H., Ohkawa, T., Kashani-Sabet, M., and Scanlon, K. J. (1996) Tissue-specific expression of an anti-*ras* ribozyme inhibits proliferation of human malignant melanoma cells. *Nucl. Acids Res.* **24**, 938–942.

38. Kashani-Sabet, M., Funato, T., Florenes, V. A., Fostad, O., and Scanlon, K. J. (1994) Suppression of the neoplastic phenotype in vivo by an anti-*ras* ribozyme. *Cancer Res.* **54**, 900–902.

39. Funato, T., Shitara, T., Tone, T., Jiao, L., Kashani-Sabet, M., and Scanlon, K. J. (1994) Suppression of H-*ras*-mediated transformation in NIH3T3 cells by a *ras* ribozyme. *Biochem. Pharmacol.* **48**, 1471–1475.

40. Pier, G. N., Nicortra, M. R, Bigotti, A., Venturo, I., Slamon, D. J., Fendly, B. M., and Ullrich, A. (1990) Expression of the p185 encoded by *HER*2 oncogene in normal and transformed human tissues. *Int. J. Cancer* **45**, 457–461.

15

Anti-K-*ras* Ribozyme Adenoviral Vector for Gene Therapy of Non-Small Cell Lung Cancer

Yu-An Zhang, John Nemunaitis, Alex W. Tong

1. Introduction

Lung cancer is the leading cause of cancer death for men and women in the United States. Several factors affect survival in nonsmall-cell lung cancer [NSCLC; i.e., stage, age, Karnofsky Performance Status (KPS)]. The 5-yr survival rate is <15% for newly diagnosed cases following conventional treatments. Tumor oncogenetic defects appear to be associated with adverse survival *(1,2)*. The presence of a *ras* mutation or p21^{ras} oncoprotein overexpression correlates with an unfavorable prognosis for patients with nonsmall-cell lung cancer *(3)*. These findings suggest that abnormal *ras* function contributes to pathophysiology, and raise the possibility that reversal of aberrant *ras* activity may serve as a viable therapeutic approach.

Mutations of the *ras* oncogene have been observed in approx 30% lung adenocarcinomas, predominantly involving codon 12 with a G→T transversion *(3)*. The *ras*-encoded p21^{ras} protein is a membrane-bound guanine nucleotide binding GTPase that relays extracellular growth and/or differentiation signals to the nucleus via the *raf* protein, MAPk (mitogen-activated protein kinase) kinase, and MAP kinase. The normal p21^{ras} cycles alternately through its inactive and active form through the catalytic exchange of GDP (inactive p21^{ras}) to GTP (active p21^{ras}). By comparison, activating *ras* mutations, invariably found in the GTP binding regions of p21^{ras}, produce a constitutively activated GTP-locked p21^{ras} that is believed to contribute to uncontrolled malignant growth.

Recently, Zhang and others have generated retroviral *(4)* and adenoviral *(5)* constructs with a 2 kb K-*ras* gene antisense DNA insert that is specific for the codon 61 mutation CAA→CAT. These antisense-viral vectors inhibited p21^{ras}

From: *Methods in Molecular Medicine, Vol. 35: Gene Therapy: Methods and Protocols*
Edited by: W. Walther and U. Stein © Humana Press, Inc., Totowa, NJ

expression specifically in NSCLC H460a cells that carry the relevant homozygous K-*ras* codon 61 mutation, and reduced their in vitro growth by up to 90%. Intratracheal instillation of this construct similarly inhibited the growth of H460a xenografts in 87% of innoculated animals *(6)*. These observations suggest that specific targeting of *ras* can collaterally suppress lung cancer cell growth.

Ribozymes (catalytic RNAs, RNA enzymes) are RNAs with intrinsic site-specific RNA cleavage or ligation activities *(7,8)*. They are attractive candidates for modulating gene expression, by virtue of their simple structure, and site-specific mRNA cleavage activity and catalytic potential that are lacking in antisense reagents *(9)*. The consensus sequences, structural and kinetic characteristics of ribozymes have been defined through mutational analysis, structural studies, and other biochemical experiments *(10)*. Thus, it is feasible to construct ribozymes that discriminate substrate RNAs with a single base mutation *(11)* as well as closely related RNAs *(12)*. The hammerhead ribozyme requires a substrate of "NUH" sequence 3′ of the cleavage site, with *N* being any nucleotide and *H* being *A*, *C*, or *U*. The GUC triplet is frequently chosen as a cleavage substrate because of its wide occurrences in natural ribozyme motifs *(12)*. Substrates containing GUA, GUU, UUC, or CUC triplets are also efficiently cleaved, whereas GAC, GUG, AUC, CGC, GGC, AGC, or UGC triplet sequences are poorly cleaved. Efficacy of cleavage seems to depend on the size and composition of the flanking sequence *(13)*.

The mutant *ras* oncogene is an attractive target for ribozyme-mediated gene modulation, in view of its high mutation incidence in NSCLC, the restricted mutational sites within the *ras* gene, and the crucial role of *ras* in signal transduction and neoplastic growth. The growth inhibitory effect of anti-K-*ras* as well as anti-H *ras* hammerhead ribozymes, has been well documented in human pancreatic carcinoma, melanoma, and bladder carcinoma *(8,14,15)*, but not in human lung cancers. The authors *(1)* and others *(3)* have found that nearly all NSCLC *ras* mutations occur in codon 12 of the K *ras* gene in the United States. Our study focuses on the use of a hammerhead ribozyme that is specific for the K-*ras* codon 12 mutant GUU. The human NSCLC cell lines H1725 and H441 were used to characterize the outcome of mutant *ras* gene modulation by the anti-K-*ras* ribozyme and its antitumor effect. Both lines express a heterozygous K-*ras* codon 12 mutation of GGT→GTT. As such, they are more likely to reflect *ras*-mutant tumors in patients, because point mutation resulting in a heterozygous single base pair mismatch is expected to be more prevalent than homozygous mutations. In earlier studies, we have utilized a plasmid construct comprised of the anti-K-*ras* mutant codon 12 (GUU) ribozyme construct (KRbz) cloned into the pHβ Apr-1-neo plasmid. The growth rate of H1725 cells was reduced by 81% following KRbz transfection, as compared with a less than 15% decrease in growth rate in mock-transfected cultures *(16)*. Thus KRbz was effective in inhibiting growth of NSCLC cells that carry the relevant heterozygous K-*ras* codon 12 mutation.

For potential clinical applications, it is necessary that the ribozyme be delivered effectively to the desired tissue in a nontoxic manner. Among viral vectors, the adenovirus has the advantages of being able to infect both dividing and nondividing cells, with a high efficacy of gene transfer in many types of human cancers. Adenoviruses are stable and can be obtained, in many systems, in higher titer than retrovirus (10^{10} vs 10^8 pfu/mL, respectively), thereby offering an advantage in clinical situations that require higher quantities of viral particles. In light of its natural tropism to respiratory tissues, the adenovirus vector may be particularly appropriate for delivery to lung cancers. Certain ribozymes could be designed with an inducible and/or tissue-specific enhancer/promoter for exclusive expression in diseased tissue. Such a sequence is currently not available for applications in NSCLC. As an alternative, the CMV promoter *(17)* used in our current KRbz-adenoviral construct provides a constitutive and high level of ribozyme RNA production *(8)*. Recently, we have examined the gene therapy applicability of an anti-K-*ras* ribozyme viral-vector construct (KRbz-ADV) for lung cancer cells. For the remaining portion of this chapter, we describe the production of this KRbz-adenoviral vector that is specific for the K-*ras* mutation GTT at codon 12, and evaluation of its in vivo effectiveness with a NSCLC xenograft expressing the relevant K-*ras* mutation in athymic mice.

2. Materials

2.1. Production of Anti-K-ras Ribozyme Adenoviral Vector by In Vivo Homologous Plasmid Recombination

1. Transfection grade pJM17 plasmid and pACCMVpLpA plasmid containing the KRbz insert *(18)*: these plasmids were provided by Dr. Kevin J. Scanlon (Berlex Bioscience, Richmond, CA), and purified by the Qiagen Plasmid Maxi Kit (Qiagen, Chatsworth, CA) *(19)*.
2. Trypsin-EDTA (Life Technologies, Grand Island, NY).
3. 293 cells (ATCC, Rockville, MD): cells with less than 35 passages.
4. Culture medium (all from Life Technologies): Dulbecco's modified Eagel's medium (DMEM) with 10% heat-inactivated (56°C, 30 min) horse serum and antibiotic/antimycotic (penicillin, 100 U/mL; streptomycin, 100 µg/mL; amphotericin B, 0.25 µg/mL).

5. 6-well (35-mm diameter) culture plate (Primaria, Becton Dickinson, Franklin Lakes, NJ).
6. DOTAP (N-[1-{2,3-dioleoyloxy}propyl]-N,N,N-trimethyl-ammonium methyl-sulfate (Cat# 1202 375, Boehringer Mannheim, Indianapolis, IN).
7. 12 × 75 mm and 15 mL sterile polypropylene tubes (Becton Dickinson, Franklin Lakes, NJ).
8. 20 mM HEPES Buffer, pH 7.4: filter-sterilized (Sigma, St. Louis, MO).

2.2. Viral Titer Determination by Plaque Assay

1. 293 cells (ATCC, Rockville, MD): cells with 31–40 passage.
2. Culture medium: 1X DMEM with 10% horse serum and antibiotic/antimycotic (*see* **Subheading 2.1.4.**); 1X, 2X DMEM medium only; fetal bovine serum (FBS: Atlanta Biologicals, Norcross, GA).
3. Filter-sterilized phosphate buffered saline (PBS: Sigma).
4. Low-melting agarose (SeaPlaque, FMC Bioproducts, Rockland, ME): 1.6% in deionized water, autoclaved and stored at room temperature.
5. 60-mm diameter culture dishes (Primaria, Beckston Dickson).
6. Sterile 15-mL and 50-mL tubes and 10-mL pipet (Becton Dicknson).
7. 10% bleach solution.
8. Equipment: vortexer; microwave oven; 44°C water bath; fluorescent light box.

2.3. Evaluation of Antitumor Efficacy with Human NSCLC Cell Line Xenograft

1. Immunodeficient athymic or SCID mice: NIH Swiss athymic nude mice (NIHS-*nuf*DF, Taconic, Germantown, NY) can be used. Four-to-six-week-old female mice should be housed in autoclaved-sterilized polycarbonate isolator cages with air filter (Lab Products). All procedures involving animal use are approved by the Institutional Animal Care and Use Committee.
2. Adenoviral vector: 1) KRbz-ADV vector (*see* **Subheading 3.1.**; **ref. *19***); 2) Control vector: adenoviral vector containing a noncatalytic antisense sequence only, a nonmutant hammerhead ribozyme insert with respect to the KRbz-ADV construct *(20)*, or an irrelevant insert (such as luciferase: *Luc*-ADV) at the multiple cloning site *(21)*.
3. NSCLC H441 cell line (Dr. Herbert Oie, National Cancer Institue, Bethesda, MD).
4. Cell-culture supplies: Trypsin/EDTA, RPMI1640 (Life Technologies) with 10% FBS (Atlanta Biologicals); sterile 50-mL conical tubes and 10-cm cell-culture dishes (Primaria, Becton Dickinson).
5. 1.0-mL sterile TB syringe (25G) (Becton Dickson).
6. Vernier caliper (General Hardware Manufacturing Co., New York, NY).
7. 10% bleach solution.
8. General purpose centrifuge (such as Beckman GPR centrifuge with GH 3.7 rotor or equivalent, Beckman, Palo Alto, CA).

3. Methods

3.1. Production of Anti-K-ras *Ribozyme Adenoviral Vector by In Vivo Homologous Plasmid Recombination*

The sequence encoding the anti-K-*ras* hammerhead ribozyme was first constructed into pACCMVpLpA plasmid as illustrated in **Fig. 1.** *(16,22)*. Adenoviral vectors are typically generated by in vivo homologous recombination between the adenoviral packaging vector and the vector carrying a desired gene insert *(23)*. We used a commercial liposome agent (DOTAP) to cotransfect the adenoviral packaging plasmid (pJM17) and the KRbz-shuttle plasmid (KRbz-pACCMVpLpA) into E1A transcomplementing low-passage 293 cells. The manufacturer's protocol was modified as described below (*see* **Note 1**):

1. At 24 h prior to transfection, trypsinize 293 cells and wash once with fresh culture medium. Inoculate 0.5×10^6 cells in 3 mL medium into each well of a 6-well plate. Culture to 60–80% confluence (approx. 24 h). Each cotransfection experiment should be carried out with a minimum of eight wells, since the plasmid recombination event is expected to be rare.
2. For each 293 cell-culture well to be transfected, mix KRbz-pACCMVpLpA DNA (1 μg), pJM17 DNA (1.5 μg), and HEPES buffer (20 mM) to a final volume 30 μL in a sterile polystyrene (12 × 75mm or smaller) tube.
3. Mix DOTAP (18 μL) with HEPES buffer (20 mM) to a final volume of 60 μL in another polystyrene tube for each well to be transfected.
4. Transfer 30 μL of the plasmid DNA preparations to the tube containing the DOTAP/HEPES buffer. Mix the transfection mixture by gentle pipetting. Do not vortex or centrifuge.
5. Incubate the transfection mixture for 10–15 min (room temperature). Clouding in the mixture does not affect transfection efficiency.
6. Aliquot 3.0 mL of fresh culture medium in a polystyrene tube. Transfer 90 μL of the DOTAP/KRbz-pACCMVpLpA/pJM17 mixture to the medium. Mix by gentle pipetting.
7. Remove existing culture medium in cell culture well and add 3.0 mL of the culture medium/DOTAP/KRbz-pACCMVpLpA/pJM17 preparation in a dropwise fashion.
8. Incubate at 37°C, 5% CO_2 for 6 h. Replace medium with the same volume of fresh culture medium.
9. Change media every 3 d until a cytopathic effect (CPE) is evident. CPE is indicated by "punched holes" in the cell monolayer that enlarge with time and is accompanied by increasing numbers of floating and rounded 293 cells. Onset of CPE occurs approximately 12 to 18 d post-transfection. CPE is complete at about 3 d after onset.
10. Collect the culture suspension in a sterile 15-mL polypropylene tube and lyse any

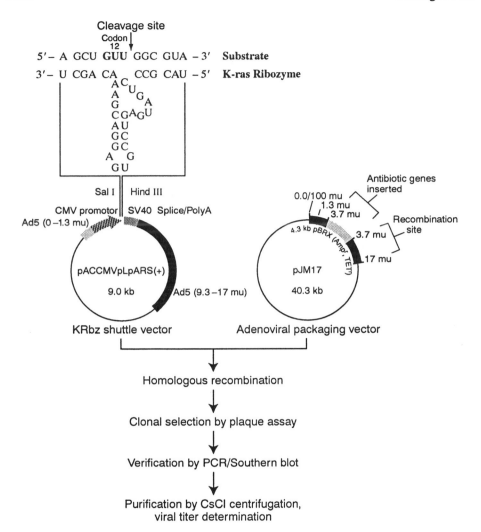

Fig. 1. Schema for the generation of the KRbz-ADV adenoviral vector. The K-*ras* ribozyme hammerhead sequence targets the GUU mutant mRNA sequence of K-*ras* 12. The ribozyme sequence was subcloned into the *Hind*III and *Sal*I site of pACCMVpLpARS(+) to form the shuttle plasmid KRbz-pACCMVpLpA. This ribozyme expression shuttle vector and the adenoviral packaging plamid pJM17 were cotransfected into 293 cells to generate the KRbz-ADV by homologous recombination.

remaining intact cells by four cycles of freeze (30 min, –70°C)-thawing (10 min, 37°C). Pellet cell debris by centrifugation and store the viral supernatant at –20°C.
11. Standard cloning protocols (*23,24*) are used for isolation and expansion of viral clones. PCR assays can be used for verification of KRbz-ADV (*see* refs. *15* and *22*; *see* **Notes 2** and **3**).

3.2. Viral Titer Determination by Plaque Assay

Viral titer of replication-defective adenoviral vector is commonly quantitated by the plaque assay with adenoviral-permissive cells such as the human embryonic kidney cell line 293 *(23,24)*. Plaque assays reflects the ability of a virus to infect, replicate in, and lyse target cells. The viral titer [plague forming unit (pfu)/mL] is determined by target cell permissibility and target cell growth phase, and efficiency of the transfection process. The transfection efficiency is affected by virus activity and concentration, volume of transfection medium, and duration of transfection *(25,26)*. To minimize the variations in quantifications, the viral titer of the anti-*ras* ribozyme adenoviral vector or control vectors should be assessed in parallel and in triplicates at any given transfection dose. Thirteen to 16 wells of 293-plated cultures are usually needed per viral stock. One should expect a viral titer of 10^8–10^9 pfu/mL for adenoviral vectors obtained from the infectious medium, and 10^{10}–10^{11} for adenoviral vectors after CsCl-purification *(23)*. Based on these considerations, we have modified the standard plaque assay *(23,24)* for titer determination of the ribozyme adenoviral vector, as described below.

1. On the day before infection, seed 2×10^6 subconfluent 293 cells onto a 60-mm diameter culture dish in 5.0 mL of complete culture medium. Culture cells for overnight at 37°C, 5% CO_2 to allow cell attachment. These cultures should attain 80% to 100% confluence, probably within 24 h.
2. Dilute the original viral stock by 1:100 (10–20 µL), followed by 1:10 serial dilutions of the viral stock in 15-mL sterile tubes (mix 0.8 mL of prediluted viral stock with 7.2 mL of 1X DMEM + 2% FBS). Mix thoroughly by gently vortexing the tubes (**Note 4**).
3. Rinse 293 cells with PBS (2.0 mL/dish) at room temperature, immediately followed by adding 2.0 mL of the diluted viral stock (or medium only as negative control). Incubate for 90 min (at 37°C; 5% CO_2) with gentle agitation (2–3 times every 30 min).
4. During incubation, heat the 1.6% low-melting agarose stock to boiling by placing in the microwave oven. Place the agarose stock in a 44°C water bath for 1 h to allow temperature equilibration.
5. Immediately before using the agarose, mix the 1.6% agarose with equal volumes of 2X concentrated DMEM + 4% FBS + 1:50 diluted antimycotics at room temperature.
6. Rinse 293 cells with PBS (2.0 mL/well). Layer 5.0 mL of the agarose-containing medium (1X DMEM, 2% FBS, 0.8% agarose and 1:100 diluted antimycotics) on each 60-mm well. Leave the dishes at room temperature for at least 15 min to allow proper agarose solidification.
7. At day 4 postinfection, layer additional 5.0 mL of the agarose-containing media to each dish. The plaques are expected to be evident visually at day 4–5, and are enumerated at day 7–8. Individually distinct plaques are counted by placing the

dishes on top of light box. The smaller ambiguous plaques require further verification by microscopy to verify the presence of cytopathic effect (rounded and lysed cells).

8. Viral titer calculations are based on infected cultures that contained between 20 and 100 plaques per plate *(27)*, based on formula: Viral titer (pfu/mL) = (Mean no. of Plaques) × *D*/2, where *D* is dilution factor and 2, volume (2.0 mL) of infective medium used. For example, when 58, 60, and 62 plaques were found in three separate plates following infection with 2.0 mL of the viral stock that had been diluted to 10^{-9}; viral titer = $[(58 + 60 + 62)/3] \times 10^9/2.0$, or 3.0×10^{10} pfu/mL.

3.3. Evaluation of Antitumor Efficacy with Human NSCLC Cell Line Xenograft

Human NSCLC line H441 was previously determined having a heterozygous GTT mutation at K-*ras* codon 12 *(16,28)*. This point mutation fulfills the theoretical substrate sequence requirement for the anti-K-*ras* hammerhead ribozyme (**Fig. 1**; *see* **ref.** *29*). KRbz-ADV significantly inhibited in vitro H441 growth (50 pfu/cell), based on ^{3}H-thymidine uptake assay *(30)*. To evaluate the tumor inhibitory activity of KRbz-ADV in vivo, we established NSCLC xenograft by subcutaneous injection of the NSCLC cell line H441 into nude mice. Antitumorigenic effect was determined by comparing the tumor growth rates of KRbz-treated, untreated, and control vector-treated xenografts as described below.

1. Seed H441 cells (3×10^6/10-cm culture dish) in 12.5 mL of RPMI1640 with 10% FBS and culture (37°C 5% CO_2) overnight. Four to five dishes are needed to generate enough cells for one mouse (*see* **Note 5**).
2. Immediately before infection, count cell number in one dish and incubate cell cultures with KRbz-ADV, or a control vector at the desired dose (pfu/cell) in 4.0 mL of RPMI1640 + 2% FBS for 90 min (37°C, 5% CO_2).
3. Add an additional 11.0 mL of RPMI1640 + 10% FBS, and culture for 20–24 h.
4. Trypsinize and collect cells together with the preexisting medium into 50-mL conical tubes. Pellet the cells by centrifugation ($300g$ 15 min). Discard supernatants into 10% bleach solution and wash pellet once with 20 mL of RPMI1640.
5. Count cell number, wash in RPMI1640, then resuspend to a final concentration of 1×10^8 cells/mL in RPMI1640. Draw the cell suspension into a 1.0-mL sterile TB syringe (25G) prior to injection into mice.
6. Inject subcutaneously onto the right flank of mice with 1×10^7 NSCLC H441 cells (0.1 mL RPMI1640) that are either untreated (Group A) or previously treated with KRbz-ADV (Group B) or control vector (Group C).
7. Observe twice weekly for tumor emergence. Measure any palpable xenograft twice a week by a vernier caliper (typically 30 d, post emergence of tumors). Tumor size can be expressed as the mean tumor diameter, as determined by the geometric mean of two perpendicular measurements. $M = \sqrt{M_1 M_2}$; where *M* is

geometric mean, M_1 and M_2 perpendicular measurements. Growth curve is plotted as tumor size vs days postinoculation.

4. Notes

1. Biosafety considerations: all procedures involving the use of 293 cells and recombinant adenoviral vectors should be carried out in accordance with the Biosafety Regulations governing the use of these agents *(24)*. Sixty-mm dishes or 6-well plates are both applicable for cotransfection with pMJ17 and KRbz-pACCMVpLpA, although we have used 6-well plates in our protocol. DOTAP and its aggregate with plasmid DNA have a tendency to adhere to polypropylene surfaces, leading to loss of reagents and a significantly reduced transfection efficiency. Therefore, polystyrene tubes are recommended for preparing cotransfection reagents for pJM17 and KRbz-pACCMVpLpA plasmids.
2. Wild-type (like) adenovirus may be produced during the cotransfection-recombination process or in increasing passage of viral stock in 293 cells *(23,24,31)*. Thus it is important to keep a stock of low-passage recombinant adenovirus as the source for large-scale recombinant adenovirus production.
3. Recombinant adenovirus was observed to be capable of inducing pancreatic islet cell death via modulating apoptosis at high viral concentration [multiplicity of infection (MOI), $1:1000$] *(32)*. The degree of cell resistance to adenvirus-inducing apoptosis may vary for different cell types. NSCLC line H1725 appears to be more sensitive to adenoviral transfection than the others (such as H441).
4. Correct determination of viral titer depends on correct serial dilution techniques. We recommend mixing sample thoroughly, and using a pipet tip only once, in the serial dilution steps of the viral stock.
5. Volume of the transfection medium may affect transduction efficiency for KRbz-ADV on H441 cells, even if the ratio of pfu vs target cell number remains unchanged *(26)*. A time-saving approach is to infect cells collectively in a large culture flask (T150 or T75) as opposed to culture dishes. However, there should be consistency with respect to the transfection process from experiment to experiment, to ensure proper correlation of adenoviral vector dose with treatment outcome.

Acknowledgments

The authors thank Drs. Kevin Scanlon and David Bouffard of Berlex Biosciences, Richmond, CA, for their technical advise, and Ms. Beverly Peters of Baylor Research Institute, Dallas, TX, for her assistance with preparation of the figure.

References

1. Nemunaitis, J., Klemow, S., Tong, W. A, Courtney, A., Johnston, W., Mack, M., et al. (1998) Prognostic value of K-*ras* mutations, *ras* oncoprotein and c-erb B-2 oncoprotein expression in adenocarcinoma of the lung. *Am. J. Clin. Oncol.* **21,** 155–160.

2. Ginsberg, R., Vokes, E. and Raben, A. (1997) Non-small cell lung cancer, in *Cancer: Principles and Practice of Oncology*, 5th ed. (DeVita, V. J., Hellman, S., and Rosenberg, S., eds.), Lippincott-Raven, Philadelphia, PA, pp. 858–911.

3. Rodenhuis, S. (1996) RAS oncogenes and human lung cancer, in *Lung Cancer: Prinicples and Practice* (Pass, H. I., Mitchell, J. B., Johnson, D. H., and Turrisi, A. T., eds.), Lippincott-Raven, Philadelphia, PA, pp. 73–82.

4. Zhang, W. W. and Roth, J. (1994) Anti-oncogene and tumor suppressor gene therapy-examples from a lung cancer animal model. *In Vivo* **8,** 755–769.

5. Alemany, R., Ruan, S., Kataoka, M., Koch, P. E., Mukhopadhyay, T., Cristiano, R. J., et al. (1996) Growth inhibitory effect of anti-K-ras adenovirus on lung cancer cells. *Cancer Gene Ther.* **5,** 296–301.

6. Georges, R. N., Mukhopadhyay, T., Zhang, Y., Yen, N., and Roth, J.A. (1993) Prevention of orthotopic human lung cancer growth by intratracheal instillation of a retroviral antisense K-ras construct. *Cancer Res.* **53,** 1743–1746.

7. Cech, T. M. (1990) Self-splicing of group Introns. *Ann Rev. Biochem.* **59,** 543–568.

8. Kijima, H., Ishida, H., Ohkawa, T., Kashani-Sabet, M., and Scanlon, K. J. (1995) Therapeutic applications of ribozymes. *Pharmacol. Ther.* **68,** 247–267.

9. Haseloff, J. and Gerlach, W. L. (1988) Simple RNA enzymes with new and highly specific endoribonuclease activities. *Nature* **334,** 585–591.

10. Cech, T. R. and Uhlenbech, O. C. (1994) Hammerhead nailed down. *Nature* **372,** 39–40.

11. Koizumi, M., Hayase, Y., Iwai, S., Kamiya, H., Inoue, H., and Ohtsuka, E. (1989) Design of RNA enzyme distinguishing a single base mutation in RNA. *Nucleic Acids Res.* **17,** 7059–7071.

12. Bennett, M. J. and Cullimore, J. V. (1992) Selective cleavage of closely related mRNA. *Nucl. Acids Res.* **20,** 831–837.

13. Ruffner, D. E., Stormo, G. D., and Uhlenbeck, O. C. (1990) Sequence requirements of the hammerhead RNA self-cleavage reaction. *Biochemistry* **29,** 10,695–10,702.

14. Ohta, Y., Kijima, H., Kashani-Sabet, M., and Scanlon, K. J. (1996) Suppression of the malignant phenotype of melanoma cells by anti-oncogene ribozymes. *J. Invest. Dermatol.* **106,** 275–280.

15. Feng, M., Cabrera G., Desane, J., Scanlon, K. J., and Curiel, D. T. (1995) Neoplastic reversion accomplished by high efficiency adenoviral-mediated delivery of an anti-ras ribozyme. *Cancer Res.* **55,** 2024–2028.

16. Zhang, Y. A., Nemunaitis, J., Mues, G., Scanlon, K. J., and Tong, A. W. (1996) In vitro suppression of human non-small cell lung cancer (NSCLC) cell growth by an anti-K-ras ribozyme (abstr.). *FASEB J.* **10,** A1409.

17. Larrson, S., Hotchkiss, G., Andang, M., Nyholm, T., Inzunza, J., Jansoon, I., and Ahrlund-Richter, L. (1994) Reduced β2-microglobulin mRNA levels in transgenic mice expressing a designed hammerhead ribozyme. *Nucl. Acids Res.* **22,** 2242–2248.

18. Kijima, H., Bouffard, D. Y., and Scanlon, K. J. (1996) Ribozyme-mediated reversal of human pancreatic carcinoma phenotype, in *Proceedings of International Symposium on Bone Marrow Transplantation* (Ikehara, S., Takaku, F., and Good, R., eds.), Springer-Verlag, Tokyo, pp. 153–163.

19. Tong, A. W., Zhang, Y. A., Nemunaitis, J., and Mues, G. (1998) K-ras ribozyme for lung cancer, in *Methods in Molecular Medicine*, Vol. 11, Therapeutic Application of Ribozymes (Scanlon, K. J., ed.), Humana, Clifton, NJ, pp. 209–222.
20. Ohkawa, T., Suzuki, T., Irie, A., Bouffard, D. Y., Kashani-Sabet, M., and Scanlon, K. J. (1997) Adenoviral-mediated delivery of an anti-H-ras hammerhead ribozyme in athymic mice bearing human malignant melanoma. *AACR Proc.* **38,** 175.
21. Toloza, E. M., Hunt, K., Swisher, S., McBride, W., Lu, R., Pang, S., et al. (1996) In vivo cancer gene therpy with a recombinant interleukin-2 adenovirus vector. *Cancer Gene Ther.* **3,** 11–17.
22. Tong, A. W., Zhang, Y. A., Bouffard, D. Y. and Nemunaitis, J. (1998) The use of ribozymes for gene therapy of lung cancer, in *Ribozyme in Gene Therapy of Cancer* (Kashani-Sabet, M. and Scanlon, K. J., eds.), RG Landes, Georgetwon, TX, pp. 151–164.
23. Becker, T. C., Noel, R. J., Coats, W. S., Gomez-Foix, A. M., Alam, T., Gerard, R. D. and Newgard, C. B. (1994) Use of recombinant adenovirus for metabolic engineering of mammalian cells. *Meth. Cell Biol.* **43,** 161–189.
24. Graham, F. L. and Prevec, L. (1991) Manipulation of adenovirus vectors, in *Methods in Molecular Biology, vol. 7: Gene Transfer and Expression Protocols* (Murray, E. J., ed.), Humana, Clifton, NJ, pp. 109–128.
25. Strayer, D. S., Duan, L. X., Ozaki, I., Milano, J., Bobraski, L. E., and Bagasra, O. (1997) Titering replication-defective virus for use in gene transfer. *BioTechniques* **22,** 447–450.
26. Johnson, L. G., Pickles, R. J., Boyles, S. E., Morris, J. C., Ye, H., Zhou, Z., et al. (1996) In vitro assessment of variables affecting the efficiency and efficacy of adenovirus-mediated gene transfer to cystic fibrosis airway epithelia. *Human Gene Ther.* **7,** 51–59.
27. Hierholzer, J. C. and Killington, R. A. (1996) Virus isolation and quantitation, in *Virology Methods Manual* (Mahy, B. W. J. and Kangro, K. O., eds.), Academic, San Diego, CA, pp. 26–46.
28. Mistudomi, T., Viallet, J., Mulshine, J. L., Linnoila, I., Minna, J. D., and Gazdar, A. F. (1991) Mutations of ras genes distinguish a subset of non-small-cell lung cancer cell lines from small-cell lung cancer cell line. *Oncogene* **6,** 1353–1362.
29. Scanlon, K. J., Ohta, Y., Ishida, H., Kijima, H., Ohkama, T., Tsai, J., et al. (1995) Oligoncleotide-mediated modulation of mammalian gene expression. *FASEB J.* **9,** 1288–1296.
30. Zhang, Y. A. (1997) Growth inhibition of human non-small cell lung cancer cells by anti-K-ras ribozyme, in Ph.D. dissertation (Zhang, Y. A.), pp. 37–54.
31. Hehir, K. M., Armentano, D., Cardoza, L. M., Choquette, T. L., Berthelette, P. B., White, G. A., et al. (1996) Molecular characterization of replication-competent variants of adenovirus and genome modifications to prevent their occurrence. *J. Virol.* **70,** 8459–8467.
32. Weber, M., Deng, S., Kucher, T., Shaked, A., Ketchum, R. J., and Brayman, K. L. (1997) Adenoviral transfection of isolated pancreatic islets: a study of progrmmed cell death (apoptosis) and islet function. *J. Surg. Res.* **69,** 23–32.

I

EXPERIMENTAL APPROACHES IN CANCER GENE THERAPY

F: Delivery Systems and Tumor Targeting

16

Green Fluorescent Protein Retroviral Vector

Generation of High-Titer Producer Cells and Virus Supernatant

Wolfgang Uckert, Lene Pedersen, and Walter Günzburg

1. Introduction

Genes-encoding marker proteins, which are easily assayable, are useful to monitor cell lineage, gene expression, or promoter activities. In gene-transfer technology such marker genes allow a direct and simple detection of successfully transduced cells. The detection of marker gene products such as β-galactosidase (β-gal), chloramphenicol acetyltransferase (CAT), alkaline phosphatase, or luciferase involves either cell fixation, which kills the cells or antibody-mediated detection, which is time consuming. Drug-resistance genes such as neomycin, puromycin, hygromycin, or zeocin allow a positive selection of transduced cells, but require days to weeks of growth in selective media. Moreover, these genes can change the growth characteristics of the transduced cells through terminal differentiation or can interfere with the expression of the gene of interest *(1)*. Therefore, a marker gene system that provides timely, accurate, and nontoxic detection of successfully transduced living cells would be of great advantage. One interesting candidate gene that fulfills these requirements is the gene-encoding green fluorescent protein (GFP). It was originally isolated from the jellyfish *Aquorea victoria*. The GFP cDNA consists of 730 bp, which encode a 238 amino acid protein with a molecular weight of 27 kD *(2)*. Wild-type GFP emits a vibrant green fluorescence upon exposure to blue light (450–490 nm). The signal is detectable by fluorescence microscopy and fluorescence-activated cell sorting (FACS) *(3)*. Because the fluorescence of wild-type GFP after excitation is not strong enough for many applications, different variants of GFP have been developed. In one such

From: *Methods in Molecular Medicine, Vol. 35: Gene Therapy: Methods and Protocols*
Edited by: W. Walther and U. Stein © Humana Press, Inc., Totowa, NJ

variant, a point mutation was introduced at amino acid 65 (GFP-S65T) leading to a "red-shifted" excitation maximum with an approximately five-fold stronger fluorescent intensity *(4)*. In a further variant, the "red-shifted" GFP was "humanized" by the introduction of numerous silent mutations that alter the codons to those more commonly used in human genes resulting in the improved translation of the gene *(5–7)*. An additional point mutation at amino acid 64 in which phenylalanine was altered to leucine (F64L) further enhances gene expression *(8)*. GFP has been expressed without cytotoxic effects in different organisms and is of special interest as a marker for monitoring cell lines and gene expression *(3)*. The application of GFP in gene-transfer protocols allows the simple detection of transduced cells and offers the possibility for immediate enrichment of viable transduced cells by FACS *(3,9,10)*. This is of great interest in gene transfer into poorly transducable cells, e.g., hematopoietic stem and progenitor cells.

For stable integration/expression of genes in mammalian cells, retroviral vectors are the transfer system of choice. Retroviral vector particles are generated by transfection of the retroviral vector DNA, harboring the sequences to be transferred, into a helper cell line. This cell line provides the replication and packaging functions, which allow the propagation of the recombinant genome. Usually, after drug selection of transfected cells, individual cell clones are expanded into cell lines. The titers obtained from packaging cell lines generated by DNA transfection vary widely on a clonal basis. Therefore, it is necessary to screen several clones to identify the highest titer-virus-producer cell line. This procedure is time consuming and often fails to establish high-titer virus producers. Alternatively, "ping-pong" transduction between ecotropic and amphotropic packaging cells has been applied to increase the virus production from packaging cell lines *(11)*, but again this procedure is very time consuming and can rapidly lead to the production of replication competent virus.

The protocol for the generation of GFP retroviral vector high-titer virus producer is based on multiple enrichment of GFP transfected packaging cells by FACS sorting with expansion of the "high" fluorescent cell fraction after each round of sorting. The subsequent propagation of these packaging cells in roller culture bottles at 32°C and the harvest of viral supernatants at 48-h intervals leads to virus titers of up to 2×10^8 green fluorescent forming units (GFU) per mL as estimated on D17 indicator cells *(12)*. Thus, the virus titer of FACS-enriched producer cells is as high as the titer of the best individually isolated packaging cell clones. Furthermore, a decrease in titer of packaging cells can be avoided by resorting of the virus producer cells and enrichment of the high-titer fraction. The methods described are using the GFP retroviral vector pLEGFPSN *(13)* and the amphotropic packaging cell line FLYA *(14)*, but can

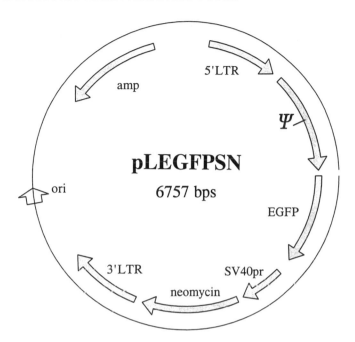

Fig. 1. Schematic structure of pLEGFPSN retrovirus vector. Structural features include long terminal repeats (LTR), packaging signal (Ψ), the cDNA encoding an enhanced green fluorescent protein gene (EGFP), the simian virus 40 early promoter (SV40pr), the neomycin resistance gene which confers G418 resistance (neomycin), the origin of replication (ori), and the ampicillin resistance gene (amp).

be applied also to other GFP encoding retroviral vectors, as well as to other packaging cell lines.

2. Materials

2.1. Cells and Vector

1. FLYA retroviral packaging cell line *(14)*.
2. D17 indicator cell line *(12)*.
3. The pLEGFPSN retroviral vector contains a humanized variant of the GFP gene cloned under the control of the Moloney murine leukemia virus promoter (**Fig. 1**) *(13)*.

2.2. Cell Culture

1. Selective and nonselective tissue-culture media.
2. D-MEM, Alpha-MEM, fetal calf serum (FCS) (Life Technologies, Gaithersburg, MD). Tissue-culture medium was always supplemented with 10% heat-inactivated (56°C, 1 h) FCS if nothing else is indicated.

3. Penicillin, streptomycin, amphotericin B (each 1 %) (Life Technologies).
4. EDTA-trypsin (Life Technologies).
5. Tissue-culture flasks, roller-culture bottles, 10-cm diameter dishes, 24-well plates (Costar, Cambridge, MA).
6. Disposable pipets (1 mL, 5 mL, 10 mL, 25 mL) (Costar).

2.3. Solutions and Kits

1. PBS: 1% NaCl, 0.025% KCl, 0.14% Na_2HPO_4, 0.025% KH_2PO_4, pH 7.3, autoclaved.
2. NaCl: 0.9%, autoclaved.
3. G418 (Sigma, St. Louis, MO): stock solution 50 mg/mL in PBS. Filter-sterilize and store at 4°C.
4. Polybrene (Sigma): stock solution 800 µg/mL in distilled water. Filter-sterilize and store at 4°C.
5. Plasmid DNA purification kit (Quiagen, Chatsworth, CA).
6. Mammalian DNA transfection kit (Stratagene, La Jolla, CA).

2.4. Equipment

1. FACS Vantage (Becton Dickinson, Rutherford, NJ).
2. Roller apparatus Cellroll (Integra Biosciences).
3. Fluorescence microscope BX50 (Olympus).
4. Flow cytometer Epics-XL2 (Coulter, Hialeah, FL).
5. Hemacytometer.

3. Methods
3.1. Transfection of Retroviral Vector DNA into Packaging Cells

1. Purify retroviral vector plasmid pLEGFPSN (or other GFP containing vectors) using a DNA purification kit according to the manufacturer's instruction.
2. Day 1: Trypsinize the packaging cell line to be transfected, e.g., FLYA and plate cells at a density of 5×10^5 per 10-cm diameter tissue-culture dish with 10 mL D-MEM.
3. Day 2: Change medium and transfect cells with 10 µg of pLEGFPSN DNA using a calcium phosphate precipitation kit according to the supplier's instruction (*see* **Note 1**).
4. Day 3: Wash cells twice with PBS, add fresh medium, and propagate cells in the presence of 1.0 mg/mL G418 (*see* **Note 2**).
5. After approximately 14 d, or when all control cells are dead, transfer bulk-culture cells into tissue-culture flasks, expand cells, and freeze cells in liquid nitrogen.

3.2. Generation of High-Titer GFP Retroviral Vector Producers by FACS

1. Thaw transfected packaging FLYA/pLEGFPSN bulk-culture cells quickly at 37°C.

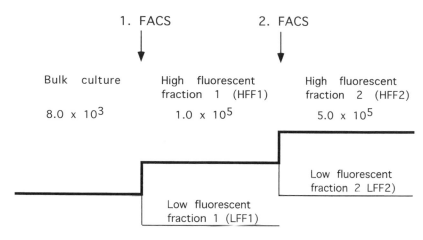

Fig. 2. Schematic representation and virus titer (GFU/mL) of FACS sorted GFP retroviral vector producers.

2. Expand FLYA/pLEGFPSN cells in T175 tissue-culture flasks. Trypsinize cells. Wash cells two times in serum-free D-MEM and resuspend cells in 5 mL of serum-free medium (*see* **Note 3**).

3. Sort 2×10^7 cells using a FACS into a "high" fluorescent fraction 1 (HFF1) and a "low" fluorescent fraction 1 (LFF1) (**Figs. 2** and **3**).

4. Transfer HFF1 cell fraction into a T25 tissue-culture flask and expand cells in D-MEM in G418 selective medium (1.0 mg/mL) in the presence of penicillin G (10,000 U/mL), streptomycin (10,000 µg/mL), and amphotericin B (25 µg/mL) (*see* **Note 4**).

5. Repeat **step 3**. FACS sort 2×10^7 cells of HFF1 generating a "high" fluorescent fraction 2 (HFF2) and a "low" fluorescent fraction 2 (LFF2) (**Figs. 2** and **3**).

6. Repeat **step 4**. Expand HFF2 fraction and freeze cells as stock in liquid nitrogen.

3.3. Production of High-Titer Virus Supernatants in Roller Culture Bottles

1. Thaw FLYA/pLEGFPSN HFF2 cells quickly at 37°C and propagate cells in a T25 tissue-culture flask with 5 mL of D-MEM and 1.0 mg/mL G418.

2. When cells reach confluence, trypsinize and transfer cells to a T75 tissue-culture flask with 15 ml D-MEM and G418 (1.0 mg/mL). When cells are 50 to 60% confluent, split 1:3 and grow until the cell monolayer is nearly confluent.

3. Trypsinize and transfer cells into three T175 tissue-culture flasks with 30 mL of D-MEM and G418 (1.0 mg/mL).

4. When cells are confluent, trypsinize and transfer all cells (approx 5×10^7 to 1×10^8 from three T175 flasks) into one roller-culture bottle with 150 mL of D-MEM, but without G418. Grow cells at 37°C, 5% CO_2, and a rotation speed of the roller-culture bottle of 0.2 rpm (*see* **Note 5**).

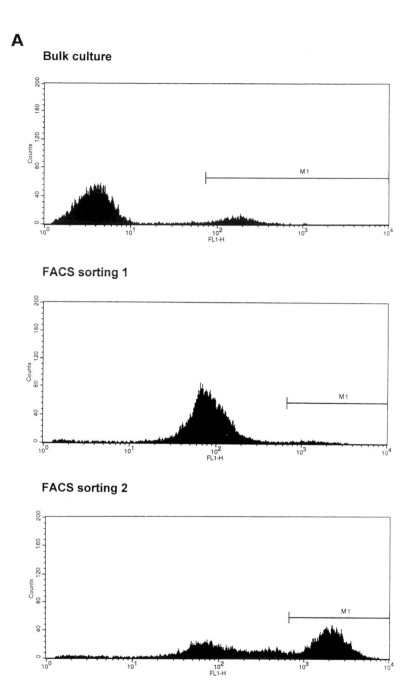

Fig. 3. **(A)** Flow cytometry profiles and **(B)** fluorescent microscopic detection (magnification 40-fold) of FACS sorted FLYA/pLEGFPSN retroviral vector producers.

B

Bulk culture

High fluorescent fraction 1

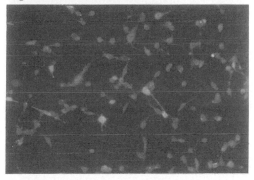

High fluorescent fraction 2

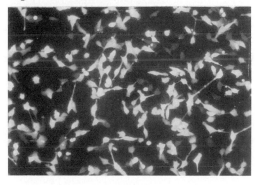

Fig. 3B

5. When the cells reach confluence (*see* **Note 6**), remove medium and add 40 mL of D-MEM without G418. Increase rotation speed of the roller-culture bottle to 0.4 rpm and decrease temperature of the incubator to 32°C (*see* **Note 7**).

6. Harvest virus containing supernatant at intervals of 48 h (*see* **Note 8**). Remove cells and debris by filtration through a 0.45 μm disposable filter. Store aliquots of viral supernatant at –80°C.

3.4. Virus Titration

1. Day 1: Seed 1×10^6 FLYA/pLEGFPSN packaging cells with 5 mL D-MEM in a T25 tissue-culture flask (*see* **Note 9**).

2. Day 2: Replace the medium on the producer cells with exactly 5 mL of D-MEM. Plate D17 indicator cells at a density of 1×10^4 cells /cm^2 into a 24-well plate with 1 mL of Alpha-MEM (*see* **Note 10**).

3. Day 3: Harvest virus containing supernatant from packaging cells and filter through a 0.45 μm disposable filter to remove cells and debris (*see* **Note 11**).

4. Use 0.5 mL of virus containing supernatant made 8 μg/mL with respect to polybrene to generate serial dilutions from 10^{-1} to 10^{-6}. To do this, pipet 4.5 ml of Alpha-MEM containing 8 μg/mL polybrene into each of six sterile 15-mL tubes labeled 10^{-1} to 10^{-6}. Pipet 0.5 mL of viral supernatant into tube 10^{-1} and mix thoroughly using a fresh pipet. Transfer 0.5 mL of the 10^{-1} virus dilution into tube 10^{-2}, mix again thoroughly and carry on until the 10^{-6} tube (*see* **Note 12**).

5. Remove medium from D17 indicator cell 24-well plate and transfer each 0.5 mL of the different virus dilutions in duplicates into the wells of the plate.

6. Incubate D17 indicator cells 4 h at 37°C and 5% CO_2, add 1.5 mL fresh Alpha-MEM and incubate D17 cells another 44 h at 37°C and 5% CO_2.

7. Count green fluorescent colonies using a fluorescent microscope and calculate virus titer (*see* **Note 13**).

8. Alternatively, estimate the percentage of GFP transduced cells by means of a flow cytometer. To do this, trypsinize cells from the two wells of the same virus dilution of the 24-well plate, combine cells, wash the cells two times with PBS, estimate the total number of cells by counting an aliquot in a counting chamber and use the remaining cells for flow cytometry (*see* **Note 14**).

4. Notes

1. Equally good results were obtained when transfection kits of other suppliers were used. Do not split cells in a ratio of 1:10 into new tissue culture plates 24 h after transfection as recommended in most transfection protocols.

2. The appropriate G418 concentration for other packaging cell lines should be determined empirically. For human cells (FLYA, BOSC23) and most NIH3T3 derivatives (ΨCRIP, ΨCRE, GP + envAm12, GP + E 86) it is between 0.4 μg/mL and 1.0 μg/mL.

3. PBS can be used instead of serum-free D-MEM.

4. Antibiotics were used in order to avoid contamination of cells, which can occur during the FACS sorting procedure. It takes approx 1–2 wk to obtain enough cells from HFF1 to perform the second round of FACS sorting.

5. Most cells settle within 48 h. Nonattached cells do not have to be removed by medium change before the cell monolayer is confluent.

6. On the average, it takes 14 d from thawing of transfected packaging cells to reach a confluent cell monolayer in roller-culture bottles.

7. Decrease of culture temperature from 37°C to 32°C results in a slower decay of virus particles *(15)*.

8. Harvests of virus containing supernatants at intervals of 48 h can be continued without decrease in virus titer until cells detach from the surface of the roller-culture bottle. If the harvested virus supernatant contains to much cell debris, a preclarification of the supernatant by low-speed centrifugation ($1000g$, 5 min) before the 0.45 μm-filtration is recommended.

9. FLYA/pLEGFPSN cells used for the estimation of virus titers were not grown in G418 selective medium to avoid the transfer of traces of G418 to the indicator cells.

10. To plate 1×10^4 cells/cm^2 into each well of a 24-well plate, 9×10^5 D17 cells have to be resuspended thoroughly in 25 mL of Alpha-MEM. 1 mL of this cell suspension is then transferred into each well of the plate. After 24 h, cells can be used for virus titration.

11. At this point, virus containing supernatant can be used directly for titration or can be stored at –80°C until further use. Be aware that one time freezing/thawing may result in a decrease of virus titer of up to one magnitude.

12. Polybrene concentrations below 8 μg/mL can also be used without influencing the infection efficiency of D17 cells; lower polybrene concentrations may be suitable for more sensitive indicator cells. Higher concentrations than 8 μg/mL are not recommended because polybrene could be harmful for the cells.

13. Green fluorescent cells can be counted upon exposure to blue light using a fluorescence microscope at 450 nm. To obtain the precise virus titer, counting of green fluorescent colonies (cells in close vicinity and with the same fluorescent appearance) should be performed in both wells of the same virus dilution and in two different, easy to count virus dilutions (number of green fluorescent colonies between 1 and 200). To obtain the virus titer in green colony forming units (GFU)/mL the number of green fluorescent colonies of each counted well has to be multiplied by the factor 2 because only 0.5 mL of viral supernatant was used for infection of indicator cells. For easier counting, it is recommended to replace the tissue culture medium with PBS or 0.9 % NaCl solution.

14. The virus titer estimated by flow cytometry is, in general, higher than that obtained by fluorescence microscopy because every green fluorescent cell is counted as a single event. Because application of flow cytometry is less time consuming and more objective, both methods should be evaluated in a direct comparison in the same titration experiment. To estimate the virus titer by flow

cytometry the total amount of indicator cells, e.g., from two wells of the same virus dilution of the 24-well plate, has to be counted. Knowing the total number of indicator cells and the percentage of fluorescent cells measured by flow cytometry, the virus titer can be calculated.

Acknowledgments

We thank P. Grasshoff (MDC) and D. Klein (UVSV) for help in FACS sorting and flow cytometry, respectively. This work was supported by the Deutsche Forschungsgemeinschaft (Bl 288/4-1), the BMBF (0311180), the Karen Elise Jensen's Fund, and the EU (B104 CT95-0100).

References

1. Valera, A., Perales, J. C., Hatzoglou, M., and Bosch, F. (1994) Expression of the neomycin-resistance (neo) gene induces alterations in gene expression and metabolism. *Human Gene Ther.* **5,** 449–456.
2. Prasher, D. C., Eckenrode, V. K., Ward, W. W., Prender-Gast, F. G., and Cormier, M. J. (1992) Primary structure of the *Aquorea victoria* green fluorescent protein. *Gene* **111,** 229–233.
3. Chalfie, M., Tu, Y., Euskirchen, G., Ward, W. W., and Prasher, D. C. (1994) Green fluorescent protein as a marker for gene expression. *Science* **263,** 802–805.
4. Heim, R., Cubitt, A. B., and Tsien, R. Y. (1995) Improved green fluorescence. *Nature* **373,** 663–664.
5. Levy, J. P., Muldoon, R. R., Zolotukhin, S., and Link, C. J. (1996) Retroviral transfer and expression of a humanized, red shifted green fluorescent protein into human tumor cells. *Nature Biotechnol.* **14,** 610–614.
6. Zolotukhin, S., Potter, M., Hauswirth, W. W., Guy, J., and Muzyczka, N. (1996) A "humanized" green fluorescent protein cDNA adapted for high level expression in mammalian cells. *J. Virol.* **70,** 4646–4654.
7. Muldoon, R. R., Levy, J. P., Kain, S. R., Kitts, P. A., and Link Jr., C. J. (1997) Tracking and quantitation of retroviral-mediated transfer using a completely humanized, red shifted green fluorescent protein gene. *BioTechniques* **22,** 162–165.
8. Cormack, B. P., Valdivia, R. H., and Falkow, S. (1996) FACS-optimized mutants of the green fluorescent protein (GFP). *Gene* **173,** 33–38.
9. Kain, S. and Ganguly, S. (1995) Use of fusion genes in mammalian transfection. Overview of genetic reporter systems, in *Current Protocols in Molecular Biology* (Ausubel, M., Rent, R., Kingston, R. E., Moore, D. D., Seidman, J. G., Smith, J. A., Struhl, K., eds.), Wiley, New York, unit 9.6.
10. Dunbar, C. E. and Emmons, R. V. B. (1994) Gene transfer into hematopoietic progenitor and stem cells: progress and problems. *Stem Cell* **12,** 563–576.
11. Riviere, I. and Sadelain, M. (1997) Methods for the construction of retroviral vectors and the generation of high-titer producers, in *Methods in Molecular Medicine: Gene Therapy Protocols* (Robbins, P. D., ed.), Humana, Totowa, NJ, pp. 59–78.

12. Riggs, J. L., Mcallister, R. M., and Lennette, E. H. (1974) Immunofluorescent studies of RD-114 virus replication. *J. gen. Virol.* **25,** 21–29.
13. Klein, D., Indraccolo, S., von Rombs, K., Amadori, A., Salmons, B., and Günzburg, W. H. (1997) Rapid identification of viable retrovirus-transduced cells using the green fluorescent protein as a marker. *Gene Ther.* **4,** 1256–1260.
14. Cossett, F. L., Takeuchi, Y., Battini, J. L., Weiss, R. A., and Collins, M. K. (1995) High-titer packaging cells producing recombinant retrovirus resistant to human serum. *J. Virol.* **69,** 7430–7436.
15. Kaptein, L. C. M., Greijer, A. E., Valerio, D., and van Beusechem, V. W. (1997) Optimized conditions for the production of recombinant amphotropic retroviral vector preparations. *Gene Ther. 4, 172–176.*

17

HSV-1 Vectors for Gene Therapy of Experimental CNS Tumors

Ulrich Herrlinger, Andreas Jacobs, Manish Aghi, Deborah E. Schuback, and Xandra O. Breakefield

1. Introduction

Gliomas account for about 60% of all primary CNS tumors; two-thirds of all gliomas comprise the most malignant form, glioblastoma multiforme, or glioma grade IV. Although much progress has been achieved in the treatment of other solid tumors over the last few decades, the median survival of patients with glioblastoma remains at around 12 mo after standard treatment, which includes bulk resection and irradiation, as well as chemotherapy in some cases *(1)*. Essentially, no patient can expect to survive 5 yr. New treatment modalities like immunotherapy have been applied so far with only limited success *(2)*. With the improvement of methods for in vivo and ex vivo gene delivery, gene therapy became a new, promising approach to glioma therapy. Gliomas appear to be a particularly good target for a gene therapy approach using locally applied vectors, as the growth of gliomas is restricted to the brain. Clinical trials are under way using retrovirus and adenovirus vectors which carry the herpes simplex virus type-1 (HSV-1) thymidine kinase gene *(HSV-tk)*. This gene encodes a prodrug-activating enzyme, which in infected cells converts the nontoxic prodrug, ganciclovir (GCV), to its cytotoxic phosphorylated form *(3–5)*. There is an ever-increasing list of other prodrug-activation systems that showed efficacy in culture and in preclinical studies using rodent glioma models. These include, for example, cytosine deaminase converting 5-fluoro-cytosine to 5-fluoro-uracil *(6)*, cytochrome P450-2B1 converting cyclophosphamide to phosphoramide mustard *(7)*, deoxycytidine kinase phosphorylating cytosine arabinoside *(8)*, and the *Escherichia coli* guanine phosphoribosyl

From: *Methods in Molecular Medicine, Vol. 35: Gene Therapy: Methods and Protocols*
Edited by: W. Walther and U. Stein © Humana Press, Inc., Totowa, NJ

transferase (*gpt*) metabolizing 6-thioxanthine and 6-thioguanine to toxic nucleoside analogs *(9)*. Moreover, gene therapy approaches to brain tumors include the viral transfer of immune-enhancing cytokines, particularly granulocyte/macrophage colony-stimulating factor *(10)*, or antisense to TGF-β to glioma cells *(11)* used for vaccination purposes. Other approaches use the transfer of genes that modulate angiogenesis *(12,13)* or are involved in apoptosis like *p53 (14)*. All aforementioned gene-transfer methods use nonreplicative viral vectors.

A mutant HSV-1 was introduced as the first replicating virus for gene therapy or so called "virus therapy" of gliomas by Martuza et al. *(15)*. The replication of HSV-1 vectors is cytotoxic, as evident by the appearance of a cytopathic effect (CPE). Thus, replication of *HSV-1* alone without adding any prodrugs is oncolytic following infection of a tumor cell. For some HSV-1 mutants, the oncolytic effect by replication has been combined with prodrug-activation using the *HSV-1-tk* gene, already a natural part of the HSV-1-genome *(16)*. In the future, additional prodrug activating systems can be recombined into the HSV-1-genome without compromising replication in tumor cells *(17)*. For this purpose, a transgene capacity of at least 30 out of the total 152 kb of the HSV-1 genome is available. HSV-1 particles are relatively stable and can be concentrated to high titers (10^{12} plaque forming units (PFU)/mL). They are highly infectious for cells in the nervous system, both glia and neurons. Intratumoral injection of HSV-1 induces an immune reaction, which may enhance the immune response against the tumor by the nonspecific release of cytokines. As illustrated in **Fig. 1**, HSV-1 consists of a capsid surrounded by a lipid bilayer envelope bearing glycoproteins with tegument proteins in between. The entry of the virion into a cell is mediated by a multistep process, which involves binding of envelope glycoproteins gC and gB to heparan sulfate on the cell surface, binding of gH to the high-affinity receptor HSV-1 entry mediator protein (HVEM) *(18)*, fusion of virus envelope and cell membrane mediated mainly by gB, and release of the capsid into the cytoplasm. The capsid and associated tegument proteins are transported to the nucleus where viral DNA enters through the nuclear pores. Viral DNA transcription is initiated mainly by the tegument protein VP16, which activates in turn the genes for viral immediate-early (IE) transcription factors, such as infected cell protein (ICP) 4, ICP0, and ICP27. Expression of these proteins alone can cause some cytotoxicity in the infected cell *(19)*. HSV-1 DNA is replicated by a rolling circle process and is packaged into capsids formed in the nucleus. After being enveloped at the nuclear membrane, infectious progeny virus particles leave the cell in an ultimately lytic process.

One major goal for gene therapy using replicating HSV-1 vectors is to render the replication specific to proliferating cells. For gene therapy of brain

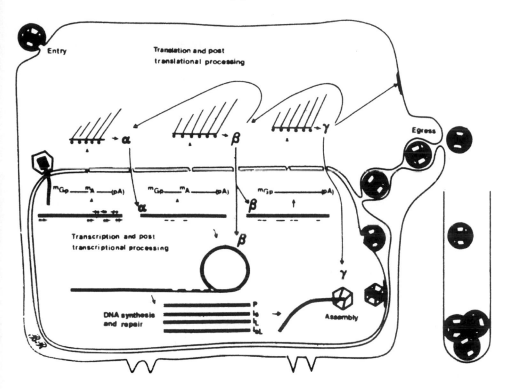

Fig. 1. Replication of HSV-1 in permissive cells. Viral envelope and cell membrane fuse after attachment of the virus to the cell membrane. The capsid is transported to the nuclear membrane and releases the viral DNA into the nucleus. Viral DNA circularizes in the nucleus. VP-16, a protein that is part of the HSV-1 tegument and is brought in by infection, is a potent transactivator and initiates the transcription of alpha (IE) genes. Alpha mRNAs are translated in the cytoplasm, their proteins transported back into the nucleus where the transcription of β-genes ensues. Viral DNA is replicated by a rolling cycle mechanism and γ-genes, coding mainly for structural proteins of the virus, are transcribed and translated. The concatemers of viral DNA are cleaved to unit-length and packaged into capsids. Capsids containing viral DNA attach to membrane patches which contain viral glycoproteins and tegument proteins and are enveloped. After passage through the endoplasmatic reticulum progeny, viral particles are released into the extracellular space. Reprinted with the permission of Roizman and Batterson (62).

tumors this is an especially appealing approach as tumor cells are—besides endothelial cells and reactive glia—the only proliferating cells within the brain, thus providing a platform for specificity. For this purpose, so-called "replication conditional" or "attenuated" HSV-1 vectors have been developed. These vectors are mutated in genes that code for proteins that are not critical to virus replication in dividing cells, but are essential for viral replication in nondividing cells such as neurons (*HSV-tk* *(15)*, ribonucleotide reductase (*RR/U$_L$39/ICP6*) *(16,20,21)*, uracil DNA glycosylase (*UNG*) *(22)*, or which are associated with neurotoxicity ($\gamma_1 34.5$) *(23)*. The first three are enzymes that are involved in increasing the pool of nucleoside precursors necessary for DNA replication. In proliferating cells undergoing DNA replication, corresponding cellular enzymes are upregulated and are thus able to complement the mutant HSV-1 vectors. In postmitotic cells, however, the expression of such complementary cellular enzymes is not sufficient and thus replication of the viral DNA is curtailed. $\gamma_1 34.5$ has several functions among them blocking the viral shutoff of host-cell protein synthesis and thus apoptosis induced by HSV-1 infection *(24)*. The mechanisms that mediate the neurotoxicity of the $\gamma_1 34.5$ gene are less well known. To increase the safety of replication-conditional HSV-1 vectors, efforts have been made to decrease the neurotoxicity while maintaining the ability of these viruses to replicate selectively in tumor cells. HSV-1 mutants have been generated that carry mutations in more than one of the aforementioned genes: $\gamma_1 34.5$ and *ung* *(25)*, RR and $\gamma_1 34.5$ [G207 *(26)*; MGH-1 *(27)*]. These second generation HSV-1 mutants are generated by deletion or disruption of the target gene by insertion of a stop codon *(28)* or a marker gene, like *lacZ* *(20)*. The genome of such a vector is exemplified by the MGH-1 vector *(27)* in **Fig. 2**. The methodology necessary for developing new HSV-1 mutants by homologous recombination is comprehensively covered by Krisky et al. *(29)*.

In cell culture, 9L rat gliosarcoma cells infected with a RR^- mutant (*hrR3*) at low multiplicity of infection (MOI of 0.1) are virtually all killed by day 6 after infection because of the replication of the virus. In this process, high titers of progeny virus are produced *(27,30,31)*. Some rodent glioma cell lines, like C6 glioma and D74/RG-2 glioma, are less susceptible to the oncolytic effects of replication conditional HSV-1 vectors *(21)*. A CPE is seen only after infection with a high MOI of 100 *(32)*. This observation may be explained by a lack of HVEM receptors, important for the entry of HSV-1, on these cells. Additionally, some cell lines might not be able to fully complement the genes mutated in the replication-conditional HSV-1 vectors. Unidentified cellular factors are thought to be responsible for the observation that $\gamma_1 34.5$ mutant vectors do not replicate or cause substantial CPE in rat glioma cells *(27,33)*. In mouse glioma cells, $\gamma_1 34.5$ mutant vectors do not replicate to a great extent, but do cause some oncolysis *(33)*. Human glioma cells are generally much more infectable with HSV-1 vectors *(32,34)* and also support replication of $\gamma_1 34.5$ mutants *(34)*.

In animal studies with Fischer rats bearing syngeneic intracerebral (ic) 9L tumors, intratumoral injection of high titers of *hrR3* (10^8 PFU) resulted in a significant prolongation of survival with long-term survival in a few animals

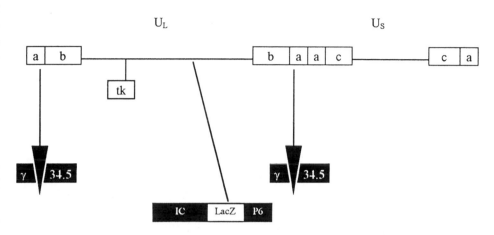

Fig. 2. Schematic map of the HSV-1 mutant *MGH-1*. The genome contains the two unique segments, U_L and U_S, each flanked by inverted repeat elements, ab and ca, respectively. The genome termini consists of the short "a" sequence, which is also present in an inverted orientation at the joint between the long and the short components of the genome. Depending on their localization, either in the unique or in the repeat segments, the HSV-1 genes exist in one or two copies. Deleted genes are marked by black boxes, intact genes by white ones (genes not drawn on scale). *MGH-1* was derived from R3616 in which both copies of the neurovirulence gene $\gamma_1 34.5$ were deleted *(23)*. In *MGH-1*, the single-copy *ICP6* gene coding for ribonucleotide reductase is additionally interrupted by insertion of the *E. coli lacZ* reporter gene as previously described for the HSV-1 mutant *hrR3 (20)*. Modified after Kramm et al. *(27)*.

(16). The mutant *R4009*, which has a stop codon inserted into both $\gamma_1 34.5$ genes also prolonged the survival of nude or scid mice inoculated intracerebrally with MT539MG mouse glioma cells *(35)* or human (U251MG or D-54MG) glioma cells *(34)*. Therapeutic effects of $RR/\gamma_1 34.5$ double mutants were dependent on the animal model studied: injection of the G207 mutant into ic human gliomas induced a significant prolongation of survival, including some long-term survivors *(26)*, whereas injection of the MGH-1 mutant into ic 9L tumors in syngeneic Fischer rats did not yield a substantial prolongation of survival *(27)*. Also, the efficacy of additional GCV treatment depended on the virus and the animal model used. Using the virus *hrR3*, which replicates well in rodent gliosarcoma cells, GCV treatment following virus injection increased median survival time and the percentage of long-term survivors significantly *(16)*. This effect was abolished using D74 rat glioma cells, which are less infectable with *hrR3* and only poorly support viral replication *(32)* or the mutants MGH-1 or G207 that replicate poorly in rodent glioma cells *(27,36)*. In the ic mouse glioma model applied by Chambers et al. *(35)*, additional GCV treatment even abolished the therapeutic effect caused by intratumoral injection of a

$\gamma_1 34.5$ mutant presumably by blocking virus replication. Beside its therapeutic effect for tumor killing, GCV thus also serves as a potential means of safety for gene therapy using HSV-1 vectors, as it stops HSV-1 replication. Staining of tumor sections for the expression of *lacZ* and *HSV-tk* as marker genes showed that these HSV-1 mutants infect mainly tumor cells, as well as some inflammatory and glia cells *(30)*. Occasionally, intratumoral hemorrhage was observed possibly resulting from the destruction of neovascularization by virus replicating in proliferating endothelial cells.

As alternative ways of vector application, the vector can reach the tumor cells through the vasculature or the cerebrospinal fluid (CSF). The *hrR3* mutant was injected into the carotid artery together with bradykinin or RMP-7, as blood-brain barrier modifying agents with substantial delivery to the periphery of ic gliomas *(37–39)*. Intrathecal combined with intratumoral injection of *hrR3* achieved long-term survival in 89% of animals bearing combined frontal/leptomeningeal 9L tumors *(40)*.

Before HSV-1 vectors reach clinical applicability, certain safety issues have to be addressed. In culture, the cytotoxicity of $\gamma_1 34.5$ mutants on normal astrocytes is markedly reduced as compared to the HSV-1 F-strain wild-type *(34)*. The *G207* virus mutated in both *RR* and $\gamma_1 34.5$ genes did not produce any cytopathic effect on rat astrocytes and cerebellar neurons *(26)*. In nude mice, the LD_{50} after ic inoculation into brains without tumors increased from $10^{2.5}$ for wild-type virus to $>10^7$ for mutant virus ($\gamma_1 34.5^-$) *(34)*. In owl monkeys (*Aeotus nancymai*), which are highly susceptible to HSV-1 infection, no substantial neurotoxicity was observed after ic inoculation of 10^7 PFU of the G207 vector into normal brain parenchyma *(26)*. Another safety concern is whether ic inoculation of HSV-1 vectors could induce a strong and neurotoxic immune response, especially in humans who in 40–80% have antibodies to HSV-1 *(41)* and thus might mount a particularly strong neurotoxic inflammatory reaction at the injection site. No neurotoxic reaction was seen, however, in Fischer rats preimmunized against HSV-1 and injected ic with a RR^- replication conditional HSV-1 mutant *(32)*. Moreover, as HSV-1 is latent in the trigeminal ganglia of about 65% of all humans and HSV-1 sequences can be found within the CNS in about one-third of human autopsy cases examined *(42)*, the problem of potentially reactivating latent HSV-1 by ic vector application has to be studied carefully. In two rat latent infection models, it was demonstrated that intracranial injection of an RR^- mutant did not reactivate latent wild-type virus *(43)*. The spread of replicating HSV-1 to other organs beyond the CNS and related toxicity also needs further evaluation. Preliminary results in a rat tumor model showed that 2 d after ic injection of *hrR3*, HSV-1 sequences can be detected in internal organs of all nonimmunized animals. In internal organs of animals that had been previously immunized against HSV-1, HSV-1 sequences were detected with much lower frequency *(32)*. Thus, preexisting immunity against HSV-1 appears to be beneficial because it limits the spread of the virus. Finally, the ability of replication-conditional vectors to be shed to the environment after ic injection needs to be evaluated.

Beyond replication-conditional HSV-1 vectors, other types of HSV-1 vectors might have future potential for gene therapy of brain tumors. (The generation and different applications of these vectors are not covered in this Methods and Protocols section.) 1) HSV-1 vectors can be mutated in their *IE* genes *(29)*. Because these genes are essential for the replication of HSV-1, such vectors do not replicate in any cells except those transfected with the respective complementing gene. The applicability of these vectors as oncolytic agents for direct intratumoral injection remains doubtful, however they might serve as means to transfer toxic genes like prodrug-activation enzymes, or cytokines. 2) A disabled infectious single-cycle herpes simplex virus (DISC-HSV) has been developed, which is mutated in the gene for glycoprotein H (*gH*) *(44)*. DISC-HSV can be grown to high titers in complementing cell lines expressing gH. This vector can only go through one further round of infection in other cell types. Thereafter, the progeny virus released is noninfectious as viral particles lack gH required for target cell entry. This vector has been already used as a tool for cytokine-enhanced immunotherapy *(45)*. 3) HSV-1 amplicon systems have been used less frequently for gene therapy of experimental glioma. A HSV-1 amplicon vector consists of a plasmid, which in its minimal version bears only a packaging signal (DNA cleavage signal), a HSV-1 origin of DNA replication, procaryotic sequences for propagation of plasmid DNA in bacteria (*E. coli* origin of DNA replication and antibiotic resistance gene) and a gene of interest. New generations of hybrid amplicon vectors contain additional sequences from adeno-associated virus that allow for amplification and potentially for chromosomal integration of the transgene in dividing human cells *(46)*, or from Epstein-Barr virus that allow the amplicon DNA to be retained as a replicating episome during cell division *(47)*. Amplicon plasmids get packaged as linear head-to-tail concatemers into infectious HSV-1 virions when all other essential functions of HSV-1 replication and packaging are provided in the same cell. These functions are typically introduced by coinfection with any of several HSV-1 mutants which can replicate only in the packaging cells. Conventional amplicon systems provide the complementary HSV-1 functions in a helper virus, which is mutated in a replication-essential IE-gene and is packaged in cells complementing this IE-gene, e.g., IE3⁻ virus in Vero cells transfected with IE3. Such systems have been used for gene transfer to neurons *(48)* and for interleukin-2 enhanced immunotherapy in a hepatocellular carcinoma model *(49)*. Injection of a replication-conditional system consisting of an amplicon coding for HSV-TK and a $\gamma_1 34.5$ mutant as helper virus into a subcutaneous (sc) glioma and subsequent GCV treatment proved to be a more effective way of treatment than treatment with the helper virus and GCV alone *(50)*. The enhanced effect was mainly attributed to the multiple copies of HSV-*tk* brought into the glioma cells by the amplicon. In the "piggyback" version of the HSV-1 amplicon system, the replication of amplicon and helper virus are mutually dependent on each other, as the amplicon plasmid carries the replication essential IE-gene for which the helper virus is mutated *(51)*. Thus, replication is only possible in cells infected with both helper and amplicon vectors. This favors propagation of both amplicon vectors and helper virus within the glioma and has proven to be effective in a sc glioma model *(52)*. As the most recent development, amplicon vectors can be packaged helper virus-free *(53)*. This is accomplished by cotransfecting packaging cells with an amplicon plasmid and an overlapping set of cosmids which covers the complete HSV-1 genome, but are mutated in their packaging signals. This process yields highly infectious, completely nonreplicating virions which express no viral genes and thus are essentially nontoxic and only poorly immunogenic. Its value for safe delivery of therapeutic genes by direct intratumoral injection and as a tool for ex vivo or *in situ* immunotherapy of glioma is under investigation.

2. Materials

1. Working with HSV-1 requires biosafety level 2 and a biocontainment hood, all cell-culture materials that have come in contact with HSV-1 particles need to be disinfected with a virucidal agent (e.g., LpHse[R], Calgon, St. Louis, MO) and/or autoclaved, sterile hoods have to be wiped with a virucidal agent. HSV-1 can only be transmitted through fluids, but eyewear and gloves should be worn for any procedures outside the biocontainment hood. Sonication is especially hazardous as it creates an aerosol containing HSV-1 virions.
2. In tissue culture, HSV-1 infected plates need not to be separated from uninfected plates. Virus transmission only occurs through fluids during sonication by the generation of an aerosol.
3. HSV-1 permissive cell lines: Vero cells (African green monkey kidney cells; ATCC# CCL81), baby hamster kidney cells (BHK; ATCC# CCL10); human glioma cell lines: U-87MG (ATCC# HTB 14) and T98G (ATCC# CRL 1690), rat 9L gliosarcoma *(54)*.
4. Phosphate-buffered saline, pH 7.4 (PBS).
5. Cell-culture media: Dulbecco's modified Eagle's medium (DMEM); DMEM + 10% fetal calf serum (FCS) + 100 U/mL penicillin + 100 mg/mL streptomycin (DMEM + 10% FCS + P/S); DMEM + 2% FCS 100 U/mL penicillin + 100 mg/ml streptomycin (DMEM + 2% FCS + P/S).

6. Agarose (IB70042, Eastman Kodak, Rochester, NY).
7. Anesthesia for rodents: ketamine (Ketalar™, Parke-Davis, Morris Plains, NJ); xylazine (Rompun™, Bayer, Shawnee Mission, KA).
8. Ganciclovir (Cytovene™, Hoffmann-LaRoche, Nutley, NJ). An aequos solution of ganciclovir (GCV) can be stored for 12 h at room temperature (RT).
9. Stereotactic apparatus and automatic drill for ic inoculation of tumors (Kopf, Tujunga, CA), Hamilton syringe (Hamilton, Reno, NV) for injection of volumes of 1–10 µL.
10. For animal perfusion and fixation of tissue: PBS pH 7.4; 4% para-formaldehyde in PBS pH 7.4, this solution is best if freshly prepared, storage at 4°C for a few days is tolerable; 30% sucrose in PBS pH 7.4.
11. Giemsa staining solution (Accustain™, Sigma GS-500), make a 1:20 dilution in deionized water before use.
12. For *LacZ* staining: substrate buffer (100 mM $K_3[Fe(CN)_6]$, 100 mM $K_4[Fe(CN)_6]$, 100 mM $MgCl_2$ in PBS, pH 7.4); X-gal solution [40 mg X-Gal] (Fisher Scientific, Pittsburgh, PA) dissolved in 1 mL DMSO; store in the dark at 4°C; to be diluted 1:40 in substrate buffer before use).
13. Antibodies to determine marker gene expression and to track the generation of HSV-1 virions:
    1. Rabbit polyclonal anti-HSV-TK Serum A (Dr. William Summers, Yale University, New Haven, CT).
    2. Antibodies against HSV-1 envelope proteins gD (H1103) or gB (H1105) (Goodwin Institute for Cancer Research, Plantation, FL).
    3. Monoclonal antibody against HSV-1 ICP4 (H1101; Goodwin Institute for Cancer Research).
14. For immunohistochemistry: PBS + 1% bovine serum albumine (BSA); peroxidase VECTASTAIN Elite ABC kit (Vector; VPK-610); 3,3'-diaminobenzidine (DAB) substrate kit (Vector, SK-4100).
15. Neutral Red staining solution and differentiator (800 mL each):1200 mL deionized H_2O, 23 ml glacial acetic acid, 2.46 g sodium acetate, 400 mL 95% ethanol; add to half of the volume (800 mL) 4 g neutral red (staining solution), the other half of the solution serves as differentiator (store at RT).
16. Harris hematoxylin staining solution (Poly Scientific, Bay Shore, NY), equal part solution (25% v/v each of deionized H_2O, acetic acid (glacial), acetone, and ethanol; store at RT).
17. For dehydration of histological sections: 70%, 95%, and 100% (v/v) ethanol solution in H_2O; xylene.

3. Methods

3.1. Generation and Titration of HSV-1 Vector Stocks

The development and testing of recombinant HSV-1 viruses mutated in one or several IE-genes of HSV-1 have been comprehensively reviewed by Krisky et al. *(29)*. The techniques used to generate such mutants can be applied likewise to the development of replication-conditional HSV-1 vectors which are mutated in early or late genes.

3.1.1. Growing Replication Conditional Virus to Achieve High-Titer Stocks

To achieve high virus titers, the virus has to be grown on highly permissive and proliferating cells that are able to provide enzymes involved in DNA synthesis (*RR*, HSV-*TK*) whose viral counterparts are mutated in replication-conditional HSV-1 vectors. Vero cells are the most-commonly used cells for this purpose. Alternatively, BHK cells can be used. Virus will be grown by infecting these permissive cells and harvesting the virus at a time when the CPE is maximal and the cells are not yet detached. The burst size, i.e., the amount of virus produced by one cell after infection with HSV-1, reaches 100–1000 PFU.

At time of infection, Vero cells should be 80–90% confluent, i.e., the cells are still proliferating but have already formed cell–cell contacts through which the infection can be spread to neighboring cells without virus shedding to the supernatant. A small volume for infection is critical, as it enhances the probability that an infectious particle will touch a cell. The CPE caused by HSV-1 is the morphological equivalent of the toxic change in intracellular metabolism because of viral replication. For most HSV-1 mutants, the CPE consists of rounding up of the cells but some HSV-1 mutants also form syncytia. The CPE is associated with the imminent death of the cell, its detaching from the plate, and the release of progeny virus to the supernatant through cell lysis. However, at the time of maximal CPE, still a considerable amount of virus is trapped within the cell. Only repeated freezing and thawing or sonication can liberate these progeny virus particles. Applying the following protocol, 7×10^6 Vero cells plated into a T175 flask and infected with 10^7 PFU *hrR3* 1 d later yield 10^9 PFU *hrR3* 36–48 h later.

1. Plate Vero cells and wait until 80–90% confluency is reached.
2. Remove the media, rinse 1X with PBS, infect with a MOI of 0.1–1 in a small volume of DMEM+2 % FCS+P/S (4 mL in T175 flask; 400 μL per 100-mm tissue-culture dish).
3. Incubate at 37°C for 1–2 h, rotating every 10–15 min.
4. Add DMEM+10% FCS + P/S (Total volume in T175 flask is 20 mL, in 100-mm tissue-culture dish 8 mL) without removing the infection medium.
5. Check the Vero cell cultures frequently for CPE. When all cells are rounded up, but still attached to the plate, virus yield is maximal (36–48 h after infection). At that time, scrape the cells and harvest the cell/media-mix.

6. Freeze and thaw the cell/media-mix three times using dry ice and a 37°C water bath.
7. Spin out remaining cell debris (~1800 rpm, 6 min, 4°C).
8. Transfer the supernatant to fresh tubes, mix well, aliquot the virus in glass vials, quick-freeze on dry ice and store at –80°C.

The virus preparation can be now titered (*see* **Subheading 3.1.2.**) and used for cell culture experiments. For animal studies, for which high titers (up to 10^{10} PFU/mL) are required and where the virus preparation has to be particularly clean, the virus can be further concentrated. By using the following protocol, virus stocks are usually concentrated 20–200-fold including the loss of 50% of the total titer.

1. Spin the virus supernatant, which is already free of cell debris, in a sterile, covered tube for 1 h at 4°C, 12,500 rpm in a Sorwall GSA rotor (~25,000g).
2. Carefully remove the supernatant from the pellet.
3. Resuspend the virus pellet in the desired volume of DMEM by repeated pipeting.
4. Aliquot the virus in glass vials and store at –80°C.

3.1.2. Titration of Virus Stocks

Titration of virus stocks can be carried out in two different ways: 1) by plaque-forming assay on cell monolayers, the results given in PFU, or 2) by staining for the expression of a transgene, such as *lacZ*, *HSV-tk*, or *HSV-1* IE-genes, after the infection of permissive cells, the results given in transducing units (TU). For a particular mutant, PFU values can be different from TU values, depending on the ability of the mutant to replicate in the cells used for titration and on the sensitivity of the enzyme assay or antibody used for immuncytochemical staining. For the purpose of gene therapy of glioma using replication-conditional vectors, it is advisable to rely on PFU values rather than tu values because a major part of the therapeutic effect depends on the CPE resulting from replication. For the *lacZ+* virus *hrR3* it has been shown *(55)* that the values of PFU obtained in a regular plaque test and TU values are similar for a wide range of titers when the LacZ staining is done at 8–10 h p.i. on Vero cells. LacZ staining at later time-points probably overestimates the titer resulting from virus spread.

To reliably compare the titers of different virus preparations, the titration should be always done on the same type of cells according to the same protocol. The most commonly used cells for titration of HSV-1 viruses in a plaque forming assay are Vero cells as these cells form confluent monolayers in which plaques are easily detectable. For plaque-forming assays, agarose is layered over the Vero cells after a brief infection period to prevent lateral spread of the virus and thus reduce the formation of plaques because of secondary infection.

1. Plate 500,000 Vero cells per well in a 6-well plate the day before the infection.
2. Prepare agarose 1.5% in distilled water, autoclave, and keep in a 50°C water bath while proceeding with the infection.
3. Make serial 1 : 10 dilutions of the virus stock (dilutions of $1 : 10^5 – 1 : 10^8$ are the most important ones for a single or double replication-conditional mutant).
4. Wash the cells once with PBS and add 400 µL of each dilution to the wells in triplicate.
5. Incubate at 37°C for 1–2 h, rotating every 10–15 min.
6. Mix equal volumes of DMEM+10% FCS + P/S (RT) and 1.5% agarose solution (50°C) and add 3 mL per well.
7. Let the agarose solidify at room temperature for 10 min before placing the plates into the incubator at 37°C.
8. 4 d after infection, plaques can be counted using a phase-contrast microscope, PFU/mL can be calculated accordingly. It is reasonable to assess the PFUs only for the virus dilutions that lead to clearly distinguishable plaques (20–200 plaques/well in a 6-well plate).
9. If the virus is *lacZ+*, plaques can also be stained by overlaying 0.7 mL of a 1 mg/mL X-gal solution in X-gal staining buffer and overnight incubation at 37°C on day 4; plaques can be counted on day 5.

3.2. In Vitro Characterization of Recombinant HSV-1 Vectors

3.2.1. Single Step Growth Analysis

Before proceeding to an in vivo application, the replication dynamics of each new HSV-1 mutant has to be determined in the tumor cells that will be used in vivo. The replication dynamics of different viruses in the same glioma cell line can differ widely as exemplified by Kramm et al. *(27)* using 9L gliosarcoma cells. Also, the replication dynamics of a particular virus in different glioma cell lines can vary considerably *(21,32)*. This depends on the infectability of the cell line which, in turn, depends on the expression of cell surface receptors (HVEM) mediating the entry of the virus particle *(18)*. Some rat glioma cells (D74/RG2 and C6) are only poorly infectable with HSV-1 vectors. Additional largely unknown cellular factors influence the fate of the virus once it has entered the cell. It has been shown, for example, that $\gamma_1 34.5$-negative mutants replicate well in human glioma cells *(26,34)*, whereas these mutants do not replicate to a significant extent in rodent glioma cells that are highly infectable with HSV-1 *(27,33)*.

The time to complete one life-cycle (infection to release of the first virus particles) is about 18 h for wild-type HSV-1 virus and also for some mutants like *hrR3*. After infection with an MOI of 1, the maximal PFU-yield is observed 36–48 h p.i. *(27)*. Thus, the time-points to choose for a single growth step analysis should at least include one early time-point (<10 h), when almost all virus is absorbed by the cells, another time point after completion of the first life-cycle, and one time-point around the expected maximum of virus yield.

1. Plate 5×10^5 9L or U87 glioma cells per 60-mm tissue-culture dish.
2. One day later (day 0) wash 1X with PBS, trypsinize, and count three representative dishes.
3. Infect the remaining dishes in triplicate for each time-point of virus harvest with the respective HSV-1 mutant at an MOI of 1 in 500 μL DMEM+2% FCS+P/S per dish; the negative controls remain uninfected.
4. Keep the dishes in the incubator at 37°C for 1–2 h and rotate every 10–15 min.
5. Add 3 mL of DMEM+10% FCS+P/S.
6. To determine the virus yield, infected cells are scraped into the medium at different time intervals after infection.
7. The harvested cell/medium mix is frozen and thawed three times and subsequently analyzed in a standard plaque test as described above.

The sensitivity of a recombinant HSV-1 vector to GCV treatment as a means to stop HSV-1 replication can be tested by treating infected cell cultures with 1 μg/mL GCV over the 2–3 d infection period and calculating the ratio of plaque formation in GCV treated cultures vs non-GCV treated cultures

3.2.2. Assessment of the Cytolytic Potential of Recombinant HSV-1 Vectors

This method can be used either for determining the oncolytic potential of the recombinant vector using glioma cells or for assessing the neurotoxic potential using primary neuron cultures or glial cultures. The remarks in **Subheading 3.2.1.** about the broad range of infectability and replication dynamics of HSV-1 mutants in rodent and human glioma cells apply even more to the cytolytic potential of these mutants.

The technique described below has been worked out for rat 9L gliosarcoma cells. When assaying the cytolytic activity of replication-conditional HSV-1 mutants on other cells, the cell numbers should be modified so that uninfected negative controls are able to grow for at least 5 d without detaching.

1. Plate 3×10^5 9L glioma cells per 60-mm tissue-culture dish.
2. One day later (day 0) wash with PBS, trypsinize, and count three representative dishes.
3. Infect with the HSV-1 mutant at MOI 0.01, 0.1, and 1 in triplicate in 500 μL DMEM+2% FCS+P/S per dish; the negative control remains uninfected.
4. Keep the dishes in the incubator at 37°C for 1–2 h and rotate every 10–15 min.
5. Add 3 mL of DMEM+10% FCS+P/S.
6. On each of the following five days, three plates per MOI are thoroughly washed three times with PBS to remove dead cells, trypsinized, and counted.

The cytolytic effect of some replication-conditional vectors can be combined with prodrug-activation therapy using ganciclovir (GCV), which becomes activated by HSV-TK. Using *hrR3* on 9L cells as described above, addition of 1 μg/mL GCV on day 3 led to significantly increased cell killing in culture *(16)*. Addition of GCV before day 3 with the goal to increase the cell killing is not advisable as it might block virus replication and thus the formation of a CPE. For *RR⁻* mutants, the effect of the prodrug-activation of GCV can be studied by infection of target cells at 39.5°C *(56)*. In contrast to HSV-1 wild-type and HSV-*TK⁻* mutants, the replication of *RR⁻* mutants is severely compromised at elevated temperatures.

3.3. In Vivo Testing

In vivo studies for gene therapy of gliomas using HSV-1 vectors can be directed toward three purposes:

1. To analyze the distribution of gene transfer to glioma cells and other cells within the CNS under anatomically correct conditions.
2. To assess the therapeutic efficacy.
3. To evaluate the neurotoxicity.

In vivo testing for the therapeutic potential of an HSV-1 mutant can be done in syngeneic or xenogeneic rodent glioma models. Studies in syngeneic models include the host's immune reaction against the vector and tumor antigens. Most rodent glioma cell lines (9L, C6, CNS-1, F98, GL261) are highly immunogeneic in their syngeneic host. The D74/RG-2 rat glioma line seems to be different in that regard *(57)*, but is unfortunately not highly infectable with HSV-1 *(21,32)*. The immunogenicity of these cell lines in their syngeneic hosts may be enhanced upon viral infection because of the nonspecific release of immunostimulating cytokines. Thus, the therapeutic efficacy determined in these models may be overestimated as compared to the clinical situation with low immunogenic human gliomas. To avoid confounding immunologic factors, a xenogeneic model using immunocompromised nude or scid mice can be used to assess the cytolytic potential of HSV-1 vectors. In this case, not only rodent glioma cell lines, but also the clinically more relevant human cell lines can be implanted.

There are two principally different ways of assessing the therapeutic efficacy of an HSV-1 vector in vivo: (1) measuring sc tumor growth by volume or (2) determining survival time in an ic tumor model. In the sc tumor model, effects can be detected at relatively high resolution and quantified as a continous variable. Less animals per treatment group are generally necessary to obtain a statistically significant effect as compared to the ic model. In the ic model, a 50% reduction in tumor size by treatment would lead only to a prolongation of survival by 1–2 d for a cell line with a doubling time of about 24 h. However, the ic tumor model provides glioma growth under anatomically correct conditions. For studies in which the immune system or the passage of pharmacological agents through the blood-brain barrier plays a major part, the correct implantation site within the brain is crucial. In the ic model, the tumor size can be determined by measuring tumor areas on serial histologic sections. This, however, is much more work-intensive than measuring tumor volumes in the sc model.

The median survival time (MST) is measured from the intracranial injection of tumor cells until the animals become moribund, cannot move or feed themselves, and thus have to be sacrificed. MST of animals injected intracranially with a defined number of glioma cells is highly reproducible, in the Fischer rat: 4×10^4 9L–MST 20 d *(16)*; 4×10^4 D74–22 d *(32)*; in the C57BL/6 mouse: 10^6 GL261 glioma– 18 d *(10)*; in the nude mouse: 2×10^4 U-87MG–30 d *(26)*; in the scid mouse 10^6 U251MG–30–35 d; 10^6 D-54MG–18–22 d *(34)*. To obtain statistically significant differences in survival between treatment groups each treatment group should at least comprise eight animals.

3.3.1. Analysis of Therapeutic Efficacy

3.3.1.1. TREATMENT STUDY USING A SC TUMOR MODEL

1. Trypsinize cells, wash in PBS and resuspend in DMEM without FCS to a concentration of $10^6/100$ μL and put on ice.
2. Inject 10^6 cells (100 μL) per animal subcutaneously into the right flank of nude mice.
3. Treatment can start when the tumors are at least 70 mm³ in diameter (after 7–14 d for 9L gliosarcoma) by injecting 50 μL DMEM containing 10^8 PFU.
4. Before treatment and at several time-points during treatment the tumor volume is measured using calipers. Animals should be marked so that tumor growth can be analyzed separately for each individual animal. The tumor volume is calculated by multiplying width × breadth × height. Tumor growth is represented as a growth ratio relative to the tumor volume on day 0 before treatment was started.

3.3.1.2. TREATMENT STUDY USING AN IC TUMOR MODEL

1. Trypsinize 9L or U87 glioma cells, wash in PBS, resuspend in DMEM without FCS to a concentration of $2 \times 10^4/$μL and hold on ice.
2. Anesthesia: prepare a 1:1:2 mixture of ketamine 100 mg/mL, xylazine 20 mg/mL, and 0.9% NaCl and inject intraperitoneally about 80 μL to an 8-wk-old nude mouse or 500 μL to a 250 g rat. After 8–10 min, animals are well anesthetized and anesthesia lasts for at least 30 min.
3. Shave the skull of anesthetized animals, fix the skull in the sterotactic frame, make a sagittal skin incision and expose the skull; prepare a burr hole 2 mm to the right and 2 mm in front of the bregma.

4. Inject 2 µL glioma cell suspension using a stereotactic apparatus and a Hamilton syringe over about 2 min; the needle is slowly retracted over another 2 min.
5. The burr hole is closed with bone wax, the skin wound disinfected with betadine solution, and stitched with a 4–0 silk suture.
6. The intratumoral virus injection ensues 5 d later using the same burr hole and the same technique and precautions. Typically, 10^8 PFU in 10 µL plain DMEM are injected.
7. The animals should be observed at least once daily; especially in the first days after virus injection some neurotoxicity, evident as increased lethargy, is regularly seen.
8. Animals should be sacrificed when they are not longer able to move or feed themselves.

As in culture, additional treatment with GCV can give an additional oncolytic, and thus survival-prolonging, effect *(16,40)* for some mutants. The optimal timing of the GCV treatment depends on the treatment strategy: both the Kramm and Boviatsis studies treated Fischer rats intraperitoneally with 7.5 mg/kg GCV twice daily. The GCV was administered in 100 µL saline. However, Kramm and colleagues who used an intrathecal as well as an ic injection of the virus started on day 2 after virus injection to reduce toxicity whereas Boviatsis and colleagues started on day 7 after ic virus inoculation where virus toxicity is less. Beyond a potential additional oncolytic effect, GCV treatment also serves as a safety measurement by completely blocking further replication of *HSV-tk+* HSV-1.

3.3.2. Assessing Gene Transfer and Virus Replication Within the Tumor

Gene transfer to tumor cells and other cells within the brain is assessed by staining for recombinant marker genes like *lacZ*. Gene transfer plus viral replication are monitored by immunohistochemistry for HSV-TK or HSV-core proteins. These early or late viral genes are well suitable for this purpose as they are almost exclusively expressed in cells in which the virus replicates.

The LacZ and HSV-TK staining described below works well on sections that are fixed with 4% para-formaldehyde (PFA). However, if the plan is also to do immunohistochemical staining against leucocyte surface antigens it must be taken into account that most commercially available antibodies against leucocyte surface antigens do not work on 4% PFA-fixed sections. For this purpose, fresh-frozen sections have to be used.

3.3.2.1. *LacZ* STAINING

1. Perfuse animals in deep anesthesia with PBS, pH 7.4, 4°C, and then with 4% PFA in PBS, pH 7.4.

2. Remove the brain, postfix for another 2 d in 4% PFA in PBS, pH 7.4, and cryopreserve the brain in 30% sucrose in PBS, pH 7.4 for 3 d.
3. Cut 10 μm cryosections and mount onto slides; if not used immediately, store the slides at −80°C.
4. For staining, equilibrate the sections in PBS, pH 7.4.
5. Prepare working solutions: dilute X-gal stock solution (*see* **Materials**) in substrate buffer to a final concentration of 1 mg/mL.
6. Incubate the sections overnight in working solution.
7. Remove the working solution and wash 2X with double-distilled water.
8. Counterstain with Neutral Red staining solution for 5 min.
9. Put into Neutral Red differentiator solution for 15–30 s.
10. Dehydrate (70%, 95%, 100% ethanol, xylene) and coverslip sections (Cytoseal 60, Stephens Scientific, Riverdale, NJ).

3.3.2.2. HSV-TK IMMUNOHISTOCHEMISTRY

1. Rinse sections in PBS.
2. Block the endogenous peroxidase by incubating the sections in 0.5% H_2O_2 in methanol for 30 min.
3. Wash twice with PBS.
4. Incubate with 10% normal goat serum in PBS+1% bovine serum albumin (BSA) for 30 min and decant excess fluid afterwards.
5. Incubate with polyclonal anti-TK Serum A 1:1000 in PBS+1%BSA overnight at 4°C.
6. Wash three times with PBS.
7. Incubate with biotinylated goat anti-rabbit antibody 1:1000 in PBS+1% BSA at RT for 45 min.
8. During the incubation time, prepare the ABC solution (Vectastain ABC kit).
9. Wash three times with PBS.
10. Incubate with ABC at RT for 45 min.
11. Wash three times with PBS.
12. Incubate with the DAB kit at RT for 45 s.
13. Stop the reaction by rinsing with double-distilled H_2O.
14. Before counterstaining, let the sections dry.
15. Put sections into a solution of water, glacial acetic acid, acetone, and ethanol (1:1:1:1) for 3 min.
16. Rinse for 1 min in water.
17. Stain with Harris hematoxylin for 30 s.
18. Destain under flowing tab water until no more stain comes off.
19. Dehydrate and coverslip.

4. Notes

4.1. Generation and Storage of HSV-1 Stocks

1. The optimal way to freeze HSV-1 stocks is to put the tube into a bath of dry ice and ethanol. Thawing should be done rapidly in a 37°C water bath with constant

swirling of the tubes to avoid warming of the medium, which would decrease the titer.

2. Even at –80°C temperature, the titer of HSV-1 vectors decreases with time. Thus, if the stocks are stored for more than 6 mo, retitering is advisable before using the stock in an experiment depending on exact titers.

3. Storage of virus stocks in glass vials is advisable as glass only minimally adsorbs viral particles.

4. Viral titers drop with repeated freezing and thawing. Five times freezing and thawing reduces the titer by 90%. Thus, for experiments depending on exact titers, aliquot the virus stocks and use a new aliquot at each time-point.

4.2. Handling of HSV-1 Virus Stocks

5. HSV-1 virions are temperature sensitive. Stocks that are not immediately used after thawing should be put on ice. At 37°C in DMEM+10% FCS, the infectious titer falls to about 10% after 6 h.

6. Other factors that may influence the stability of the virus: at highly alkaline pH, the virus might aggregate and loose its infectability. To prevent this, tissue-culture media can be additionally buffered with 20 mM HEPES.

4.3. Infecting Cells with HSV-1 Vectors

7. As an alternative way of infecting cells with HSV-1, let the virus adsorb to the cells for 1 h at 4°C, then put back at 37°C in DMEM+10% FCS. At 4°C, the virus attaches to the cell, but does not enter. Switching later to 37°C, triggers the internalization of the cell-bound virus particles.

8. As a general rule, the smaller the infection volume used, the more efficient is the infection. However, the infecting volume should cover the whole plate, so that the plate does not dry out during the infection process. In our experience, minimal infection volumes that require rotation of the plate every 10–15 min, are: 35-mm tissue-culture dish—200–400 µL; 60-mm tissue-culture dish—400–800 µL; 100-mm tissue-culture dish—1–2 mL. Infections with 250 µL in a 24-well plate do not need rotation.

4.4. Concentration and Purification

9. As an alternative way of concentrating and purifying virus, HSV-1 stocks can be run over a sucrose, cesium chloride, or ficoll density gradient. For a sucrose gradient centrifugation, place 3 mL each of a solution of 60% sucrose in PBS, pH 7.4, 30% sucrose in PBS, and 10% sucrose in PBS on top of each other, load the virus stock and spin for 1 h at 82,700g (25,000 rpm for a Beckman SW-28 rotor) in an ultracentrifuge. Harvest the virus containing interface between the 30% and 60% sucrose phase. An average of 50% of the original total titer will be lost by the procedure; the virus can be concentrated about 100-fold.

4.5. Titration of HSV-1 Vector Stocks

10. For the titration of virus stocks, an adequate agar temperature is crucial (put the previously autoclaved agar solution at least for 2 h to a 50°C water bath). Too high a temperature precipitates proteins in the DMEM/agar-mix and may harm the cells that are overlaid with the agarose. Subconfluency of Vero monolayers (60–80% confluency) at the time of infection is important, as some viruses (e.g., *hrR3*) do not replicate as well in slowly growing confluent or overconfluent monolayers. The time frame of the assay as described is 5 d (for *hrR3*) although some slower replicating viruses may take longer to form recognizable plaques. Plaques may already be distinguishable at day 2 p.i., but it is easier to count plaques at day 4 or 5.

11. There are two alternative ways of titration: 1) instead of overlaying the infected Vero cells with agarose, cells are cultured further in DMEM+10%FCS. Two days after infection, the media is removed, cells are fixed with methanol for 5–10 min, then the methanol is removed and the dishes are kept at RT until the remainder of the methanol has evaporated. Giemsa stain, diluted 1:20 in deionized water, is added for 45 min. Afterwards, plates are washed once with deionized water and plaques counted in water. This method can be also adjusted to 24-well plates (100,000 Vero cells plated the day before, infection with 100 µL virus supernatant and further dilutions +100µL DMEM+10% FCS for 1 h). The disadvantage of this method is that secondary infections cannot be excluded. The incubation time of 2 d applies to the *hrR3* mutant. Other mutants might take longer to cause recognizable plaques. 2) For *lacZ+* viruses the titer can be also determined by LacZ staining. For correct titers, expressed in tu/mL, all single LacZ+ cells have to be counted; multiple contiguous LacZ+ cells are counted as one tu as they probably originate from a single particle infecting one cell with subsequent spread of the infection to neighboring cells. To obtain tu values that correspond with PFU values it has been shown for the *lacZ+* mutant *hrR3* that LacZ staining has to be carried out 8–11 h after infection of permissive-cell monolayers (*55*).

12. If the mutant virus carries a marker gene, the titer (transducing units) should be determined on both Vero cells and the glioma cells, which are used in further studies. This will give an idea how infectable these glioma cells are in comparison to highly permissive Vero cells.

4.6. Cytotoxicity Assays

13. The cytolytic potential of a replication-conditional HSV-1 vector has to be tested on several cell lines as their susceptibility to HSV-1 oncolysis may vary considerably. Besides counting viable cells, the CPE can be quantitated by measuring mitochondrial function in a tetrazolium salt (MTT) or alamarBlue assay (*34*).

4.7. In Vivo Experiments

14. Anesthetized nude mice have to be put on a warm pad and wrapped in aluminum foil to maintain their body temperature. Instruments should be autoclaved for surgery of nude mice.

15. Slow ic injection of virus and cells and slow needle retraction from the injection site are important to allow the pressure to equilibrate and to avoid reflux out of the needle track. According to our experience, injection of up to 10 µL cell suspension into a mouse brain is well tolerated.

16. Aliquot the amount of virus to be injected into each animal in advance and store it so that each aliquot can be thawed immediately before injection.

17. For the sc implantation of tumors to both flanks, it is suggested to anesthetize the animal as it allows a more reproducible injection of the tumor cells. The measurement of only one dimension vs measurement of all three dimensions of a tumor is not advisable as tumors may grow irregularly.

18. GCV is cytotoxic for cells expressing HSV-TK over a wide range of doses administered intraperitoneally (ip). The suggested 15 mg/kg GCV/d is in the higher part of the range. Experiments with sc 9L tumors, which stably express HSV-TK, showed that with ip GCV doses as low as 1 mg/kg a considerable oncolytic effect is achieved *(58)*. With ip administration of 30 mg/kg/d GCV to nude mice over 1 wk no toxicity has been observed.

4.8. Histology and Immunohistochemistry

19. Mice do not have to be perfused to preserve LacZ staining if after sacrificing by cervical dislocation the animal the brain is quickly removed and put into 4% PFA solution, 4°C.

20. Make sure that for the LacZ staining the pH of the PBS solution used for perfusion, all washing steps and staining is 7.4 or higher. With lower pH, it is more likely to produce artifactual X-gal staining *(59)*. In the brain, artifactual reaction with the X-gal substrate can especially arise in the hippocampus, nucleus basalis Meynert, ventral pallidum, hypothalamic nuclei, red nucleus, and certain pontine nuclei *(59)*. Artifactual X-gal reaction can also be oberved in endothelial cells *(59)* and macrophages *(60)*. Artifactual LacZ staining is usually fainter and has a more granular appearance in macrophages than in cells transduced with the bacterial *lacZ* gene.

21. So far, the polyclonal anti-HSV-TK Serum A has worked best for HSV-TK detection, but is of limited availability. Dr. F. Burrows (Chiron Viagen, San Diego, CA) described a set of two monoclonal anti-HSV-TK antibodies, which are also suitable for immunocytochemistry and immuohistochemistry *(61)*.

22. If the sections to be stained with hematoxylin are equilibrated in the equal part solution of water, acetic acid (glacial), sodium acetate, and ethanol before staining, the nuclear hematoxylin staining will be greatly enhanced. Instead of hematoxylin, HSV-TK-stained sections can also be counterstained with methylgreen (1 min).

23. Cryosections can be double-stained for LacZ and HSV-TK. LacZ staining has to be followed by HSV-TK, but in contrast to the aforementioned protocol, LacZ staining is terminated with PBS and not with water. Hematoxylin is used as a counterstain. The purplish blue of the hematoxylin staining is easily distinguishable from the blue of the LacZ staining.

24. An alternative to the immunohistochemical demonstration of viral replication is described by Andreansky et al. *(34)*. Animals injected with HSV-1 are sacrificed, the brains are harvested and homogenized. Brain homogenates were assayed in a standard plaque assay for replication competent virus.

4.9. Evaluation of Neurotoxicity

25. The neurotoxicity of HSV-1 vectors can be tested in vivo by determining the LD_{50} of recombinant viruses in nude or scid mice, or by determining the median survival time after ic injection of different virus doses. The same tools as described for treatment studies are used for this purpose. Histology should be analyzed at different time points after ic injection.

References

1. Damck, D. M. and Hochberg, F. H. (1997) Clinical aspects of brain tumor. *Curr. Opin. Neurol.* **10,** 452–458.
2. Sampson J. H., Bigner D. D., and Dranoff G. (1998) Cytokine-based gene therapy of brain tumors, in *Gene Transfer and Therapy of Neurological Disorders* (Chiocca, E. A. and Breakefield, X. O., eds.). Humana, Totowa, NJ, pp. 227–290.
3. Eck, S. L., Alavi, J. B., Alavi, A., Davis, A., Hackney, D., Judy, K., et al. (1996) Treatment of advanced CNS malignancies with the recombinant adenovirus H5.010RSVTK: a phase I trial. *Hum. Gene. Ther.* **7,** 1465–1482.
4. Berger, M. S., Prados, M. D., Van Gilder, J. C., Warnick, R. E., McDermott, M. W., Marcus, S. G., and Kapcala, L. P. (1997) Phase II trial of GLI 328 HSV-TK gene therapy in recurrent glioblastoma. *Cancer Gene Ther.* **4,** S42.
5. Ram, Z., Culver, C. W., Oshiro, E. M., Viola, J. J., DeVroom, H. L., Otto, E., et al. (1997) Therapy of malignant brain tumors by intratumoral implantation of retroviral vector-producing cells. *Nat. Med.* **12,** 1354–1361.
6. Huber, B. E., Austin, E. A., Goode, S. S., Knick, V. C., Tibbels, S., and Richards, C. A. (1993) In vivo antitumor activity of 5-gluorocytosine on human colorectal carcinoma cells genetically modified to express cytosine deaminase. *Cancer Res.* **53,** 4619–4626.
7. Wei, M. X., Tamiya, T., Chase, M., Boviatsis, E. U., Chang, T. K. H., and Hochberg, P., et al. (1994) Experimental tumor therapy in mice with the cyclophosphamide-activating cytochrome P450 2B1 gene. *Hum. Gene Ther.* **5,** 969–978.
8. Manome, Y., Wen, P. Y., Dong, Y., Tanaka, T., Mitchell, B. S., Kufe, D. W., and Fine, H. A. (1996) Viral vector transduction of the human deoxyxytidine kinase cDNA sensitizes glioma cells to the cytocoxic effects of cytosine arabinoside in vitro and in vivo. *Nat. Med.* **2,** 567–573.

9. Tamiya, T., Ono, Y., Wei, M. X., Mroz, P., Moolten, F. L., and Chiocca, E. A. (1996) The Escherichia coli gpt gene sensitizes rat glioma cells to killing by 6-thioxanthine or 6-thioguanine. *Cancer Gene Ther.* **3,** 155–162.

10. Herrlinger, U., Kramm, C. M., Johnston, K. M., Louis, D. N., Finkelstein, D., Reznikoff, G., et al. (1997) Vaccination for experimental gliomas using GM-CSF transduced glioma cells. *Cancer Gene Ther.* **4,** 345–352.

11. Fahkrai, H., Dorigo, O., Shawler, D. L., Lin, H., Mercola, D., Black, K. L., et al. (1996) Eradication of established intracranial rat gliomas by transforming growth factor beta antisense therapy. *Proc. Natl. Acad. Sci. USA* **93,** 2909–2914.

12. Millauer, B., Shawyer, L. K., Plate, K. H., Risau, W., and Ullrich, A. (1994) Glioblastoma growth inhibited in vivo by a dominant-negative Flk-1 mutant. *Nature* **367,** 576–578.

13. Saleh, M., Stacker, S. A., and Wilks, A. F. (1996) Inhibition of growth of C6 glioma cells in vivo by expression of antisense vascular endothelial growth factor sequence. *Cancer Res.* **56,** 393–401.

14. Gomez-Manzano, C., Fueyo J., Kyritsis, A. P., Steck, P. A., Roth J. A., McDonell, T. J., et al. (1996) Adenovirus-mediated transfer of the p53 gene produces rapid and generalized death of human glioma cells via apoptosis. *Cancer Res.* **56,** 694–699.

15. Martuza, R. L., Malick, A., Markert, J. M., Ruffner, K. L., and Coen, D. M. (1991) Experimental therapy of human glioma by means of a genetically engineered virus mutant. *Science* **252,** 854–856.

16. Boviatsis, E. J., Park. J. S., Sena-Esteves, M., Kramm, C. M., Chase, M., Efird, J. T., et al. (1994) Long-term survival of rats harbouring brain neoplasms treated with ganciclovir and a herpes simplex virus vector that retains an active thymidine kinase gene. *Cancer Res.* **54,** 5745–5761.

17. Chase, M., Chung, R. Y., and Chiocca, E. A. (1998) An oncolytic viral mutant that delivers the CVP2B1 transgene and augments cyclophosphamide chemotherapy. *Nat. Biotechnol.* **16,** 444–448.

18. Montgomery, R. I., Warner, M. S., Lum, B. J., and Spear, P. G. (1996) Herpes simplex virus-1 entry into cells mediated by a novel member of the TNF/NGF receptor family. *Cell* **87,** 427–436.

19. Wu, N., Watkins, S. C., Schaffer, P. A., and DeLuca, N. A. (1996) Prolonged gene expression and cell survival after infection by a herpes simplex virus mutant defective in the immediate-early genes encoding ICP4, ICP27, and ICP22. *J. Virol.* **70,** 6358–6369.

20. Goldstein, D. J. and Weller, S. (1988) Herpes simplex virus type 1-induced ribonucleotide reductase activity is indispensable for virus growth and DNA synthesis: isolation and characterization of an ICP6 *lacZ* insertion mutant. *J. Virol.* **62,** 196–205.

21. Kaplitt, M. G., Tjuvajev, J. G., Leib, D. A., Berk, J., Pettigrew, K. D., Posner, J. B., et al. (1994) Mutant herpes simplex virus induced regression of tumors growing in immunocompetent rats. *J. Neuro-Oncol.* **19,** 137–147.

22. Pyles, R. B. and Thompson, R. L. (1994) Evidence that Herpes simplex virus type 1 uracil DNA glycosylase is required for efficient viral replication and latency in the murine nervous system. *J. Virol.* **68,** 4963–4972.

23. Chou, J., Kern, E. R., Whitley, R. J., and Roizman, B. (1990) Mapping of herpes simplex virus-1 neurovirulence to $\gamma_l 34.5$, a gene nonessential for growth in culture. *Science* **250,** 1262–1266.

24. Chou, J., Chen, J.-J., Gross, M., and Roizman, B. (1995) Association of a novel M_r 90,000 phosphoprotein with PKR kinase in cells exhibiting enhanced phosphorylation of EIF-2alpha and premature shut-off of protein synthesis after infection with $\gamma_l 34.5^-$ mutants of herpes simplex virus. *Proc. Natl. Acad. Sci. USA* **92,** 10,516–10,520.

25. Pyles, R. B., Warnick, R. E., Chalk, C. L., Szanti, B. E., and Parysek, L. M. (1997) A novel multiply-mutated HSV-1 strain for the treatment of human brain tumors. *Hum. Gene Ther.* **8,** 533–544.

26. Mineta, T., Rabkin, S. D., Yazaki, T., and Hunter, W. D. (1995) Attenuated multi-mutated herpes simplex virus-1 for the treatment of malignant gliomas. *Nat. Med.* **1,** 938–943.

27. Kramm, C. M., Chase, M., Herrlinger, U., Jacobs, A., Pechan, P. A, Sena-Esteves, M., et al. (1997) Therapeutic efficiency and safety of a second-generation replication-conditional HSV1 vector for brain tumor gene therapy. *Hum. Gene Ther.* **8,** 2057–2068.

28. Chou, J., Poon, A. P. W., Johnson, J., and Roizman, B. (1994) Differential response of human cells to deletions and stop codons in the $\gamma_l 34.5$ gene of herpes simplex virus. *J. Virol.* **68,** 8304–8311.

29. Krisky, D., Marconi, P., Goins, W. F., Glorioso, J. C. (1997) Development of replication-defective herpes simplex virus vectors, in *Methods in Molecular Medicine, Gene Therapy Protocols* (Robbins, P., ed), Humana, Totowa, NJ, pp. 79–102.

30. Boviatsis, E. J., Scharf, J. M., Chase, M., Harrington, K., Kowall, N. W., Breakefield, X. O., and Chiocca, E. A. (1994) Antitumor activity and reporter gene transfer into rat brain neoplasms inoculated with herpes simplex virus vectors defective in thymidine kinase or ribonucleotide reductase. *Gene Ther.* **1,** 323–331.

31. Jacobs, A., Tjuvajev, J. G., Joshi, A., Joshi, R., Herrlinger, U., Avril, N., et al. Quantitative kinetics of HSV1-*tk* gene delivery by a recombinant HSV-1 virus vector in tumor cells: implications for imaging rHSV-1 mediated gene transfer in vivo. Submitted.

32. Herrlinger, U., Kramm, C. M., Aboody-Guterman, K. S., Silver, J. S., Johnston, J. M., Pechan, P., et al. (1998) Pre-existing Herpes simplex virus-1 (HSV-1) immunity decreases but does not abolish gene transfer by a HSV-1 mutant vector. *Gene Ther.* **5,** 809–819.

33. Andreansky, S. S., He, B., Gillespie, G. Y., Soroceanu, L., Markert J., Chou J., et al. (1996) The application of genetically engineered herpes simplex viruses to

the treatment of experimental brain tumors. *Proc. Natl. Acad. Sci. USA* **93,** 11,313–11,318.

34. Andreansky, S., Soroceanu, L., Flotte, E. R., Chou, J., Markert, J. M., Gillespie, G. Y., et al. (1997) Evaluation of genetically engineered herpes simplex viruses as oncolytic agents for human malignant brain tumors. *Cancer Res.* **57,** 1502–1509.
35. Chambers R., Gillespie, G. Y., Soroceanu, L., Andreansky, S., Chatterjee, S., Chou, J., et al. (1995) Comparison of genetically engineered herpes simplex viruses for the treatment of brain tumors in a scid mouse model of human malignant glioma. *Proc. Natl. Acad. Sci. USA* **92,** 1411–1415.
36. Toda, T., Rabkin, S. D., and Martuza, R. L. (1997) Lack of ganciclovir-mediated antitumor effect when thymidine kinase is present in a replication-competent herpes simplex virus. *Proc. Am. Assoc. Cancer Res.* **38,** 14.
37. Rainov, N. G., Zimmer, C., Chase, M., Kramm, C. M., Chiocca, E. A., Weissleder, R., and Breakefield, X. O. (1995) Selective uptake of viral and monocrystalline particles delivered intra-arterially to experimental brain tumors. *Hum. Gene Ther.* **6,** 1543–1552.
38. Rainov, N. G., Dobberstein, K. U., Heidecke, V., Dorant, U., Chase, M., Kramm, C. M., et al. (1998) Long-term survival in a rodent brain tumor model by bradykinin-enhanced intra-arterial delivery of a therapeutic herpes-simplex virus vector. *Cancer Gene Ther.* **5,** 158–162.
39. Barnett, F. H., Ikeda, K., Rainov, N. G., Schuback, D. E., Elliott, P., Kramm, C., et al. Selective delivery of herpes virus vectors to experimental brain tumors using RMP-7. *Cancer Gene Ther.* **6,** 14–20.
40. Kramm, C. M., Rainov, N. G., Sena-Esteves, M., Barnett, F. H., Chase, M., Herrlinger, U., et al. (1996) Long-term survival in a rodent model of disseminated brain tumors by combined intrathecal delivery of herpes vectors and ganciclovir treatment. *Hum. Gene Ther.* **7,** 1989–1994.
41. Corey, L. and Spear, P. G. (1986) Infections with Herpes simplex viruses. *N. Engl. J. Med.* **314,** 686–691.
42. Baringer, J. R. and Pisani, P. (1994) Herpes simplex virus genomes in human nervous system tissue analyzed by polymerase chain reaction. *Ann. Neurol.* **36,** 823–829.
43. Wang, Q., Guo, J., and Jia, W. (1997) Intracerebral recombinant HSV-1 vector does not reactivate latent HSV-1. *Gene Ther.* **4,** 1300–1344.
44. Forrester, A., Farrell, H., Wilkinson, G., Kaye, J., Davis-Poynter, N., and Minson, T. (1992) Construction and properties of a mutant of herpes simplex virus type I with glycoprotein H coding sequences deleted. *J. Virol.* **66,** 341.
45. Dilloo, D., Rill, D., Entwisle, C., Boursnell, M., Zhong, W., Holden, W., et al. (1997) A novel herpes vector for the high-efficiency transduction of normal and malignant human hematopoetic cells. *Blood* **89,** 119–127.
46. Johnston, K. M., Jacoby, D., Pechan, P. A., Fraefel, C., Borghesani, P., Schuback, D., et al. (1997) HSV/AAV hybrid amplicon vectors extend transgene expression in human glioma cells. *Hum. Gene Ther.* **8,** 359–370.

47. Wang, S. and Vos, J. (1996) A hybrid herpesvirus infectious vector based on Epstein-Barr virus and herpes simplex virus type I for gene transfer into human cells in vitro and in vivo. *J. Virol* **70**, 8422–8430.
48. Ho, D. (1994) Amplicon-based herpes simplex vectors. *Meth. Cell. Biol.* **43**, 191–210.
49. Tung, C., Federoff, H. J., Brownlee, M., Karpoff, H., Weigel, T., Brennan, M. F., and Fong, Y. (1996) Rapid production of interleukin-2-secreting tumor cells by herpes simplex virus-mediated gene transfer: implications for autologous vaccine production. *Hum. Gene Ther.* **7**, 2217–2224.
50. Miyatake, S., Martuza, R. L., and Rabkin, S. D. (1997) Defective herpes simplex virus vectors expressing thymidine kinase for the treatment of malignant glioma. *Cancer Gene Ther.* **4**, 222–228.
51. Pechan, P. A., Fotaki, M., Thompson, R. L., Dunn, R., Chase, M., Chiocca, E. A., and Breakefield, X. O. (1996) A novel 'piggyback' packaging system for herpes simplex virus amplicon vectors. *Hum. Gene Ther.* **7**, 2003–2013.
52. Pechan, P. A., Herrlinger, U., Aghi, M., Jacobs, A., Johnston, K., Dunn, R., and Breakefield, X. O. (1999) Enhanced therapeutic efficacy of combined HSV-1 recombinant and amplicon vectors for experimental glioma tumors. *J. Gene Med.* **1**, 176–185.
53. Fraefel, C., Song, S., Lim, F., Lang, P., Yu, L., Wang, Y., et al. (1996) Helper virus-free transfer of herpes simplex virus type 1 plasmid vectors into neural cells. *J. Virol.* **70**, 7190–7197.
54. Weizsaecker M., Deen, D. F., Rosenblum, M. L., et al. (1981) The 9L rat brain tumor: description and application of an animal model. *J. Neurol.* **224**, 183–192.
55. Jacobs, A., Herrlinger, U., Chiocca, E. A., and Breakefield, X. O. Rapid titration of replication-conditional HSV-1 vectors: implications for the comparison of infectious units between different viral vectors. Submitted.
56. Preston V. G., Darling, A. J., and McDougal, I. M. (1988) The herpes simplx virus type 1 temperature-sensitive mutant ts1222 has a single base pair deletion in the small subunit of ribonucleotide reductase. *Virology* **167**, 458–467.
57. Tzeng, J., Barth, R. F., Grosz, C. G., and James, S. M. (1991) Phenotype and functional activity of tumor-infiltrating lymphocytes isolated from immunogenic and non-immunogenic rat brain tumors. *Cancer Res.* **51**, 2373–2378.
58. Aghi, M., Kramm, C. M., Chou, T.-C., Breakefield, X. O., and Chiocca, E. A. (1998) Synergistic anticancer effects of ganciclovir/thymidine kinase and 5-gluorocytosine/cytosine desaminase gene therapies. *J. Natl. Cancer Inst.* **90**, 370–380.
59. Rosenberg, W. S., Breakefield, X. O., DeAntonio, C., and Isacson, O. (1992) Authentic and artifactual detection of the E. coli *lacZ* gene product in the rat brain by histochemical methods. *Mol. Brain Res.* **16**, 311–315.
60. Rhodes, J. M., Rasmussen, S. E., Burchardt, S., and Larsen S. O. (1987) Modulation of beta-galactosidase activity in peritoneal macrophages from C57B1 mice after exposure to Propionibacterium acnes. *Acta Pathol. Microbiol. Immunol. Scand.* **95**, 213–220.

61. Kruse, C. A., Roper, M. D., Kleinschmidt-DeMasters, B. K., Banuelos, S. J., Smiley, W. R., Robbins, J. M., and Burrows, F. J. (1996) Purified herpes simplex thymidine kinase Retrovector™ particles. I. In vitro characterization, in situ trasnduction efficiency, and histopathological analyses of gene therapy-treated brain tumors. *Cancer Gene Ther.* **4,** 118–128.
62. Roizman, B. and Batterson, W. (1985) Herpesviruses and their replication, in *Virology* (Fields, B. N., ed.), Raven, New York, pp. 497–526.

18

Intratumoral Injection of Naked DNA

Jingping Yang

1. Introduction

Direct injection of naked DNA into tissues as a gene-delivery method has been extensively studied for genetic immunization and gene therapy *(1)*. When naked plasmid DNA was used as a negative control while cationic liposomes were studied, it was surprisingly found that direct injection of naked DNA into skeletal muscle resulted in higher gene expression than injection of cationic liposomes *(2)*. Naked DNA was reported as more efficient than retroviral and adenoviral vectors following direct injection into adult mouse skeletal muscle *(3)*. Subsequently, cardiac muscles, thyroid, joint, liver, lung, brain, kidney, as well as solid tumors were found capable of taking up and expressing naked DNA *(4–10)*. In some tumors, gene expression following intratumoral injection of naked DNA was higher than that of DNA associated with cationic liposomes (**Fig. 1**) *(7)*. This is probably because of the faster dessimination rate of naked plasmid DNA in the tumor than that of DNA complexed with cationic liposomes *(11)*.

The most-used route to deliver naked DNA is via direct injection into target tissues. Via vascular injection, efficient gene expression in the local tissues was recently reported. The intraillac artery injection into all the muscles of a rat hindlimb resulted in as high as 20% muscle cells tranfected, and intraportal vein injection of naked DNA was also reported to result in gene expression in hepatocytes. However, extremely large injection volume, 10 mL injected into rat illac artery and 1 mL into murine portal vein, was critical for high gene expression in the cases of intravascular injection *(12–14)*. There is a recent report about high gene expression in the liver following tail vein injection of naked DNA in a large volume, 1.6 mL *(15)*. DNA entry into cells may be

From: *Methods in Molecular Medicine, Vol. 35: Gene Therapy: Methods and Protocols*
Edited by: W. Walther and U. Stein © Humana Press, Inc., Totowa, NJ

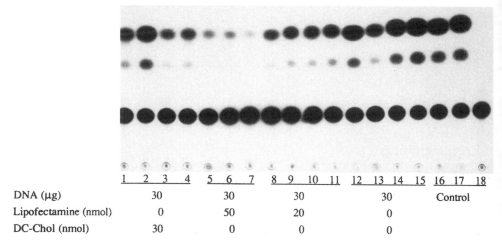

DNA (µg)	30	30	30	30	Control
Lipofectamine (nmol)	0	50	20	0	
DC-Chol (nmol)	30	0	0	0	

Fig. 1. CAT reporter gene expression in murine BL6 melanoma. pUCCMVCAT plasmid DNA was injected into the tumor. Mice were sacrificed 2 d later and tumor protein extracts were assayed for CAT activity. Lanes 16 and 17: 0.005 and 0.01 units of purified CAT standard enzyme, respectively. Lane 18: extracts from tumors injected with 5% glucose only [with the permission from (7)].

limited to situations of physical damage of targeting a cell's membrane. After direct injection, most transfected cells are found around the injection site, and only a few transfected cells were away from the injection site in muscles and solid tumors (7,16). In tumors, a low concentration of detergent in the injection solution significantly enhanced trasfection efficiency probably because of detergent permeabilization of the cell membrane. Endocytosis also maybe involved in the naked DNA entry into cells. Cells actively engaged in pinocytosis, such as follicular cells and synovial cells, are easier to be transfected (6,8). Endocytosis maybe mediated by DNA receptors, which have been reported (17,18).

All tumors tested exhibited uptake and expression with directly injected naked DNA (7), whereas the level of gene expression varied greatly in different types of tumors (**Table 1**). In mice bearing murine melanoma BL6, human cervical carcinoma, and breast tumors, injection of naked DNA was more efficient than cationic liposome associated DNA (unpublished data). However, with murine melanoma B16-F0 or B16 F10, and human melanoma, cationic liposome mediated transfection was higher than directly injected naked DNA. Murine melanoma BL6 produced about 2 ng of foreign protein following injection of 30 µg naked DNA. The foreign gene expression lasted for 10 d in murine melanoma BL6, unlike the skeletal muscle in which transgene could last for 19 mo (7,19). This is probably explained by differences in the cell state; muscle cells are differentiating and tumor cells are proliferating.

Table 1
CAT Gene Expression in Different Types of Tumor

Tumor	CAT activity (% conversion)[a]		
	Plasmid DNA	DNA/DC-chol liposome	DNA/Lipofectamine
HeLa	3, 4	46.2, 8	nd^c
852	5.6, 1.2	11.4, 15	nd^c
983B	2.2, 25	10.6, 76	40, 77
CL8-1	$2 \pm 0.7 \ (n = 4)^b$	nd^c	nd^c
F0	$2.7 \pm 1.6 \ (n = 5)^b$	nd^c	nd^c
F10	5, 0.5, 0.7	nd^c	nd^c
BL6	$72.5 \pm 4.4 \ (n = 13)^b$	$28.4 \pm 12.9 \ (n = 4)^b$	$21 \pm 7.4 \ (n = 4)^b$

[a]Thirty µg of pUCCMVCAT dissolved in 50 µl of 5% glucose were injected into the tumor. The ratio of DNA/DC-chol liposome and DNA/Lipofectamine was 1 µg : 1 nmol and 3 µg : 2 nmol, respectively. CAT assay was performed 2 d later.
[b]Mean ± SD.
[c]Not done.
[with the permission from (7)]

In this chapter, we describe the general principles and basic protocols of intratumoral injection of naked DNA plasmids. The factors influencing transfection efficiency will be discussed in **Subheading 4.**

2. Materials

2.1. Animals

Female C57BL/6 mice, 4–5 wk old, were from Charles River Breeding Laboratories (Raleigh, NC). Animal care was according to the institutional guidelines.

2.2. Cell Culture

1. Murine melanoma BL6 and B16-F0 cells were kindly provided by Dr. E Gorelik, University of Pittsburgh, PA. The BL6 cell was selected by screening a subline of B16-F10 for higher invasiveness through the bladder membrane (20). The B16-F10 cell line was obtained from ATCC (Rockville, MD).
2. RPMI 1640, DMEM, penicillin, streptomycin, glutamine, trypsin-EDTA, Hank's balanced salt solution (HBSS) were from Life Technologies (Gaithersburg, MD).
3. Fetal bovine serum (FBS) was from Hyclone (Logan, UT).

2.3. Syringe and Dissecting Tools

1. One cc syringe, insulin syringe, and 27-1/2-gauge needle were from Becton Dickinson (Franklin Lakes, NJ). The insulin syringe has low dead volume.
2. Dissecting board, dissecting pans with wax, dissecting pins, scissors, forceps, 12 × 75-mm glass tube, and homogenizer purchased from Fisher, (Pittsburgh, PA).

2.4. Plasmid DNA

1. Plasmid pCMVCAT is constructed by inserting cDNA of CAT under the control of CMV promoter. Plasmid pCMV-*luc* was constructed by inserting a fragment of luciferase cDNA into *Hind*III-XbaI sites of pCDNA3 vector. pCDNA3 vector was from Invitrogene (Carlsbad, CA).
2. Purified plasmid DNA containing the report gene was prepared by cesium chloride gradient centrifugstion or Qiagen (Chatsworth, CA) column chromatography, precipitated in 75% ethanol, redissolved in distilled water, aliquoted, and then stored at –20°C. Multiple freeze and thaw cycles should be avoided. Because EDTA inhibits naked DNA expression in tumors, TE buffer is not recommended to store DNA.
3. 50% glucose: dissolve 50 g glucose in endotoxin-free distilled water by heating in a boiling water bath and adjust volume to 100 mL, and sterilize by filtering through 0.22-μm filter before it cools. It can be stored at room temperature for 6 mo.
4. DNA solution for injection: a 50 μg of stock DNA and 5 μL of 50% glucose were diluted with endotoxin-free distilled water to a final volume of 50 μL.

2.6. Report Gene Assay Equipment and Reagents

2.6.1. CAT TLC Assay

1. Equipment: Whatman Thin-layer chromatography (TLC) and chromatographic tank were from VWR Scientific Products (Willard, OH) and PhosphorImager from Molecular Dynamics (Sunnyvale, CA).
2. Extraction buffer: 40 mM Tris-HCl, pH 7.5, 10 mM EDTA, 150 mM NaCl.
3. Protein assay reagent: Coomassie Plus Protein Assay Reagent was from Pierce (Rockford, IL).
4. CAT assay cocktail solution: 10 μL of 40 mM acetyl CoA (Sigma, St. Louis, MO), 1 μL of 100 μCi/μL ^{14}C-chloramphenicol (ICN, Irvine, CA), 37.5 μL of 1M Tris-HCl buffer, pH 7.5, 1.5 μL of distilled water.
5. Ethyl acetate.
6. Development solution: 190 mL chloroform and 10 mL methanol.

2.6.2. CAT ELISA Assay

CAT ELISA kit was from Boehringer Mannheim (Indianapolis, IN).

2.6.3. X-gal Assay

1. Fixation solution: 5% glutaraldehyde.
2. Wash buffer: PBS, pH 7.5, 1 mM MgCl$_2$.
3. X-gal solution: 1 mg/ml X-gal (Sigma), 1 mM MgCl, 5 μM K$_3$Fe(CN)$_6$:3H$_2$O, PBS, pH 7.5.

2.6.4. Luciferase Assay

1. Extraction buffer: 200 mM Tris-HCl, pH 7.8, 2 mM EDTA, 0.05% Triton X-100.
2. Luciferase assay substrate reagent kit was from Promega Corporation (Madison, WI).

3. Autolumat LB 953 Luminometer was from EG&G berthold (Bad Wildbad, Germany).

3. Methods

3.1. Cell Culture

Murine melanoma BL6 cells were cultured in RPMI 1640 medium. Murine B16-F0 and B16-F10 cells were cultured in DMEM medium. Media were supplemented with 10% FBS, penicillin (100 U/mL), streptomycin (100 mg/mL), and glutamine (0.292 mg/mL).

3.2. Tumor Implantation

1. Harvest cells with trypsin-EDTA. Wash cells with HBSS twice to remove serum proteins and then count.
2. 2×10^5 murine melanoma BL6, B16-F0, or B16-F10 cells resuspended in 50 μL of HBSS were injected subcutaneously to the flank of C57BL/6 mice by using a 27-1/2-gauge needle. Gently vortex the tumor cell solution to make sure the same amount of cells are implanted in each mouse.

3.3. Intratumoral Injection

When tumors reach 3×3 mm, anesthetize mice. Let the mouse lay on a dissecting board. Fix the mouse on the board by taping the feet. Use one hand to hold the tumor and one hand to hold the syringe. Push the needle directly into the tumor. Let the needle go into the tumor as deeply as possible, but not through the tumor. Push the solution smoothly into the tumor. After injection, leave the needle in the tumor for about 20 s, and then slowly pull the needle out. A small drop of injected solution usually comes out with the needle. If the needle went completely through the tumor before being pulled back, much of the injected solution will leak from the injection site. If multiinjection sites are required, after the first injection, slowly pull the needle back, but not out of tumor, change the direction of the needle inside the tumor and then push in for additional injection sites. If the needle is pulled completely out and then returned for a new injection, the injected solution will leak from the first injection site.

3.4. Tumor Preparation for Reporter Gene Assay

1. One day after injection, sacrifice the mouse by cervical dislocation. Let the mouse lay on the several tissues that were placed in a dissecting pan with wax. Fix the foot of the mouse on the pan by pins. Cut the skin longitudinally in the middle of the front of the mouse. Clip the skin with forceps and pull it to the side. The tumor stays attached to the skin. Fix the skin on the pan with pins. Carefully cut out the tumor from the skin.

2. Weight the tumor. Put the tumor in a glass test tube and add cold extraction buffer for the assay to be performed according to the tumor weight (1 mL/200 mg tumor). Homogenize the tumor. Transfer the homogenized tumor mixture to a 1.5-mL centrifuge tube. Keep the sample at 4°C. If the reporter gene assay cannot be done right way, tumors or tumor extractions can be frozen with dry ice and stored at –70°C up to 1 yr if CAT gene is used, up to 1 wk if luciferase is used as reporter gene.

3.5. Reporter Gene Assay

3.5.1. CAT Assay by TLC

1. Freeze the homogenized tumor mixture in liquid nitrogen and thaw in 37°C water bath 3X. Heat at 60°C in a water bath for 10 min to inactivate deacetylase activity. Spin in a microcentrifuge for 5 min at 16,000*g* at 4°C. The protein concentration in the supernatant is determined by Coomassie blue assay.
2. A volume corresponding to 100 µg of sample protein is diluted with the extraction buffer to a final volume of 100 µL in 1.5-mL centrifuge tube. Add 50 µL of cocktail solution. Mix and incubate at 37°C for 2–5 h.
3. Add 1 mL of ethyl acetate to stop the reaction. Vortex the mixture and spin for 10 s at 16,000*g*.
4. The radioactive substrate is in the top organic layer. Transfer 800 µL of the top organic layer to centrifuge tubes and evaporate to dryness in a speedvac evaporator for 30 min or by placing opened tubes in a hood.
5. Add 30 µL of ethyl acetate to the dried centrifuge tube to redissolve the radioactive substrate, vortex and spin for 2 s at 16,000*g*.
6. Spot all of redissolved substrate drop by drop (about 5 µL) 2 cm above the bottom edge of a TLC sheet. Use a hair dryer to evaporate the spotting solution.
7. Develop the TLC in an equilibrated chromatographic tank. The tank was equilibrated with developing solution at least 2 h before development.
8. Dry the TLC plate, wrap with plastic wrap, expose it on the Phosphoimager screen overnight.

3.5.2. CAT Assay by ELISA

Prepare tissue extract as in the **Step 1** of **Subheading 3.5.1.** Perform the ELISA assay according to the manufacturer's instructions.

3.5.3. Luciferase Assay

Spin the homogenized tumor mixture for 5 min at 4°C. Place 10 µL of the supernatant in the bottom of 12 × 75 mm glass tube. Place the tube in the luminometer and measure the relative light units by adding 100 µL of substrate reagent.

3.5.4. X-Gal Staining

1. Freeze the tumor with liquid nitrogen. Slice the tumor into 8-μm sections.
2. Fix tumor sections with 5% glutaraldehyde for 10 min at RT. Wash 2X with wash solution.
3. Stain with X-gal solution for 4 h.

4. Notes

1. The number of cells to implant is related to the growth rate of tumor. Murine melanoma BL6 grows very fast, therefore, only 2×10^5 BL6 cells are implanted. For growth of human cervical carcinoma (by injection of skov3 cell line) in SCID mice, 2×10^6 cells are implanted.
2. Gene expression from naked plasmid DNA directly injected into tumor is dose-dependent. Optimal dosage is 30 to 70 μg of DNA. Exceeding this range can result in lower gene expression.
3. A larger injection volume results in higher and less-variable gene expression in tumors. Gene expression with a 100-μL injection volume was almost fourfold of that with a 10-μL injection volume. However, mice bearing BL6 tumor some times died immediately, probably because of pulmonary embolism from the damaged tumor tissue. However, this phenomena was observed only in this particular tumor. For other tumors such as cervical carcinoma and breast cancer, we could inject 100 μL without immediate deaths. Consequently, a 100-μL injection volume is recommended for other tumors.
4. The osmolarity of the plasmid buffer can influence the transfection efficacy of directly injected naked DNA. Isotonic buffer resulted in higher transfection efficiency than hypotonic buffer (distilled water). Hypotonic buffer (25% glucose) gave the similar resuls as isotonic buffer. Among the four isotonic buffers tested, saline, PBS, HBSS, and 5% glucose, there was no significant differences in transfection. Differences of ion composition in these buffers, Na^{2+}, Ca^{2+}, K^+, Mg^{2+}, did not affect transfection efficiency. However, the presence of 10 mM EDTA inhibited the transfection, probably by chelating calcium vital for normal cellular functions. In addition, 0.01% Triton-X 100 in the injection buffer significantly increased the transfection efficiency. This implies that the permeabilization of cell membrane enhances the entry of naked DNA into cells.
5. Injection of a constant 30 μg of DNA into different tumor sizes ranging from 150 to 1500 mg, gave no significant difference in gene expression per miligram tumor protein. On the other hand, larger tumors gave higher gene expression per tumor. This implies that the percentage of transfected tumor cells is same regardless of the tumor size.
6. Multiple injection sites initially was thought to result in higher transfection efficiency because most transfected cells are located around the injection site. However, recent results from tumors do not show this phenoma. Multiple injection and single injection sites result in similar gene expression in tumors.

7. The plasmid structure affects the gene expression greatly. It has been shown that the promoter plays any important role in the level and persistence of transgene expression, in skeletal muscle. The CMV promoter produces the highest gene expression but is less persistent compared to the RSV promoter. In tumors, the CMV promoter produces a much higher gene expression than either the SV40 or the T7 promoters.

References

1. Davis, H. L., Michel, M. L., Whalen, R. G. (1995) Use of plasmid DNA for direct gene transfer and immunization. *Ann. NY Acad. Sci.* **772**, 21–29.
2. Wolff, J. A., Malone, R. W., Williams, P., et al. (1990) Direct gene transfer into mouse muscle in vivo. *Science* **247**, 1465–1468.
3. Davis, H. L., Demeneix, B. A., Quantin, B., Coulombe, J., and Whalen, R. G. (1993) Plasmid DNA is superior to viral vectors for direct gene transfer into adult mouse skeletal muscle. *Hum. Gene Ther.* **4**, 733–740.
4. Acsadi, G., Jiao, S. S., Jani, A., et al. (1991) Direct gene transfer and expression into rat heart in vivo. *New Biol.* **3**, 71–81.
5. Malone, R. W., Hickman, M. A., Lehmann-Bruinsma, K., et al. (1994) Dexamethasone enhancement of gene expression after direct hepatic DNA injection. *J. Biol. Chem.* **269**, 29,903–29,907.
6. Sikes, M. L., O'Malley, B. W., Jr., Finegold, M. J., and Ledley, F. D. (1994) In vivo gene transfer into rabbit thyroid follicular cells by direct DNA injection. *Hum. Gene Ther.* **5**, 837–844.
7. Yang, J. P. and Huang, L. (1996) Direct gene transfer to mouse melanoma by intratumor injection of free DNA. *Gene Ther.* **3**, 542–548.
8. Yovandich, J., O'Malley, B., Jr., Sikes, M., and Ledley, F. D. (1995) Gene transfer to synovial cells by intraarticular administration of plasmid DNA. *Hum. Gene Ther.* **6**, 603–610.
9. Schwartz, B., Benoist, C., Abdallah, B., Rangara, R., Hassan, A., Scherman, D., and Demeneix, B. A. (1996) Gene transfer by naked DNA into adult mouse brain. *Gene Ther.* **3**, 405–411.
10. Lin, K. F., Chao, J., and Chao, L. (1995) Human atrial natriuretic peptide gene delivery reduces blood pressure in hypertensive rats. *Hypertension* **26**, 847–853.
11. Nomura, T., Nakajima, S., Kawabata, K., Yamashita, F., Takakura, Y., and Hashida, M. (1997) Intratumoral pharmacokinetics and in vivo gene expression of naked plasmid DNA and its cationic liposome complexes after direct gene transfer. *Cancer Res.* **57**, 2681–2686.
12. Budker, V., Zhang, G., Danko, I., Williams, P., and Wolff, J. A. (1998) The efficient expression of intravascularly delivered DNA in rat muscle. *Gene Ther.* **5**, 272–276.
13. Budker, V., Zhang, G., Knechtle, S., and Wolff, J. A. (1996) Naked DNA delivered intraportally expresses efficiently in hepatocytes. *Gene Ther.* **3**, 593–598.
14. Zhang, G., Vargo, D., Budker, V., Armstrong, N., Knechtle, S., and Wolff, J. A. (1997) Expression of naked plasmid DNA injected into the afferent and efferent

vessels of rodent and dog livers [In Process Citation]. *Hum. Gene Ther.* **8,** 1763–1772.

15. Liv, F., Song, Y. K., and Liv, D. (1999) Hydrodynamics-based transfection in animals by systemic administration of plasmid DNA. *Gene Ther.* **6,** 1258–1266.
16. Wolff, J. A., Dowty, M. E., Jiao, S., et al. (1992) Expression of naked plasmids by cultured myotubes and entry of plasmids into T tubules and caveolae of mammalian skeletal muscle. *J. Cell Sci.* **103,** 1249–1259.
17. Loke, S. L., Stein, C. A., Zhang, X. H., et al. (1989) Characterization of oligo-nucleotide transport into living cells. *Proc. Natl. Acad. Sci. USA* **86,** 3474–3478.
18. Yakubov, L. A., Deeva, E. A., Zarytova, V. F., et al. (1989) Mechanism of oligo-nucleotide uptake by cells: involvement of specific receptors? *Proc. Natl. Acad. Sci. USA* **86,** 6454–6458.
19. Wolff, J. A., Ludtke, J. J., Acsadi, G., Williams, P., and Jani, A. (1992) Long-term persistence of plasmid DNA and foreign gene expression in mouse muscle. *Hum. Mol. Genet.* **1,** 363–369.
20. Hart, I. R. (1979) The selection and characterization of an invasive variant of the B16 melanoma. *Am. J. Pathol.* **97,** 587–600.

19

Cationic Liposome Gene Transfer

Kyonghee Kay Son

1. Introduction

Development of safe and effective technology for delivering functional DNA into cells in an intact organism is crucial to broad applications of gene therapy to human disease. Both viral and nonviral vectors have been developed. Of the technologies currently being studied, liposomal delivery system is particularly attractive. Cationic liposome mediated gene transfection (lipofection), a relatively new technique pioneered by Felgner and coworkers *(1)*, was highly efficient for transfecting cells in culture. The liposomes were composed of an equimolar mixture of a synthetic cationic lipid N-[1-(2,3,-dioleyloxy)propyl]-N,N,N,-trimethyl-ammonium chloride (DOTMA) and a helper lipid dioleoylphosphatidylethanolamine (DOPE). The DOTMA/DOPE mixture (Lipofectin™) forms complexes with DNA by charge interaction upon mixing at room temperature. Other cationic lipids commercially available are DOTAP, DOSPER, LipofectAMINE™, Lipofectam™, Tfx™, and DC-chol. DOTAP is a diester analog of DOTMA. DOSPER differs from DOTAP in that the fatty acids are connected to the 1- and 3-position of the structure's propane backbone. LipofectAMINE and Lipofectam are polycationic lipids with a spermine head group that show increased frequency and activity of eukaryotic cell transfection *(2,3)*. Tfx is N,N,N′,N′-tetramethyl-N,N′-bis(2-hydroxyethyl)-2,3,-dioleoyloxy-1,4-butanediammonium iodide. 3β-[N-(N′,N′-dimethy-aminoaminoethane) carbamoyl] cholesterol (DC-chol), a cationic cholesterol derivative, was introduced by Gao and Huang *(4)* and is routinely used in our laboratory. DC-chol can be easily synthesized with a single step reaction from N,N-dimethylethylenediamine and cholesterol chloroformate *(4)*, and improves the efficiency of transfection with minimal toxicity. Liposomes prepared with DC-chol and DOPE (3:2 molar ratio) are stable at 4°C for at least 1 yr *(4)*.

From: *Methods in Molecular Medicine, Vol. 35: Gene Therapy: Methods and Protocols*
Edited by: W. Walther and U. Stein © Humana Press, Inc., Totowa, NJ

Complexes of plasmid DNA and DC-chol/DOPE liposomes can be easily prepared by simple mixing. A plasmid containing a reporter gene such as *Escherichia coli* chloramphenicol acetyltransferase (CAT) *(5)*, β-galactosidase *(6)*, or luciferase *(7)*, under the control of a promoter of interest, is introduced into eukaryotic cells. Within a few days after transfection, the cells are harvested and the amount of reporter gene protein in the lysate is measured. This is usually done with a simple enzymatic assay. The transfection activity of the complex tested with many cell lines and primary cells depends on the cell type. Transformed epithelial cells such as epidermal carcinoma A431 cells, lung epithelial carcinoma A549 cells, embryonic kidney epithelium 293 cells, and airway epithelium IB3-1 cells are readily transfected, but fibroblast and endothelial cells are less efficiently transfected *(8)*. Suspension cells including lymphoid cells are difficult to transfect using cationic liposomes, in general. Human ovarian carcinoma cells grown as subcutaneous solid tumor in SCID mouse can be transfected by directly injecting plasmid DNA/liposome complex into the tumor. The level of CAT reporter gene expression in the tumor cells was significantly elevated if the animal received a single ip injection of cisplatin 1 wk before the intratumor lipofection *(9)*. Likewise, murine ovarian carcinoma grown as ascitic tumors in the peritoneal cavity was also significantly transfectable with both liposomal CAT and a target gene interferon-gamma: the expression of interferon-gamma gene reached a peak at day 11 after cisplatin treatment and lasted over 1 wk *(10)*. Cisplatin followed by liposomal interferon-gamma gene treatment suppressed tumor growth (or killed tumor cells) and increased the long-term survival of animals (at least 80 d) without tumors *(10)*. This observation has a profound clinical implication as a sequential and combination therapy.

Because of the apparent safety and the versatility offered by liposomal delivery system, this technology has proven important in delivering DNA for therapeutic purposes in human. DC-chol/DOPE liposomes have been used in clinical trials for cancer *(11)* and cystic fibrosis transmembrane conductance regulator (CFTR) *(12)* gene therapy.

2. Materials

1. DC-chol (Sigma, St. Louis, MO)/DOPE (Avanti Polar Lipids) liposomes (2 nmol/μL).
2. Plasmids pSV2CAT (constructed by Dr. Mark Magnuson, Vanderbilt University) or pCMVCAT (constructed by Dr. Hassan Farhood, University of Pittsburgh), pCMVβgal, and pRSVLuc at 1 μg/μL in TE buffer (10 mM Tris-HCl, pH 7.4, 0.1 mM EDTA) was amplified in *E. coli* and purified as described in the instruction manual of DNA-Pure™ plasmid mega-prep kit (CPG).

3. Sterile tissue-culture flasks, dishes and tubes, plates, and pipets.
4. Autoclaved pasteur pipets, microcentrifuge tubes (1.5 mL), yellow and blue tips, phosphate buffered saline (PBS).
5. Tissue-culture medium supplemented with penicillin (100 U/mL)/ streptomycin (100 mg/mL) (Life Technologies, Gaithersburg, MD) with or without 10% fetal bovine serum (FBS) (Life Technologies).
6. 0.05% trypsin + 0.53 mM EDTA in Ca^{++} or Mg^{++} free sterile saline (Life Technologies).
7. Lysis buffer: 0.1% Triton X-100 in 0.25M Tris-HCl, pH 7.8.
8. Sterile disposable 20-, 25-, and 27-gauge needle.
9. Sterile disposable 1.0- and 5.0-mL syringe.
10. Sterile disposable cell scraper (handle length: 25 cm).
11. Sterile Hanks' Balanced Salt Solution (HBSS).
12. Tissue-Tearor Homogenizer (Biospec Product Corp., Racine, WI).
13. Sterile dimethyl sulfoxide (DMSO).
14. Tumor extraction buffer: 40 mM Tris-HCl, pH 7.5, 10 mM EDTA, and 150 mM NaCl.
15. Benchtop centrifuge and Eppendorf microcentrifuge.
16. Water bath.
17. Mice of interest (animal care in accordance with the AAALAC guidelines).

3. Methods
3.1. Purification of Plasmid DNA

Growth of the bacterial culture is as described by Sambrook et al *(13)*. Harvesting and lysis of the bacteria and purification of plasmid DNA are performed based on a standard alkaline lysis procedure utilizing a special DNA binding resin and vacuum filtration according to the manufacturer's protocol (CPG).

3.2. Tissue Culture Cells and In Vitro Transfection

1. Culture cells of interest in defined medium supplemented with 10% fetal bovine serum (FBS) at 37°C with 5% CO_2.
2. Trypsinize cells and plate them into 24-well plates the day before transfection such that the culture is 60–80% confluent.
3. Add appropriate quantity of cationic liposomes (10–20 nmols) to the bottom of a 1.5-mL microcentrifuge tubes.
4. Add 200 µL plasmid DNA (0.5–2.0 µg) diluted with serum-free culture medium to the liposomes.
5. Incubate for 10 min at room temperature to form liposome/DNA complex.
6. Remove serum-containing medium from each well and wash the cells once with serum-free medium.

7. Add the liposome/DNA mixture to each well and incubate cells for 5 h at 37°C in 5% CO_2 (transfection).
8. Remove the serum-free medium and add 0.5 mL of serum-containing medium to each well.
9. Incubate the cells in 5% CO_2 for 2 d (posttransfection).
10. Remove serum-containing medium and wash once with PBS.
11. Add 200 µL of lysis buffer to each well and incubate 10–15 min at room temperature or freeze at –80°C.
12. Collect the lysed cells in microcentrifuge tubes (ready for CAT, β-galactosidase, and luciferase assay as well as for protein assay).

3.3. Tumor Inoculation on Mice and Intratumor Transfection

3.3.1. Subcutaneous Solid Tumor

1. Seed a tumor cell line in 150-mm tissue-culture dish and grow to confluency in complete medium.
2. Harvest cells with cell scraper, centrifuge and wash with HBSS, and resuspend in HBSS at 2×10^7 cells/mL.
3. Inject 0.1-mL aliquots sc to the flanks and back of mice using a 25-gauge needle.
4. Grow solid tumors to about 8 mm in diameter.
5. Mix 30 µg of pUCCMVCAT in 1X TE buffer (1 µg/µl) with 30 nmols of DC-chol/DOPE liposomes (3:2, mol/mol) in water (2 nmol/µl). Total volume equals to 45 µL.
6. Directly inject the DNA/liposome complex into the tumor in three different sites using a 27-gauge needle.
7. After 48 h, sacrifice the animal and excise the tumor.
8. Homogenize the tumor in extraction buffer.
9. Lyse cells by three cycles of freeze/thawing.
10. Heat the lysate at 65°C for 10 min and centrifuge at 14,000 rpm for 10 min.
11. The supernatant is ready for protein and CAT assay, or it can be frozen at –80°C for at least 7 d.

3.3.2. Peritoneal Ascitic Tumor

1. Grow and harvest murine or human ovarian carcinoma cells as described in **steps 1** and **2** in **Subheading 3.3.1.**
2. Inject 0.5-mL aliquots into the peritoneum of mice using a 25-gauge needle.
3. Grow ascitic tumors and take ascites from the peritoneal cavity using a 20-gauge needle and 5-mL syringe.
4. Ascites can be frozen in the presence of DMSO (10%) at –80°C for at least 6 mo.
5. Inject 0.2–0.5 mL aliquots into the peritoneum of mice.
6. Grow ascitic tumors. After 10 and 40 d for fast- and slow-growing cells, respectively, directly inject ip a mixture of 200 µg of pUCCMVCAT and 200 nmols of DC-chol/DOPE liposomes using a 27-gauge needle. Total volume equals to 300 µL.

7. After 72 h, take ascites (1 mL) from animal and centrifuge at 3000 rpm for 5 min to separate ascitic tumor cells from ascitic fluid.
8. Process tumor cells as described in **steps 8–11** in **Subheading 3.3.1.**

4. Notes

1. Anion-exchange purification of plasmid DNA is safe, effective and time-saving alternative to CsCl purification. Plasmid DNA isolation kit is also available from Qiagen (Chatsworth, CA), Clontech (Palo Alto, CA), (NucleoBond), and Boehringer Mannheim (Mannheim, Germany) (High Pure™). Different cell lines require different optimal liposome/DNA ratio and different total amounts of complex. Defining and optimizing transfection conditions are important. In vitro transfection protocol of DC-chol/DOPE liposomes should be optimized with respect to the ratio of liposome/DNA, dose of the complex, the incubation time with cells for transfection and post transfection, and serum concentration *(14)*. In vivo transfection protocol of DC-chol/DOPE liposomes on sc solid tumor directly should be optimized with respect to tumor size, number of injections on tumor, and injection volume and the ratio of liposome/DNA. In vivo transfection protocol of DC-chol/DOPE liposomes on the peritoneal ascitic tumor directly should be optimized with respect to dose of DNA/liposome, injection volume, and the ratio of liposome/DNA.
2. The transfection activity of cell line depends on both DC-chol and DNA concentration, showing a bell-shaped curve *(15)*. Thus, it is important to define the optimal concentrations of liposomes and DNA. The optimal ratio of DC-chol (nmol)/DNA (µg) is between 10 to 20 for a variety of transformed epithelial cells and tumor cell lines.
3. The transfection activity increases with the amount of liposome/DNA complex added to the cells at a complex of liposome/DNA ratio of 1 (nmol/µg). This is a suboptimal ratio, which allows transfections with high complex doses and minimal toxicity. As the ratio of liposome/DNA complex increases, the toxicity of liposome to cells increases and affects the transfection activity.
4. Cell density (the status of the cultured cells that are seeded on plate) is another factor for a successful transfection and high level expression of foreign DNA. The efficiency reduces greatly if transfection is performed on the confluent cells *(15)*. To achieve high transfection efficiency, transfection may be performed at a confluency of approx 60% and 80% for fast-and slow-growing cells, respectively.
5. The toxicity varies among cell types, and is dependent on the confluency of the cell culture. Confluent cells are more resistant to the toxicity of the liposome/DNA complex. As a compromise between high transfection activity and low toxicity, cells with 60% to 80% confluency are the optimum.
6. Supercoiled DNA gives higher transfection efficiency compared to nicked, covalently closed, or linear DNA.
7. pCMVCAT (an expression plasmid of CAT gene under the control of CMV early promoter) is more efficient for high level of expression than pSV2CAT (an expression plasmid of CAT gene under the control of SV40 early promoter).

8. Use a serum-free medium, or a very low concentration of serum, if cells are not stable for at least 4 to 5 h in the absence of serum because the transfection activity is strongly inhibited by the presence of high concentrations of serum component. DC-chol liposomes can tolerate up to 2% FBS without significantly reducing activity *(4)*.
9. DC-chol/DOPE liposomes and plasmid DNA should be sterile for in vitro tissue-culture work.
10. Transfection on different-sized culture wells gives similar results when volumes were adjusted in proportion to surface area of the wells.
11. Transfectability decreases with increase in tumor size.
12. There is dose limitation of liposome/DNA complex because of the limitation of injection volume.
13. More injection sites on a single tumor increases the transfection efficiency.
14. The best transfection is obtained when the ratio of liposome/DNA complex is 1 nmol/μg. This is because injection volume increases with an increase in the ratio of liposome/DNA complex.
15. Tumors (size ranging from 8 to 10 mm) have difficulty taking injection volumes of liposome/DNA complex greater than 200 μl.
16. Preinjection of cisplatin to mice 1 wk before lipofection greatly increases the transfection efficiency of solid tumors (in situ lipofection) *(9)*. Tumor cells taken from animals injected with cisplatin are also more transfectable in vitro as compared to cells taken from animals injected with PBS *(15)*.
17. Transfection efficiency is related to DNA dose *(16)*. 100 μg to 1000 μg of DNA can be injected. However, injection volume should be kept less than 500 μL. Lyophilization of liposome/DNA (1:1, nnole:μg) did not affect transfection activity. To achieve high transfection efficiency with high dose (i.e., 1000 μg DNA and 1000 nmol liposome), a complex may be prepared as a lyophilized form and injected after reconstituting with small volume of water before use *(16)*.
18. Higher liposome/DNA ratio gives higher transfection efficiency *(16)*. It is noted, however, that injection volume increases and affect the transfection activity as the ratio and dose of liposome/DNA complex increase.
19. Preinjection of cisplatin to mice before lipofection also greatly increases the transfection efficiency of ascitic tumors: this enhanced lipofection is tumor-specific and prolongs for at least 10 d *(10)*.
20. Anticancer drugs sensitize ascitic tumor cells for lipofection, although the level of sensitization varies *(16)*. It is important to optimize dose of each drug to be preinjected as the sensitization is greater with subtoxic dose *(16)*.
21. Cisplatin-sensitized lipofection is observed to be host-independent *(16)*.

References

1. Felgner, P. L., Gadek, T. R., Holm, M., Roman, R., Chan, H. W., Weinz, M., et al. (1987) Lipofectin: a highly efficient, lipid-mediated DNA-transfection procedure. *Proc. Natl. Acad. Sci. USA* **84,** 7413–7417.

2. Hawley-Nelson, P., Ciccarone, V., Gebeyehu, G., Jesee, J., and Felgner, P. (1993) LipofectAMINE™ reagent: a new, higher efficiency polycationic liposome transfection reagent. *Focus* **15,** 73–79.

3. Behr, J. P., Demeneix, B., Loeffler, J.-P., and Perez-Mutul, J. (1989) Efficient gene transfer into mammalian primary endocrine cells with lipopolyamine-coated DNA. *Proc. Natl. Acad. Sci. USA* **86,** 6982–6986.

4. Gao, X. and Huang, L. (1991) A novel cationic liposome reagent for efficient transfection of mammalian cells. *Biochem. Biophys. Res. Commun.* **179,** 280–285.

5. Sankaran, L. (1992) A simple quantitative assay for chloramphenicol acetyltransferase by direct extraction of the labeled product into scintillation cocktail. *Anal. Biochem.* **200,** 180–186.

6. Lim, K. and Chae, C.-B. (1989) A simple assay for DNA transfection by incubation of the cells in culture dishes with substrates for β-galactosidase. *BioTechniques* **7,** 576–579.

7. DeWet, J. R., Wood, K. V., DeLuca, M., Helinski, D. R., and Subramani, S. (1987) Firefly luciferase gene: structure and expression in mammalian cells. *Mol. Cell. Biol.* **7,** 725–737.

8. Gao, X. and Huang, L. (1993) Cationic liposomes and polymers for gene transfer. *J. Liposome Res.* **3,** 17–30.

9. Son, K. and Huang, L. (1994) Exposure of human ovarian carcinoma to cisplatin transiently sensitize the tumor for liposome mediated gene transfer. *Proc. Natl. Acad. Sci. USA* **91,** 12,669–12,672.

10. Son, K. (1997) Cisplatin-based interferon γ gene therapy of murine ovarian carcinoma. *Cancer Gene Ther.* **4,** 391–396.

11. Nabel, G. J., Chang, A., Nabel, E. G., Plautz, G., Fox, B. A., Huang, L., and Shu, S. (1992) Clinical Protocol: immunotherapy of malignancy by in vivo gene transfer into tumors. *Human Gene Ther.* **3,** 399–410.

12. Gill, D. R., Southern, K. W., Mofford, K. A., Seddon, T., Huang, L., Sorgi, F., et al. (1997) A placebo-controlled study of liposome-mediated gene transfer to the nasal epithelium of patients with cystic fibrosis. *Gene Ther.* **4,** 199–209.

13. Sambrook, J., Fritsh, E. F., and Maniatis, T. (1989) Plasmid vectors, in *Molecular Cloning: A Laboratory Manual*, vol. 1, ch. 1, Cold Spring Harbor Laboratory, Cold Spring Harbor, NY.

14. Farhood, H., Bottega, R., Epand, R. M., and Huang, L. (1992) Effect of cationic cholesterol derivatives on gene transfer and protein kinase C activity. *Biochim. Biophy. Acta* **1111,** 239–246.

15. Son, K., Sorgi, F., Gao, X., and Huang, L. (1997) Cationic liposome-mediated gene transfer to tumor cells in vitro and in vivo, in *Gene Therapy Protocol. Methods in Molecular Medicine* (Robbins, P., ed.), Humana, Totowa, NJ, pp. 329–337.

16. Son, K. (1999) Chemical toxicants activate murine ovarian ascitic tumor cells for *in situ* lipofection. *Drug Delivery* **6,** 75–79.

20

In Vivo Particle-Mediated Gene Transfer
for Cancer Therapy

Alexander L. Rakhmilevich and Ning-Sun Yang

1. Introduction

During the past several years, particle-mediated delivery techniques have been developed as a nonviral technology for gene transfer (1–7). For mammalian somatic tissues, this technology, popularly known as the gene gun method, has been shown effective for transfection of skin, liver, pancreas, muscle, spleen, and other organs in vivo (3,4), brain, mammary, and leukocyte primary cultures or tissue explants ex vivo (2,5–7), and a wide range of cell lines in vitro (3,6,7). In this chapter, we describe the general principles, mechanisms, protocols, and uses of the particle-mediated gene transfer technology for in vivo gene transfer, mainly into skin tissues. Specific applications of this technology to basic studies in molecular biology as well as to gene therapy and genetic immunization against cancer are addressed.

1.1. Principles of the Particle-Mediated Gene Transfer

The general principles of particle-mediated gene transfer are illustrated in **Fig. 1A**. Microscopic gold particles are coated with transgenes of interest and accelerated by a helium shock wave to sufficient velocities to penetrate the target cells, resulting in intracellular delivery of the DNA molecules. Using DNA/gold particles loaded within a small teflon tube as a cartridge, the hand-held helium pulse gun can hold 12 cartridges in a revolving cylinder. Each gene transfer can be performed in less than 5 s, thus making the gene gun a highly efficient device for repeated, multiple-gene deliveries. This design may be especially desirable in clinical applications for gene therapy and DNA vaccination.

From: *Methods in Molecular Medicine, Vol. 35: Gene Therapy: Methods and Protocols*
Edited by: W. Walther and U. Stein © Humana Press, Inc., Totowa, NJ

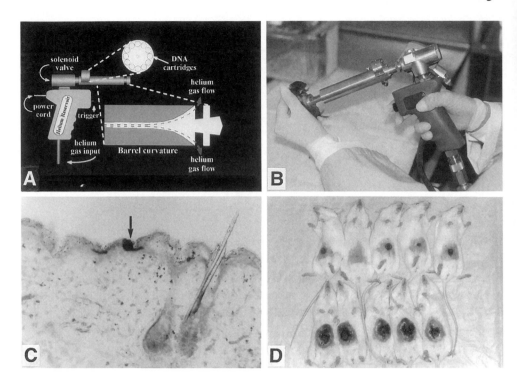

Fig. 1. Design, operation, and biological action of the gene gun. (**A**) Diagram of the Dermal PowderJect-XR (formerly Accell) gene gun and particle-mediated gene delivery mechanism (artwork of Dr. K. Barton); (**B**) Gene gun-mediated gene transfer to mouse-skin tissue. Before transfection, the abdominal area is shaved. Epidermal transfections can be conveniently performed at a rate of 5 s per mouse. (**C**) Detection of transgenic IL-12 protein in gene gun-treated skin tissues at 24 h after IL-12 cDNA delivery. Immunoperoxidase assay demonstrates the presence of IL-12 protein (arrow) in the epidermal cell layers of the test mice. (**D**) Regression of established SA-1 sarcoma following IL-12 gene delivery in the skin. Mouse skin overlying and surrounding established (0.8 cm in diameter) tumor was transfected with IL-12 (upper row) or Luciferase (lower row) cDNA expression vectors on day 7 after intradermal tumor cell implantation, following by three additional treatments on days 8, 10, and 11. At each treatment, mice received four transfections (5 µg plasmid DNA/treatment). The photograph of the mice was taken on day 20 posttumor cell implantation.

1.1.1. Operational Parameters for Gene Transfer

Functional parameters that can be modified to optimize particle-mediated gene transfer into skin include the following: physical acceleration rate for particle penetration, shape form and size of particles, particle loading rate per target surface area, and DNA loading rate per particle. For transfecting appropriately treated skin tissues, a pressure of 300–500 psi for the helium pulse gun *(8)* has been found to confer high levels of transgene expression in mouse skin. Particles made from dense materials, including gold, tungsten, iridium, and platinum are all capable of effective delivery of DNA via the gene gun-mediated gene transfer. However, gold particles are most commonly chosen for two reasons: elemental gold is chemically inert with no cytotoxic effects, and, owing to its common use in the electronics industry, uniform-sized gold particles are commercially available.

A wide range of gold particle sizes have been evaluated for gene transfer via particle-mediated gene transfer. These include 0.95-, 1–3-, 5–7-, and ≥15-μm diameter gold particles. For mammalian skin tissues, the 2–3-μm gold particles are recommended *(3,4,8)*. Some gold particles are readily available in different forms (e.g., as round particles, crystals, or even aggregates). For gene transfer into skin epidermal cells, crystal and spherical gold particles were found to be similarly useful in gene delivery.

1.1.2. Molecular and Cell Biology Considerations

A major advantage of the particle-mediated gene delivery method for gene transfer is its capacity for intracellular delivery of high copy numbers of DNA into target tissues in vivo. Onto a single 1–3-μm gold particle, more than 5000 copies of 5–10 kb plasmid DNA can be effectively coated with a Ca^{2+}/ spermidine or PEG formulation in precipitated form. With a predetermined gold-particle loading rate of 0.1 mg/cm^2, approximately 1–2 gold particles (1–3 μm) per cell can be delivered via random distribution into the epidermis containing stratified epithelial cells on the order of 15 μm in diameter. Excessive particle loading rates (e.g., >5 particles/cell) can often cause trauma to transfected tissues. On the other hand, too low a particle load (e.g., 1 particle/3 cells) often results in low gene-transfer efficiency. A preliminary gene transfer to any tissue tested using a reporter gene assay can effectively determine the optimal particle loading rate and the DNA dosage. Use of a reporter gene capable of histological assay can greatly facilitate the optimization of transfection efficiency.

Another important feature of particle-mediated gene delivery is the much reduced restriction on the size of the DNA vectors. Plasmid DNA, genomic DNA (≥23 kb), and reporter genes cloned in lambda phage genomic libraries (~44 kb) can all be effectively delivered into mammalian cells by gene gun techniques for transgene expression *(2)*. This capability offers new opportunities for transferring multiple genes, large-size genomic DNA sequences, or multiple-tandem genes into mammalian somatic tissues. In addition, cotransfection of multiple genes on different plasmids has also been shown to be efficiently achieved by using the particle-mediated gene transfer method *(4,9)*. Furthermore, we have shown that RNA molecules can be similarly delivered as DNA vectors via the gene gun delivery system *(10)*.

1.2. General Applications of the Particle-Mediated Gene Transfer Approach

Among the applications of gene gun technology, transfection of the skin tissues of live animals (**Fig. 1B**) has resulted in some most interesting findings, enabling a series of transgenic studies with applications to both basic research and gene therapy experiments. Briefly, high levels of transgene expression have been demonstrated by in vivo particle-mediated gene transfer of skin epidermal tissues *(11)*. This result was shown to be highly reproducible for virtually all tested animal species, including mouse, rat, pig, dog, and rhesus monkey. The adaptability of a skin gene-transfer protocol across a broad range of experimental animal systems illustrates the capability and versatility of the gene gun transfection method. Efficient delivery and expression of transgenes in skin tissues have been extended to several reporter genes *(2,3)*, a number of candidate therapeutic genes *(12–15)*, various cytokine genes *(16–18)*, and some viral antigens *(19,20)*, demonstrating the wide ranging applicability of this gene transfer strategy. In vivo gene gun-mediated DNA delivery into skin tissues has been used for developing genetic immunization technology *(12–15,19,20)*, for gene therapy of subcutaneous (sc) tumors *(16–18)*, for wound healing *(21)*, for delivery of RNA as transgenes or immunogens *(10)*, for analysis of transcriptional promoters and other regulatory sequences in gene expression vectors *(4,22)*, and for studying different cell types in transgene expression and migration following DNA immunization *(23,24)*.

Histological studies show that cDNA expression vectors can be introduced into and expressed in different cell layers of epidermal or dermal tissues by adjusting the ballistic variables. These include the motive force for particle acceleration, gold particle size, pretreatment and manipulations of epidermal and dermal tissues prior to blasting, and the DNA formulations for coating gold particles. In general, topical skin gene delivery results in high-level transient expression almost exclusively in the epidermal cell layers *(3,4,17)*, which may vary considerably in different animals, e.g., 3–4 cell layers and 10–30 cell layers for mouse and pig skin, respectively. Treatment of dermal tissues via exposure of the underside of a skin flap can result in long-term transgene expression, though at a much reduced level *(4,16)*. Because the epidermis is exquisitely competent for eliciting both a humoral and a cell-mediated immune response, highly efficient in synthesis and secretion of transgenic proteins, and is easily accessible, it has been shown as an attractive target for gene transfer, particularly for vaccine and cancer gene immunotherapy approaches.

1.3. Antitumor Efficacy of Particle-Mediated Gene Transfer In Vivo

Because particle-mediated gene transfer into skin has many advantages as a simple and efficacious in vivo gene delivery method, it has been recently applied to cancer research, mainly for two purposes: DNA vaccination and gene therapy *(11)*. The first approach involved the delivery into the skin of genes coded either for model "tumor antigens" such as β-galactosidase *(12,15)* or ovalbumin *(15)*, or natural tumor-associated antigens, such as mutant p53 oncoprotein *(13)* or carcinoembrionic antigen *(14)*, in attempts to induce antitumor immune responses. Indeed, successful vaccinations against tumors have been achieved in these cases, resulting in genetic priming of mice to generate a cytolytic T-cell response in vitro and to resist tumor challenge in vivo *(12,13,15)*. Importantly, in the study of Ross et al. *(15)*, particle-mediated gene vaccination was found to be more effective than vaccination with a peptide even in the combination with an adjuvant. Transfection of skin cells in vivo with the gold particle-coated cDNA, followed by trafficking of dendritic cells carrying the DNA/gold beads to draining lymph nodes, has been recently demonstrated *(23)*. These results suggest that the enhanced antigen presentation by bone marrow-derived *(24)* dendritic cells to T lymphocytes is responsible for induction of the antitumor immunity in cutaneous gene-immunization experiments. Successful use of the gene gun method for a codelivery of adjuvant cytokine genes with a tumor-antigen DNA, resulting in enhanced antitumor immunity, has also been recently reported *(12,14)*.

A second approach involved the treatment of already established sc tumors with cytokine genes. As we have recently reported *(17)*, a powerful immunologically mediated tumor regression was observed following skin transfection with an interleukin 12 (IL-12) gene in several mouse tumor models (**Fig. 1D**). Moreover, the localized IL-12 gene delivery into the skin overlaying the immunogenic tumor have resulted in a systemic effect against visceral metastases *(17)* and a distant solid tumor *(18)*. Histological analysis showed that IL-12 transgene expression was readily detectable in the epidermis (**Fig. 1C**), although the DNA-coated gold beads did not reach the implanted tumor. The data suggest, therefore, that a gradual, continuous release of small doses of transgenic IL-12 protein by transfected epidermal cells in the vicinity of test tumor can effectively result in activation of a local, regional, and then systemic antitumor immunity. Although several other cytokine genes have also been employed in a therapeutic strategy by the particle-mediated gene transfer *(16,18)*, IL-12 was shown to be the most effective one tested thus far *(18)*. This gene therapy approach using a gene gun technology was later shown to be applicable and effective not only against cutaneous tumors, but also against tumors in visceral organs such as the liver *(25)*.

We have recently observed a new phenomenon related to the particle-mediated gene transfer for treatment of established tumors. Namely, IL-12 gene transfer into the skin surrounding and overlaying an apparently non-immunogenic 4T1 mouse mammary adenocarcinoma has resulted in a significant reduction of spontaneous lung metastases and had no effect on the growth of the primary intradermal tumor *(26)*. In contrast to the aforementioned anti-tumor effect of IL-12 gene therapy, this antimetastatic effect was not mediated by T cells. The mechanisms of this effect is currently under investigation.

2. Materials

2.1. Instrumentation

1. The Dermal PowderJect-XR helium pulse gun (trademark of PowderJect Vaccines, Inc., Madison, WI), formerly known as the Accell® gene gun, is now commercially available from Bio-Rad Laboratories, Inc. (Hercules, CA) as the Helios gene gun. Mechanical operation and/or manipulation of gene gun devices are relatively straightforward, as detailed by the manufacturer's manual.
2. Compressed helium gas, grade 4.7.
3. Ultrasonic cleaner.
4. Personal hearing-protection device.

2.2. Elemental Gold-Particle Preparations

Microscopic gold particles of different sizes (e.g., 0.95, I-3, 5-7 µm) and in different shapes (e.g., spherical particles, crystals, aggregates, etc.) can be purchased from the Degussa Corporation (South Plainfield, NJ). Gold particles with sizes of 2 to 3 µm was found to be the best for in vivo gene transfection into the skin *(8)*. It is important that these gold particles be obtained as elemental gold, not as gold salt or colloidal gold. If necessary, the gold particles can be washed and cleaned by rinsing them in distilled water, 70% ethanol, and 100% ethanol in sequence prior to use. The particles can also be sterilized in phenol or $CHCl_3$ if necessary. It is important to microscopically examine each newly purchased gold-particle preparation, making sure that the lot, particle size, and form are correct and appropriate as desired for the test systems. It is also useful to test each new lot of gold particles in a standardized gene transfer and expression assay, as some lots may not perform satisfactorily for reasons that are currently not clear to us.

2.3. DNA Vectors

A clean plasmid DNA preparation purified from CsCl gradient or Qiagen (Chatsworth, CA) columns, ethanol precipitated, and redissolved in TE buffer (10 mM Tris-HCI, pH 7.0, 1 mM EDTA), or distilled water should be used for coating particles. We have not observed significant differences in transfection efficiencies between supercoiled and linear plasmid DNAs, in contrast to some published reports using other methods. Genomic DNA preparations, genomic DNA clones in lambda phage or cosmid libraries, or cocktails of different DNA vector systems or preparations can be mixed in desired molar ratios in aqueous solution, and then effectively loaded onto gold particles.

For exploratory gene-transfer experiments, convenient and sensitive reporter gene systems that have low endogenous activity background and are inexpensive, are recommended for verification of transient gene-expression systems. A vital assay is a distinct plus.

2.4. Coating DNA onto Gold Particles and Gene Transfer

1. 0.05M spermidine in H$_2$O. Use fresh spermidine made weekly from a free-base solution (Sigma, St. Louis, MO), or make and freeze aliquots.
2. 2.5M CaCl$_2$ in H$_2$O.
3. 100% ETOH kept at −20°C.
4. I mg/mL PVP (polyvinylpyrrolidone, Sigma).

2.5. Treatment and Care of Skin

1. Oster electric hair clippers with no. 40 blade (Fisher, Pittsburgh, PA).
2. Depilatory (i.e., Nair), if needed.
3. Tegaderm adhesive (3M, St. Paul, MN).

2.6. Tissue Extraction Buffers and Enzyme Assay Systems

2.6.1. Luciferase Assay

1. Extraction buffer: 34 mL H$_2$O, 10 mL 0.5M potassium phosphate buffer (pH 7.5), 5 mg BSA, 6 mg Pefabloc SC, 5 mL 10% TX-100.
2. 5X reaction buffer: 0.46 gm glycylglycine, 0.7 gm MgCl$_2$ · 6H$_2$O, add to 20 mL H$_2$O while stirring; 0.540 gm ATP; 0.225 mL 2M Tris-HCl pH 7.5. Adjust pH to 7.8, bring up to 30 mL, then add 15 mg BSA.
3. Luciferin solution: dissolve 14 mg luciferin in one drop of 1M NaOH. Immediately add to 50 mL H$_2$O with 566 µL 7.5% NaHCO3. Adjust pH to 6.0. Protect from light.
4. Luminometer (Lumat LB 9501, Berthold Systems, Pittsburgh, PA).

2.6.2. X-Gal Assay

1. X-gal substrate (5-bromo-4-chloro-3-indolyl-,8-D-galactoside): dissolve X-gal into dimethyl formamide at a concentration of 40 mg/mL.
2. Buffer solution: 44 mM HEPES buffer, 3 mM K$^+$ ferricyanide, 3 mM K$^+$ ferrocyanide, 15 mM NaCl, 1.3 mM MgCl$_2$, pH 7.4.
3. X-gal buffer: Add X-gal substrate to buffer solution to make a final 1 mg/mL solution.

2.6.3. Cytokine Assay and Other Assays

General extraction buffer: 9.5 mL PBS (0.2 gm potassium chloride, 0.2 gm potassium phosphate monobasic, 8.0 gm NaCI, 1.15 gm sodium phosphate dibasic to 1 L distilled H$_2$O), 2.4 mg Pefabloc, 0.5% Triton X-100.

3. Methods
3.1. Coating DNA onto Gold Particles

1. Purify plasmid DNA or other DNA vectors via CsCl gradient centrifugation or Qiagen columns, followed by ethanol precipitation, and redissolve in TE buffer. Prepare DNA solution at a concentration of ~1 µg/µL, and store at 4°C.
2. Decide how many cartridges ("bullets") will be needed. One cartridge (conferring one transfection) contains ~ 0.5 mg of gold.
3. Assuming that 40 cartridges will be needed, weigh 21 mg of gold particles into a 1.5-mL microcentrifuge tube.
4. Add 250 µL of 0.05M spermidine in the tube with gold (for 20–50 mg of gold use 200–300 µL spermidine, for 120 mg of gold use 400–450 µL spermidine).
5. Vortex and sonicate 3–5 s to break up gold clumps.
6. Add DNA at 2.5 DNA/gold loading rate (2.5 µg DNA/mg gold) to 21 mg of gold (e.g., at DNA concentration 1 µg/mL, add 52.5 µL DNA). For transfecting mammalian skin tissues, DNA dosages at 0.1, 0.5, 1, and 2.5 µg plasmid DNA/mg gold have been found to exhibit a linear relationship with transgene expression levels.
7. Add 250 mL of 2.5M CaCl$_2$ (or the same volume as spermidine) dropwise while vortexing the tube at a low speed.
8. Incubate at room temperature for 10 min. While waiting, prepare a culture tube with 3 mL of 100% ETOH (gold/ETOH ratio of 7 mg/ml).
9. Microcentrifuge 3–5 s. Remove supernatant and discard. Break up the pellet by flicking the tube. Add 0.5 ml of cold 100% ETOH dropwise while gently vortexing the tube, and then 0.5 mL more of 100% ETOH. Mix by inversion. Repeat this washing procedure two more times. Remove ETOH after the third wash.
10. Transfer particles into the culture tube containing 3 mL of 100% ETOH (*see* **step 8**). Sonicate briefly to disperse particles. Add PVP at 0.01 mg/ml. Particle suspensions can be used immediately, or stored at 4 or –20°C if precautions are taken to exclude moisture.

3.2. Prepare DNA Cartridges

1. Sonicate for 2–3 s, vortex, and immediately load the DNA-coated gold particle suspension into the Tefzel tubing following the manufacturer's instructions (Bio-Rad).
2. Discard unevenly coated ends of the tubing and cut the tubing into 0.5-in (~1.25-cm) pieces. Cartridges may be stored desiccated in a tightly sealed container at 4°C for several weeks.

3.3. Animal Care and Skin Treatment

1. Small experimental animals (including mouse, rat, hamster, and rabbit) usually do not need to be anesthetized for particle-mediated gene transfer into the skin. If desired, a mixture of ketamine 70 mg/kg and xylazine 17 mg/kg may be used. Large animals including dogs, pigs, and rhesus monkeys may be anesthetized under the guidance of the consulting veterinarian as required by the Animal Welfare Act and administered by the institution's IACUC.
2. Animal hair in the target area is removed with clippers. A depilatory such as Nair can be used to remove residual stubble, but this treatment is not necessary. If using a depilatory, animals should be anesthetized. Care also should be taken not to allow prolonged treatment by Nair, as it may damage the target tissue.

3.4. Epidermis and Dermis Gene Transfer

1. Allow the container with the DNA-gold cartridges to reach room temperature before opening.
2. Attach the regulator to the compressed helium tank. Connect the feed hose to the regulator and gene gun, then plug in the device.
3. Load the prepared cartridges into the 12-chambered cartridge holder, following the manufacturer's instructions.
4. Put on a hearing-protection device. Insert the loaded cartridge holder into the barrel of the gene gun device. Open the helium tank valve and the regulator valve.
5. Adjust the discharge pressure to the desired setting (usually 250–400 psi).
6. Restrain a mouse in a hand. Hold the nozzle of the device against the target skin area, as shown in **Fig. 1B**, and discharge the device. If several skin transfections are required, turn the cartridge holder clockwise and discharge at another target skin area.
7. If desired, apply semiocclusive skin dressings such as Tegaderm (3*M*, St. Paul, MN) or Opsite (Smith and Nephew, Hull, UK) to transfected epidermis. This protective application often results in higher transient gene expression.
8. To transfect dermal tissues, anesthetize a mouse, make an incision, and dissociate the full thickness skin tissue of the target size (~3.2 cm^2) from the facies and muscle tissue using standard surgical procedures and tools. Flip the skin flap over, exposing the dermal tissue and transfect the fibroblasts, muscle cells, and other stromal cell types. Moisten dermal tissues with sterile saline before closing. Close incision with sutures or wound clips.

9. Sacrifice the animals at designated time-points after gene transfer. Excise the skin target and assay for transgene activities or sequences as described in **Subheading 3.5.**

3.5. Reporter Gene-Expression Assays

3.5.1. Tissue Extraction

1. Collect transfected skin tissues from test animals by excising a small uniform portion of the targeted skin area. A piece as small as 1–2 mm^2 can be enough for Luc or β-gal reporter gene-expression assays.
2. Drop the freshly excised skin piece into a tube with the appropriate buffer (0.2–0.5 mL) and put on ice if performing assay right away, or freeze at –20°C.
3. Immediately before performing the assay, grind, scissors mince, or homogenize the frozen skin, keeping it as cold as possible. Avoid foaming the tissue. Sonicate.
4. Centrifuge the sample at a high speed to separate the tissue from the lysate. Soluble crude tissue extracts are used in microliter quantities for various reporter gene assays.

3.5.2. Luciferase Assay

1. After lysate has been collected, prepare dilutions in PBS if necessary.
2. Add 80 μL reaction buffer, 1–10 μL lysate, and 310 μL distilled H$_2$O into reaction tube and vortex.
3. Read relative light units in a luminometer (e.g., Lumat LB 9501, Wallac, Gaithersburg, MD) and run a standard curve to quantify results.

3.5.3. X-Gal Staining

1. Perform a whole-mount tissue staining by simply placing the excised skin target into X-gal buffer. For best results, we suggest gluing the skin to a 35-mm dish to keep the skin stretched out for better examination. The tissue can also be fixed in methanol:acetone (1:1) for 10 min and then stained with X-gal buffer.
2. For microscopic examination at the cellular level, make tissue sections using a cryostat microtome or paraffin sectioning. After the tissue has been sectioned into ~10 μm-sections, place the slide in ice-cold 1.5% glutaraldehyde solution for 10 min, and wash in ice-cold PBS 5X for 5 min each. The tissue slides are then stained with X-gal buffer for 1 h. Avoid prolonged staining because a blue background can develop in hair follicles of certain skin tissues.

3.5.4. ELISA and RIA

Enzyme-linked immunosorbent assay (ELISA) tests are most commonly used for cytokine quantification. They may be purchased as a kit or antibody pairs may be purchased, and used in a sandwich-style assay (i.e., capture Ab-cytokine-detecting Ab-conjugate-substrate). The ELISAs may be run on serum, plasma, skin extract (using general extraction buffer), or tegadermstripped cell extract. Some transgenes such as hGH can be detected using a radioimmunoassay (RIA). This assay can also be used with serum, plasma, skin extract, or tegaderm extract.

3.6. Summary

The epidermis plays a key role in providing first-line immunological responses. The immune and inflammatory processes now clearly demonstrated in cutaneous tissue make it a suitable target for gene transfer-based vaccines. In addition to keratinocytes, the epidermis contains Langerhans cells, a subset of dendritic cells, both of which can serve as professional antigen-presenting cells. Particle-mediated gene transfer to skin has been shown to result in induction of high level and durable humoral and cytotoxic immune responses *(12–20)*. These immune responses were shown to be fully protective in DNA-immunized mice subjected to a lethal tumor challenge *(12,13,15)*. The DNA cancer vaccination studies and the studies demonstrating regression of established primary and metastatic tumors following epidermal cytokine gene transfer *(17,18,25,26)* suggest the potential of a particle-mediated gene delivery approach for cancer therapy.

4. Notes

1. Particle-mediated gene transfer provides a physical means of delivering biologically active molecules, including DNA, RNA, and proteins intracellularly. Because of its physical nature, this method displays properties distinct from those characteristic of chemical and biological gene transfer agents, and it may prove advantageous in many cases. The method is readily adaptable to a wide range of mammalian cells and organs *(2)*. A major advantage of particle-mediated gene transfer is its applicability to cells in vivo. Its effectiveness in vivo has also been demonstrated in several animal species including large size animals as dogs, pigs, and rhesus macaques *(19)*, which is especially significant for extrapolation of experimental results in laboratory animals to human population.

2. No restrictions on the size or form of the DNA have been encountered thus far, other than those inherent in the need to prepare the DNA and perform routine manipulations, like pipeting. The amount of DNA required fo particle-mediated gene transfer is relatively low; for example, nanogram amount of DNA per cm^2 of target area have been shown effective for DNA vaccine applications *(27)*. This amount corresponds to 10~500 plasmid molecules per particle, on average, assuming a uniform distribution of DNA on the particles. In other studies, an amount of 5000 copies of cDNA delivered per cell was found to be optimal for commonly used reporter genes *(3,4)*.

3. The current devices for particle delivery can achieve penetration depths up to a few hundred micrometers depending on the target tissue, corresponding to a depth of 20–30 cell layers in a stratified tissue, like the epidermis. This depth of

penetration, though not sufficient to reach internal organs, is greater than that typically achieved with viral vectors or chemical gene transfer agents where solid tissue penetration is often limited to only one or two cell layers.

4. Skin is an attractive target tissue for gene therapy and DNA-vaccination applications, and appears particularly amenable to particle-mediated gene transfer. One striking advantage of skin is its accessibility. One can conduct gene transfer to skin without resorting to any invasive procedures. The organization and dimensions of the epidermis are also a good fit with the penetration capabilities of the current particle-acceleration devices. A second advantage of skin derives from its continuous and consistent turnover. A vast majority of epidermal keratinocytes are differentiated nondividing cells destined to eventually exfoliate from the body. Gene transfer to these cells is thus temporary and self-reversing, unless the gene transfer itself disrupts their normal differentiation process. Gene transfer to the basal cells that repopulate the epidermis, although conceptually possible, is currently unlikely owing to the scarcity of these cells and their position in the deepest regions of the epidermis. We have not yet observed sectors of permanent transgenic epidermal cells as a result of epidermal gene transfer. Approaches seeking to transfect these generative cells to produce stable transgenic skin will thus probably require special targeting strategies to be successful.

5. The major current disadvantages of particle-mediated gene transfer in vivo are the limited transfection efficiency for certain tissue systems (particularly if permanent gene transfer to the target cells is necessary) and the depth of tissue that can be accessed. Although transient transfection efficiencies from 5–15% can frequently be obtained in vivo, and efficiencies approaching 3~50% are possible in vitro, efficiencies for stable (i.e., integrative) gene transfer in vivo are apparently low, and have not been clearly established in various transfected somatic tissues. Long-term transgene expression following particle-mediated gene transfer has been observed in muscle and dermis, but these tissues seem to be the exception rather than the rule. More general long-term gene expression may be possible through a combination of particle-mediated gene transfer and replicating or actively integrating vector systems, but for the present it appears that the technique is most suitable in applications where short- to medium-term transgene expression is sufficient or desirable, such as DNA-vaccine applications. The gene gun method at present also cannot deliver genes systemically to cell fractions scattered in large, three-dimensional tissues like the liver or brain as can certain other gene transfer systems that can be administered through the circulatory system *(28)*.

Acknowledgments

We thank our colleagues, D. McCabe and C. Emler (Agracetus, Inc.), and Dr. W. Swain, J. Burkholder, and J. Culp (PowderJect Vaccines, Inc.), for their valuable discussions during developing the particle-mediated gene transfer technique and the gene gun device. We also thank Dr. L. Payne (PowderJect Vaccines, Inc.) for editing the manuscript. Part of this work was supported by the U.S. Army Medical Research Acquisition Activity Grant to the authors, under DAMD17-96-2-6017, subcontracted to the University of Wisconsin-Madison by PowderJect Vaccines, Inc.

References

1. Christou, P. (1994) Application to plants, in *Particle Bombardment Technology for Gene Transfer* (Yang, N.-S. and Christou, P., eds.), Oxford University Press, New York, pp. 71–99.
2. Yang, N.-S. and Ziegelhoffer, P. (1994) The particle bombardment system for mammalian gene transfer, in *Particle Bombardment Technology for Gene Transfer* (Yang, N.-S. and Christou, P., eds.), Oxford University Press, New York, pp. 117–141.
3. Yang, N.-S., Burkholder, J., Roberts, B., Martinell, B., and McCabe, D. (1990) In vivo and in vitro gene transfer to mammalian somatic cells by particle bombardment. *Proc. Natl. Acad. Sci. USA* **87**, 9568–9572.
4. Cheng, L., Ziegelhoffer, P., and Yang, N.-S. (1993) In vivo promoter activity and transgenic expression in mammalian somatic tissues evaluated by using particle bombardment. *Proc. Natl. Acad. Sci. USA* **90**, 4454–4459.
5. Jiao, S., Cheng, L., Wolff, J., and Yang, N.-S. (1993) Particle bombardment-mediated gene transfer and expression in rat brain tissues. *Bio/Technology* **11**, 497–502.
6. Thompson, T. A., Gould, M. N., Burkholder, J. K., and Yang, N.-S. (1993) Transient promoter activity in primary rat mammary epithelial cells evaluated using particle bombardment gene transfer. *In Vitro Cell Dev. Biol.* **29A**, 165–170.
7. Burkholder, J. K., Decker, J., and Yang, N.-S. (1993) Transgene expression in lymphocyte and macrophage primary cultures after particle bombardment. *J. Immunol. Meth.* **165**, 149–156.
8. Yang, N-S., Burkholder, J., McCabe, D., Neumann, V., and Fuller, D. (1997) Particle-mediated gene delivery in vivo and in vitro, in *Curr. Protocols Hum. Genet.* John Wiley and Sons, pp. 12.6.1–12.6.14.
9. Williams, R. S., Johnston, S. A., Riedy, M., DeVit, M. J., McElligot, S. G., and Sanford, J. C. (1991). Introduction of foreign genes into tissues of living mice by DNA-coated microprojectiles. *Proc. Natl. Acad. Sci. USA* **88**, 2726–2730.
10. Qiu, P., Ziegelhoffer, P., Sun, J., and Yang, N.-S. (1996) Gene gun delivery of mRNA in situ results in efficient transgene expression and immunization. *Gene Ther.* **3**, 262–268.
11. Rakhmilevich, A. L. and Yang, N-S. (1997) Particle-mediated gene delivery system for cancer research, in *Concepts in Gene Therapy* (Strauss, M. and Barranger, J. A., eds.), Walter de Gruyter-Berlin, New York, pp. 109–120.
12. Irvine, K. R., Rao, J. B., Rosenberg, S. A., and Restifo, N. P. (1996) Cytokine enhancement of DNA immunization leads to effective treatment of established pulmonary metastases. *J. Immunol.* **156**, 238–245.
13. Ciernik, F., Berzofsky, J. A., and Carbone, D. P. (1996) Induction of cytotoxic T lymphocytes and antitumor immunity with DNA vaccines expressing single T cell epitopes. *J. Immunol.* **156**, 2369–2375.

14. Conry, R. M., Widera, G., LoBuglio, A. F., et al. (1996) Selected strategies to augment polynucleotide immunization. *Gene Ther.* **3,** 67–74.

15. Ross, H. M., Weber, L. W., Wang, S., et al. (1997) Priming for T-cell-mediated rejection of established tumors by cutaneous DNA immunization. *Clinical Cancer Res.* **3,** 2191–2196.

16. Sun, W. H., Burkholder, J. K., Sun, J., Culp., J., Turner, J., Lu, X. G., et al. (1995) In vivo cytokine gene transfer by gene gun suppresses tumor growth in mice. *Proc. Natl. Acad. Sci. USA* **92,** 2889–2893.

17. Rakhmilevich, A. L., Turner, J., Ford, M. J., et al. (1996) Gene gun-mediated skin transfection with interleukin 12 gene results in regression of established primary and metastatic murine tumors. *Proc. Natl. Acad. Sci. USA* **93,** 6291–6296.

18. Rakhmilevich, A. L., Janssen, K., Turner, J., Culp, J., Yang, N-S. (1997) Cytokine gene therapy of cancer using gene gun technology: superior antitumor activity of IL-12. *Hum. Gene Ther.* **8,** 1303–1311.

19. Fuller, D. H., Corb, M. M., Barnett, S., Steimer, K., and Haynes, J. R. (1997). Enhancement of immunodeficiency virus-specific immune responses in DNA-immunized rhesus macaques. *Vaccine* **15,** 924–926.

20. Feltquate, D. M., Heaney, S., Webster, R. G., and Robinson, H. L. (1997). Different T helper cell types and antibody isotypes generated by saline and gene gun DNA immunization. *J. Immunol.* **158,** 2278–2284.

21. Andree, C., Swain, W. F., Page, C. P., Macklin, M. D., Slama, J., Hatzis, D., and Eriksson, E. (1994) In vivo transfer and expression of an EGF gene accelerates wound repair. *Proc. Natl. Acad. Sci. USA* **91,** 12,188–12,192.

22. Rajagopalan, L. E., Burkholder, J. K., Turner, J., Culp, J., Yang, N.-S., and Malter, J. S. (1995) Targeted mutagenesis of GM-CSF cDNA increases transgenic mRNA stability and protein expression in normal cells. *Blood* **86,** 2551–2558.

23. Condon, C., Watkins, S. C., Celluzzi, C. M., et al. (1996) DNA-based immunization by in vivo transfection of dendritic cells. *Nature Medicine* **2,** 1122–1128.

24. Iwasaki, A., Torres, C. A. T., Ohashi, P. S. Robinson, H. L., and Barber, B. H. (1997) The dominant role of bone marrow-derived cells in CTL induction following plasmid DNA immunization ar different sites. *J. Immunol.* **159,** 11–14.

25. Weber, S. M., Shi, F., Heise, C., Warner, T., and Mahvi, D. M. (1999) IL-12 gene transfer results in CD8-dependent regression of murine CT26 liver tumors. *Annals of Surg. Oncol.* **6,** 186–194.

26. Rakhmilevich, A. L., Janssen, K., and Yang, N-S. (1999) Interleukin 12 gene therapy of an apparently nonimmunogenic mouse mammary carcinoma results in reduction of spontaneous lung metastases. Submitted.

27. Eisenbraun, M. D., Fuller, D. H., and Haynes, J. R. (1993) Examination parameters affecting the elicitation of humoral immune responses by particle bombardment mediated genetic immunization. *DNA Cell Biol.* **12,** 791–797.

28. Perales, J. C., Perkol, T., Beegen, H., Ratnoff, O., and Hanson, R. W. (1994) Gene transfer in vivo: sustained expression and regulation of genes introduced into the liver by receptor-targeted uptake. *Proc. Natl. Acad. Sci. USA* **91,** 408–4090.

21

Gene Targeting to Hepatomas (AFP)

Shotaro Tsuruta, Akio Ido, and Shigenobu Nagataki

1. Introduction

Hepatocellular carcinoma (HCC) is one of the most common malignancies with poor prognosis worldwide, especially in eastern Asia and Africa *(1)*. Recent advances in delivering genes to mammalian cells stimulate the possibility of gene therapy for human diseases, including cancer gene therapy *(2)*. One approach of gene therapy for cancers is the transduction of the herpes simplex virus thymidine kinase *(HSV-tk)* gene in tumor cells, because the killing effect of the *HSV-tk* product on the virus-infected cells is seen in only proliferating cells *(3)*. *HSV-tk* can efficiently phosphorylate nucleoside analogs, and the phosphorylated products act as a chain terminator of DNA synthesis, leading to cell death *(4)*. In addition, successful application of suicide gene therapy for cancer, in part, relies on the bystander effect, where the active chemotherapeutic agent produced in target cells diffuses from cells to neighboring malignant cells in sufficient concentrations to induce growth inhibition *(5)*.

The tissue- or tumor-specific promoter sequence is useful for the selective expression of the *HSV-tk* gene in tumor cells. Many cancers often reexpress fetal or embryonic genes. Most HCC cells express α-fetoprotein (AFP) *(6–8)*. There has been much progress in characterization of *cis-* and *trans*-acting elements regulating the human AFP gene *(9–12)*. It has been shown that the hepatocyte-specific enhancers and promoter exist in 5'-flanking region of AFP gene, and that the position-dependent silencer elements are located between the enhancer region and the promoter region *(10)*. The 0.3 kb human AFP promoter sequence (–230 to +29 bp relative to the cap site) contains the glucocorticoid responsive element (GRE) and hepatocyte nuclear factor-1 (HNF-1) binding sites *(11,12)*. This sequence is suitable for HCC-specific expression of the *HSV-tk* gene *(13,14)*.

From: *Methods in Molecular Medicine, Vol. 35: Gene Therapy: Methods and Protocols*
Edited by: W. Walther and U. Stein © Humana Press, Inc., Totowa, NJ

In this chapter, we describe the experimental approach of gene therapy for hepatomas in the following fashion:

Cell culture
Construction of the plasmid pLNAF0.3TK
Production of recombinant retrovirus
Retroviral infection
GCV-, ACV-mediated growth inhibition

2. Materials

2.1. Cell Culture

2.1.1 Cell Lines

1. PA317; the amphotropic retrovirus packaging line *(15)*, available from the American Type Cell Collection (ATCC Number: CRL-9078).
2. Psi-2; the ecotropic retrovirus packaging line *(16)*.
3. NIH3T3; the mouse fibroblast cells, available from the ATCC (ATCC Number: CRL-1658).
4. HepG2; the human hepatoma cell line, available from the ATCC (ATCC Number: HB-8065).
5. PLC/PRF/5; the human hepatoma cell line, available from the ATCC (ATCC Number: CRL-8024).
6. HuH-7; the human hepatoma cell line, a generous gift from Dr. H. Nakabayashi *(17)* available from the Japanese Collection of Research Bioresources (JCRB0403).
7. huH-1/cl.2; the human hepatoma cell line, a generous gift from Dr. H. Nakabayashi *(18)*.
8. HeLa; the human cervical adenocarcinoma cell line, available from the ATCC (ATCC Number: CCL-2).

2.1.2. Culture Medium

1. Dulbeco's modified Eagles medium (DMEM); commercially available.
2. IS-RPMI; chemical difined medium established by Dr. H. Nakabayashi et al. *(19)*. The components are listed in **Tables 1** and **2**.
3. Fetal bovine serum (FBS); commercially available.
4. Trypsin.
5. All media are sterilized by membrane filtration using 0.45-μm pore size filter and stored at 4°C.

2.2. Quantitative Analysis of AFP Secretion

1. RIA kit for AFP assay.
2. α-FETO-RIABEAD; a commercially available RIA kit (Dainabot, Tokyo, Japan).

Table 1
Composition of Chemically Defined Medium, IS-RPMI

Components	mg/L	Final concentrations
RPMI-1640	10400.00	
HEPES	1190.00	$5 \times 10^{-3}M$
Na_2SeO_3	0.00387	$3 \times 10^{-8}M$
$(NH_4) 6M_o7O_{24}.4H_2O$	0.00371	$3 \times 10^{-9}M$
$FeSO_4.7H_2O$	0.0278	$1 \times 10^{-7}M$
$MnCl_2.4H_2O$	0.000059	$3 \times 10^{-10}M$
NH_4VO_3	0.00117	$1 \times 10^{-8}M$
linoleic acid	0.00084	$3 \times 10^{-9}M$
oleic acid	0.00085	$3 \times 10^{-9}M$
$NaHCO_3$	1300.00	$1.55 \times 10^{-2}M$

Table 2
Composition of Stock Solutions for Preparing IS-RPMI

Solution	Components	mg/L	Final conconcentrations
No. 1 $(1000X)^a$	Na_2SeO_3	3.87	$3 \times 10^{-5}M$
No. 2 $(1000X)^b$	$FeSO_4.7H_2O$	27.8	$1 \times 10^{-4}M$
No. 3 (1000X)	$(NH_4) 6M_o7O_{24}.4H_2O$	3.71	$3 \times 10^{-6}M$
	$MnCl_2.4H_2O$	0.0594	$3 \times 10^{-7}M$
	NH_4VO_3	1.17	$1 \times 10^{-5}M$
No. 4 $(10000X)^c$	linoleic acid	8.4	$3 \times 10^{-5}M$
No. 5 $(10000X)^c$	oleic acid	8.5	$3 \times 10^{-5}M$

[a] Na_2SeO_3 is nutralized with $4M$ NaOH.
[b] One drop of concentrated HCl is added.
[c] Pure linoleic and oleic acids are dissolved in absolute ethanol and stored in the dark at $-20°C$ for up to 1 mo.

2.3. Construction of the Plasmid pLNAF0.3TK

2.3.1. Plasmids

1. pTK4; the plasmid contains 2-kb PvuII fragment of the *HSV-tk* gene in pBR322 *(20)*.
2. pLNCX; MLV-based retroviral vector, pLNCX is provided by Dr. A. D. Miller *(21)*.
3. pAF1.0-CAT; AFP-CAT plasmid, expression of CAT gene is driven by 1.0 kb AFP promoter, pAF1.0-CAT is provided by Dr. T. Tamaoki *(9)*.
4. pBluescripts II/KS(+); commercially available from Stratagene (La Jolla, CA).

2.3.2. Restriction Enzymes and Buffers

1. *Bg*lII, *Pvu*II, *Hind*III, *Cla*I, *Ssp*I, *Eco*RV, and *Bam*HI are used.
2. All restriction enzymes are commercially available, and stored at −20°C.
3. Buffers for restriction enzymes are prepared at 10X concentration and stored at −20°C.
4. Buffer components (final concentrations in m*M*) are indicated in **Table 3**.

2.3.3. Kit for Recovering of DNA

1. QIAEX II; commercially available from Qiagen GmbH, Hilden, Germany.

2.3.4. Linker Ligation and Subcloning

1. *Hind*III linker and *Cla*I linker; commercially available.
2. T4 DNA ligase; commercially available, stored at −20°C.
3. Buffers for ligation are prepared at 10X concentration (composition: 100 m*M* Tris-acetate, 100 m*M* magnesium acetate, and 500 m*M* potassium acetate, pH 7.5), stored at −20°C.
4. ATP; commercially available, stored at −20°C.

2.3.5. Amplification and Examination of Plasmid

1. DH5α; competent bacteria; commercially available, stored at −70°C.
2. Wizard MiniPreps DNA purification system; a commercially available kit for DNA purification (Promega, Madison, WI).

2.3.6. Other Solutions Used for Construction of Plasmid

All solutions are prepared as described in "Molecular Cloning" *(22)*.

1. ddH2O; stored at room temperature.
2. ethanol; stored at room temperature.
3. 3*M* sodium acetate, pH 5.2; stored at room temperature.
4. TE buffer (10 m*M* Tris-Cl, 1 m*M* EDTA, pH 8.0); stored at room temperature.
5. TAE buffer (40 m*M* Tris-acetate, 1 m*M* EDTA, pH 8.0); stored at room temperature.
6. phenol; stored at 4°C in dark glass bottle, harmful (phenol can cause severe burns).
7. chloroform; stored at room temperature.
8. SOB medium; stored at 4°C.
9. 2*M* MgCl$_2$; stored at −20°C.
10. 2*M* Glucose; stored at −20°C.
11. LB medium (Luria-Bertani medium); stored at 4°C.

2.4. Production of Recombinant Retrovirus

2.4.1. Production of Ecotropic Retrovirus

1. Cell: Psi-2.
2. Medium: DMEM with 5% FBS.

Table 3
Buffers for Restriction Enzymes (Final Concentrations in m*M*)

	Tris-HCl	MgCl$_2$	NaCl	Dithioerythritol	2-Mercaptoethanol	pH
*Bgl*II	50	10	100	1	—	7.5
*Pvu*II	10	10	50	1	—	7.5
*Hind*III	10	5	100	—	1	8.0
*Cla*I	50	10	100	1	—	7.5
*Ssp*I	50	10	100	1	—	7.5
*Eco*RV	10	5	100	—	1	8.0
*Bam*HI	10	5	100	—	1	8.0

3. Solutions used for transfection:
   –2.5*M* CaCl$_2$, stored at –20°C.
   –2X HBS (280m*M* NaCl, 50 m*M* HEPES and 2.8 m*M* Na$_2$HPO$_4$, pH 7.10), filtrated, stored at –20°C

2.4.2. Production of Amphotropic Retrovirus

1. Cell: Psi-2/pLNAF0.3TK transfected packaging cells PA317
2. Medium: DMEM with 5 or 10% FBS.
3. Polybrene [hexadimethrine bromide] (commercially available), soluble in water, stored at 4°C, not hazardous.
4. G418 [Geneticin] (commercially available), stored at room temperature as powder, soluble in water (dissolve to 1*M*), and stored at 4°C as liquid, harmful by inhalation, in contact with skin, and if swallowed.

2.4.3. The Titration of the Recombinant Retrovirus

1. Cell: NIH3T3 cells.
2. Medium: DMEM with 10% FBS.
3. Polybrene.
4. G418.

2.4.4. Southern Blot Analysis

1. Probe: The 1.8-kb *HSV-tk* gene, which is released from pLNCTK by *Hind*III-*Cla*I double digestion, is used as a probe.

2.5. Retroviral Infection

2.5.1. Infection of the Amphotropic Recombinant Retrovirus to the Target Cells

1. Cell: PA317/pLNAF0.3TK transduced packaging cells target cells (HepG2, PLC/PRF/5,HuH7, huH1/cl.2 and HeLa).
2. Medium: DMEM with 10% FBS IS-RPMI with 1, 5, or 10% FBS.
3. Polybrene.

2.5.2. Selection of G418-resistant Pooled Population of the Virus-Infected Cells

1. Cell: pLNAF0.3TK-transduced target cells.
2. Medium: IS-RPMI with 1, 5, or 10% FBS.
3. G418.

2.5.3. Northern Blot Analysis

1. Probe: The 1.8-kb *HSV-tk* gene, which is released from pLNCTK by *Hind*III-*Cla*I double digestion, is used as a probe.

2.6. GCV-, ACV-Mediated Growth Inhibition

2.6.1. Treatment of the Virus-Infected Target Cells with Varying Concentrations of GCV or ACV

1. Cell: pLNAF0.3TK-transduced target cells.
2. Medium: IS-RPMI with 1, 5, or 10% FBS.
3. GCV [gancyclovir] (available from F. Hoffmann-La Roche Ltd., Basel, Switzerland), dissolved in 10*N* NaOH, then filled up to final concentration (10 m*M*), and stored at 4°C. Hazardous; reduction in numbers of platelets and white blood cells.
4. ACV [acyclovir] (available from Welcome Japan, Osaka, Japan), dissolved in 10N NaOH, then filled up to final concentration (10 m*M*), and stored at 4°C. Hazardous; reduction in numbers of platelets and white blood cells.

2.6.2. Cell Viability Quantified by MTT Assay

1. MTT [3-(4,5-dimethylthiazol-2-yl)-2,5-diphenyltetrazolium bromide], commercially available, dissolved in PBS, then filled up to final concentration (5 mg/mL), and the solution is filtered through a 0.2-µm pore size cellulose acetate filter, stored at 2–8°C for frequent use or frozen for extended periods.
2. NP-40; polyglycol ether (nonionic) surfactants, commercially available, stored at room temperature.
3. n-propyl alcohol.
4. HCl.
5. Automatic plate reader (Bio-Rad, Model 450).

2.7. Modulation of ACV-Mediated Cytotoxicity by Dexamethasone

1. Cell: pLNAF0.3TK transduced target cells.
2. Medium: IS-RPMI with 1, 5, or 10% FBS.
3. ACV.
4. MTT.
5. NP-40.
6. n-propyl alcohol.
7. HCl.
8. Automatic plate reader.

3. Methods
3.1. Cell Culture

1. The amphotropic retrovirus packaging line PA317 and ecotropic packaging line Psi-2 are maintained in DMEM with 5% FBS.
2. The mouse NIH3T3 fibroblast cells are cultured in DMEM supplemented with 10% FBS.
3. The human hepatoma and nonhepatoma cell lines are maintained in IS-RPMI with 5% (HepG2, PLC/PRF/5), 1% (HuH7, huH1/cl.2), or 10% (HeLa) FBS.

3.2. Quantitative Analysis of AFP Secretion

1. The human hepatoma cells are plated at a density of 4×10^4 cells/well in 24-well multiplates and then incubated at 37°C in 5% CO_2 for 2 d.
2. At the end of the incubation period, the numbers of cells are counted, and the medium AFP is assayed by a commercially available radioimmunoassay kit (Dainabot, Tokyo, Japan).

3.3. Construction of the Plasmid pLNAF0.3TK

3.3.1. Insertion of the HSV-tk Gene Isolated from pTK4 into the MLV-Based Retroviral Vector to Generate pLNCTK

1. pTK4 is digested with *Bgl*II and *Pvu*II to release 1.8 kb of *HSV-tk* fragment.
2. The 1.8 kb fragment is isolated by gel electrophoresis.
3. Both ends of this fragment are changed to *Hind*III and *Cla*I site with linkers, respectively.
4. pLNCX (**Fig. 1A**) is digested with *Hind*III and *Cla*I.
5. *Hind*III/*Cla*I fragment of *HSV-tk* gene is inserted into *Hind*III-*Cla*I site of pLNCX to make pLNCTK (**Fig. 1B**).

3.3.2. Construction of pLNAF0.3TK Expressing the HSV-tk Gene Under the Control of the Human AFP Promoter

1. The 0.3-kb *Ssp*I-*Hind*III fragment between −230 and +29 base pairs relative to the cap site of the human AFP gene (**Fig. 2**) is released from pAF1.0-CAT.
2. pBluescripts II/KS(+) is digested with *Eco*RV and *Hind*III.
3. The 0.3-kb *Ssp*I-*Hind*III fragment of AFP promoter is inserted into *Eco*RV/*Hind*III site of pBluescripts II/KS(+) to make pBS-AF0.3 (**Fig. 1C**).
4. The 0.3 kb of the human AFP gene-promoter sequence is released from pBS-AF0.3 by *Bam*HI/*Hind*III double digestion.
5. The CMV promoter is removed from pLNCTK by *Bam*HI/*Hind*III digestion.
6. The CMV promoter in pLNCTK is replaced with the 0.3 kb AFP promoter sequence to make pLNAF0.3TK (**Fig. 1D**).
7. The 5′ MLV-LTR constitutively regulates the *neo* gene expression, whereas the synthesis of the HSV-TK protein largely depends on the human AFP 0.3-kb promoter-mediated transcription in this construct.

A : pLNCX

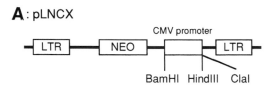

B : pLNCTK

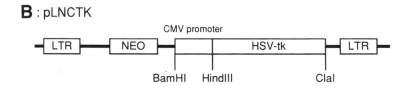

C : pBS-AF0.3

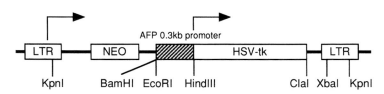

D : pLNAF0.3TK

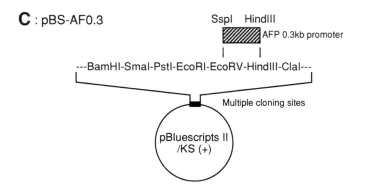

Fig. 1. **(A)** The structure of the pLNCX, MLV-based retroviral vector. NEO; Neo-mycin-resistance gene. **(B)** The structure of the pLNCTK retroviral vector containing the *HSV-tk* gene under the control of the CMV promoter. **(C)** The structure of the pBS-AF0.3, the 0.3 kb AFP promoter is inserted into pBluescript II/KS(+). The 0.3-kb AFP promoter is shown hatched. **(D)** The structure of the pLNAF0.3TK retroviral vector containing the *HSV-tk* gene under the control of the human AFP gene promoter. The CMV promoter in pLNCTK is replaced with the 0.3 kb AFP promoter. The 0.3-kb AFP promoter is shown hatched. Arrows indicate the transcription start sites and the direction of transcriptions.

```
-240 TGAGGAGAAT ATTTGTTATA TTTGCAAAAT AAAATAAGTT
            SspI

-200 TGCAAGTTTT TTTTTTCTGC CCCAAAGAGC TCTGTGTCCT

-160 TGAACTAAAA ATCACAATAA CCGCTATGCT GTTAATTATT

-120 GGCAAATGTC CCATTTTCAA CCTAAGGAAA TACCATAAAG

 -80 TAACAGATAT ACCAACAAAA GGTTACTAGT TAACAGGCAT

 -40 TGCCTGAAAA GAGTATAAAA GAATTTCAGC ATGATTTTCC

 +1 ATATTGTGCT TCCACCACTG CCAATAACA
```

Fig. 2. The nucleotide sequence of the human AFP gene promoter. GRE and two HNF-1 binding sites are indicated by double- and single-underlines, respectively. TATA is indicated by a box.

3.4. Production of Recombinant Retrovirus

3.4.1. Production of Ecotropic Retrovirus

1. 3×10^6 Psi-2 cells are placed on 100-mm tissue-culture plates in DMEM with 5% FBS.
2. Twenty hours later, the retroviral vector, pLNAF0.3TK, is transfected into Psi-2 ecotropic packaging cells using the calcium phosphate precipitation method.
   a. 10 µg/500µl of DNA solution and 50 µl of 2.5M CaCl$_2$ are mixed.
   b. The DNA mixture is dropped to 500 µl of 2X HBS and incubated at room temperature for 30 min.
   c. The final mixture is added to cultured Psi-2 cells.
   d. Four hours later, the cells are exposed to 1.5 mL of glycerol-HBS for 10 s.
   e. The cells are washed with PBS twice, and the fresh medium is added to the plate.
3. Two days later, the cultured supernatant containing ecotropic recombinant retroviruses is harvested and filtered through a 0.45-µm pore size cellulose acetate filter.

3.4.2. Production of Amphotropic Retrovirus

1. 3×10^6 PA317 cells are placed on 100-mm tissue-culture plates in DMEM with 10% FBS 1 d before the infection.
2. PA317 cells are infected by 5–10 mL of viral supernatant in the presence of 8 µg/mL of polybrene. Four hours later, the medium is aspirated and replaced with the flesh medium.
3. Two days later, the culture medium is aspirated and replaced with the culture medium containing 800 µg/mL G418 to obtain G418-resistant cells.

4. The medium containing 800 μg/mL G418 is changed at 3-d intervals. After 10 d following selection, G418-resistant colonies are cloned using cloning rings.
5. PA317/LNAF0.3TK clones are cultured in 24-well multiplates in DMEM with 10% FBS containing 800 μg/mL G418. After cell growth reaches a confluence, cells are transferred to 6-well multiplates, and consequently to 100-mm tissue-culture plates.
6. 3×10^6 PA317/LNAF0.3TK clones are placed on 100-mm dishes in DMEM with 10% FBS containing 800 μg/mL G418 and allowed to become confluent.
7. The cells are maintained at the confluent condition for 4 d, and the culture medium is replaced with the fresh G418-free culture medium.
8. One day later, the cultured supernatant containing amphotropic recombinant retroviruses is harvested and filtered through a 0.45-μm pore size cellulose acetate filter, and stored at –70°C.

3.4.3. The Titration of the Recombinant Retrovirus

1. NIH3T3 cells (1×10^5 cells/well) are placed on 6-well multiplates in DMEM with 10% FBS 1 d before the infection. Two mL of viral supernatant samples serially diluted (10^{-3}-, 10^{-4}-, 10^{-5}-, and 10^{-6}-fold) with the flesh medium is added to the wells. Polybrene is also added to each well to a final concentration of 8 μg/ml.
2. After 4 h-infection, the medium is aspirated and replaced with the fresh medium, and the cells are incubated under the same condition for a period when cell growth reaches a confluence (about 2 d). After then, the medium is replaced with the medium containing 800 μg/mL G418. The medium containing 800 μg/mL G418 is changed at 3-d intervals.
3. After 10 d following selection, numbers of G418 resistant colonies are counted, and the virus titer is expressed as a number of CFU/mL.

3.4.4. Southern Blot Analysis

1. High molecular weight cellular DNA is isolated from established producer cell, PA317/LNAF0.3TK.
2. Aliquots (10 μg) of DNA are digested with *Kpn*I, *Eco*RI/*Xba*I, or *Hind*III.
3. The resultant fragments are analyzed on the electrophoresis in a 0.9% agarose gel according to the method of Southern *(12)*.
4. The 1.8-kb *HSV-tk* gene, which is released from pLNCTK by *Hind*III-*Cla*I double digestion, is used as a probe.

3.5. Retroviral Infection

3.5.1. Infection of the Amphotropic Recombinant Retrovirus to the Target Cells

1. 5×10^6 target cells (hepatoma or nonhepatoma cells) are placed on 100-mm tissue-culture plates in each recommended culture medium.

2. One day later, the medium is replaced with 10 mL of the fresh medium or the fresh medium plus the stored virus supernatant containing 8 µg/mL of polybrene and further incubated at 37°C in 5% CO_2 for 24 h.

3.5.2. Selection of G418-Resistant Pooled Population of the Virus-Infected Cells

1. The cells are cultured in the complete medium containing G418 for about 2 wk. The medium is changed at 3-d intervals.
2. The concentrations of G418 used for each cell line are 600 µg/mL for HepG2, HuH7, PLC/PRF/5, and huH1/cl.2, and 400 µg/mL for HeLa.
3. G418-resistant pooled populations are collected.

3.5.3. Northern Blot Analysis

1. Total cellular RNA is isolated by the guanitidium isothiocyanate method.
2. *HSV-tk* transcripts are detected using a 1.8-kb *HSV-tk* gene, released from pLNCTK by *Hind*III-*Cla*I double digestion.
3. Glyceraldehyde-3-phosphate dehydrogenase (GAPDH) cDNA is used as a control probe.

3.6. GCV-, ACV-Mediated Growth Inhibition

3.6.1. Treatment of the Virus-Infected Target Cells with Varying Concentrations of GCV or ACV

1. 1×10^4 virus-infected cells are placed on 48-well multiplates. One day later (day 0), the cells are treated with 500 µL of the fresh medium in the absence or presence of varying concentrations of GCV or ACV.
2. Each medium is replaced with a corresponding fresh medium on day 2 and 4.

3.6.2. Cell Viability Quantified by MTT Assay

1. GCV- or ACV-mediated cell growth inhibition is determined by the colorimetrical quantitation of the viable cell number.
2. To quantify the cell viability, 50 µL of 5 mg/mL MTT [3-(4,5-dimethylthiazol-2-yl)-2,5-diphenyltetrazolium bromide] in phosphate-buffered saline is added to each well.
3. The cells are further cultured for 2 h at 37°C. The supernatants are aspirated, and 150 ml of n-propyl alcohol containing 0.1% NP-40 and 4×10^{-3} M HCl is added to each well.
4. The color reaction is quantitated using an automatic plate reader at 570 nm with a reference filter of 630 nm.
5. Percent growth inhibition is calculated with the following formula: % growth inhibition = $(1-B/A) \times 100$, where A is absorbance from the cells incubated with medium alone, and B is absorbance from the cells incubated with the medium containing varying concentrations of GCV or ACV.

3.7. Modulation of ACV-Mediated Cytotoxicity by Dexamethasone

1. 1×10^4 virus-infected cells are placed on 48-well multiplates. One day later (day 0), the cells are treated with 500 μL of fresh media containing $3 \times 10^{-6}M$ dexamethasone in the absence or presence of varying concentrations of ACV.
2. Each medium is replaced with a corresponding fresh medium or fresh medium containing $3 \times 10^{-6}M$ dexamethasone on day 2 and 4.
3. The effect of dexamethasone on ACV-mediated cell growth inhibition is determined by the colorimetrical quantitation of the viable cell number.

4. Notes

4.1. Alternative Protocols

4.1.1. Incubation of the Producer Cells at 32°C to Enhance the Production of Retroviral Vector

1. The method to establish PA317/LNAF0.3TK clones is same as mentioned in **Subheading 3.4.2.**
2. 3×10^6 PA317/LNAF0.3TK clones are placed on 100-mm dishes in DMEM with 10% FBS containing 800 μg/mL G418 at 37°C and allowed to become confluent.
3. The cells are maintained at the confluent condition at 37°C for 4 d. The culture medium is replaced with the fresh G418-free culture medium and then, the cells are incubated at 32°C.
4. One day later, the cultured supernatant containing amphotropic recombinant retroviruses is harvested and filtered through a 0.45-μm pore size cellulose acetate filter, and stored at μ70°C.
5. The titer of the recombinant retroviral vectors is determined as mentioned in the **Subheading 3.4.3.** This can result in fivefold increase in the virus titer.

4.1.2. Use of Sodium Butyrate to Enhance the Production of Retroviral Vector

1. The method to establish PA317/LNAF0.3TK clones is same as mentioned in **Subheading 3.4.2.**
2. Additional reagent sodium butylate; commercially available, stocks of sodium butylate (100 mM) are made up in water, sterilized by filtration using a 0.22-μm pore size filter, stored at –20°C.
3. 3×10^6 PA317/LNAF0.3TK clones are placed on a 100-mm dish in DMEM with 10% FBS containing 800 μg/mL G418 and allowed to become confluent.
4. The cells are maintained at the confluent condition for 4 d, and the culture medium is replaced with the fresh G418-free culture medium containing 5 mM sodium butyrate.
5. One day later, the cultured supernatant containing amphotropic recombinant retroviruses is harvested and filtered through a 0.45-μm pore size cellulose acetate filter, and stored at –70°C.

6. This can result in about 10-fold increase in the virus titer of the recombinant retroviral vectors.

4.1.3. Concentration of Viral Supernatant
Using Polyethilene Glycol (PEG)

1. The method to obtain the cultured supernatant containing amphotropic recombinant retroviruses is same as mentioned in **Subheading 3.4.2.**
2. Additional reagent Polyethilene glycol (PEG-8000); commercially available, 32% (w/w) stock solution of PEG-8000 is prepared in ddH$_2$O, stock solution is sterilized by autoclaving and stored at 4°C.
3. The viral supernatant in a 50-mL polystyrene tube is centrifuged at 3000 rpm for 20 min at 4°C and filtered through a 0.45-μm pore size filter to remove the cell debris.
4. The supernatant is transferred to a new 50-mL polystyrene tube, and PEG is added to the tube to a final concentration of 8% and mixed gently. The mixture is maintained at 4°C for at least 12 h.
5. The mixture is centrifuged at 2500 rpm for 45 min and the resultant supernatant is completely aspirated because of the cytotxicity of PEG. The recombinant retroviral vectors in the precipitate are dissolved in 1/10 to 1/30 volumes of DMEM.
6. The titer of the retroviral vector can increase 10- to 30-fold.

4.1.4. Concentration of Viral Supernatant
by Relatively Low Speed Centrifugation

1. The method to obtain the cultured supernatant containing amphotropic recombinant retroviruses is same as mentioned in **Subheading 3.4.2.**
2. The viral supernatant in a 50-mL polystyren tube is centrifuged at 3000 rpm for 20 min at 4°C and filtered through a 0.45-μm pore size filter to remove the cell debris.
3. The supernatant is transferred to a new tube, and then the precipitate is collected by centrifugation at 7000 rpm for 16 h at 4°C. The supernatant is decantated, and the recombinant retroviral vectors in the precipitate are dissolved in 1/50 to 1/100 volumes of DMEM, pass through a 26G needle 3X and filtered through a 0.45-μm pore size filter.
4. The titer of the recombinant retroviral vector can increase up to 20-fold.

References

1. Levin, B. and Amos, C. (1995) Therapy of unresectable hepatocellular carcinoma. *N. Engl. J. Med.* **332,** 1294–1296.
2. Gutierrez, A. A., Lemoine, N. R. and Sikora, K. (1992) Gene therapy for cancer. *Lancet* **339,** 715–721.
3. Miller, D. G., Adam, M. A., and Miller, A. D. (1990) Gene transfer by retrovirus vectors occurs only in cells that are actively replicating at the time of infection. *Mol. Cell. Biol.* **10,** 4239–4242.

4. Moolten, F. L. (1986) Tumor chemosensitivity conferred by inserted herpes thymidine kinase genes: paradigm for a prospective cancer control strategy. *Cancer Res.* **6,** 5276–5281.

5. Bi, W. L., Parysek, L. M., Warnick, R., and Stambrook, P. J. (1993) Invitro evidence that metabolic cooperation is responsible for the bystander effect observed with HSV tk retroviral gene therapy. *Hum. Gene Ther.* **4,** 725–731.

6. Tamaoki, T. and Fausto, N. (1984) Expression of the α-fetoprotein gene during development, regeneration, and carcinogenesis, in *Recombinant DNA and cell proliferation* (Stein, G. S. and Stein, J. L. eds.), Academic, New York, pp. 145–168.

7. Urano, Y., Sakai, M., Watanabe, K., and Tamaoki, T. (1984) Tandem arrangement of the albumin and α-fetoprotein genes in the human genome. *Gene* **32,** 255–261.

8. Nakata, K., Motomura, M., Nakabayashi, H., Ido, A., and Tamaoki, T. (1992) A possible mechanism of inverse developmental regulation of α-fetoprotein and albumin genes: studies with epidermal growth factor and phorbol ester. *J. Biol. Chem.* **267,** 1331–1334.

9. Watanabe, K., Saito, A., and Tamaoki, T. (1987) Cell-specific enhancer activity in a far upstream region of the human α-fetoprotein gene. *J. Biol. Chem.* **262,** 4812–4818.

10. Nakabayashi, H., Hashimoto, T., Miyao, Y., Tjong, K. Chan, J., and Tamaoki, T. (1991) A position-dependent silencer plays a major role in repressing α-fetoprotein expression in human hepatoma. *Mol. Cell. Biol.* **11,** 5885–5893.

11. Nakabayashi, H., Watanabe, K., Saito, A., Otsuru, A., Sawadaishi, K., and Tamaoki, T. (1989) Transcriptional regulation of α-fetoprotein expression by dexamethasone in human hepatoma cells. *J. Biol. Chem.* **264,** 266–271.

12. Sawadaishi, K., Morinaga, T., and Tamaoki, T. (1988) Interaction of a hepatoma-specific nuclear factor with transcriptional-regulatory sequences of the human α-fetoprotein and albumin genes. *Mol. Cell. Biol.* **8,** 5179–5187.

13. Ido, A., Nakata, K., Nakao, K., Murata, K., Fujita, M., Ishii, N., et al. (1995) Gene therapy for hepatoma cells using a retrovirus vector carrying herpes simplex virus thymidine kinase gene under the control of human α-fetoprotein gene promoter. *Cancer Res.* **55,** 3105–3109.

14. Mawatari, F., Tsuruta, S., Ido, A., Ueki, T., Nakao, K., Kato, Y., et al. (1998) Retrovirus-mediated gene therapy for hepatocellular carcinoma: Selective and enhanced suicide gene expression regulated by human α-fetoprotein enhancer directly linked to its promoter. *Cancer Gene Ther.* in press.

15. Miller, A. D. and Buttimore, C. (1986) Redesign of retrovirus packaging cell lines to avoid recombination leading to helper virus production. *Mol. Cell. Biol.* **6,** 2895–2902.

16. Mann, R., Mulligan, R. C., and Baltimore, D. (1983) Construction of a retrovirus packaging mutant and its use to produce helper free defective retrovirus. *Cell* **33,** 153–159.

17. Nakabayashi, H., Taketa, T., Miyano, K., Yamane, T., and Sato, J. (1982) Growth of human hepatoma cell lines with differentiated functions in chemically defined medium. *Cancer Res.* **42,** 3858–3863.
18. Huh, N. and Utakoji, T. (1981) Production of HBs-antigen by two new human hepatoma cell lines and its enhancement by dexamethasone. *Gann* **72,** 178–179.
19. Nakabayashi, H., Taketa, K., Yamane, T., Oda, M., and Sato, J. (1985) Hormonal control of alpha-fetoprotein secretion in human hepatoma cell lines proliferating in chemically defined medium. *Cancer Res.* **45,** 6379–6383.
20. Wagner, M. J., Sharp, J. A., and Summers, W. C. (1981) Nucleotide sequence of the thymidine kinase genc of herpes simplex virus type 1. *Proc. Natl. Acad. Sci. USA* **78,** 1441–1445.
21. Miller, A. D. and Rosman, G. J. (1989) Improved retroviral vectors for gene transfer and expression. *BioTechniques* **7,** 980–990.
22. Sambrook, J., Fritsch, E. F., and Maniatis, T. (1989) *Molecular Cloning: A laboratory manual,* second edition (Nolan, C., ed.), Cold Spring Harbor Laboratory, New York.

22

Adenovirus-Mediated Targeted Gene Therapy for Breast Cancer and for Purging Hematopoietic Stem-Cell Sources

Ling Chen

1. Introduction

Gene therapy provides a potentially powerful approach for cancer treatment. One strategy is based on direct transfer of a suicide gene, which encodes enzymes that can activate a prodrug within tumor cells and thereby render the tumor cells sensitive to agents that are otherwise nontoxic to the cell. For example, introduction of the herpes simplex virus thymidine kinase gene (HSV-*tk*) or the bacterial cytosine deaminase (CD) gene, which respectively render mammalian cells sensitive to the otherwise nontoxic antiviral agent ganciclovir *(1,2)* and to the antifungal drug 5-fluorocytosine *(3,4)*. Another novel prodrug activation system is the activation of conventional anticancer prodrug cyclophosphamide and ifosphamide by intratumor expression of mammalian cytochrome *P450*, such as rat 2B1 or human 2B6 to further sensitize cancer cells *(5,6)*. Whereas gene therapy may provide a new therapeutic approach, clinical efficacy will require gene delivery systems, which possess both high gene-transduction efficiency and target-cell specificity.

Human adenoviruses are nonenveloped double-stranded DNA viruses with a genomic size of approx 36 kb. The *E1* gene-deleted adenoviruses are replication defective and can be grown in a packaging cell line transformed with the *E1*a and *E1*b genes. Moreover, adenovirus-mediated gene transfer is a highly efficient means for delivery of genetic material into a wide spectrum of cells both in vitro and in animals. First generation adenoviral vectors deleted at the *E1* and *E3* regions are capable of accommodating DNA inserts up to 8 kb *(7,8)*.

From: *Methods in Molecular Medicine, Vol. 35: Gene Therapy: Methods and Protocols*
Edited by: W. Walther and U. Stein © Humana Press, Inc., Totowa, NJ

Although recombinant adenoviruses hold promise for in vivo gene therapy, one of the limitations of this vector system for cancer therapy may be the non-specific transduction of therapeutic genes into nontarget cells. Whereas strategies to redirect viral tropism by modifying adenoviral fiber or penton base are being developed, one strategy to circumvent this limitation would be to use a tumor-tissue specific/selective DNA regulatory element to direct the expression of a therapeutic gene in the desired target tumor cells.

DF3 (MUC1) is a member of a family of high molecular weight glycoproteins that are aberrantly overexpressed in 75–90% of primary human breast carcinomas *(9)*. Overexpression of the *DF3* gene in human MCF-7 and ZR-75 breast cancer cells is regulated at the transcriptional level *(10–12)*.

In this chapter, we describe the use of replication-defective adenoviral vectors containing the *Escherichia coli* β-galactosidase gene (Ad.DF3-βgal) or the *HSV-tk* gene (Ad.DF3-*tk*) under control of the DF3 promoter for treating breast carcinomas in a preclinical model *(13)*. Furthermore, because tumor contamination of bone marrow (BM) and peripheral blood (PB) can potentially affect the outcome of breast cancer patients receiving high-dose chemotherapy with autologous transplantation of their BM or PB *(14–16)*, we herein describe a feasible application for purging breast cancer cells in hematopoietic stem-cell sources *(17,18)*.

2. Materials

2.1. Cell Lines

Most cell lines can be obtained from American Type Culture Collection (ATCC, Rockville, MD). The MCF-7, ZR-75-1, and BT-20 are DF3/MUC1-positive breast cancer cells. The MDA-*MB231* is a DF3/MUC1-negative breast cancer and the Hs578*Bst* is a DF3/MUC1-negative myoepithelial cell line derived from normal breast tissue adjacent to a infiltrating ductal carcinoma. Cells are grown as monolayers in recommended culture medium supplemented with 10% heat-inactivated fetal bovine serum (FBS), 2 mM L-glutamine, 100 U/mL penicillin, and 100 mg/mL streptomycin. All cells are cultured in a 5% CO_2-humidified atmosphere at 37°C.

2.2. Recombinant Adenoviruses

2.2.1. Recombinant Adenoviruses

Ad.CMV-βgal, *Ad.CMV-tk*, Ad.DF3-βgal, and *Ad,DF3-tk* are structurally similar replication-deficient recombinant adenoviruses in which the β-galactosidase and *HSV-tk* genes, respectively, are under the control of cytomegalovirus (CMV) immediate-early promoter and DF3 promoter *(13)*.

2.2.2. Preparation of Adenoviruses

Recombinant adenoviruses are constructed by homologous recombination in the human embryonic kidney cell line 293 (obtained from ATCC). Large-scale production of recombinant adenovirus was accomplished by growth in 293 cells and purification by double-cesium gradient ultracentrifugation. Titers of purified adenovirus can be determined by a spectrophotometer as particles per mL and by plaque assays as plaque forming units (PFU) per mL. One O.D. equals 1×10^{12} particles per ml. In general, the particle number is about 100-fold higher than the number of PFU.

2.3. Animals

Female athymic nude mice (Swiss-nu/nu) 20–25 g at 8–10 wk of age are used for implantation of human breast cancers.

3. Methods

3.1. Evaluation of Adenovirus-Mediated Selective Reporter Gene Expression in Tumor Cell Lines

3.1.1. Adenovirus Infection of Cultured Cells

1. Seed 1×10^6 cells per well in 30-mm plates about 12–18 h before adenoviral infection.
2. Add Ad.DF3-βgal or Ad.CMV-βgal at a multiplicity of infection (MOI) range from 0, 1, 10, 50, and 100 into cultured cells.
3. At 24 h or at a specified time postinfection, perform assays to determine the expression of β-galactosidase.
4. The expression of DF3/MUC1 antigen in breast cancer cells can be determined by FACS analysis using a monoclonal antibody that detects DF3/MUC1 *(9)*.
5. Evaluate the correlation of reporter-gene expression mediated by Ad.DF3-βgal or Ad.CMV-βgal in different cell lines.

3.1.2. Assays for β-galactosidase

1. Histochemical staining with 5-bromo-4-chloro-3-indolyl β-D-galactoside (X-Gal). Fix cells or sections of fresh frozen tissue (5–12 mm) with 0.5% glutaraldehyde in phosphate-buffered saline (PBS) containing 1 mM MgCl$_2$ for 10 min, rinse with PBS, and then incubate with X-Gal (1 mg/mL), 5 mM K$_3$Fe(CN)$_6$, 5 mM K$_4$Fe(CN)$_6$, 1 mM MgCl$_2$ in PBS for 4 h at 37°C.
2. FACS-GAL assay *(19)*. Suspend 1×10^6 cells in 50 mL of serum-free culture medium and warm to 37°C. Add an equal volume of 2 mM fluorescein di-b-D-galactopyranoside (FDG; Molecular Probes, Eugene, OR) to each aliquot of cells. Mix rapidly, but gently, and incubate for 1 min at 37°C. Thereafter, wash cells once with 4 mL ice-cold PBS and maintain in ice-cold PBS until analysis on a flowcytometer.

3. Chemiluminescence assay. Quantitation of enzyme activity can be determined by a chemiluminescence assay using Galacto-Light system (Tropix, Inc., Bedford, MA) that detects 2 fg to 20 ng of β-galactosidase. Activity is presented as relative luminescent units (RLU) in an indicated number of cells.

3.2. Evaluation of Adenovirus-Mediated Selective β-galactosidase Gene Expression in Human Tumor Xenografts

1. Subcutaneous Tumor Model. Inject tumor cells that are in exponential growth phase (1×10^7 in 0.2 mL serum-free medium) subcutaneously in the flanks of the animals. For mice bearing MCF-7 or ZR-75-1 breast carcinomas, a single pellet of 17 β-estradiol (1.7 mg/60-d release, Innovative Research, Toledo, OH) need to be implanted subcutaneously 1 d before tumor inoculation.
2. At 4 to 6 wk after tumor implantation, use a Hamilton syringe with a 26 gauge to inject adenovirus Ad.DF3-βgal or Ad.CMV-βgal ($1-10 \times 10^9$ PFU in 20–50 μL) into DF3/MUC1-positive MCF-7 or ZR-75-1 tumors, and DF3/MUC1-negative MDA-MB231 or T98G tumors.
3. Two days, or at a desired time after adenoviral infection, sacrifice the animals and evaluate the expression of the reporter gene in tumor xenografts and host tissues.
4. Freeze samples at –70°C.
5. Section tissues with a cryostat microtome at 5–12 μM per slice.
6. Fix with 0.5% glutaraldehyde in PBS containing 1 mM $MgCl_2$ for 10 min, rinse with PBS, and then incubate with X-Gal (1 mg/mL), 5 mM $K_3Fe(CN)_6$, 5 mM $K_4Fe(CN)_6$, 1 mM $MgCl_2$ in PBS for 4 h at 37°C.
7. Observe under a microscope for β-galactosidase expression.

3.3. Tumor Killing by Selective Prodrug Activation

3.3.1. Tumor Cell Growth Inhibition Assay

1. Seed 1×10^6 cells/well in 30-mm 6-well plates about 12–18 h before adenoviral infection.
2. Add Ad.DF3-*tk* or Ad.CMV-*tk* or control vectors at an MOI range from 0, 10, 50, and 100 into cultured cells.
3. At 24 h or at a specified time postinfection, replate cells at 4×10^4 cells/well in duplicate in 30-mm 6-well plates.
5. Prepare ganciclovir (GCV) in serum-free medium as 10-fold concentrated stock before use.
6. Add GCV to the cultured cells at various final concentrations range from 0 250 mM.
7. After 6–7 d of incubation, trypsinize cells and suspend cells in an equal volume (1–2 mL).
8. Count the number of viable cells with a hemocytometer under a microscope by Trypan blue exclusion method.

3.3.2. Tumor Cell Clonogenic Assay

1. At 24 h after adenovirus (Ad.DF3-*tk*, Ad.CMV-*tk*, and control) infection, add GCV to cells and incubate for 24 h.
2. Replate cells in duplicate at serial dilutions ranging from 500 to 10^6 cells per well onto 30-mm culture dishes. Culture cells for 2 wk.
3. Stained cells with crystal violet and count colonies with >50 cells. Results can be expressed as the surviving cell fraction ± SEM for the treated groups compared to controls.

3.3.3. Intraperitoneal Breast Cancer Carcinomatosis Model

1. Inject MCF-7 cells (1×10^7 in 0.2 mL serum-free medium) i.p. for the development of intraperitoneal tumors (day 0).
2. On days 4 and 5 after tumor cell injection, inject 1×10^9 PFU adenoviruses (Ad.DF3-*tk*, Ad.CMV-*tk*, or reporter vectors) in 0.5 mL PBS i.p. into the mice.
3. On day 7, treat the animals with either PBS or GCV (100 mg/kg) daily for 4 d by i.p. injection.
4. Sacrifice the mice at 5–6 wk after tumor inoculation.
5. Examine peritoneal cavity for the ascites and tumor clusters. Measure the volume of ascite, collect and weigh tumors for each animal.
6. Alternatively, the survival of animals can be followed after treatment.

3.4. Selective Transgene Expression for Detection and Elimination of Contaminating Breast Cancer Cells in Hematopoietic Stem-Cell Sources

3.4.1. Preparation of Human Hematopoietic Cells from Healthy Donors and Patients

1. BM mononuclear cells and human PB mononuclear cells are isolated by Ficoll-Paque (Pharmacia, Piscataway, NJ) density gradient centrifugation ($d = 1.077$, 400g) from leukocyte-enriched leukopaks of healthy donors. Suspend cells in MyeloCult medium (Stem Cell Technologies, Vancouver, Canada).
2. CD34+ cells can be isolated using the Ceprate LC cell separation system (CellPro Inc., Bothell, WA). In brief, incubate BM cells with a biotinylated mouse anti-CD34+ MAb, wash once and then pass through an avidin column. Nonadsorbed cells are removed by washing, and the CD34+ cells can be eluted from the column. The enriched cells (80–90% CD34+) are maintained in Iscove's MEM containing 12.5% FBS, 12.5% horse serum, and 1 mM hydrocortisone.

3.4.2. Adenovirus-Mediated Reporter Gene Expression in Hematopoietic Stem-Cell Sources

1. To assess if the level of adenovirus-mediated reporter-gene expression correlates with the number of contaminating breast cancer cells, MCF-7 or ZR-75 breast

cancer cells can be premixed with PB or BM obtained from healthy donors at ratios of $1:10^6$ to $1:10^3$.

2. Add Ad.DF3-βgal or Ad.CMV-βgal at MOIs of 1 to 10 in an equal volume (e.g., 10^6 in 1.0 mL) into samples prepared as described in **Subheading 3.4.1.** from patients or healthy donors premixed with breast cancer cells

3. At 24 h postinfection, evaluate β-galactosidase expression by chemiluminescence assay or FACS as described in **Subheading 3.1.2.**

3.4.3. Gene Therapy for Purging Contaminating Cancer Cells in Hematopoietic Stem Cell Sources

1. Add Ad.DF3-*tk* at MOIs of 1 to 10 to samples (e.g., 10^6 BM cells in 1.0 mL volume) prepared from patients or healthy donors premixed with breast cancer cells.

2. Incubate cells in a 5% CO_2 humidified atmosphere at 37°C.

3. At 12 h postinfection, add GCV prepared as 10X stock (1 m*M*) into samples to a final concentration of 100 μ*M*.

4. Incubate cells in a 5% CO_2 humidified atmosphere at 37°C for 24 h.

5. Determine the survival of tumor cells by PCR for the presence of tumor-specific antigen (DF3/MUC1) or by clonogenic assay as described in **Subheading 3.3.2.**

3.4.4. Hematopoietic Progenitor Cell Assays

1. Erythroid burst-forming units (BFU-E) and granulocyte-monocyte colony-forming units (CFU-GM) are assayed in a methylcellulose culture system (MethoCult) containing recombinant human stem-cell factor (50 ng/mL), GM-CSF (10 ng/mL), IL-3 (10 ng/mL), and erythropoietin (EPO) (3 U/mL) according to a detail instruction provided by the manufacture (Stem Cell Technologies, Vancouver, Canada). The numbers of colonies can be determined after 2 wk.

2. For evaluating more primitive progenitor cells, the number of long-term culture-initiating cells (LTC-ICs) can be determined by culturing serial dilutions of CD34+ cells on irradiated BM stromal cells in 96-well plates for 5 wk. The number of wells containing colonies can then be assessed by growth in MyeloCult medium (Stem Cell Technologies) *(20)*. The frequency of LTC-ICs is calculated by plotting the input cell number against the proportion of negative wells *(21)*. A software provided by StemCell Technologies can facilitate the analysis.

4. Notes

1. Expression of β-galactosidase can be observed in MCF-7, ZR-75-1, and BT-20 cells infected with Ad.DF3-βgal, whereas no or little β-galactosidase activity could be detected in similarly infected Hs578Bst, MDA-MB231, and T98G cells. Expression of β-galactosidase in Ad.DF3-βgal infected cells correlates with the expression of DF3. All of these cell lines showed strong expression of β-galactosidase when infected with Ad.CMV-βgal.

2. For evaluation of intratumor injection of adenovirus expressing a reporter gene such as β-galactodisae, the needle can be coated with fine charcoal particles to

mark the needle tract in order to verify colocalization of the expression of the reporter gene with the viral injection.

3. Ad.DF3-*tk* sensitizes DF3-positive MCF-7 and ZR-75-1 breast cancer cells to GCV. Nude mice inoculated i.p. with MCF-7 cells developed tumor masses throughout the peritoneal cavity and 2–4 mL of bloody ascites that contained tumor cells in 6–8 wk. Mice treated with Ad.DF3-*tk* plus GCV showed no grossly identifiable tumor mass or only a few small tumor clusters.

4. Adenovirus-mediated gene transfer is markedly inefficient in the transduction of BM, PB, and purified CD34+ cells, as compared to breast carcinoma cells. The use of the DF3/MUC1 promoter in the context of adenoviral vector further assure the maximal selectivity of targeting DF3/MUC1-positive breast cancer cells in hematopoietic stem-cell sources.

5. The selective expression of HSV-TK followed by GCV treatment can achieve elimination of 6-logs of contaminating breast cancer cells. There was little adverse effect on recovery of CFU-GM, BFU-E, and LTC-ICs of hematopoietic progenitor cells.

6. The differential sensitivity of hematopoietic as compared to carcinoma cell by Ad.DF3-*tk* and GCV treatment supported the use of this approach to purge contaminating tumor cells. Recently, other adenoviral gene therapy approaches for BM purging have been explored, such as the delivery of wild-type p53 to induce apoptosis of contaminating tumor cells (*22,23*). However, in order to maximize therapeutic index, it is desirable to employ a tumor-specific promoter to direct the expression of these therapeutic genes.

References

1. Moolten, F. L. and Wells, J. M. (1990) Curability of tumors bearing herpes thymidine kinase genes transferred by retroviral vectors. *J. Natl. Cancer Inst.* **82,** 297–300.
2. Culver, K. W., Ram, Z., Wallbridge, S., Ishii, H., Oldfield, E. H., and Blaese, R. M. (1992) In vivo gene transfer with retroviral vector-producer cells for treatment of experimental brain tumors. *Science* **256,** 1550–1552.
3. Mullen, C. A., Kilstrup, M., and Blaese, R. M. (1992) Transfer of the bacterial gene for cytosine deaminase to mammalian cells confers lethal sensitivity to 5-fluorocytosine: a negative selection system. *Proc. Natl. Acad. Sci. USA* **89,** 33–37.
4. Huber, B. E., Richards C. A., and Krenitsky, T. A. (1991) Retroviral-mediated gene therapy for the treatment of hepatocellular carcinoma: an innovative approach for cancer therapy. *Proc. Natl. Acad. Sci. USA* **88,** 8039–8043.
5. Chen, L. and Waxman, D. J. (1995) Intratumoral activation and enhanced chemotherapeutic effect of oxazaphosphorines following cytochrome P450 gene transfer: development of a combined chemotherapy/cancer gene therapy strategy. *Cancer Res.* **55,** 581–589.
6. Chen, L., Waxman, D. J., Chen, D., and Kufe, D. W. (1996) Sensitization of human breast cancer cells to cyclophosphamide and ifosphamide activation by transfer of a liver cytochrome P450 gene. *Cancer Res.* **56,** 1331–1340.

7. Graham, F. L. and L. Prevec. (1991) Manipulation of adenvirus vectors, in *Methods in Molecular Biology: Gene Transfer and Expression Protocols* (Murray, E. J., ed.) Humana, Clifton, NJ.

8. Bett, A. J., Haddara, W., Prevec, L., and Graham, F. L. (1994) An efficient and flexible system for construction of adenovirus vector with insertions or deletions in early regions 1 and 3. *Proc. Natl. Acad. Sci. USA* **91,** 8802–8806.

9. Kufe, D. W., Inghirami G., Abe M., Hayes D., Justi-Wheeler H., and Schlom J. (1984) Differential reactivity of a novel monoclonal antibody (DF3) with human malignant versus benign breast tumors. *Hybridoma* **3,** 223–232.

10. Abe, M. and Kufe, D. W. (1990) Transcriptional regulation of DF3 gene expression in human MCF-7 breast carcinoma cells. *J. Cell. Physiol.* **143,** 226–231.

11. Kovarik, A., Peat, N., Wilson, D., Gendler, S. J., and Taylor-Papadimitriou, J. (1993) Analysis of the tissue-specific promoter of the MUC1 gene. *J. Biol. Chem.* **268,** 9917–9926.

12. Abe, M. and Kufe, D. W. (1993) Characterization of cis-acting elements regulating transcription of the human DF3 breast carcinoma-associated antigen (MUC1) gene. *Proc. Natl. Acad. Sci. USA* **90,** 282–286.

13. Chen, L., Chen, D., Manome, Y., Dong, Y., Fine, H. A., and Kufe, D. W. (1995) Breast cancer selective gene expression and therapy mediated by recombinant adenoviruses containing the DF3/MUC1 promoter. *J. Clin. Invest.* **96,** 275–2782.

14. Ross, A. A., Cooper, B. W., Lazarus, H. M., Mackay, W., Moss, T. J., Ciobanu, N., et al. (1993) Detection and viability of tumor cells in peripheral blood stem cell collections from breast cancer patients using immunocytochemical and clonogenic assay techniques. *Blood* **82,** 2605–1210.

15. Cote, R. J., Rosen, P. P., Lesser, M. L., Old, L. J., and Osborne, M. P. (1991) Prediction of early relapse in patients with operable breast cancer by detection of occult bone marrow micrometastases. *J. Clin. Oncol.* **9,** 1749–1756.

16. Diel, I. J., Kaufmann, M., Goerner, R., Costa, S. D., Kaul, S., and Bastert, G. (1992) Detection of tumor cells in bone marrow of patients with primary breast cancer: a prognostic factor for distant metastasis. *J. Clin. Oncol.* **10,** 1234–1539.

17. Wilson, J. M (1997) When bad gene transfer is good. *J. Clin. Invest.* **98,** 2435.

18. Chen, L., Pulsifer, D., Chen, D., Sieff, C., Elias, A., Fine, H. A., and Kufe, D. W. (1997) Selective transgene expression for detection and elimination of contaminating carcinoma cells in hematomoietic stem cell sources. *J. Clin. Invest.* **98,** 2539–2548.

19. Nolan, G. P., Fiering, S., Nicolas, J. F., and Herzenberg, L. A. (1988) Fluorescence-activated cell analysis and sorting of viable mammalian cells based on beta-D-galactosidase activity after transduction of Escherichia coli lacZ. *Proc. Natl. Acad. Sci. USA* **85,** 2603–2607.

20. Sutherland, H. J., Lansdorp, P. M., Henkelman, D. H., Eaves, A. C., and Eaves, C. J. (1990) Functional characterization of individual human hematopoietic stem cells cultured at limiting dilution on supportive marrow stromal layers. *Proc. Natl. Acad. Sci. USA* **87,** 3584–3588.

21. Taswell, C. (1981) Limiting dilution assays for the determination of immunocompetent cell frequencies. I. data analysis. *J. Immunol.* **126,** 1614–1619.
22. Seth, P., Brinkmann, U., Schwartz, G. N., Katayose, D., Gress, R., Pastan, I., and Cowan, K. (1996) Adenovirus-mediated gene transfer to human breast tumor cells: an approach for cancer gene therapy and bone marrow purging. *Cancer Res.* **56** 1346–1351.
23. Wroblewski, J. M., Lay, L. T., Van Zant, G., Phillips, G., Seth, P., Curiel, D., and Meeker, T. C. (1996) Selective elimination (purging) of contaminating malignant cells from hematopoietic stem cell autografts using recombinant adenovirus. *Cancer Gene Ther.* **3,** 257–264.

23

Chemotherapy-Inducible Vector for Gene Therapy of Cancer

Wolfgang Walther, Ulrike Stein, Robert H. Shoemaker, Peter M. Schlag

1. Introduction

A great variety of viral and nonviral expression systems has been developed and assessed for their ability to transfer genes into somatic cells. In particular, retroviral and adenoviral mediated gene transfer has been extensively studied and improved at least because of their capability to efficiently infect the targeted cells. However, the lack of cell type specificity of viral and nonviral vectors still represents one major obstacle for appropriate and controlled expression of foreign genes. Many attempts have been made to achieve efficient gene delivery by targeting, e.g., retroviral integration via modifications in viral envelope protein sequences, using antibodies as specific mediators in viral infection and pseudotyped viruses, and so on (1,2,3,4).

All of these strategies are based on the targeting of gene delivery by restricting the viral infection or liposomal binding to a specific cell type. Alternatively, or in addition to these delivery technologies, regulated conditional expression of therapeutic genes is of great interest for cancer gene therapy. The identification of responsive/inducible elements within promoter sequences created the basis for the applicability of these elements in construction of viral and nonviral vectors for the conditional expression of the desired gene.

Numerous promoters and enhancers that have been identified and characterized, can be activated via responsive elements by certain inducing factors such as steroid hormones, growth factors, cytokines, cytostatic drugs, irradiation, or heat shock. Using such regulatory elements as internal promoters to drive the expression of therapeutic genes in vector constructs, a controlable and restricted expression of these genes can be achieved. In addition to high-level and

From: *Methods in Molecular Medicine, Vol. 35: Gene Therapy: Methods and Protocols*
Edited by: W. Walther and U. Stein © Humana Press, Inc., Totowa, NJ

efficient gene expression, minimizing inappropriate gene expression in surrounding nontarget cells is of great importance for numerous gene therapeutic approaches, particularly if tumor cell killing is attempted in cancer gene therapy. Therefore, vector systems harboring elements that respond to regulatory signals represent an important component for selective and safe expression of therapeutic genes associated with regulated gene expression at therapeutically relevant levels.

1.1. "Therapy-inducible" Promoters for Controlled Gene Expression

In a search for conditionally active promoters, several groups have focused their attention on genes that are induced in their expression by factors or modalities that act on tumor cells during certain therapeutic treatments such as chemotherapy, irradiation, or hyperthermia. Originally, such promoters regulate the induction of protective mechanisms in the cell. The usefulness of these promoters is based on their inducibility by factors that are components of established clinical cancer-treatment settings like cytostatic drugs, irradiation, hyperthermia, or those that represent specific metabolic situations in solid tumors (e.g., hypoxia). They provide the potential for the construction of "therapy-inducible" vectors to express auxiliary therapeutic genes that might act synergistically with chemotherapy, radiotherapy, or hyperthermy of tumors *(5,6)* (**Fig. 1**).

The investigation of gene regulation of the multidrug resistance gene (MDR1), the X-irradiation induced tissue-type plasminogen activator (t-PA) or the early growth response gene *(Egr-1)*, the human heat-shock protein HSP70, the glucose-regulated protein (GRP78), or the hypoxia-inducible element (HRE) of the phosphoglycerate kinase-1 gene led to the discovery of a class of promoter sequences being inducible by defined therapy-associated conditions or conditions associated with tumor physiology *(7–11)*. Such promoter elements perfectly fulfill the criteria for their utilization in "therapy inducible" vector constructs. Recently, a growing number of studies is employing radiation- or heat shock-inducible promoters for the expression of therapeutic genes. To approach this, X-irradiation responsive elements were isolated from the t-PA promoter, which was inducible after X-irradiation in radioresistant human melanoma cells *(7)*. Similar X-irradiation responsive elements were identified in the 5'-untranslated region of the *Egr-1* gene. The *Egr-1* gene promoter/enhancer element was utilized for the TNFα gene expression in a adenoviral vector. Delivery of the vector to human tumors growing in nude mice resulted in an up-to-10-fold increase in TNFα production after irradiation of the transduced tumors causing an up-to-21-d lasting cytokine accumulation within the irradiated tumor tissue *(8)*.

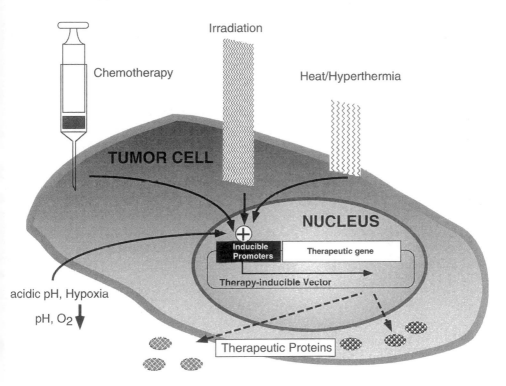

Fig. 1. Schematic representation of the strategy for utilization of therapy-inducible vectors in gene therapy of cancer. Such vectors harbor regulatable promoters, which are responsive to factors associated with conventional tumor therapies (chemotherapy, radiation, hyperthermia). These vectors can be employed for the conditional expression of therapeutic genes, which in addition can augment the conventional therapy to improve antitumor efficacy.

Another stress-induced protein is the HSP70. The HSP70 promoter harbors elements that respond to normal conditions of cell growth and, more interestingly, to stress factors including heat shock and heavy metals. Examination of the HSP70 promoter revealed a single heat-shock element required for the heat shock-induced activity of the promoter *(9)*. In conjunction with hyperthermia treatment of solid tumors, such promoters will be useful for the heat-inducible expression of therapeutic genes within defined tumor areas, as was recently attempted by Blackburn and colleagues for the heat-induced expression of reporter and suicide genes *(12)*.

Abnormal physiological conditions occuring in solid tumor environments or provoked by certain cancer-treatment modalities can also act as inducers for the expression of particular genes. The Grp78 protein is induced about 10-fold under stress situations, such as glucose deprivation, chronic anoxia, and acidic pH, conditions known to exist in poorly vascularized tumors. Therefore, the employment of the Grp78 promoter may offer advantages for high level expression in solid tumors in a pathology-dependent fashion. Fusion of the 600 bp portion of the Grp78 promoter to the neomycin reporter gene in a retroviral vector and transduction of the vector into the murine fibrosarcoma B/C10ME caused high-level neomycin gene expression in the tumors in vivo *(10)*. Highest expression levels were observed in the tumor center, conferring the inducibility of the promoter under glucose-starved stress conditions. Dachs and collegues employed the hypoxia-responsive element (HRE) of the mouse phosphoglycerate kinase-1 for the expression regulation of the cytosine deaminase gene in vitro and in vivo *(11)*. They showed strong inducibility of the system under hypoxic conditions leading to significant increase in sensitivity of transduced tumor cells towards the prodrug 5-fluorocytosine.

1.2. MDR1 Gene Promoter and Drug Inducibility

Following this line of therapy-inducible promoters, the human MDR1 promoter may be employed for a temporally activated chemotherapy-inducible expression system. Numerous studies have shown that the expression of the *MDR1* gene is inducible by different stress factors (UV irradiation, heat shock, arsenite, and so on) including cytostatic drugs *(13,14,15)*. This leads to the upregulation of MDR1 gene expression in drug-treated cells causing resistance to chemotherapy of tumors resulting in the multidrug resistance (MDR) phenotype *(16,17)*. The promoter of the human *MDR1* gene consists of two regions, the upstream and the downstream (proximal) promoter. Particularly, the proximal promoter harbors essential regulatory elements that mediate reponsiveness toward different factors for constitutive basal and induced conditional expression of the *MDR1* gene.

In this context, it has been shown that the MDR1 promoter harbors defined drug-responsive elements in the downstream promoter region. The drug-inducible elements of the proximal human MDR1 promoter are located within a region spanning from −136 to +121. These elements are inducible by MDR-associated cytostatic compounds, such as vincristine, adriamycin, or actinomycin D, which are part of chemotherapeutic treatment schedules in tumor therapy *(18,19)*. Detailed characterization of the MDR1 promoter in transient CAT-reporter assays revealed the applicability of these elements for the construction of conditional expression vectors responding to anticancer drug treatments. In vitro studies demonstrated that the MDR1 promoter induction by cytostatic drugs is time and also drug-concentration dependent. For the utilization of the human MDR1 promoter in a chemotherapy-regulatable vector we have isolated a defined promoter fragment from human osteosarcoma specimen by PCR *(19)*. This fragment encompasses the promoter region from –207 to +158, which includes the drug-responsive elements.

The methods described in this chapter are based on our experiments that led to the isolation characterization and utilization of the MDR1 promoter for drug-inducible gene therapy of tumor cells. These methods and procedures are examples for how we approached the construction of such a conditional vector system that can be utilized for the expression of any therapeutic gene in combination of chemotherapeutic treatments. The methodology can be adapted for research and development of similar strategies in cancer gene therapy.

2. Materials
2.1. Cell Lines and Cell Culture

1. The human colon carcinoma cell lines HCT15 *(20)* and KM12 *(21)* and the human mammary carcinoma cell line MCF-7 *(22)* were maintained in RPMI-1640 medium (Life Technologies, Gaithersburg, MD) supplemented with 10% fetal calf serum (FCS, HyClone, Logan, UT) and 5 mM L-glutamine (Life Technologies) at 37°C, 5% CO_2. The cell-culture medium did not contain antibiotics (*see* **Note 1**).
2. EDTA-trypsin (Life Technologies).
3. G418 (Life Technologies) stock solution 50 mg/mL in distilled sterile water (storage at 4°C).
4. Tissue-culture flasks, 10-cm diameter Petri dishes, 24- and 96-well plates (Costar, Cambridge, MA).
5. Disposable 1mL, 5 mL , 10 mL and 25 mL pipets (Costar).
6. Disposable cell scraper for cell harvesting (Falcon, Los Angeles, CA).
7. Drugs for induction experiments: vincristine (Sigma, St. Louis, CA), adriamycin (Sigma) (*see* **Note 2**).

2.2. DNA and RNA Isolation

2.2.1. Solutions and Reagents for Isolation of High Molecular Weight DNA

1. Proteinase K solution: stock solution, 2 mg/mL proteinase K in water, store in aliquots at –20°C.
2. Lysis buffer: 10 mM Tris-HCl, pH 7.4, 50 mM NaCl, 5 mM EDTA.
3. 10% SDS solution in water.
4. Phenol-chloroform (1:1) solution saturated with TE (0.01M Tris-HCl, 0.001M EDTA) buffer, pH 7.0.
5. Chloroform.
6. Dialysis tubing, flat width 76 mm.
7. RNase A solution: stock solution 10 mg/mL RNase A in TE buffer with 15 mM NaCl.

2.2.2. Solutions and Reagents for Isolation
of Total Cellular RNA (see **Note 3**)

1. Lithium chloride-urea solution: 3M LiCl, 6M urea in autoclaved diethyl-polycarbonate (DEPC) water.
2. TES buffer: 10 mM Tris-HCl pH 7.6, 1 mM EDTA, and 0.5% SDS.
3. Phenol-chloform isoamyl alcohol (25:24:1) solution (*caution: corrosive*), saturated with TE.
4. Absolute ethanol.
5. 3M sodium acetate solution in DEPC-water, pH 7.0 (autoclaved).
6. 70% ethanol in DEPC-water.

2.3. PCR and RT-PCR Solutions, Kits, and Primers

The performance of PCR and RT-PCR requires access to thermocycler equipment. In our studies the DNA Thermal Cycler 480 (Perkin-Elmer, Norwalk, CT) was used.

2.3.1. Kits and Reagents for PCR

1. Gene Amp PCR Reagent kit with Ampli Taq DNA Polymerase (Perkin-Elmer, Foster City, CA).
2. Human specific oligonucleotides (primers) for PCR (23): sense primer; 5′-GAATTC-CTTGCCCTTTCTAG-3′ (including the *Eco*RI-site) antisense primer; 5′-GGATCC-AGTAGCTCCCAGCTT-3′ (including the *Bam*HI-site) These primers amplify a 374 bp PCR product of the human mdr1 promoter.

2.3.2. Kits and Reagents for RT-PCR

1. Gene Amp RNA PCR kit (Perkin-Elmer).
2. Human TNFα-specific oligonucleotides (primers) for RT-PCR (24): sense primer; 5′-ATGAGCACTGAAAGCATGATC-3′, antisense primer; 5′-TCAC AGGGCAATGATCCCAAAGTAGACCTGCCC-3′. These primers amplify a 702 bp TNFα-specific PCR product.
3. Human β-actin specific oligonucleotides (primers) for RT-PCR (25): sense primer; 5′-ATCATGTTTGAGACCTTCAA-3′, antisense primer; 5′-CATCTCT TGCTCGAAGTCCA-3′. These primers amplify a 316 bp β-actin-specific PCR product.

2.4. Plasmid and Vector Construction

1. Restriction enzymes as needed for the desired cloning strategy (*see* **Subheading 3.**), T4 DNA-Ligase (Promega, Madison, WI) and buffers supplied by the manufacturer.
2. Plasmid DNA purification kit (Qiagen, Chatsworth, CA).
3. Plasmids pBluescript IISK$^{+/-}$ (Stratagene, La Jolla, CA), pSP72 (Promega), pCAT-Basic (Promega), and the retroviral vector pM3-hTNF (*26*).

4. Luria-Bertani (LB) medium: 5 g trypton, 2.5 g yeast extract, 5 g NaCl in 500 mL water, adjust to pH 7.5 and autoclave.
5. Subcloning efficiency DH5α-competent cells (Life Technologies).
6. GeneClean kit (Dianova, Hamburg, Germany).

2.5. CAT Assay Solutions and Kits

In all CAT-experiments, the control plasmids pCAT-Basic (negative control) and pSV2CAT (positive control) were used (Invitrogen, San Diego, CA).

2.5.1. Material for Thin Layer Chromatography (TLC) CAT-Assay

1. CAT enzyme assay kit (Promega).
2. TE buffer containing protease inhibitors (10 mg/mL aprotinin and 100 mg/mL PMSF).
3. [^{14}C]-labeled chloramphenicol (0.05 mCi/mL, NEN Du Pont, Bad Homburg, Germany).
4. Coomassie Plus protein assay reagent (Pierce, Rockford, IL).
5. Ethyl acctate (Sigma).
6. TLC silica gel plates (Analtech Inc., Newark, DE).
7. Phospho Imager SF (Molecular Dynamics, Sunnyvale, CA).

2.5.2. Material for Liquid Scintillation Counting (LSC) CAT-Assay

1. Xylene (Sigma).
2. Ready-Safe Scintillant (Promega).
3. Scintillation Counter LS 6000 LL (Beckman Instruments, Palo Alto, CA).

2.6. Transfection and Drug-Induced Gene Expression

For all transfections, the electroporation apparatus Electroporator II from Invitrogen (San Diego, CA) was utilized.

1. Phosphate-buffered saline (PBS) (Life Technologies).
2. Electroporation cuvettes, gap size 0.4 cm (Invitrogen).
3. Cytostatic drugs (*see* **Note 2**): Vincristine, adriamycin (Sigma).

2.7. Cytotoxicity MTT-Assay

For both, the cytotoxicity assay and the cytokine ELISAs microtiterplate-reader from SLT-Labinstruments, Salzburg, Austria, was used. The measurements of the two methods were calculated and normalized to the respective controls (MTT-assay) or standard curves (ELISA) by the EasySoftG200/Easy-Fit (MTT-assay) or EasySoft/G200Easy-Base (ELISA) software, respectively (SLT-Labinstruments, Crailsheim, Germany).

1. MTT: 3-(4,5-dimethyl-2-thioazolyl)-2,5-diphenyl-2(H)-tetrazolium bromide (Serva); 0.4% stock solution in PBS, store at 4°C and protect from light.
2. 10% SDS solution in water.

2.8. TNFα-ELISA

1. TNF-ELISA kit (Biosource, Camarillo, CA).

3. Methods

3.1. PCR-isolation of the mdr1 Promoter Fragment

To perform PCR amplification of human mdr1 promoter sequences, high molecular weight DNA had to be isolated from tumor samples. For the isolation of the DNA, tumor samples were obtained from osteosarcoma surgery. These samples were shock frozen in liquid nitrogen during surgery and crysections were evaluated by pathologists. Portions of the samples were then subjected to high molecular weight DNA preparation.

1. Homogenize the tumor tissue (approximately 0.125 cm^3) in 1 mL ice cold lysis buffer in a Dounce-homogenizer (*see* **Note 4**).
2. Add to the tumor homogenate proteinase K solution to a final concentration of 100 µg/mL and SDS solution to a final concentration of 0.5% and incubate at 37°C, overnight (ON).
3. Then, treat the homogenate with phenol/chloroform, shake thoroughly, centrifuge at 3000 rpm, transfer the supernatant to another tube and treat the supernatant with chloroform.
4. After 15 min of centrifugation at 4500g at 3.1., transfer the DNA containing supernatant into dialysis tubes and dialyze in TE-buffer for 3 h at room temperature (RT).
5. Transfer the DNA solution to an Eppendorf tube and add RNase A solution to a final concentration of 100 µg/mL and incubate for 3 h at 37°C. Thereafter, repeat **steps 3** and **4**.
6. Take the DNA solution and determine the DNA concentration in a spectrophotometer at 260 nm.
7. For the PCR take 100 ng of high molecular weight DNA and perform the PCR by using the Ampli Taq DNA Polymerase kit and the mdr1 promoter specific primers at the following conditions: 94°C 1 min, 45°C 1min, 72°C 2 min for 30 cycles. After the PCR clean the PCR products with the GeneClean kit.
8. Digest the PCR products (*see* **Note 5**) and the pBluescript plasmid with *Eco*RI and *Bam*HI (Boehringer Mannheim, Mannheim, Germany) at 37°C for 2 h (*see* **Fig. 2**).
9. Ligate the PCR product and the pBluescript plasmid at 14°C for 4 h by using T4 DNA Ligase (*see* **Note 6**).
10. Take the ligation mix and transform 50 µL DH5α-competent cells (subcloning efficiency DH5α-competent cells, Life Technologies) for 30 min on ice. Grow the transformed cells in 1 mL LB-medium at 37°C for 1 h and plate cells (100–200 µL) on agar containing 100 µg/mL ampicillin.
11. Select white colonies for plasmid-minipreparation *(27)*.
12. Digest the plasmid DNA with *Eco*RI/*Bam*HI (Boehringer Mannheim) to select mdr1 promoter haboring clones after gel electrophoresis.

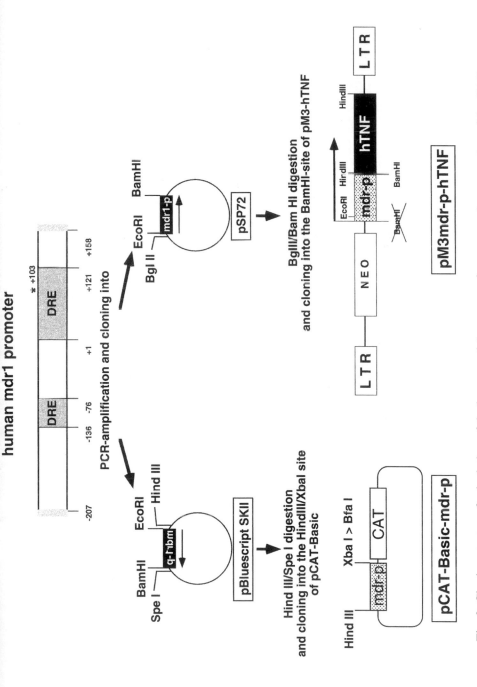

Fig. 2. Cloning strategy for isolation of the human mdr1 promoter fragment and construction of the CAT-reporter plasmid and the drug-inducible retroviral vector pM3mdr-p-hTNF (*see* **Subheadings 3.1, 3.2,** and **3.4.**).

The pBluescript mdr1 promoter plasmid was used for sequencing to confirm the correct sequence of the mdr1 promoter fragment spanning from –207 to +158. The promoter harboring pBluescript plasmid was used for the contruction of the pCAT-Basic-mdr-p plasmid.

3.2. Construction of CAT-Reporter Plasmids

1. For the construction of the CAT-reporter plasmid digest 5 µg of the mdr1 promoter harboring pBluescript with *Hind*III/*Spe*I (Boehringer Mannheim) and digest 1 µg of the pCAT-Basic plasmid with *Hind*III/*Xba*I at 37°C for 2 h (**Fig. 2**).
2. For purification of the digested pCAT-Basic plasmid treat the reaction mix with the same volume of chloroform, centrifuge at 10,000 rpm for 5 min, remove the aqueous supernatant and precipitate the DNA by adding 1/10 vol 5*M* sodium acetate and 2.5 vol absolute ethanol for 2 h at –20°C. Then centrifuge at 12,000 rpm for 10 min, wash the DNA pellet once with 0.5 mL 70% ethanol and redissolve the DNA in 5 mL TE buffer.
3. To isolate the mdr1 promoter fragment, run the digested DNA in gel electrophoresis, cut the promoter fragment representing band out of the gel under UV light, and purify the DNA with GeneClean.
4. Ligate the GeneClean-purified *Hind*III/*Spe*I mdr1 promoter fragment into *Hind*III/*Xba*I site of the pCAT-Basic plasmid by T4 DNA Ligase at 14°C for 4 h (*see* **Note 7**).
5. For transformation and plasmid minipreparation, follow **step 10** of **Subheading 3.1.** and digest the plasmid DNA with *Hind*III/*Bfa*I to release the mdr1 promoter fragment for identification of the promoter carrying clones in gel electrophoresis (owing to the cloning strategy the *Xba*I site of pCAT-Basic was altered to an *Bfa*I site).

In the resulting pCAT-Basic-mdr-p plasmid, the CAT expression is under the transcriptional control of the human mdr1 promoter fragment that harbors drug responsive elements. This construct was employed for the CAT-assays to evaluate the promoter efficacy and the drug-inducibility of the human mdr1 promoter sequence in vitro.

3.3. Testing of mdr1 Promoter Activity and Drug Inducibility in CAT-Reporter Assay

For the CAT-reporter assays the human colon carcinoma cell lines HCT15 and KM12 were used.

1. Harvest exponentially growing cells by trypsinization and centrifuge the cells at 800 rpm for 5 min at 4°C. Resuspend cell pellets in ice-cold PBS and adjust the cell concentration to 1×10^6 cells/mL.
2. Place 0.8-mL aliquots of the cell suspensions in electroporation cuvets and add 20 µg of the control plasmids pCAT-Basic (negative control), pSV2CAT

(positive control), and the plasmid pCAT-Basic-mdr-p. Keep the cells on ice for 10 min.

3. Electroporate the cells at 1000 µF, 300 V in an Electroporator II apparatus and keep the cells on ice for another 10 min.
4. Split the cells into cell-culture flasks (*see* **Note 8**) and grow cells for 48 h before starting the induction experiments with the cytostatic drug.
5. For induction, treat the cells with 0.4, 4, 40, and 400 ng/mL vincristine for 24 h at 37°C.
6. After the drug incubation, remove the medium, wash twice with 2 mL ice-cold PBS, and add 1 mL ice-cold TE containing protease inhibitors (*see* **Note 9**).
7. Harvest cell lysates by performing three cycles of freeze-thawing: place cells for 5 min into a –70°C freezer and transfer to a water bath for 5 min at 37°C. Collect the lysates in Eppendorf tubes on ice.
8. Determine the protein concentrations of the cell lysates by using the Coomassie Plus protein assay reagent following the recommendations of the manufacturer (Pierce, Rockford, IL).
9. For the CAT-assay use the CAT-enzyme assay kit (Promega) (*see* **Note 10**). For each CAT-assay, place 50 µg protein of lysates, 5 µL n-Butyryl Coenzyme A and 3 µL [^{14}C]-chloramphenicol (0.05 mCi/mL) in a 1.5-mL Eppendorf tube. Adjust with distilled water to final volume of 125 µL.
10. Prepare also positive controls (e.g., lysates of pSV2CAT-transduced cells) as well as negative controls (cell lysates of empty plasmid pCAT-Basic transduced cells and aliquots w/o cell lysates).
11. Prepare standard curves using CAT enzyme dilutions of the stock solution (Promega) in 0.25M Tris-HCl buffer, pH 8.0 to the final CAT enzyme concentrations of 0.1, 0.05, 0.025, 0.0125, and 0.00625 U CAT-enzyme.
12. Incubate samples for 3 h at 37°C.
13. After a brief spin, divide reaction mixture for thin-layer chromatography (TLC; 100 µL aliquotes of the reaction mixture) and for liquid scintillation counting (LSC; 25 µL aliquots of the reaction mixture).

3.3.1. Thin-Layer Chromatography (TLC)

1. Add 400 µL ethyl acetate to 100 µL of the reaction mixture to stop the reaction.
2. Vortex for 1 min and spin 3 min at 14,000 rpm in a microcentrifuge.
3. Transfer upper, organic phase into another Eppendorf tube.
4. Evaporate the ethyl acetate in nitrogen flow.
5. Resuspend the residue in 30 µL ethyl acetate.
6. Spot 10 µL of each sample onto a silica gel TLC plate using glass capillaries (Analtech Inc., Newark, DE) and dry (*see* **Note 11**).
7. Perform TLC in a tank that was equilibrated with chlorophorm/methanol (97:3) for 3 h.
8. Dry the TLC plate, cover with Saran Wrap, and expose the X-ray film (Kodak safety film AR) ON.

9. Use a computer-aided Phospho Imager SF (Molecular Dynamics, Sunnyvale, CA) for quantitation of the metabolized butyrylated derivatives of $[^{14}C]$-chloramphenicol (this is an alternative to CAT quantitation using liquid scintillation counting).

3.3.2. Liquid Scintillation Counting (LSC)

1. Terminate CAT-assay reaction by adding 300 µL xylene to 25 µL of the reaction mixture.
2. Vortex for 30 s and spin at 14,000 rpm in a microcentrifuge for 3 min.
3. Transfer 225 µL of the upper phase into another Eppendorf tube and add 100 µL 0.25M Tris buffer.
4. Repeat vortexing and spinning, and transfer 150 µL of the upper phase again in a fresh tube.
5. Add again 100 µL of 0.25M Tris buffer and repeat the vortexing and spinning steps.
6. Add 75 µL of the upper phase to 12 mL scintillation liquide (Ready-Safe scintillant, Promega) in a scintillation vial.
7. Measure the dpm of $[^{14}C]$ for 5 min by at least 5 cycles in a liquide scintillation counter (LS 6000 LL apparatus, Beckman Instruments).

The CAT-reporter experiments revealed that the mdr1 promoter-driven CAT expression is inducible by the addition of cytostatic drugs as shown for vincristine in transduced HCT15 (A) and KM12 (B) colon carcinoma cells. **Figure 3** depicts concentration dependence of the drug-induced CAT expression in the TLC (CAT-TLC, **Fig. 3A** and **B**) and LSC (CAT-LSC, **Fig. 3A** and **B**) assay after addition of vincristine.

3.4. Construction of the Drug-Inducible Retroviral Vector

For the construction of the drug-inducible retroviral vector, we used the mdr1 promoter PCR product as described in **Subheading 3.1.** for the cloning into the pSP72 (Promega) plasmid (*see* **Fig. 2**).

1. Digest the PCR amplified mdr1 promoter fragment with *Eco*RI/*Bam*HI as described in **Subheading 3.1.**
2. Digest 1 µg of the pSP72 plasmid DNA with *Eco*RI/*Bam*HI for 2 h at 37°C.
3. For ligation, purify the plasmid DNA as described in **Subheading 3.2.**
4. Ligate the *Eco*RI/*Bam*HI digested mdr1 promoter fragment into the *Eco*RI/*Bam*HI digested pSP72 plasmid with T4 ligase for 4 h at 14°C.
5. Follow **Subheading 3.1., step 10.** for minipreparation of plasmid DNA.
6. After isolation of mdr1 promoter harboring bacterial clones, grow a 500 µL LB culture in the presence of 100 mg/mL ampicillin. Perform large-scale preparation of the plasmid DNA for further cloning procedures using the Plasmid DNA purification kit (Quiagen).
7. Digest 5 µg of the mdr1 promoter harboring pSP72 plasmid with *Bgl*II/*Bam*HI for 2 h at 37°C to release the 374 bp mdr1 promoter fragment and run the

A

CAT-TLC

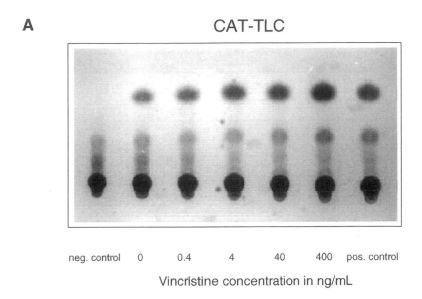

| neg. control | 0 | 0.4 | 4 | 40 | 400 | pos. control |

Vincristine concentration in ng/mL

CAT-LSC

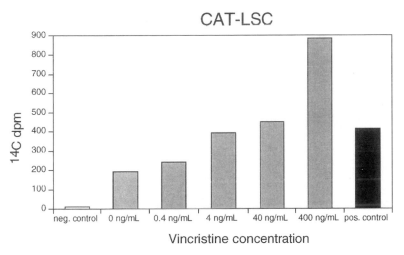

Vincristine concentration

Fig. 3. CAT-reporter assay in pCAT-Basic-mdr-p transduced HCT15 (**A**) and KM12 (**B**) human colon carcinoma cells. The cells were treated with different concentrations of vincristine (*see* **Subheading 3.3.**) and CAT-activity was determined in the thin layer chromatogaphy (CAT-TLC) and liqud scintillation counting (CAT-LSC). Both assays indicate the inducibility of the CAT expression in the two cell lines, which increases with elevating drug concentrations. pCAT-Basic transduced cells served as negative control (neg. control) and pSV2CAT transduced cells represent the positive control (pos. control). The [^{14}C]dpm values were normalized to the respective protein concentration of the cell lysates.

digested DNA on a 1% agarose gel. Prepare the promoter DNA as described in **Subheading 3.2.3.**

8. Take 1 µg of the pM3-hTNF retroviral vector *(26)* and digest with *Bam*HI at 37°C for 2 h. Purify the vector DNA as described in **Subheading 3.2.2.**

9. Ligate the *Bgl*II/*Bam*HI digested mdr1 promoter fragment into the *Bam*HI site of the pM3-hTNF retroviral vector at 14°C for 4 h using T4 DNA ligase.

10. After ligation, transform DH5α competent cells and follow **Subheading 3.1., steps 10** and **11.** for minipreparation of vector DNAs.

11. For identification of mdr1 promoter carrying clones in the miniprep plasmid, DNAs digest the DNA with *Eco*RI/*Bam*HI to release the promoter fragment if inserted in the correct orientation (*see* **Fig. 2**). Run the digested DNAs on 1% agarose gel and select positive clones.

12. Prepare sufficient vector DNA in large-scale preparations for the further transfection experiments.

The resulting pM3mdr-p-hTNF retroviral vector harbors the human mdr1 promoter, which drives the expression of the human TNFα gene. This construct was employed for detailed studies to achieve cytostatic drug-inducible expression of the cytokine gene in transduced human tumor cell lines.

3.5. Transfection and Drug-Inducible Gene Expression in Tumor Cells

3.5.1. Establishment of TNFa Expressing Cell Clones

The neomycin resistance gene in the retroviral vector pM3mdr-p-hTNF allows selection of stably transduced cell clones using G418.

1. Trypsinize exponentially growing MCF-7 human mammary carcinoma cells and perform transfection of these cells using 20 µg pM3mdr-p-hTNF vector DNA. Follow the transfection protocol described in **Subheading 3.3.**

2. Start selection of vector harboring cell clones 48 h after transfection by adding 0.5 mg/mL G418 (Life Technologies) to the cell-culture medium (*see* **Note 12**).

3. Isolate G418 resistant cell clones by ring cloning and transfer the isolated clones into 24-well plates. Grow the clones in the presence of G418.

4. When these clones reach almost confluence, take 100 µL aliquots of the cell-culture medium, which should have been on the cells for at least 24 h. Use these aliquots for screening of TNFα expression by TNF-ELISA (BioSource).

5. Select TNFα expressing cell clones (*see* **Note 13**) and expand them for further studies. These cell clones have to be treated repeatedly with G418 (every 2 to 4 wk) to prevent potential outgrowth of nontransduced cells.

3.5.2. Drug-Inducible TNFα Expression in Transduced Tumor Cells

The drug-induced TNFα expression of pM3mdr-p-hTNF transduced MCF-7 mammary carcinoma cells was determined at mRNA and at protein levels by

B

CAT-TLC

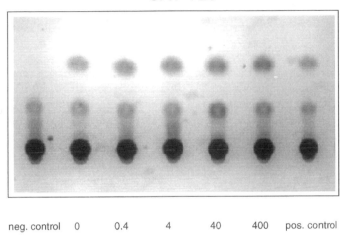

| neg. control | 0 | 0.4 | 4 | 40 | 400 | pos. control |

Vincristine concentration in ng/mL

CAT-LSC

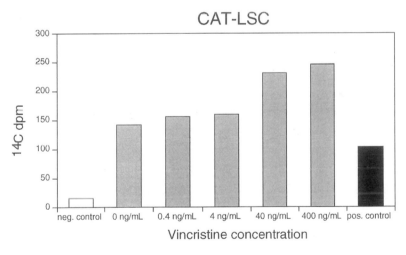

Fig. 3B.

using TNFα-specific RT-PCR and TNFα-specific ELISA. These studies included the evaluation of time- and drug-concentration dependence of the drug-inducible expression mediated by the mdr1 promoter in the pM3mdr-p-hTNF retroviral vector. Both methods, RT-PCR and the ELISA allow the semiquantitative or quantitative analysis of TNFα expression to evaluate the efficacy of the mdr1 promoter mediated drug inducibility.

1. Seed 5×10^4 pM3mdr-p-hTNF transduced cells into a 12-well plate and grow the cells for 24 h at 37°C.

2. Add the cytostatic drugs adriamycin or vincristine to the cells for the induction of cytokine expression: final concentrations for vincristine are 25, 50, and 100 ng/mL and for adriamycin 400, 800, and 1200 ng/mL (*see* **Note 14**). Incubate the cells for the desired time at 37°C.

3. Harvest cells 0, 2, 4, 6, 12, and 24 h after drug addition for total cellular RNA isolation: remove the medium, wash the cells once with 1 mL ice cold PBS, and add 500 µL LiCl/urea solution for RNA isolation. Transfer this viscous solution to an Eppendorf tube and let stand on ice for 20 min. Centrifuge at 14,000 rpm for 20 min at 4°C, discard the supernatant and redissolve the viscous pellet in 250 µL TES buffer and vortex. Add 250 µL phenol/chloroform, vortex and centrifuge at 14,000 rpm for 10 min. Transfer the supernatant to another Eppendorf tube add 1/10 vol 3*M* sodium acetate and 2.5 vol ethanol and precipitate the RNA a −70°C for 20 min. Spin at 14,000 rpm for 15 min at 4°C, wash the pellets with 500 µL 70% DEPC-ethanol, dry the pellets, and redissolve in 10 mL DEPC-water.

4. Take 1 µg of total cellular RNAs and random hexamer primers, run the RT-reaction at 42°C for 15 min, denaturate at 95°C for 15 min, and cool at 5°C for 5 min.

5. Use the TNFα-specific and β-actin specific primers for the PCR. Perform the PCR with amplification at 95°C for 2 min and 35 cycles of melting (95°C, 1 min), annealing-extending with *Taq* polymerase (60°C, 1 min) and a final step at 72°C for 7 min.

6. Run the PCR products on a 1.5% agarose gel (**Fig. 4A**) and semiquantify densities of DNA bands from video images by densitometry using the Image 1.44b11 program (obtained from Wayne Rasband, NIMH, Bethesda, MD). The semiquantification is normalized to the expression level of β-actin and is compared to the expression level of the nontreated transduced cells.

7. For the TNFα-ELISA, harvest the supernatants of drug-treated cells 0, 4, 6, 24, 48, 72, 96, and 120 h after drug addition, collect in Eppendorf tubes and freeze at −70°C until the ELISA is performed. Take transduced but non-induced cells as controls and collect the supernatants at the same time-points.

8. Take 2×100 µL aliquots as duplicates for each time-point of drug induction and perform the TNFα-ELISA using the Cytoscreen ELISA kit.

9. Read absorbance at 450 nm in a microplate reader and determine the TNFα values by using the EasySoftG200/Easy-Fit software. Calculate the TNFα amount in pg/mL (**Fig. 4B**).

In these studies of drug-induced TNFα expression in MCF-7 cells, we demonstrated that the human mdr1 promoter mediates the upregulation of the cytokine expression during the treatment with the cytostatic drugs adriamycin, vincristine, but also by taxol. All these drugs are known to be related to the multidrug resistance phenomenon (MDR). **Fig. 4A** shows a representative

A

time of vincristine induction

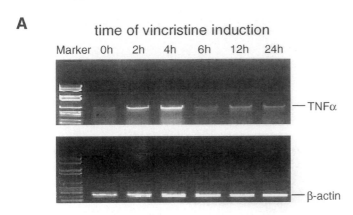

B

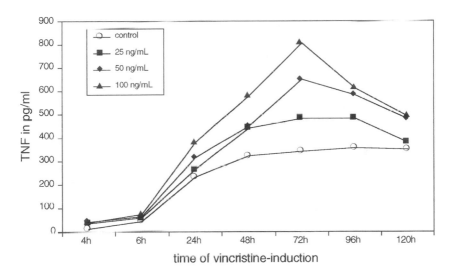

Fig. 4. Expression of TNFα in vincristine-induced pM3mdr-p-hTNF transduced MCF-7 cells. Cells were treated with different concentrations of vincristine (25, 50, 100 ng/mL) and TNFα mRNA and protein expression was analyzed by TNFα-specific RT-PCR (**A**) or ELISA (**B**) at indicated time-points (*see* **Subheading 3.5.2.**).

experiment in pM3mdr-p-hTNF transduced MCF-7 cells: the TNFα mRNA expression is induced 2 to 4 h after addition of the drug vincristine (**Fig. 4A**), whereas secretion of the TNFα protein increases 24 to 120 h after drug application (**Fig. 4B**). We observed that this type of induction kinetic can also be seen in other transduced tumor cell lines and for other inducing drugs *(28)*.

3.6. Analysis of the Antitumor Effect
of Drug-Induced TNFα Expression

To evaluate the therapeutic potential of the drug-induced expression of the chemosensitizing cytokine TNFα, cytotoxicity assays with pM3mdr-p-hTNF transduced and nontransduced tumor cells were performed. The intended therapeutic concept aims at the drug induction of the cytokine expression at nontoxic drug concentrations to sensitize the tumor cells for the subsequent treatment with therapeutically relevant doses of the respective cytostatic drug. In the present protocol, adriamycin was used for drug induction and subsequent chemotherapeutic treatment.

1. Plate 5×10^3 pM3mdr-p-hTNF transduced and nontransduced MCF-7 cells into each well of 96-well microtiter plates and grow the cells for 24 h.
2. For drug induction of TNFα expression, incubate the cells with 800 ng/mL adriamycin for 24 h at 37°C (*see* **Note 15**).
3. Then, remove the medium from treated, but also from untreated control cells, wash cells with 200 µL medium and add another 200 µL medium containing adriamycin at the final concentration of 1600 ng/mL.
4. Incubate the cells for 3 d at 37°C.
5. Remove the medium, wash the cells once with 200 µL PBS, and add 100 µL MTT solution to each well.
6. After incubation with MTT for 3 h at 37°C, solubilize the formazan dye with 150 µL SDS solution.
7. Measure the absorbance at 450 nm in a microplate reader (SLT Labinstruments) (*see* **Note 16**). The absorbance of untreated control cells was taken as 100% survival and the percentage of growth inhibition was calculated using the EasySoftG200/Easy-Base software (SLT Labinstruments).

The cytotoxicity studies have shown that the combination of drug-induced TNFα expression and subsequent treatment with therapeutic doses of the respective cytostatic drug produces higher chemosensitivity of the transduced tumor cells (*see* **Fig. 5**).

In summary, all these studies demonstrate that the human mdr1 promoter is suitable for the construction of a conditional drug-inducible vector system, which can be employed for gene therapy of cancer. The regulation of gene expression by chemotherapy of tumors is an attractive concept combining gene therapy approaches with conventional chemotherapy. Using this approach, we have shown that mdr1 promoter-mediated temporal expression of genes can be utilized to augment efficacy of chemotherapy such as chemosensitization of tumor cells by the expression of TNFα (*28,29*).

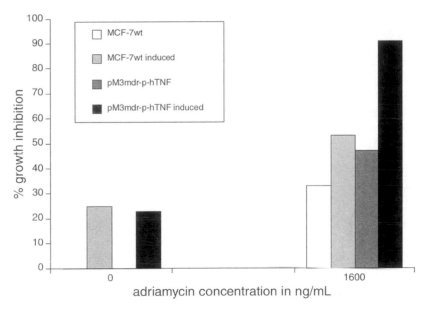

Fig. 5. Combined effects of drug-induced TNFα expression and adriamycin application on tumor cell growth. The pM3mdr-p-hTNF transduced MCF-7 cells were induced for TNFα expression by addition of 800 ng/mL adriamycin for 24 h at 37°C. Then, cells were either treated with 1600 ng/mL adriamycin (right panel) or were incubated in drug-free medium (left panel) for 3 d at 37°C. Thereafter, the MTT cytotoxicity assay was performed (*see* **Subheading 3.6.**).

4. Notes

1. We do not use antibiotics as additives for cell-culture medium, because substances such as penicillin, streptomycin, amphotericin, and so on could interfere in cytotoxicity assays or with activities of substances like cytokines used in our studies. To ensure quality of utilized cell lines, cells are routinely tested for sterility and potential mycoplasma infection.
2. Use caution when cytostatic drugs are involved in the studies; these are toxic and/or mutagenic compounds. It is important, to make up all diluted working solutions of the drugs freshly at the time when they are needed, because during time, these drugs can lose activity, particularly if the drugs are dissolved in cell-culture medium. Stock solutions of the drugs should be stored at 4°C.
3. For preparation of RNA, it is essential to autoclave all glassware and plasticware (if not provided sterile from the manufacturer) to prevent possible RNase contamination.

4. Because the sarcoma tissue can be very solid and rigid material, it may be necessary to pulverize the tissue in a homogenizer in liquid nitrogen before transferring to the Dounce homogenizer. This procedure will improve the yield of DNA.

5. When using PCR primers with restriction sites at the respective ends, it is important to make sure to add sufficient flanking bases close to the respective restriction endonuclease recognition site (cleavage close to the end of DNA fragments). This is essential to ensure complete digestion of the required restriction sites by the enzymes in a given incubation time.

6. Meanwhile, there are very fast and efficient cloning kits available (Invitrogen) making the direct cloning of PCR products faster and easier. These kits utilize the topoisomerase I as the ligating enzyme.

7. When performing ligations, it is of essential importance to chose the right ratio of insert and vector DNA in the ligation mix. If the insert is relatively small, a three- to fourfold excess of insert DNA will improve ligation efficiencies.

8. After the electroporation, many cell lines tend to form viscous cell suspensions and it is important to resuspend the cells thoroughly in medium for better attachment of the cells.

9. Because of our observation, protease inhibitors prevent the degradation of the CAT-protein, which results in better measurements for the CAT-assay.

10. For a nonradioactive method, alternatively the CAT-ELISA assay (Boehringer Mannheim) can also be employed. This system generates reproducible results and allows quantitation of CAT enzyme amounts in the lysates.

11. For better orientation after development of the exposed X-ray film, mark definite spots onto the plate with 1.5 µL of ^{14}C-chloramphenicol.

12. We observed that in most transduced cell lines, which have been treated with G418 resistant colonies start to appear after 14 d of treatment. It is useful to isolate colonies with reasonable size (50 to 100 cells), because during the ring cloning with sterile stainless steel or glass cylinders (diameter approximately 5 mm) loss of cells can occur.

13. We preferably selected clones expressing a minimum TNFα concentration of 100 pg TNF/mL secreted by 1×10^6 cells in 24 h. The expression of TNFα was confirmed by TNF-specific RT-PCR using total cellular RNA from these cell clones.

14. Before we used these concentration ranges for adriamycin and vincristine, these drugs had to be tested for their cytotoxicities in the MTT assay to estimate the IC_{50} for the respective cell line. In the drug-induction experiments, drug concentrations were used which did not exceed 20% of growth inhibition.

15. The drug concentration we used for the drug induction of TNFα expression was chosen, because this concentration exerted only minimal cytotoxic effects of 20% to 30% growth inhibition. This is a good basis to evaluate possible synergistic effects between the drug and the antitumor activity of the cytokine.

16. The formazan dye forms small crystals at the bottom of the well. To dissolve these crystals, SDS or DMSO has to be added. The microtiter plates should be shaken before measurement.

Acknowledgment

This study was supported by Feodor-Lynen Fellowships (to W. Walther and U. Stein) of the Alexander von Humboldt Foundation (Bonn, Germany), the Office of International Affairs, National Cancer Institute (Bethesda, MD) and the Boehringer Mannheim GmbH (Penzberg, Germany).

References

1. Bushman, F. (1995) Targeting retroviral integration. *Science* **267,** 1443–1444.
2. Friedmann, T. and Yee, J.-K. (1995) Pseudotyped retroviral vectors for studies of human gene therapy. *Nature Med.* **1,** 275–277.
3. Kasahara, N., Dozy, A. M., and Kan Y. W. (1994) Tissue-specific targeting of retroviral vectors through ligand-receptor interactions. *Science* **266,** 1373–1376.
4. Salmons, B. and Günzburg, W. H. (1993) Targeting of retroviral vectors for gene therapy. *Hum. Gene Ther.* **4,** 129–141.
5. Walther, W. and Stein, U. (1996) Cell type specific and inducible promoters for vectors in gene therapy as an approach for cell targeting. *J. Mol. Med.* **74,** 379–392.
6. Miller, N. and Whelan, J. (1997) Progress in transcriptionally targeted and regulatable vectors for genetic therapy. *Hum. Gene Ther.* **8,** 803–815.
7. Boothman, D. A., Lee, I. W., and Sahijdak, W. M. (1994) Isolation of an X-ray-responsive element in the promoter region of tissue-type plasminogen activator: potential uses of X-ray-responsive elements for gene therapy. *Radiat. Res.* **138 (1Suppl.),** S68–71.
8. Hallahan, D. E., Mauceri, H. J., Seung, L. P., Dunphy, E. J., Wayne, J. D., Hanna, N. N., et al. (1995) Spatial and temporal control of gene therapy using ionizing radiation. *Nature Med.* **1,** 786–791.
9. Williams, G. T. and Morimoto, R. I. (1990) Maximal stress-induced transcription from the human HSP70 promoter requires interactions with the basal promoter elements independent of the rotational alignment. *Mol. Cell. Biol.* **10,** 3125–3136.
10. Gazit, G., Kane, S. E., Nichols, P., and Lee, A. S. (1995) Use of the stress-inducible grp78/BiP promoter in targeting high level gene expression in fibrosarcoma in vivo. *Cancer Res.* **55,** 1660–1663.
11. Dachs, G. U., Patterson, A. V., Firth, J. D., Ratcliffe, P. J., Townsend, K. M. S., Stratford, I. J., and Harris A. L. (1997) Targeting gene expression to hypoxic tumor cells. *Nature Med.* **3,** 515–520.
12. Blackburn, R. V., Golaforo, S. S., Corry, P. M., and Lee, Y. J. (1998) Adenoviral-mediated transfer of a heat-inducible double suicide gene into prostate carcinoma cells. *Cancer Res.* **58,** 1358–1362.
13. Chin, K. V., Tanaka, S., Darlington, G., Pastan, I., and Gottesmann, M. M. (1990) Heat shock and arsenite in rease expression of the multidrug resistance (MDR1) gene in human renal carcinoma cells. *J. Biol. Chem* **256,** 221–226.
14. Chaudhary, P. M. and Roninson, I. B (1992) Activation of MDR1 (p-glycoprotein) gene expression in human cells by protein kinase C agonists. *Oncol. Res.* **4,** 281–290.
15. Uchiumi, T., Kohno, K., Tanimura, H., Matsuo, K., Sato, S., Uchida Y., and

Kuwano, M. (1993) Enhanced expression of the human multidrug resistance 1 gene in response to UV light irradiation. *Cell Growth Differ.* **4,** 147–157.

16. Licht, T., Fiebig, H. H., Bross, K. J., Herrmann, F., Berger, D. P., Shoemaker, R., and Mertelsmann, R. (1991) Induction of multiple drug resistance during antineoplastic chemotherapy in vitro. *Int. J. Cancer* **49,** 630–637.
17. Chaudhary, P. M. and Roninson, I. B. (1993) Induction of multidrug resistance in human cells by transient exposure to different chemotherapeutic drugs. *J. Natl. Cancer Inst.* **85,** 632–639.
18. Kohno, K., Sato, S.-I., Takano, H., Matsuo, K.-I., and Kuwano, M. (1989) The direct activation of human multidrug resistance gene (MDR1) by anticancer agents. *Biochem. Biophys. Res. Comm.* **165,** 1415–1421.
19. Stein, U., Walther, W., and Wunderlich, V. (1994) Point mutations in the mdr1 promoter of human osteosarcomas are associated with in vitro responsiveness to multidrug resistance relevant drugs. *Eur. J. Cancer* **30A,** 1541–1545.
20. Iwahashi, T., Okochi, E., Ono, K., Sugawara, I., Tsuruo, T., and Mori, S. (1991) Establishment of multidrug resistant human colorectal HCT-15 cell lines and their properties. *Anticancer Res.* **11,** 1309–1312.
21. Morikawa, K., Walker, S. M., Nakajima, M., Pathak, S., Jessup, J. M., and Fidler I. J. (1988) Influence of organ environment on the growth selection, and metastasis of human colon carcinoma cells in nude mice. *Cancer Res.* **48,** 6863–6871.
22. Soule, H. D., Vasquez, J., Long, A., Albert, S., and Brennan, M. (1973) A human cell line from a pleural effusion derived from a breast carcinoma. *J. Natl. Cancer Inst.* **51,** 1409–1416.
23. Kohno, K., Sato, S.-I., Uchiumi, T., Takano, H., Kato, S., and Kuwano, M. (1990) Tissue specific enhancer of the human multidrg-resistance (MDR1) gene. *J. Biol. Chem.* **265,** 19,690–19,696.
24. Brenner, C. A., Daniel, S. L., and Adler, R. R. (1989) Cytokine mapping: observation and quantification of cytokine mRNA in small numbers of cells using the polymerase chain reaction, in *Cytokines-A Practical Approach* (Balkwill, F. R., ed). Oxford University Press, Oxford, pp. 51–59.
25. Wu, L., Smythe, A. M., Stinson, S. F., Mullendore, L. A., Monks, A., Scudiero, D. A., et al. (1992) Multidrug resistant phenotype of disease-oriented panels of human tumor cell lines used for anticancer drug screening. *Cancer Res.* **52,** 3029–3034.
26. Walther, W., Fichtner, I., and Uckert, W. (1993) Retrovirus-mediated gene transfer of tumor necrosis factor alpha into colon carcinoma cells generates a growth inhibition. *Anticancer Res.* **13,** 1565–1574.
27. Sambrook, J., Fritsch, E. F., and Maniatis, T. (1989) *Molecular Cloning*, 2nd ed., Cold Spring Harbor Laboratory, Cold Spring Harbor, pp. 1.26–1.28.
28. Walther, W., Wendt, J., and Stein, U. (1997) Employment of the mdr1 promoter for the chemotherapy-inducible expression of therapeutic genes in cancer gene therapy. *Gene Ther.* **4,** 544–552.
29. Stein, U., Walther, W., and Shoemaker R. H. (1996) Reversal of multidrug resistance by transduction of cytokine genes into human colon carcinoma cells. *J. Natl. Cancer Inst.* **88,** 1383–1392.

I

EXPERIMENTAL APPROACHES IN CANCER GENE THERAPY

G: Alternative Approaches in Cancer Gene Therapy

24

Oncolytic Adenoviral Vectors

Ramon Alemany and Wei-Wei Zhang

1. Introduction

After an initial attempt to use adenoviruses as lytic agents for the treatment of cancer in the 1950's, and many cancer gene therapy attempts in the 1990's using replication-deficient adenoviruses as vectors of transgenes, a new wave of replication-competent adenoviruses have been recently developed for cancer treatment *(1–3)*. This virotherapy revival has been stirred up by the difficulty of nonreplicating vectors to reach all tumor cells, even when the vectors carry transgenes that produce a bystander effect in proximal nontransduced cells. This new generation of replication-competent viruses differs from the previously used wild-type adenoviruses in that they replicate selectively in tumors cells, but not in normal cells. One of the approaches in the design of conditionally replication-competent adenoviruses is to delete viral genes used to inactivate the brakes of the cell cycle in normal cells *(4,5)*. Another approach is to regulate viral replication in tumor cells by controlling the expression of early viral genes with promoters of tumor-associated proteins *(6,7)*. A different strategy to confine viral replication is to use a plasmid-based transcomplementation of E1A to support one replication round of an E1A-deleted adenovirus in the cotransduced cells *(8)*. Further development along this line is to design complementary vectors, which allow viral replication in coinfected cells (**Fig. 1**).

It is important to analyze to what extent these random or designed mutations abrogate viral replication in normal cells because a tightly controlled vector could be injected at higher doses intratumorally or even systemically. On the other hand, it is also important to analyze to what extent these mutations affect the amount of virus produced per infected tumor cell (burst size) compared to wild-type virus because lower yields will result in a slower propagation throughout the tumor. Finally, as concluded from the clinical trials with wild-

From: *Methods in Molecular Medicine, Vol. 35: Gene Therapy: Methods and Protocols*
Edited by: W. Walther and U. Stein © Humana Press, Inc., Totowa, NJ

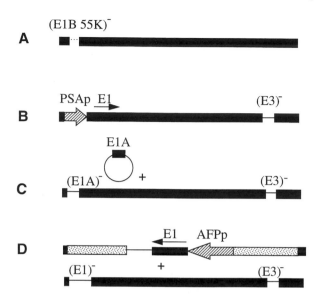

Fig. 1. Four current adenoviruses designed for tumor-specific oncolysis. (**A**) Onyx-O15 (dl1520) contains a 827-bp deletion in E1B and a point mutation at codon 2022 that prevents expression of this gene *(4)*. (**B**) CN706 contains an enhancer/promoter element from the prostate-specific antigen inserted upstream the E1A gene *(7)*. (**C**) Ionic linkage of a plasmid containing E1A to the capsid of an E1A-deleted virus enables one round of replication of the virus. Tumor-specificity could be easily designed in this system deleting the Rb-binding domain of E1A or inserting a tumor-specific promoter in front of E1A. (**D**) A gutless or miniAd vector containing E1 under the control of the AFP promoter is designed to complement an E1-deleted vector in cells that express AFP.

type adenoviruses, the most crucial element in the outcome of the oncolysis is the host immune response to the virus. This response can block the viral spread before all tumor cells have been infected and allow the tumors to relapse. Further manipulations of the adenoviral vectors are needed to make them not only oncolytic, but also effective in interacting with host immune responses. This chapter describes protocols to analyze these safety and efficacy aspects of oncolytic adenoviral vectors that are conditionally replication-competent.

2. Materials
2.1. Production and Characterization of Vectors

1. NaNO$_2$ solution: 0.7 M NaNO$_2$ in 1 M sodium acetate buffer, pH 4.6.
2. CaCl$_2$ 2.5M: 36.75 g in 100 mL, filter (0.22 μm) and aliquot. Store at –20°C.
3. 2XBBS:50 mM BES pH 6.95 (pH is important), 280 mM NaCl, 1.5 mM Na$_2$HPO$_4$. Prepared with "Cell culture tested" Sigma reagents by mixing BES

2.132 g, NaCl 3.27 g, 1M Na$_2$HPO$_4$ 300 μL, H$_2$0 to 200 mL. Adjust pH, filter, and store aliquots at –20°C.

4. 10X first strand buffer: 500 mM Tris-HCl pH 8.3, 500 mM KCl, 100 mM MgCL$_2$, 5 mM spermidine, 100 mM DTT.
5. DOC lysis buffer: 20 % EtOH, 100 mM Tris-HCl pH 9.0, 0.4% sodium deoxicholate.
6. SDS-PAGE sample buffer: 0.125M Tris-HCl, pH6.8, 2% SDS, 10% 2-mercapto-ethanol, 10% glycerol, 10 μg/mL Bromophenol blue.

2.2. Tumor Specificity and Efficiency of Propagation

1. Psoralen: Prepare a 100X stock (33 mg/mL) of 8-Methoxypsoralen (Sigma, St. Louis, MO) in dimethylsulfoxide.
2. Peroxidase developing solutions: 3-amino-9-ethylcarbazole (Sigma) in 0.05M acetate buffer, pH 5.0. 3,3′-diaminobenzidine (Sigma) in Tris-HCl pH 7.3 with 0.006% H$_2$O$_2$.
3. Lysis buffer: 10 mM EDTA, 10 mM Tris-HCl pH 7.4, 0.6% SDS.
4. SSC 10 X: 1.5M NaCl, 0.15M sodium citrate.
5. Nitrocellulose blocking buffer: 50 mM Tris-HCl (pH 7.5), 150 mM NaCl, 5% dry milk, 0.1% Tween 20.

2.3. Immune Responses

1. Coating buffer: 50 mM NaHCO$_3$/Na$_2$CO$_3$ pH 9.6.
2. Digestion buffer: 1 mg/mL Type IV collagenase, 50 U/mL DNase I (Sigma) in DMEM.

3. Methods
3.1. Production and Characterization of Vectors

The genomic changes to achieve tumor-specific replication can be obtained by random mutagenesis and selection or can be designed based on the molecular alterations of the target tumor cells. In the case of designed modifications of the viral DNA, the virus can then be generated in 293 cells or directly in the target tumor cells. In the latter case, different tumor cell lines can be analyzed for promoter activity, infectivity, and virus yields in order to choose the best cell line for the generation and propagation of the vector. Besides these three factors, when generating a vector by transfection the transfection efficiency of the target tumor cell lines should also be considered to choose the initial target cell line. **Notes 1–6** give some guidelines on the design of mutations.

3.1.1. Construction of Vectors by Random Mutagenesis (see **Notes 7** and **8**)

Mutagenesis of a purified virus stock (*see* **Note 3** as an alternative method):

1. Mix 0.1 mL of virus stock with 1.9 mL of $NaNO_2$ at RT for 8 min.
2. Stop the reaction by adding four volumes of cold $1M$ Tris-HCl pH 7.9.
3. Dilute the final mixture 50 times with culture medium.

Mutagenesis in infected cultures:

1. Infect monolayers at 10 multiplicity of infection (MOI).
2. Add medium without serum, but containing 50 μg/mL of 5-fluorouracil or 5 μg/mL of N-methyl-N'-nitro-N-nitrosoguanidine.
3. Incubate until cytophatic effect (CPE).

3.1.2. Vector Generation in 293 Cells by Cotransfection (see **Notes 10–12**)

1. Prepare a 50–60% confluent monolayer of cells in 6-well plates.
2. For each well of a 6-well plate, mix in order: 2 μg of shuttle plasmid + 2 μg of pJM17 (or other) + H_2O to 110 μL + 12.5 μL of 2.5M $CaCl_2$.
3. Add 125 μL of 2X BBS and mix.
4. Incubate 10 min at RT to allow DNA precipitate to form.
5. Add dropwise the 250 μL DNA precipitate into the well onto a 50–60% confluent monolayer in which medium has been changed (DMEM 10% FCS, 2 mL/well) 2 h before transfection.
6. Incubate overnight in 3% CO_2 (no 5%) incubator.
7. Next day, precipitate should be visible. Coarse precipitate indicates not enough DNA and extremely fine precipitate indicates too much DNA was used.
8. Change medium every day and monitor the monolayer for the onset of plaques (if overlaid with agarose) or appearance of CPE (if no overlay).

3.1.3. Vector Generation Directly in Target Tumor Cells (see **Note 13**)

3.1.3.1. RT-PCR TO CHECK PROMOTER ACTIVITY (SEE **NOTE 14**)

1. Wash cell monolayer ($\sim 3 \times 10^6$ cells) once with PBS, scrape the cells and pellet them in an Eppendorf tube.
2. Resuspend cells in 1 mL of Trizol (Life Technologies, Gaithersburg, MD) and incubate at RT 15 min.
3. Add 200 μL chloroform, shake 10 s, incubate RT 3 min, and microfuge at 9000 rpm (7500g), 4°C, 15 min.
4. Transfer the supernatant to a new Eppendorf and add 0.5 mL of isopropanol to precipitate the RNA.
5. Spin at 9000 rpm in a microcentrifuge (7500g), 15 min, 4°C to pellet the RNA.
6. Wash pellet with 75% ethanol and resuspend it in 50 μL of DEPC-H20 / 1 mM EDTA.
7. Heat at 55°C for 10 min and measure RNA concentration by OD.
8. To 2.5 μg RNA, add H_2O-DEPC to 19 μL and 1.5 μL of oligo-dT (0.1 μg/μL).

9. Mix and incubate in a heat block at 65°C for 5 min.
10. Cool down slowly to RT placing the block on the bench.
11. Add 2.5 μL of 10X first strand buffer, 0.5 μL RNase inhibitor (40 U/μL), 1 μL of a solution of 25 mM of each dNTP, and 0.5 μL of MMLV-RT (50 U/μL).
12. Mix and incubate at 37°C for 1 h.
13. Heat at 90°C for 5 min.
14. Cool on ice and store at –80°C.
15. To 1 μL of reverse-transcribed product, add 14 μL of H$_2$O, 2 μL of 10X *Taq* buffer, 0.5 μL of primers (20 μM), and 0.25 μL of *Taq*.
16. Cycle: 95°C for 30 s, 55°C for 30 s, 72°C for 1 min; 30 cycles.
17. Separate the PCR product in a 2% agarose gel.

3.1.3.2. INFECTIVITY TEST (*SEE* NOTES 15 AND 16)

1. Infect cells with a serial dilution of the vector in the corresponding medium/serum used for each cell line using the same conditions of confluence (90%), volume (1 mL/well in 6 well-plates) and adsorption time (2 h).
2. Count the number of cells transduced for each cell line at 48 h postinfection (use A549 cells as standard cell line).

3.1.3.3. PRODUCTION OF VIRUS/BURST SIZE (*SEE* NOTES 17 AND 18)

1. Extract virus from the cells that were initially used to generate the virus by three cycles of quick freeze-and-thaw of the cell pellets at 48 h postinfection.
2. Starting from undiluted crude extract, use the same standard conditions of infections and serial dilution as above (1 mL per 9.6 cm^2 well; 2 h adsorption time) to determine the titer of the crude extract.
3. If the vector contains a reporter gene the easiest way to determine the titer is by counting the A549-transducing units 48 h after infection.
4. For vectors without reporter genes and based on E1 regulation, titer is estimated in a 293 plaque assay.
5. Taking into account the titer and the infectivity of each cell line, infect different cell lines with a MOI that will transduce all cells.
6. Per each cell line to be compared, prepare 21 wells of a 24-well plate so that cells are 90% confluent at the time of infection.
7. Use three wells to count the cell number and 18 to inoculate the vector (200 μL/well; 2 h adsorption).
8. Next day, rinse cells twice with fresh medium and then from day 0 to day 5 harvest the cells (per triplicate) and extract the virus by three freeze-and-thaw cycles.
9. Determine the number of tu or PFU in the crude extracts by infecting A549 or 293 cells, respectively, with serial dilution. An increase over time in these numbers indicate the production of new virus.

3.2. Stability of the Vector

3.2.1. Spermine Precipitation Method
to Isolate Encapsidated Viral DNA (**Fig. 2**)

1. At CPE, harvest and pellet the infected cells and resuspend them in TE pH 9.0 (400 μL per 10-cm dish).
2. Add 1 vol of DOC lysis buffer and mix by pipeting.
3. Transfer to an Eppendorf and add 8 μL of 500 mM spermine-HCl, mix and incubate for 10 min on ice. It will turn white as a precipitate of proteins, cellular DNA, and unpackaged viral DNA forms.
4. Microcentrifuge at maximal speed for 4 min at 4°C and transfer the supernatant to a new tube.
5. Add 40 μg RNase A and incubate 10 min at 37°C.
6. Add 60 μL of 10% SDS, 20 μl of 0.5 mL EDTA, and 2 mg of pronase and incubate for 1 h at 37°C.
7. Extract once with phenol/chloroform, add ammonium acetate to 2M, and precipitate with EtOH.
8. Resuspend the viral DNA in TE (10^7 infected cells yield approximately 15 μg of DNA.)

3.2.2. Metabolic Labeling to Analyze Virion Protein Composition

1. Incubate cells 24 h pi with met-cys free medium (Life Technologies) (met or cys alone can also be used) for 30 min.
2. Add ^{35}S-*met* and ^{35}S-*cys* (*trans*^{35}Slabel-ICN or Express-Dupont) (50 μCi/mL) for 1–2 h.
3. At the end of this labeling period, remove the medium, wash the cells with PBS, lyse cells with SDS-PAGE sample buffer (0.5 mL per 60-mm dish).
4. Heat for 5 min at 100°C, cool on ice, and spin for 15 min in microcentrifuge.
5. Run samples in a 12–17% polyacrylamide gel (50:0.235 acrylamide/bisacryl) overlaid by a 5% stacking gel (50:1.33 acrylamide/bisacrylamide).
6. Dry gel under vacuum, and expose to film.

3.3. Tumor Specificity and Efficiency of Propagation

The extent in which an oncolytic virus propagates in tumor cells vs normal cells is important to avoid a possible viremia after treatment, especially if the treatment is systemic and the cancer patient is immuno-compromised. Propagation in tumor vs normal cells can be compared using cell lines that present the tumor features to be targeted (such as the tumor-suppressor inactivation or promoter expression) vs cell lines or primary cells that do not present these features. Viral propagation can be analyzed at different levels: viral protein production, viral DNA replication, and production of viruses.

For these assays use a negative control vector prepared by UV inactivation as follows:

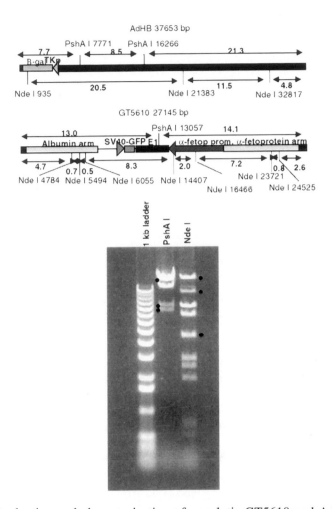

Fig. 2. Production and characterization of oncolytic GT5610 and AdHβ complementary vectors. A system of two adenoviral vectors that complement each other in
cells that express AFP is shown. The controlled vector GT5610 contains the minimal
adenoviral *cis* elements for replication and packaging and the E1 region of adenovirus
5 under the control of a 5 kb AFP promoter. GT5610 also contains the GFP reporter
gene and stuffer genomic sequences from the human albumin and AFP genes. The
supplemental vector AdHβ contains a β-galactosidase expression cassette replacing
the E1 adenoviral genes. After cotransfection and three passages in Hep G 2 cells,
*PshA*I and *Nde*I were used to perform a restriction analysis of spermidine-purified
viral DNA. Dots indicate bands derived from AdHβ.

1. Expose the purified virus in PBS/glycerol to three cycles of 120,000 µJ in a UV Stratalinker (model 1800, Stratagene, La Jolla, CA). In the presence of 330 µg/mL of psoralen, UV-inactivation can be achieved with 180 J/cm2 for 30 min. Psoralen must be removed by dialysis or chromatography (Sephadex G25 or G50).
2. Confirm inactivation in a 293 plaque assay.

3.3.1. Detection of Viral Genome Activity

3.3.1.1. IMMUNOHISTOCHEMISTRY OF HEXON/GENE EXPRESSION (SEE NOTE 19)

1. Grow cells in slide chambers and infect them with a MOI of 3.
2. Rinse cells 24 h postinfection with PBS and fix them with 10% formalin. A cell pellet of infected cells can also be frozen and cryosectioned in OCT to make slides.
3. Permeabilize cells in methanol for 30 s and wash in PBS. Incubate the sections in 1% (w/v) solution of BSA/PBS for 30 min at room temperature to block nonspecific binding of antibodies.
4. Incubate for 1 h at 37°C with anti-hexon antibody (MAB805, Chemicon International, Temecule, CA. 1:1000 dilution in BSA/PBS).
5. Wash twice with PBS and incubate for 1 h at 37°C with a biotinilated antimouse secondary antibody.
6. Add streptavidin-horseradish peroxidase conjugate (StrepABComplex, DAKO A/S, Glostrup, Denmark) and incubate for 10 min at 37°C.
7. Develop with 3-amino-9-ethylcarbazole or diaminobenzidine.
8. Counterstain with Harris' hematoxylin (Merk, Darmstadt, Germany) and coverslip with a mixture of PBS/Glycerol and Mowiol (Hoesch, Germany).

3.3.1.2. VIRAL DNA REPLICATION ASSAY WITH HIRT'S DNA (SEE NOTE 20)

1. Wash 10^7 cells with PBS and lyse them with 1 mL of lysis buffer for 10 min.
2. Add proteinase K (50 µg) and incubate for 1 h at 37°C.
3. Add NaCl to $1M$ and incubate for at least 4 h on ice (or overnight at 4°C).
4. Microcentrifuge at maximal speed for 30 min at 4°C and collect the supernatant.
5. Extract with phenol/chloroform twice and add 2 vol of ethanol to precipitate Hirt's DNA.
6. Resuspend the DNA in 50 µL of TE.
7. Treat 20 µL with the appropriate restriction enzymes, separate the fragments in a gel, transfer them to a nylon membrane, and carry out the hybridization using a viral DNA probe.

3.3.2. Quantification of In Vitro Propagation (see Note 21)

3.3.2.1. END-POINT CPE ASSAY

1. Prepare 10-fold dilutions of the virus stocks in DMEM/10% FCS.
2. Per triplicate add 100 µL to a 96-well flat-bottom microtiter plate.
3. Add 100 µL containing 10^5 cells of the cell lines to be analyzed.
4. Incubate at 37°C for 4 d and count dead cells by Trypan blue exclusion.

5. Express the virus titer for each cell line (which reflects its oncolytic potency) as the dilution that gives 50% of cell lysis.

3.3.2.2. PLAQUE ASSAY (*SEE* **NOTES 22** AND **23**)

1. Per triplicate, inoculate the monolayers with 1 mL/well (6-well plates) of the serial virus dilution prepared as above and incubate at 37°C for 2 h.
2. Melt 1% agarose (in H_2O) in a microwave or by autoclaving for 20 min and cool it to 45°C in a water bath.
3. Remove the virus and add 2.5 mL per well of a mixture of equal volumes of agarose and DMEM/ 20% FCS.
4. Let it solidify and add 1 mL of DMEM/ 10% FCS on top of the overlay.
5. Transfer the plates to the incubator and wait for plaques, changing the top medium when acidified. Addition of 0.034 % neutral red (Life Technologies) to the medium helps to visualize the plaques.
6. Over time, measure the plate size with a caliper to estimate the spread of the virus. Plaques are measured more accurately if the agarose is removed and the monolayer is fixed with 100% methanol or ethanol for 10 min and stained with 0.2% crystal violet in 2% ethanol for 5 min. Agarose can be more easily removed if final percentage is 0.9% instead of 0.5%.

3.3.3. Quantification of In Vivo Propagation (see **Notes 21**, **24** and **25**)

3.3.3.1. INTRATUMORAL VECTOR DETECTION (*SEE* **NOTE 26**)

1. Inject tumors with 10^5–10^6 transducting units (tu) of the vector in 20 μL. Use UV-inactivated vector or a nonreplicative vector as negative controls.
2. At different times, tumors are snap frozen in cold isopentane, cryosectioned to 6 μm, and mounted on silanized slides.
3. If the vectors contain reporter genes, detection is straightforward (**Fig. 3**). Vectors without reporter genes are detected by imunostaining the tumor sections as described in **Subheading 3.3.1.1.**
4. Quantitation can be attempted by processing entire tumors taking a section every 0.5 mm.

3.3.3.2. VECTOR EXTRACTION FROM TISSUES

1. Resect a piece of tumor and weigh it.
2. Homogenize the tissue with an ice-cold Teflon pestle in PBS and transfer it to a 15-mL tube containing 5 mL of plain medium (DMEM).
3. Vortex the mixture, freeze/thaw it twice, and spin it for 20 min at 1000g to separate the cellular debris from the homogenate.
4. Quantitate the viral titer in the supernatant by plaque assay on the appropriate tumor cells or in 293 cells as described in **Subheading 3.1.3.3.**

3.3.3.3. INTRATUMORAL DNA REPLICATION BY IN VIVO METABOLIC LABELING

1. Inject 200 μL of *Brd*U (RPN 201; Amersham, Arlington Heights, IL) intraperitoneally.

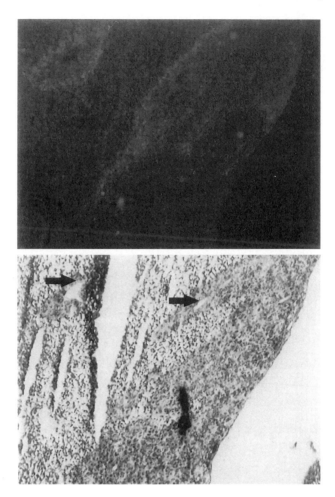

Fig. 3. Intratumoral detection of oncolytic vectors containing a reporter gene. Established hepatocellular carcinomas (HuH7, AFP+) were injected with purified GT5610/AdHβ following the protocol presented in **Subheading 3.3.4.** Twenty days after injection, one of the tumors in regression was resected for histological observation. Two serial sections are shown under fluorescence microscopy and hematoxylin/ eosin staining. Fluorescence is confined to the distal area of living cells surrounding the blood vessels (arrows). This pattern suggest that the viruses are spreading towards the proliferating cells around the blood vessels. Fluorescence filter: FITC (Fryer Company Inc. Huntley, IL); Camera Optronics DEI-750; exposure 2 s; magnification, ×100.

2. Three hours later, sacrifice the mice and extract genomic DNA from 100 mg of tumors (and other tissues to be analyzed) by the standard SDS/proteinase K method.
3. Digest 50 μg of DNA and separate the fragments on a 0.8% agarose gel.
4. Depurinize with HCl and transfer in 10X SSC to a nitrocellulose filter.

5. Immobilize DNA by UV or vacuum oven and block filter for 3 h at RT in nitro-cellulose blocking buffer.
6. Incubate overnight with anti-*BrdU* antibody (M0744; DAKO) diluted 1:50 in blocking buffer.
7. Wash twice and incubate for 2 h at RT with biotinylated anti-mouse IgG antibody (BA-2001; Vector Laboratories) diluted 1:100 in blocking buffer.
8. Wash, incubate for 1 h at RT with avidin-peroxidase (A-2004; Vector Laboratories, Burlingame, CA) diluted 1:2000 in blocking buffer.
9. Develop with an Enhanced Chemiluminiscent kit (ECL; Amersham).

3.3.4. Effect on Tumor Growth

3.3.4.1. MIXED CELL TUMORIGENICITY ASSAYS

1. Infect tumor cells with a MOI of 3 tu per cell.
2. Next day, mix infected cells with different amounts of uninfected cells (1:10 to 1:10,000).
3. Inject these mixtures of cells subcutaneously into the flanks of 6–8-wk-old SCID mice or nude mice. Inject 10^7 cells/100 µL per site and inject at least three mice per group with two injections per mice. Include 100% infected and 100% uninfected cells as controls.
4. Determine the highest ratio that prevents tumor growth.
5. Plot results as increase in tumor volume vs time and the fraction of animals remaining tumor-free vs time.

3.3.4.2. TREATMENT OF ESTABLISHED TUMORS (SEE NOTE 27)

1. Tripsinize tumor cells and wash them twice with PBS.
2. Inject 10^7 cells in 100 µL per site in both flanks of SCID or nude mice.
3. When tumors reach about 500 mm³, inject inactivated or active oncolytic vectors (10^5–10^6 tu in 20 µL) directly into the tumors. As above, use at least three mice (six tumors) per group.
4. Measure tumors with a caliper every other day and estimate the volume as length × width × thickness / 2. To correct for the differences in tumor sizes at the time of injection, calculate these volumes as relative to the volume at the time of injection for each tumor.
5. Compare tumor volumes for the respective groups using the Wilcoxon rank sum test ($p < 0.01$ is considered significant).

3.4. Immune Responses

The most important factor in the outcome of viral oncolysis is the host immune response against the virus. This response should be analyzed in detail in human clinical trials and in immunocompetent animal models. Here, we provide some basic protocols to analyze this response at humoral and cellular levels. A detailed analysis of the response against E1-deleted vectors have been presented recently *(14)*.

3.4.1. Serum Neutralization Assay to Measure Anti-Ad5 Antibodies

1. Incubate triplicate serial two-fold dilutions (in DMEM; starting with a 1:20) of heat-inactivated test serum (56°C, 30 min) with 100 tu of a reporter vector (E1-GFP or E1-βgal) for 1 h at 37°C in 100 μL.
2. Titer the mixtures in A549 cells.
3. The serum neutralizing titer is the log10 of the inverse of the highest dilution that reduced by 50% the number of vector tu in preimmune serum.

3.4.2. ELISA to Measure Anti-Ad5 Antibodies

1. Coat Immulon-2 microtitre plates (Dynatech, Chantilly, VA) with purified Ad5 (0.5 μg/well or 1.5×10^{10} virion particles) in coating buffer at 4°C overnight.
2. Use PBS/0.05% Tween-20 to wash twice (repeat washes between each step).
3. Dilute serially the samples in PBS/0.5% BSA and incubate overnight at 4°C.
4. Detect bound IgG or IgA using horse-radish peroxidase-conjugated goat anti-mouse (or antihuman) IgG or IgA, respectively.
5. Develop color with a peroxidase substrate and determine the absorbency in a microtiter reader at the appropriate wave length.
6. Present the Ab titer as the log10 of the inverse of the highest dilution of the sample, which is higher than the sum of the mean background absorbency and three standard deviations.

3.4.3. Enzyme-Linked Immunospot Assay (ELISPOT) to Quantitate Adenovirus-Specific Antibody (IgG) Secreting Lymphocytes

1. Coat nitrocellulose-based, hydrophobic, 96-well microtitre plates with purified Ad5 (1 μg/well) as above.
2. Wash with PBS (sterile) and incubate with complete medium for 1 h at RT.
3. Add 10^6 lymphocytes (isolated from the spleen, lymph nodes, or bone marrow) per well and incubate at 37°C for 8 h.
4. Wash plates with H_2O, then with PBS/0.05% Tween-20.
5. Incubate with antimouse IgG (or antihuman IgG) in PBS/0.5% BSA for 2 h, wash twice with PBS/Tween.
6. Incubate another 2 h with biotinylated goat antirabbit antibody and 1 h with streptavidin-alkaline phosphatase.
7. Develop the spots with BCIP-NBT and count them under the microscope.

3.4.4. Characterization of Tumor-Infiltrating Lymphocytes by Flow Cytometric Analysis

See **Note 28** as alternative methods and **Notes 29** and **30** as complementary methods.

1. Mince the tumor and incubate for 30 min at 37°C in digestion buffer.
2. Disrupt tissue by aspirating and expelling it 30 times through a 10-mL plastic syringe.

3. Centrifuge cells at 500g for 10 min, lyse erythrocytes in cold 0.17M NH₄Cl, and stain with fluoresceinated MAbs (PharMingen, San Diego, CA).

3.4.5. Contribution of Different Lymphocyte Populations

3.4.5.1. DEPLETION OF CD4 AND CD8

1. Inject ip 0.5-mL aliquots of 1:10 dilutions of ascites containing anti-CD4 GK 1.5 (ATCC) or anti-CD40L MR1 (ATCC) MAb at days −1, 0, +3, and +6 of vector injection.
2. To produce ascites, inject incomplete Freund's adjuvant ip in SCID mice. Two days and 1 wk later, inject ip 1 × 10⁶ and 5 × 10⁶ hybridoma cells, respectively. Centrifuge (10,000xg), purify on sepharose G column (Pharmacia, Uppsala, Sweden), and dialyze against PBS for 3 d.

3.4.5.2. TRANSFER OF SPECIFIC LYMPHOCYTE POPULATIONS

1. Incubate lymphocytes separated on a ficoll gradient with fluorescent tagged mAb to CD4 or CD8 to separate these populations by FACS.
2. Inject 2 × 10⁶ CD4+ or CD8+ T-cells in 200 μl of serum-free DMEM into the tail vein of recipient mice to test their effects in the oncolytic process.

4. Notes

1. The current detailed knowledge of the adenoviral life cycle and its interactions with the cell cycle allows the design of deletions or insertions to achieve tumor-specific propagation. E1 genes are the first to be expressed in the viral life cycle, and E1A has a regulatory function on the rest of early viral genes, thus placing E1A under the control of a tumor-specific promoter can control viral replication *(7)*. On the other hand, E1 proteins ignite cell cycle in resting cells by blocking tumor-supressor genes as *p53* or *Rb*, and the deletion of the E1 protein domains responsible for these interactions results in virus selective replication in tumor cells that have lost these tumor-supressor genes *(4)*. Once a promoter has been inserted upstream of E1A or certain E1A or E1B domains have been deleted in a plasmid containing the E1 region (shuttle plasmid) the construction of the virus follows the same protocols as for regular E1-deleted vectors *(10–13)*.
2. E1a can be placed under the control of a desired promoter by assembling an expression cassette composed of the promoter, E1 coding sequence, and a polyadenylation signal, and then transferring this cassette into the viral genome of an E1-deleted shuttle vector like pdE1sp1A (Microbix Biosystems Inc. Toronto, Ontario, Canada *[11]*). To prepare a cassette, the promoter can be amplified by PCR from genomic DNA and cloned into a plasmid upstream of a subcloned E1 region (*Afl* III-*Afl* II, *Ad*5 nt 462-3533). This region contains E1A TATA box so the promoter TATA box should be excluded from the PCR product.
3. Alternatively, the promoter can be inserted directly in front of E1A (*Ad*5 nt 475-550) into an E1 containing shuttle vector like pXC1 (Microbix *[7,11]*).

4. The maximum size allowed for the exogenous promoter is approx 1.8 kb, 4.4 kb, and 4.9 kb when using *pJM17* (or a wild-type Ad5 fragment), pBHG10, or pBHG11 (Microbix *[11]*) respectively, to generate viruses. For genomic stability, the final recombinant virus should be as long as possible (105% of wt size or 37.8 kb).

5. The E1 cassette construction approach has the advantage that the cassette can be subcloned into a gutless or miniAd vector to render an adenovirus that can support the propagation of E1-deleted vectors. The gutless vector and the E1-deleted vector complement each other in tumor cells that transcribe the controlling promoter. We have constructed, for example, one vector (named GT5610) containing the minimal viral *cis* elements for replication and packaging (i.e., ITRs and packaging signal), the E1 genes with *E1a* under the control of a 5 kb AFP promoter, and human genomic DNA as "stuffer." This vector propagates selectively in cells that express AFP and that are concurrently infected by an E1-deleted vector (**Fig. 2**).

6. Domain deletions can be performed easily in an E1-containing shuttle vector like pXC1 (Microbix *[9]*) by site-specific mutagenesis by digestion with restriction enzymes, and then incorporated into the viral genome by plasmid homologous recombination. For example, in pXC1 an E1b55K deletion spanning from *Sau*3A1 (Ad5 2426) to *Bgl* II (Ad5 3328) can be constructed by ligation of 1 kb *Xba*I-*Sau*3A1 fragment with 7.9 kb *Xba*I-*Bgl*II fragment. Alternatively, the deletion can be performed in an E1-expression cassette, which allows the construction of gutless/E1-deleted complementary vectors.

7. We can obtain mutants that only grow in tumor cells if we have a cell-culture system to select them. For example, tetracycline-regulated or temperature-sensitive mutants of *p53* that lead to G1 arrest when expressed can be used to select mutants that only grow in *p53*-negative cells. After mutagenesis and infection, cells are shifted to permissive conditions so noninfected cells or cells infected by mutants that affect *p53*-inactivating functions will stop in G1. On the contrary, cells infected by wild-type Ad5 or by mutants of genes not necessary for in vitro propagation (e.g., E3) will pass to S phase. G1 cells can be sorted out and shifted to nonpermissive conditions where the cell cycle resumes and mutants that only affected the *p53*-blocking functions, but not other vital functions are released. This selection cycle can be repeated as many times as necessary to further purify and amplify the mutants.

8. Alternatively, mutagenesis of the stock can be done by incubating with 0.1*M* hydroxylammonium chloride in PBS for 20 min at 37°C, followed by 100-fold dilution with cold cell-culture medium.

9. When adenovirus can be obtained by plasmid transfection, mutagenesis can be performed in *Escherichia coli* mutator strains (Stratagene). This can be done with plasmids such as *pJM17* (**10**), with *Xba*I restriction followed by religation to remove the plasmid backbone from the adenoviral genome. The ligation mixture can be used directly for transfection.

10. Any vector with with E1 deletions or with E1 controlled by tumor-specific promoters can be generated in 293 because these cells express E1. The advantage is

that these cells are commonly used to generate E1-deleted vectors by $CaPO_4$ cotransfection *(10–13)*.

11. As soon as the recombinant virus is generated, it should be plaque-purified and amplified in the tumor target cells to avoid recombination between the E1 viral and cellular sequences.

12. For complementary viruses, miniAd plasmid and viral DNA from E1-deleted vector are also cotransfected by calcium phosphate precipitation (e.g., 2 µg GT5610 + 0.2 µg of viral DNA per 1×10^6 cells in 9.6-cm² wells) *(14)*.

13. This is the method of choice to avoid recombinations in E1 region. First, we need to identify the target cells and then determine how sensitive these cells are to Ad5 infection and then optimize the transfection. Among the several cell lines that present the desired phenotype (lack of tumor supressor function or expression of a tumor-associated antigen), the best candidates will be the ones that are more efficiently infected and transfected.

14. Primers (20–22mer) for tumor-associated antigen detection should be chosen with no stable duplexes or hairpins, spanning several exons to avoid gene amplification, and with an optimal annealing temperature of 55–60°C. As a control, β-actin should be amplified with primers: 5′ GACGACATGGAGAAA ATCTGGCAC 3′ and 5′ GGCGACGTAGCACAGCTTCTCCTT 3′ which yield a 423 bp product.

15. An E1-deleted vector carrying a reporter gene such as GFP is the easiest way to compare the infectivity of each cell line. Use MOI from 1000 to 0.1. To achieve these MOIs use the transducing titer, that is, the number of transducing units per mL as determined in A549 cells. This titer is usually higher (2- to 5-fold) than the number of PFU/mL estimated in 293 cells presumably because not all transduced cells can develop plaques. Titration as tu/mL is quicker to estimate and better reflects the infectitvity process that we want to address.

16. To optimize transfections in the cell lines that have shown a certain sensitivity of infection, $CaPO_4$ (as described above for 293) and lipofections with different lipids should be compared using a plasmid containing a reporter gene. Lipid Perfect (Invitrogen, San Diego, CA) provides different lipids for comparison. The optimal transfection conditions are then used to cotransfect the shuttle vector and the large plasmid (pJM17 or other) to generate the desired virus. Onset of plaques could be delayed in comparison to virus generation in 293 because of a lower number of viruses produced per cell. We have observed plaques as late as 1 mo after $CaPO_4$ cotransfection of HepG2 cells with an AFP-E1 miniAd and an E1-deleted vector.

17. The amount of virus produced per cell or burst size is the most important factor to choose a cell line to further propagate it. These numbers will indicate the specificity of viral propagation. The easiest and most conclusive way to quantify it is to measure the amount of vector produced in each cell line in a time-course study.

18. The number of tu or PFU produced per infected cell will peak in a day between 2 and 5 dpi. The cell line with a higher and earlier peak is the best candidate to further propagate the oncolytic virus. As a reference, an E1-deleted vector grown

in 293 cells has a burst peak of 1000 tu/cell at day 2. Once we have determined the most sensitive cell line for propagating a particular vector, this cell line can be also used for titration.

19. For immunochemistry, the most commonly detected gene is the hexon protein because it is made in large quantities and is very immunogenic.

20. For viral DNA replication assays, we prefer Southern blot over metabolic labeling because it does not require to separate host and viral DNA. Instead of Hirt's DNA, we use total cellular DNA prepared by the standard SDS/proteinase K method when high sensitivity is not required. The signal observed at 2 h postinfection represents unreplicated input DNA. An increase over time indicates viral replication.

21. A control to be included in these assays is the wild-type Ad5 as a reference for maximum potency relative to the potency of the designed oncolytic virus in each cell line.

22. The titer determined in a plaque assay under the conditions of 2 h of adsorption time and 1 mL of adsorption volume (per 9.6 cm^2 well) is about 10-fold lower than the titer determined under optimal conditions *(15)*.

23. Plaque assays give a more quantitative determination of the oncolytic potency than CPE assays. Plaques will increase in size at a rate that will be directly proportional to the amount of vector produced per cell. However, the most accurate method to quantify the efficiency and selectivity of the propagation of viruses is to directly measure the burst size in a time course as described in **Subheading 3.1.3.3.**

24. From burst size and plaque assays we can obtain quantitative information about the lytic potency of the engineered virus. Intratumoral injection of the virus into established tumors is the easiest way to obtain this information in vivo. Differences in growth rate, angiogenicity, cell density, and so on, that shape the architecture of a established tumor will have an impact on the viral spread. Therefore, a lack of correlation can exist between the sensitivity of cell lines to in vitro and in vivo oncolysis. On the other hand, the specificity of viral propagation can be different in vitro and vivo because growth factors and cytokines secreted in response to the virus could complement their mutations and allow their propagation in certain cell types. Therefore, it would be desirable to have an animal model that would allow the propagation of adenovirus in tumor as well as in normal cells. Immunocompetency is imperative if we want to evaluate the efficacy of an oncolytic virus because antitumoral and antiviral immune responses will dictate the outcome of this treatment.

25. Tumors in pigs or cotton rats could be good models to test viruses derived from human Ad5 because of the permisivity of these species to the replication of this virus. However, the lack of tumor models in these animals and an incomplete permisivity are two major drawbacks. Another possibility would be to use engineered adenoviruses from other hosts, such as the mouse adenovirus (MAV 1), with the same mutations as the Ad5 counterpart. As MAV1 and Ad5 share the genetic structure and function, the information obtained from treating murine

tumors in immunocompetent mice could help to elucidate the efficacy of each mutation. In the meantime, we can try to get as much information from the xenogenic tumors models available, keeping in mind the limitations of the results.

26. By intratumoral detection of reporter genes or by immunostaining usually nonreplicating vectors are not detected after 2 wk of injections.

27. Treatment of established tumors is a more realistic model to evaluate the oncolytic potency than mixed cells tumorigenicity assays. When possible, orthotopic models are preferred over sc.

28. As an alternative to the flow cytometric analysis, frozen sections can be immunostained with antimouse CD4 Ab (anti-L3T4; 10 µg/mL; Boehringer) or antimouse CD8 Ab (anti-Ly-2; 50 µg/mL; Boehringer).

29. The specific activation or cytotoxicity of CTLs isolated from tumors, draining lymph nodes, spleen, and peripheral blood can be analyzed using Ad-infected (1 dpi) and uninfected tumor cells as stimulators (irradiated or mitomycin-inactivated for a ^{3}H-Thymidine uptake assay) or as targets (labeled or not for a ^{51}Cr or lactate dehydrogenase release assays).

30. The pattern of cytokines present in the tumor and lymph nodes or secreted by lymphocytes cultured from these sites at RNA levels can be quantified by RT-PCR (*see* **Subheading 3.1.3.1.**) or RNA-protection assays (PharMingen). Protein levels are usually analyzed by ELISA from cultured lymphocytes.

5. Conclusion

From the virology, tumorigenicity, and immunology standpoints, many different techniques can be applied to the study of oncolytic viruses. We have tried to summarize some of those that can be performed easily in any molecular biology laboratory because they do not require special equipment. The most important questions about the potential use of viruses for treatment of cancer remain open: how tumor-selective propagation and oncolytic potency, or which type of immune responses generated against tumor and virus correlate with an effective eradication of tumor cells? We hope that the technical approaches to these problems that we have discussed here will help those attempting to solve them.

References

1. Sinkovics, J. and Horvath, J. (1993) New developments in the virus therapy of cancer: a historical review. *Intervirology*, **36**, 193–214.
2. Russell, S. J. (1994) Replicating vectors for cancer therapy: a question of strategy. *Sem. Cancer Biol.* **5**, 437–443.
3. Kirn, D. H. and McCormick, F. (1996) Replicating viruses as selective cancer therapeutics. *Mol. Med. Today.* **2**, 519–527.
4. Bischof, J. R., Kirn, D. H., Williams, A., Heise, C., Horn, S., Muna, M., et al. (1996) An adenovirus that replicates selectively in p53-deficient human tumor cells. *Science* **274**, 373–376.

5. Heise, C., Sampson-Johanes, A., Williams, A., McCormick, F., Von Hoff, D. D., and Kirn, D. H. (1997) Onyx-015, an E1B gene-attenuated adenovirus, causes tumor-specific cytolysis and antitumoral efficacy that can be augmented by standard chemotherapeutic agents. *Nature Med.* **3,** 639–645.

6. Hallenbeck, P. L., Chang, Y-N., Hay, C., Golightly, D., Stewart, D., McGarrity, G., and Chiang, Y. (1996) Novel tumor specific replication competent adenoviral vectors for gene therapy of cancer. Abstract O-36. *Cancer Gene Ther.* **3,** s19.

7. Rodriguez, R., Schuur, E. R., Lim, H. Y., Henderson, G. A., Simons, J. W., and Henderson, D. R. (1997) Prostate attenuated replication competent adenovirus (ARCA) CN706: a selective cytotoxic for prostate-specific antigen-positive prostate cancer cells. *Cancer Res.* **57,** 2559–2563.

8. Lion, L. D., Goldsmith, K. T., Strong, T. V., Bilbao, G., Curiel, D. T., and Garver Jr., R. I. (1996) E1A RNA transcripts amplify adenovirus-mediated tumor-reduction. *Gene Ther.* **3,** 1021–1025.

9. van Ginkel, F. W., McGhee, J. R., Liu, C., Simecka, J. W., Yamamoto, N., Frizzell, R. A., et al. (1997) Adenoviral gene delivery elicits distinct pulmonary associated T helper cell responses to the vector and to its transgene. *J. Immunol.* **159,** 685–693.

10. Graham, F. L. and Prevec, L. (1991) Manipulation of adenovirus vectors. *Meth. Molec. Biol.* **7,** 109–128.

11. Bett, A. J., Haddara, W., Prevec, L., and Graham, F. L. (1994) An efficient and flexible system for construction of adenovirus vectors with insertions or deletions in early regions 1 and 3. *Proc. Nat. Acad. Sci. USA* **91,** 8802–8806.

12. Becker, C. T., Noel, R. J., Ward W. S., Gomez-Foix, A. M., Alam, T., Gerard, R. D., and Newgard, C. B. (1994) Use of Recombinant adenoviruses for metabolic engineering of cells. *Meth. Cell Biol.* **43,** 161–189.

13. Ragot, T., Opolon, P., and Perricaudet, M. (1998) Adenoviral gene delivery. *Meth. Cell Biol.* **52,** 229–260.

14. Alemany, R., Dai, Y., Lou, Y. C., Sethi, E., Prokopenko, E., Josephs, S. F., and Zhang, W-W. (1997) Complementation of helper-dependent adenoviral vectors: size effects and titer fluctuations. *J. Virol. Meth.* **68,** 147–159.

15. Mittereder, N., March, K. L., and Trapnell, B. (1996) Evaluation of the concentration and bioactivity of adenovirus vectors for gene therapy. *J. Virol.* **70,** 77,498–7509.

25

Genetically Modified Clostridium for Gene Therapy of Tumors

Mary E. Fox, Marilyn J. Lemmon, Amato J. Giaccia, Nigel P. Minton, and J. Martin Brown

1. Introduction

Many murine and human tumors contain hypoxic or necrotic regions in which the oxygen tension is abnormally low. For example, >50% of primary tumors of the breast, cervix, and head and neck contain areas that are hypoxic. Because hypoxic regions are not present in normal tissue, this provides the potential for selectively targeting gene therapy to tumor cells.

Certain species of obligate anaerobic bacteria, such as clostridia, have been shown to localize and germinate specifically in the hypoxic regions of tumors, resulting in tumor lysis. We have developed an innovative approach to cancer gene therapy in which genetically engineered clostridia are used to achieve tumor-specific drug activation (1). The overall strategy is one of enzyme/prodrug therapy, in which a nontoxic prodrug is enzymatically activated to give an active chemotherapeutic agent (2). Tumor specificity is provided by genetically engineered bacteria, which express the enzyme needed for prodrug activation only in hypoxic areas of tumors. *Clostridium beijerinckii* is amenable to genetic manipulation and has sucessfully been modified to express several enzymes, which activate different prodrugs. Many enzyme/prodrug combinations are available for such an approach including nitroreductase/CB1954, cytosine deaminase/5-fluorocytosine, and glucuronidase/glucuronide conjugates.

The overall strategy for gene therapy is outlined in **Fig. 1** using tumor-bearing mice as a model system. Clostridia are genetically modified to express the enzyme that activates the prodrug of interest. Spores from these bacteria are injected intravenously and will localize and germinate only in hypoxic

From: *Methods in Molecular Medicine, Vol. 35: Gene Therapy: Methods and Protocols*
Edited by: W. Walther and U. Stein © Humana Press, Inc., Totowa, NJ

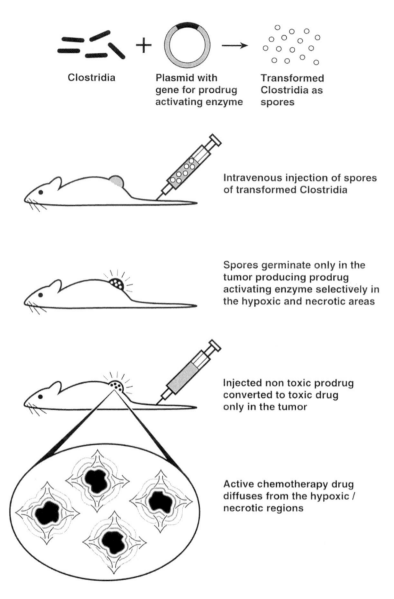

Clostridia

Plasmid with
gene for prodrug
activating enzyme

Transformed
Clostridia as
spores

Intravenous injection of spores
of transformed Clostridia

Spores germinate only in the
tumor producing prodrug
activating enzyme selectively in
the hypoxic and necrotic areas

Injected non toxic prodrug
converted to toxic drug
only in the tumor

Active chemotherapy drug
diffuses from the hypoxic /
necrotic regions

Fig. 1. A schematic of gene therapy using genetically transformed clostridia, an obligate anaerobe. The transformed clostridia are injected intravenously as spores, which distribute throughout the body, but only germinate in the hypoxic/necrotic areas of the tumor, thereby generating the prodrug activating enzyme in the tumor, which can subsequently activate a prodrug to a toxic drug in these areas. Toxic drug will diffuse from the necrotic/hypoxic areas with the highest concentrations of drug in these areas. This would be expected to produce cytotoxicity complementary to that of conventional therapy.

regions of tumor tissue. Subsequent administration of prodrug will result in tumor-specific drug activation. Because this approach is still in developmental stages, and the details of drug administration will vary between enzyme-prodrug combinations, we describe here only the techniques that are common to all agents used. Further details on specific enzyme-prodrug combinations are available upon request.

2. Materials

1. For maintenance of bacteria—Anaerobic chamber: Bacterial media: LB (10 g/L tryptone, 5 g/L yeast extract, 10 g/L NaCl), 2 X YTG (16 g/L tryptone, 10 g/L yeast extract, 5 g/L NaCl, 0.5% glucose). Antibiotics: ampicillin, erythromycin.
2. Plasmid DNA in TE.
3. For electroporation of *Bacillus subtilis*: 1 mM HEPES, pH 7.0. PEB (272 mM sucrose, 1 mM MgCl$_2$, 7 mM potassium phosphate, pH 7.4).
4. For electroporation of *C. beijerinckii*: Clostridia electroporation Buffer (270 mM sucrose, 1 mM MgCl$_2$, 7 mM NaPO$_4$, pH 7.4). Just before use, add catalase to 0.2 mg/mL and store on ice in anaerobic chamber.
5. For plasmid minipreps from *C. acetobutylicum*: Cell resuspension buffer (50 mM Tris, pH 7. 5, 25% sucrose, 5 mM EDTA). Lysozyme. Lysis buffer (0.2M NaOH, 1% SDS, made fresh). Potassium acetate solution (60 mL 5M potassium acetate, 11.5 mL glacial acetic acid, 28.5 mL H$_2$O). Phenol/Chloroform.
6. Renografin.

3. Methods

3.1. Maintenance of Clostridia

Clostiridia are maintained under anaerobic conditions (90% N$_2$, 5% CO$_2$, 5% H$_2$) in an anaerobic culture chamber. All media, plasticware, and solutions are equilibrated within the chamber for at least 24 h prior to use. All manipulations (with the exception of electroporation and centrifugation) are performed under anaerobic conditions.

3.2. Construction of Cloning Vectors

Two vectors are currently in use, pMTL500F *(3)* and pMTL540FT (**Fig. 2**); both are *clostridia-Escherichia coli* shuttle vectors so that initial manipulations can be performed in *E. coli* using standard techniques *(4)* and the final vector transferred to clostridia by electroporation. All genes expressed from these vectors have been inserted into the *Nde*I site of the multicloning site (*see* **Note 1**). Plasmids are transformed into *E. coli* using standard protocols and high quality plasmid preparations (such as Qiagen preparations, Chatsworth, CA) are used for electroporation of *B. subtilis* *(5)* or *C. beijerinckii* *(6)*.

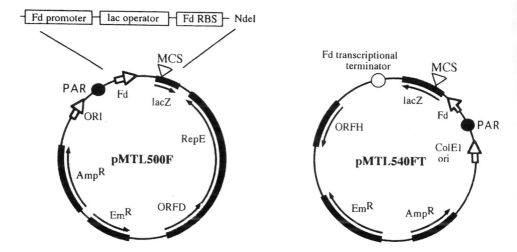

Fig 2. Structures of the *E. coli*-Clostridia shuttle vectors pMTL500F *(3)* and pMTL540FT. The clostridial replicon, which encompasses ORFH, of pMTL540FT was derived from the *C.butyricum* plasmid pCB102 *(7)*. The region containing the ferredoxin promoter and ribosome binding site (RBS) is shown in detail for pMTL500F and is identical in pMTL540FT. The *Nde*1 site shown is the first restriction site of the MCS, and is the cloning site used for insertion of the cytosine deaminase gene.

3.3. Electroporation of B. Subtilis (see **Note 2**)

1. Grow overnight culture of *B. subtilis* in LB at 37°C with vigorous aeration.
2. Inoculate 1/100 dilution into fresh LB and grow shaking until OD_{600nm} ~ 0.6.
3. Harvest cells by centrifugation at 4°C.
4. Wash once with cold 1 m*M* HEPES, pH 7.0, and twice with cold PEB buffer. Resuspend final pellet in 1/30 original culture volume of PEB.
5. Freeze-thaw cells twice on EtOH/dry ice.
6. Add 50 µL cell suspension to 0.1–0.1 µg plasmid DNA on ice. Transfer to cold 0.2-cm cuvets and pulse at 200 Ω, 25 µF, 1.5 kV (the time constant will be ~4 ms).
7. Add 1 mL LB and transfer to 15 mL tubes. Incubate shaking at 37°C for 1 h.
8. Plate 200 µL onto selective plates (LB with 5 µg/mL erythromycin) and incubate at 37°C for 24–48 h.
9. Plasmid can be isolated from *B. subtilis* using Qiagen columns and the provided protocol, except that Buffer P1 contains 2 mg/mL lysozyme and 800 µg/mL RNascA, and cells are incubated at 37°C for 15 min in modified buffer P1 prior to addition of buffer P2.

3.4 Electroporation of Clostridia

1. Set up overnight cultures with serial dilutions (neat to 10^{-5}) in 5-mL volumes of 2X YTG using a loopful from a fresh plate for the neat culture.

2. Dilute the highest two dilutions (i.e., lowest cell density), which have grown into 100 ml 2X YTG and grow to OD 600 nm ≥ 0.6 (midexponential phase, *see* **Note 3a**).
3. Harvest by centrifugation, wash in 10 mL ice-cold electroporation buffer and resuspend pellet in 5 mL ice-cold electroporation buffer. Hold on ice 10 min.
4. Add 1 µg DNA to 0.2-cm cuvete, followed by 300 µL cell suspension. Seal cuvets with both closure and cap (*see* **Note 3b**).
5. Pulse at 100 Ω, 25 µF, 1.25 kV (time constant will be ~1.7 ms).
6. Add cells to 3 mL 2X YTG and incubate 37°C for 3 h.
7. Divide cells between two Eppendorf tubes and harvest cells in microfuge. Resuspend each cell pellet in 100 µL 2X YTG and plate onto selective media (2X YTG with 20 µg/mL erythmomycin).
8. Transformants should be visible after 24–48 h incubation at 37°C.

3.5. Plasmid Minipreps from Clostridia

1. Grow 10-mL cultures overnight in anaerobic chamber with selection for plasmid.
2. Harvest cells by centrifugation, and resuspend in 100-µL cell resupsension solution containing 10 mg/mL lysozyme.
3. Incubate 37°C for 1 h.
4. Add 200 µL lysis buffer and mix by inversion. Incubate on ice 10 min.
5. Add 150 µL ice-cold potassium acetate solution. Incubate on ice 5 min.
6. Centrifuge 10 min at 4°C in microfuge. Transfer supernatant to fresh tube and extract with phenol/chloroform.
7. Transfer aqueous phase to a fresh tube and add 2 volumes ethanol.
8. Stand at room temperature for at least 10 min.
9. Centrifuge 10 min, wash pellet with 70% ethanol and air-dry pellet. Resuspend in 50 µl TE (*see* **Note 4**).

3.6. Purification of Spores from C. Beijerinckii

Spores can be separated from vegetative rods by centrifugation through Renografin (*see* **Note 5**).

1. Sporulate cultures on 2X YTG plates for 1 wk at 37°C.
2. Wash 1–2 times with water and resuspend in sterile distilled water at ≤10⁹ spores/mL.
3. Place 15-mL of 45–50% Renografin in 35-mL centrifuge tube and carefully layer 5 mL spore suspension onto the Renografin.
4. Centrifuge 20,000*g* for 30 min at 4°C.
5. Remove the vegetative rods, which are trapped at the interface, with a Pasteur pipet and decant the Renografin. Resuspend the pellet containing the spores in water. Wash spores three times with sterile water and resuspend in PBS for injection.
6. Spores can be stored at 4°C for at least 2 mo.
7. Heat shock the spores at 70°C for 10 min just prior to injection into mice to enhance spore germination.

4. Notes

1. Although the plasmids used contain a multicloning site, efficient expression of inserted DNA was achieved only when DNA was cloned into *Nde*I site. This can be conveniently achieved through the creation of a *Nde*I site over the ATG initiation codon of the gene to be inserted using PCR.
2. pMTL540FT-derived plasmids can be directly transformed into *C. beijerinckii* following isolation from *E. coli*. However, for constructs derived from pMTL500F it is necesary to transform *B. subtilis*, and use bacillus-derived plasmid to transform clostridia.
3a. For electroporation of clostridia the OD600 of the starting culture must be above 0.6.
3b. The efficiency of electroporation of clostridia is enhanced if cuvets are sealed with both the caps provided and with cuvette closures (available from Elkay Plastics, Los Angeles, CA) to minimize exposure to air during electroporation.
4. The yield of plasmid minipreps from *C. beijerinckii* will be too low to visualize ethidium bromide stained DNA on an agarose gel, but 1–2 µL should be sufficient to transform *E. coli* if it is necesary to check the plasmid by restriction digestion.
5. Vegetative rods are more immunogenic than spores, and should be removed prior to injection. Purification of spores using renografin will increase the percentage of spores in the culture from ~40% to >95%, but will result in the loss of at least 50% of the spores.

References

1. Minton, N. P., Mauchline, M. L., Lemmon, M. J., Brehm, J. K., Fox, M. E., Michael, N. P., et al. (1995) Chemotherapeutic tumour targeting using clostridial spores. *FEMS Microbiol. Rev.* **17**, 357–364.
2. Deonarain, M. P. and Epenetos, A. A. (1994) Targeting enzymes for cancer therapy: old enzymes in new roles. *Br. J. Cancer* **70**, 786–794.
3. Minton, N. P., Brehm, J. K., Swinfield, T-J., Whalen, S. M., Mauchline, M. L., Bodsworth, N., and Oultram, J. D. (1993) Clostridial cloning vectors, in *The Clostridia and Biotechnology* (Woods, D. R., ed.), Butterworth-Heinemann, Boston, MA, pp. 119–150.
4. Sambrook, J., Fritsch, E. F. and Maniatis, T. (1989) *Molecular Cloning. A Laboratory Manual.* 2nd ed., Cold Spring Harbor, Cold Spring Harbor, New York.
5. Brigidi, P., DeRossi, E., Bertarini, M. L., Riccardi, G., and Matteuzzi, D. (1990) Genetic transformation of intact cells of *Bacillus subtilis* by electroporation. *FEMS Microbiol. Letts.* **67**, 135–138.
6. Oultram, J. D., Loughlin, M., Swinfield, T-J., Brehm, J. K., Thompson, D. E., and Minton, N. P. (1988) Introduction of plasmids into whole cells of *Clostridium acetobutylicum* by electroporation. *FEMS Microbiol. Letts.* **56**, 83–88.
7. Minton, N. P. and Morris, J. G. (1981) Isolation and partial characterisation of three cryptic plasmids from strains of *Clostridiium butyricum*. *J. Gen. Microbiol.* **127**, 325–331.

26

Tumor-Targeted *Salmonella: Strain Development and Expression of the* HSV-tK *Effector Gene*

David Bermudes, Brooks Low, and John M. Pawelek

1. Introduction

Gene therapy approaches to cancer treatment have been limited by the ability of the delivery vectors to achieve specific high-level expression within tumor cells or the tumor environment following systemic administration. Numerous physical barriers exist in the delivery of therapeutic agents (including drugs, viruses, and liposomes) to solid tumors that can compromise the effectiveness *(1)*, thus stimulating the search for alternative methods of delivery. Whereas it has been known for some time that spores of anaerobic *Clostridium* can germinate within the necrotic spaces of human tumors, they are limited to larger hypoxic tumors and are inaccessible to smaller metastases *(2,3)*. The ability of motile, facultatively anaerobic *Salmonella* to target tumors following systemic administration, preferentially amplify within them, and express effector genes such as the herpes simplex virus thymidine kinase (HSV-TK) makes them an attractive alternative to *Clostridia*, liposome and viral-based delivery vectors *(4)*. These *Salmonella* were attenuated by poly-auxotrophic mutations, which limited their pathogenesis in normal tissues, but retained high-level replication within tumors, resulting in tumor suppression of both primary and metastatic tumors *(4,5)*. The attenuating mutations were added stepwise following in vitro and in vivo selection and screening methods. Although live-attenuated vectors for use in humans requires defined genetic mutations, our experience has shown that combinations of point-mutations and frame-shift mutations allows for rapid isolation of strains with multiple mutations having desirable properties, which can later be defined and/or stabilized. Bearing this in mind, we present the basic methodology for the

From: *Methods in Molecular Medicine, Vol. 35: Gene Therapy: Methods and Protocols*
Edited by: W. Walther and U. Stein © Humana Press, Inc., Totowa, NJ

development of tumor-targeting facultative anaerobes with effector gene delivery capabilities that we applied to *Salmonella*.

1.1 Tumor-Targeted Salmonella

For a pathogen such as *Salmonella* to be useful as an anticancer vector, it must both target tumors and be attenuated in virulence so that potential harm to the host is minimized. Previous work demonstrated that attenuation of *Salmonella* can be achieved through auxotrophic mutations such as those affecting the biosynthesis of purines *(6,7)*, aromatic amino acids *(8)*, or combinations of such mutations *(9)*. Because auxotrophs depend upon exogenous nutrients for growth, it seems that these might have advantages as tumor vectors because the environment of the tumor could in theory provide the missing nutrients, for example in necrotic spaces or within actively dividing cells of the tumor. Thus, mutation of organisms such as *Salmonella* to auxotrophy not only reduces their virulence, but may provide an enhancement of their selective colonization and amplification within solid tumors.

Because of the potential for biospecificity of parasites, such vectors could, in theory, deliver therapeutic agents specifically to tumors, overcoming a variety of obstacles. For example, in order for chemotherapeutic agents to eradicate metastatic tumor cells, they must *(1)*:

1. travel to the tumors via the vasculature;
2. extravasate from the small blood vessels supplying the tumor;
3. traverse through the tumor matrix to reach those tumor cells distal to the blood supply; and
4. interact effectively with the target tumor cells (adherence, invasion, prodrug activation, and so on).

Bacterial vectors not only fulfill these requirements, but they exhibit other properties that support their usefulness as gene therapy agents, including antibiotic sensitivity that allows for eradication of the parasite from the cancer patient's body upon completion of the therapeutic protocol, amenability to a variety of genetic manipulations, with stable introduction of genetic constructs, and replication within targeted environment and target cells allowing amplification of the therapeutic vector and the therapeutic agent within them. In theory, a single tumor-invading self-replicating parasite could, through its progeny, infect and eradicate every tumor cell in a patient's body.

We have realized many of these advantages, and detail below the development of aerobically invasive *Salmonella* auxotrophs that are attenuated in mice yet show pronounced tumor targeting and amplification capabilities. In addition, we provide an example of engineering these strains to express a foreign gene, HSV TK, for the conversion of an inactive prodrug, ganciclovir (GCV), into its activated phosphorylated form with antitumor activity.

1.2. Strain Properties and Requirements

For any parasite to be effective as a therapeutic vector, the benefit of the parasite as a vector must outweigh its risk as a pathogen to the patient. For example, Pidherney et al. *(10)* and Alizadeh et al. *(11)* demonstrated cytotoxicity of pathogenic amoebae toward tumor cells, but the inherent pathogenecity of these organisms was not overcome, nor was specificity for the therapeutic target obtained. The usefulness of parasites as vectors in therapy of cancer depends on both their ability to specifically recognize cancerous tumors in the body as potential hosts, as well as replicate within them. If specific recognition of neoplastic tissue can be achieved coordinately with safety, then the parasites can be employed as vectors to deliver to the tumor therapeutic proteins such as prodrug converting enzymes capable of metabolically converting nontoxic prodrugs into toxic drugs, resulting in a high degree of specificity for killing of cancerous cells.

The general in vivo properties of tumor-specific *Salmonella* strains are not fully understood, but apparently include:

1. Serum resistance, allowing the parasite to pass through the vasculature and lymphatic system in the process of seeking tumors;
2. Susceptibility to the host's defensive capabilities, limiting replication in normal tissues, but not within tumors where the host defensive capabilities may be impaired;
3. Attenuation of virulence, whereby the parasite is tolerated by the host, but does not limit intratumoral replication;
4. Facultative anaerobiasis, allowing amplification in large necrotic tumors which are hypoxic as well as small metastatic tumors that may be more aerobic;
5. Invasive capacity toward tumor cells, aiding in, but not necessary for, tumor targeting and antitumor activity;
6. The ability to express and secrete heterologous proteins having anticancer therapeutic effects;
7. Motility, aiding in permeation throughout the tumor; and
8. Antibiotic sensitivity for control during treatment and for posttreatment elimination (e.g., ampicillin, chloramphenicol, ciprofloxacin).

2. Materials
2.1. Bacterial Strains

The bacteria are representative of *Salmonella* spp, such as wild-type *Salmonella typhimurium* strain 14028 (American Type Culture Collection (ATCC),

CDC6516-60), or LB5010 (*Salmonella* Genetic Stock Center, Calgary, Canada) which lacks restriction endonuclease functions yet retains methylation ability and is highly useful for DNA transformations. *Escherichia coli*, K-12 strains for use as controls are available from the ATCC as well as other sources. These strains are grown on Luria-Bertani (LB): 1% Bactotryptone (Difco, E. Molesly, Surrey, UK), 0.5% Bacto-yeast extract (Difco), 1.0% NaCl, which is sterilized by autoclaving and can be made as solid media by the addition of 1.5% agar (Life Technologies, Gaithersburg, MD). Auxotrophic mutants are determined on minimal media 56 (M56): $0.037M$ KH_2PO_4, $0.06M$ Na_2HPO_4, 0.02% $MgSO_4 \cdot 7H_2O$, 0.2% $(NH_4)_2SO_4$, 0.001% Ca $(NO_3)_2$, 0.00005% $FeSO_4 \cdot 7H_2O$, with a carbon source (e.g., glucose 0.1 to 0.3%) as a sterile-filtered additive, and further supplemented with the appropriate nutrients, 0.1 µg/mL thiamine or 50 µg/mL each of adenine, isoleucine, valine, arginine, or uracil. Solid M56 media is made by preparing separate autoclaved 2X concentrates of the mineral salts and the agar, which are combined after sterilization. Carbon source utilization can be determined on MacConkey agar prepared using 40 g of MacConkey base (Difco) per liter H_2O sterilized by autoclaving, and supplemented with sterile-filtered sugars such as maltose or galactose (0.1% final concentration). Media are also supplemented with antibiotics used as needed to select for plasmid-based resistance markers, including tetracycline (Sigma, St. Louis, MO) at 10 µg/mL from a stock: 10 mg/mL in 70% ethanol stored in darkness at $-20°C$ or ampicillin at 100 µg/mL from a stock: 100 mg/mL in H_2O, sterile filtered and stored at $-20°C$.

2.2. Mutagenesis

Isolation of mutants requires the parental bacterial strains such as ATCC 14028 and a mutagen such as nitrosoguanidine (NG): 50 µg/mL in H_2O for 20' at 37°C (Sigma), or UV irradiation (50 J/m², λ = 254 nm) (*12,13*) described further below.

2.3. Tumor Cells

A variety of tumor cells from murine and human origins may be used in vitro and in vivo, such as human melanoma M2 (*14*) and murine melanoma B16F10 (Dr. I. J. Fidler, M.D., Anderson Cancer Center), or murine melanoma Cloudman S91, human colon cancer (HTB 39 and HCT 116), human hepatoma (HTB 52), human renal carcinoma (CRL 1611), or human breast carcinoma (BT20), obtained from the ATCC, and maintained on the specifically recommended tissue-culture medium (TCM), usually with 10% fetal bovine serum (FBS, Life Technologies) and 5% CO_2 in humidified air at 37°C. Antibiotics such as penicillin (Sigma): 100 U/mL, and streptomycin (Sigma): 100 µg/mL, may be added to aid in maintaining bacteria-free cultures. For assays of tumor cell invasion by *Salmonella*, an aqueous solution of gentamicin sulfate (Sigma) is added to the cell-culture media at a final concentration of 50 µg/mL and used in eliminating extracelluar bacteria. Mammalian cells can be freed from the culture dish using 1% EDTA or a solution of trypsin and EDTA (Sigma).

2.4. Tumor Models

Establishment of transplantable tumors requires either mice syngenic with the tumor cell line (e.g., C57B6 mice and B16F10 melanoma or DBA/2J mice and Cloudman S91 melanoma) or T-cell deficient, athymic *(nu/nu)* mice. The tumor cells should always be inoculated in the same position, e.g., sc in the left shoulder region with 5×10^5 B16F10 or Cloudman S91 mouse melanoma cells for syngenic mice or 2×10^7 cells (e.g., human colon carcinoma HCT 116, human breast carcinoma BT20, human renal carcinoma CRL 1611, or human hepatoma HTB 52) for human xenografts. Mice treated with *Salmonella* may be administered enrofloxicin (Bayer, 0.2 µg/mL drinking water) after the first 2-week period. For prodrug conversion and antitumor activity studies, a ganciclovir (GCV; ganciclovir sodium, Cytovene™, Syntex Laboratories) stock solutions is made by dissolving 25 mg/mL in 0.9% saline which can be stored frozen and redisolved at 37°C.

2.5. Plasmid Vectors and Effector Genes

Gene expression vectors for prodrug converting enzymes, such as HSV-TK, are being widely employed for use in gene therapy of malignant cancers *(15,16)*. HSV-TK phosphorylates the nontoxic substrates acyclovir (acycloguanosine; Sigma) and GCV, rendering them toxic when incorporated into genomic DNA. Radiolabeled acyclovir and GCV are available from Moravek Biochemicals. Pawelek et al. *(4)* generated an HSV-TK secreted into the periplasm by introducing into the DNA construct a secretory signal sequence from the β-lactamase gene in a derivative of pBR322 *(17)*; *see* **Subheading 3.8.**). Alternative signal sequences, which could also be employed for inclusion into DNA constructs, are also known. Bacteria have several means for secretion into the periplasm and into the outside milieu. The most typical secretion sequences are N-terminal signal sequences containing hydrophobic transmembrane spanning domains *(18)*. Some bacterial proteins utilize a secretion signal which is located at the C-terminus. The uropathogenic *E. coli* hemolysin A *(hly*A) is the best-studied member of this group *(19,20)*. It has been shown that the secretion signal is present in the last 60 amino acids of that protein and that transfer of this domain to other proteins can result in their direct secretion into the media when the accessory proteins from the hemolysin operon *(hylC*, A, B, and D) are present *(21)*. A few examples of secreted pro-

Table 1
Potential Sources of Secretion Signals for Proconverting Enzymes

Protein	Organism	Location in Transfected *E. coli* and type of signal	Ref No.
Chitinase	*Serratia marcescens*	released into medium N-terminal signal	*(22)*
α-Hemolysin	*E. coli*	released into medium C-terminal signal	*(23)*
Heat-stable enterotoxin I	various *E. coli* strains	N-terminal signal peptide; secreted into the media	*(24,25)*
Pullulanase	*Klebsiella pneumoniae*	Release into the medium; N-terminal signal peptide	*(18,26,27)*
Serine protease	*S. marcencens*	Secreted into the medium; N-terminal signal peptide	*(28)*
Pectate lyase	*Erwinia carotovara*	Periplasm	*(29–32)*
Protease	*E. chrysanthemi*	Secreted into the medium	*(33)*

teins reviewed by Pugsley *(18)* are presented in **Table 1** (*see* **refs. 22–34**). These secreted proteins as well as others constitute potential sources of secretion signals for prodrug converting enzymes. HSV-TK activity from extracts can be measured in phosphate buffered saline pH 7.2 (PBS): 8.0 g NaCl, 0.2 g KCl, 1.15 g Na_2HPO_4, 0.2 g NaH_2PO_4 per liter H_2O. PBS can be supplemented with 1 mg/mL lysozyme (Sigma) and 1% w/v TX100 (Sigma) to form a bacterial cell lysis buffer. Additional materials include stock solutions of 5-iodo-2′-deoxycytidine (IdC; Sigma): 20 mM; ^{125}I-labeled 5-iodo-2′-deoxycytidine (New England Nuclear, Boston, MA): 250 μCi/mL; ATP: 10 mM; bovine serum albumin: 0.6 mg/mL; $MgCl_2$: 10 mM; NaF: 25 mM; DE81 paper (Whatman, Clifton, NJ); and a gamma counter.

3. Methods

3.1. Mutagenesis

In any of the below described methods for attenuating bacteria for use as tumor-specific therapeutic vectors, the bacteria may be subjected to mutagenesis before enrichment procedures such as infection into mammalian cells or reisolation from tumors. For example, a wild-type strain of *Salmonella typhimurium* may be subjected to mutagenesis using both nitrosoguanidine (NG) and ultraviolet B irradiation. Other approaches such as transposon mutagenesis are not covered here, although any mutagen may be used to aid in the creation of mutant strains of bacteria.

NG and UV irradiation may be used jointly to mutagenize the bacteria.

1. The bacteria are grown exponentially at 37°C in minimal medium 56 plus glycerol (0.5%) to $OD_{600} = 0.3$, and chilled on ice.
2. Colony-forming units (CFU) of the above are determined by plating serial dilutions onto LB agar plates for determining initial CFU.
3. The bacteria are washed and resuspended in sodium citrate ($0.1M$, pH 5.5), incubated with fresh NG: 50 µg/mL, 37°C for 20 min.
4. The NG-treated bacteria are washed once by centrifugation, resuspended in medium 56, chilled, and titered again for CFU on LB agar plates.
5. An aliquot of the NG-treated bacteria can be diluted (1:5) into LB broth and grown to stationary phase for storage frozen at –80°C in 12% glycerol for later use as an NG-treatment only sample.
6. The remaining bacteria are irradiated with UV light, at a dose = 50 J/m², λ = 254 nm, whereby the time is dependent upon the output of the UV source. The cells are then titered for CFU on LB agar plates, with an aliquot diluted 1:4 into LB broth, grown to stationary phase, and stored frozen at –80°C in 12% glycerol.

A further description of monitoring mutagenesis by determining auxotrophic frequencies is described in **Subheading 3.4.**

3.2. Selection of Hyperinvasive Mutants In Vitro

A modified method of Elsinghorst *(34)* and Lee and Falkow *(35)* using melanoma cells as a novel target is employed (*see* **Note 1**). *S. typhimurium* ATCC strain 14028 is grown on LB agar and a single clone picked and designated "ATCC 14028 wild-type" ("wild-type"). *Salmonella* mutagenized with nitrosoguanidine and UVB irradiation as described may be grown as a population, or from individual colonies.

1. Prior to infection by *Salmonella*, mammalian cells are inoculated into Corning Tissue Culture flasks (25 cm²) at ~2 × 10⁵ cells/flask in 4-mL TCM (differing for different cell lines) containing penicillin (100 U/mL), and streptomycin (100 µg/mL), and incubated overnight in a 37°C gassed (5% CO_2 in air), humidified incubator. The day of the infection, the cells are rinsed twice with prewarmed TCM supplemented with 10% fetal bovine serum (FBS) and no antibiotics.
2. *Salmonella* are cultured on LB agar overnight at 37°C.
3. The following day the *Salmonella* are transferred with a platinum wire loop to LB broth or to TCM/FBS, adjusted in concentration to $OD_{600} = 0.1$ (~2 × 10⁸ CFU/mL), and subjected to further growth at 37°C on a rotator.
4. Following growth to the desired population density monitored at an optical density at 600 nm (*see* **Note 2**). These cultures are then diluted to a concentration of 10⁶ CFU/mL in TCM/FBS, and incubated at 37°C an additional 20 min.
5. The bacteria are then added to mammalian cell cultures in 25 cm² tissue-culture flasks at 4 mL/flask, and incubated with the mammalian cells in a gassed (5% CO_2/95% air), humidified incubator at 37°C for 15 min.

6. After incubation with the mammalian cells, the bacteria-containing medium is poured off, the cultures are rinsed gently with warmed TCM/FBS (4 mL) containing gentamicin sulfate (50 µg/mL, Sigma), an antibiotic that kills extracellular, but not intracellular bacteria. The gentamicin sulfate-containing medium is poured off, fresh TCM/FBS/gentamicin sulfate medium is added, and the cells are incubated for 30 min at 37°C.

7. Following incubation with gentamicin sulfate, the medium is poured off, the flasks are rinsed once with TCM/FBS (without gentamicin sulfate), and 1 mM EDTA or an EDTA/trypsin solution (Sigma Chemicals) in Ca^{++}-Mg^{++}-free physiological saline (4 mL) is added.

8. After incubating with EDTA or EDTA/trypsin (20 min, 37°C), the flasks are shaken to suspend the animal cells, and aliquots removed for quantitation. Mammalian cells are quantitated in a Coulter Counter (Coulter Electronics, Inc., Hialeah, FL) and bacteria are quantitated by liberating them from the mammalian cess by the addition of 10% TX100 (Sigma) to a final concentration of 0.1% and plating aliquots on LB agar, incubating at 37°C, and counting colonies. Quantitation is expressed as the number of infecting (gentamicin resistant) bacteria/10^6 mammalian cells.

9. Isolation of hyperinvasive, tumor-cell-specific *Salmonella* involves repeated cycles of infection into human melanoma cells, **steps 1 –7** above, with the bacterial cells from **step 8** used as the starting material for **step 2**. After the completion of four such cycles, the population of melanoma-cycled bacteria is then plated on agar and individual clones were picked and tested for their relative ability, compared to wild-type bacteria, to infect tumor cells such as M2 melanoma.

An example of our results is detailed in **Table 2**. The mixed population of four times cycled *Salmonella* cells showed three-fold increased infectivity of melanoma cells over that of the starting mutagenized population of wild-type bacteria. Of 100 clones isolated from the four times cycled population of *Salmonella*, two of them, YS6 and YS72, were found to be significantly more invasive towards melanoma cells. The remaining bacterial clones showed infectivity that was similar to, or below that of, the wild-type strain. In the experiment presented in **Table 2**, clone YS6 was 23-fold, and clone YS72 was 55-fold more infective than the mutagenized wild-type strain during a 15 min infection period. *E. coli*, strain K-12, was at least two orders of magnitude less infective than wild-type *S. typhimurium* (*see* **Note 1**).

3.3. Determinations of Intracellular Growth In Vitro

Hyperinvasive *S. typhimurium* clones, such as YS72 shown in **Table 2**, can be compared to the nonmutagenized wild-type strain ATCC 14028 for relative ability to proliferate within cancerous cells such as melanoma.

Table 2
**Internalization of *Salmonella* Populations and Clones
into M2 Human Melanoma Cells in Culture**

Strain	Infecting Bacteria/10^6 Melanoma Cells	Melanoma cells (% wild-type)
Wild-type *S.typhimurium* 14028 (mutagenized)	$3.8 \pm 3.0 \times 10^4$	100
Cycle #4 (mixed population)	$1.1 \pm 0.4 \times 10^5$	290
Cycle #4–Clone YS6	$8.6 \pm 1.0 \times 10^5$	2260
Cycle #4–Clone YS72	$2.1 \pm 0.2 \times 10^6$	5500
E. coli K-12	$<10^2$	<1

Results represent averages ± SD for triplicate infections.

Steps 1–5 as aforementioned are performed in triplicate for each strain and time-point to be determined, with **steps 6–8** performed in a time-dependent manner.

3.4. Selection of Auxotrophic Mutants

The mutagenesis procedure described above produces an increase in the number of mutations in the strain by initial criteria as assayed by decreased survival of the bacteria following mutagenesis (e.g., nitrosoguanidine = six-fold; UV B irradiation = 400-fold). Additional criteria are: 1) increased frequency of auxotrophic (nutritional requiring) mutants; 2) increased frequency of maltose mutants; 3) increased frequency of galactose⁻mutants. Determinations of auxotrophy are made as follows:

1. Cells are plated to rich media such as LB agar (approximately 300 CFU/plate) and allowed to grow at 37° C.
2. These colonies are then replica plated onto maltose-MacConkey and galactose-MacConkey plates and then LB-agar and then minimal medium. White colonies on MacConkey indicate *mal⁻* or *gal⁻* mutations, and colonies which grow on LB plates, but not minimal medium indicate auxotrophs. The observation of a reasonable frequency of these muatations (see below) in the mutagenized culture justifies its use in subsequent extensive mutant searches. Such determinations of auxotrophy are used to select for strains in order to determine if mutation in a given allele results in attenuation (**Subheading 3.5.**) and retains in vivo tumor targeting (**Subheading 3.6.**). An example of auxotrophic frequencies from our studies are detailed in **Table 3**. Multiple rounds of mutation and selection may be used to generate polyauxotrophic strains. It should be remembered, however, that each round of such mutagenesis introduces many undetected mutations which

Table 3
Mutagenesis of *Salmonella Typhimurium*

	Mutation frequency in *S. typhimurium*, strain ATCC 14028	
Genetic Marker	No mutagenesis	Mutagenesis (NG, UVB)
maltose (*mal⁻*)	$<1 \times 10^{-6}$	2×10^{-2}
galactose (*gal⁻*)	$<1 \times 10^{-6}$	0.5×10^{-2}
auxotrophy	$<1 \times 10^{-6}$	2×10^{-2}
(e.g., *met⁻*, *ade⁻*, *his⁻*)		

may or may not affect the subsequent behavior of any mutant later selected (*see* **Note 3**.)

3.5. Determination of Attenuation

In our studies, the hyperinvasive clone YS72 was also found to be Pur⁻ when assayed for auxotrophy as above, requiring adenine and thiamine (vitamin B1), although no selective pressure had been applied for isolation of the Pur⁻ phenotype. This phenotype and other auxotrophies are known to reduce virulence of *Salmonella* in mice (**7–9**) and can be determined in standard LD$_{50}$ assays (**36,37**). An alternative approach, time to death, is described which yields relative, reproducible numerical values that require fewer animals in order to determine.

1. *Salmonella* are cultured on LB agar overnight at 37°.
2. The following day they are transferred to LB broth, adjusted in concentration to OD$_{600}$ = 0.1 (~2 × 10⁸ CFU/mL), and subjected to further growth at 37° on a rotator to OD$_{600}$ = 0.8, and placed on ice.
3. Following growth, they are diluted to a concentration of 10⁷or 10⁸ CFU/mL in PBS on ice, warmed to room temperature, and 0.2 mL injected ip into C57B6 mice (*n* = 5–10).
4. Death of the animals is monitored daily, and attenuation level expressed as increased time of the mean survival as compared to the parental strain.

3.6. In Vivo Tumor-Targeting: Tumor to Normal Tissue Ratios

Strains derived from the methods described above can be assayed for their ability to target tumors, and their tumor to normal tissue ratios. Normal tissues primarily infected by *Salmonella* include the spleen and liver. Because of the size and accessibility of the liver, we generally use this organ as an indicator of the highest level CFU in normal tissues.

1. C57BL6 mice are implanted sc with 5 × 10⁵ B16F10 mouse melanoma cells, and staged until the appearance of palpable tumors (approx 2 wk).

2. *Salmonella* are cultured on LB agar overnight at 37°.
3. The following day they were transferred to LB broth, adjusted in concentration to $OD_{600} = 0.1$ (~2×10^8 CFU/mL), and subjected to further growth at 37° on a rotator to $OD_{600} = 0.8$, and placed on ice.
4. Following growth, they are diluted to a concentration of 10^4 to 10^7 CFU/mL in PBS on ice, warmed to room temperature, and 0.2 mL injected ip or iv into C57B6 mice ($n = 5$–10).
5. After subsequent time-periods, usually 1 to 7 d of infection, mice are euthanized. Tumors and livers are removed aseptically, rinsed with sterile PBS, weighed, and homogenized with LB broth at a ratio of 5:1 (vol broth:wt tumor).
6. Serial dilutions to LB agar plates are used to determine the CFU per gram of tissue.

In our preliminary studies, the wild-type and hyperinvasive, auxotrophic strains were examined for tumor and liver distribution after ip inoculation into mice bearing B16F10 melanoma. Tests of 10^1 to 10^8 CFU/mouse indicated 10^6 CFU was most useful for observing tumor and liver infectivity for at least 2d, while at the same time maintaining the viability of mice injected with partially or fully virulent strains such as ATCC 14028 and YS72. Our results have consistently shown tumor to liver ratios in excess of 1000:1 *(4)* (*see* **Note 4**).

3.7. Determination of Antitumor Activity

Experimental determination of antitumor activity follows the same general protocol for determinations of tumor-targeting described above. However, because of the rapid growth of many tumor models, and the lack of necessity for external recognition of tumors at early time-points, tumors are staged earlier; usually at 5–12 d . Tumor measurements should always made by the same person in order to compensate for any individual biases and assure consistency.

1. C57BL6 mice are implanted sc with 5×10^5 B16F10 mouse melanoma cells, and staged between day 5 and day 12.
2. *Salmonella* are cultured on LB agar overnight at 37°.
3. The following day, the bacteria are transferred to LB broth, adjusted in concentration to $OD_{600} = 0.1$ (~2×10^8 CFU/mL), and subjected to further growth at 37° on a rotator to $OD_{600} = 0.8$, and placed on ice.
4. Following growth, they are diluted to a concentration of 10^4 to 10^8 CFU/mL (usually 10^7) in PBS on ice, warmed to room temperature, and 0.2 mL injected ip or iv into C57B6 mice ($n = 5$–10).
5. After the appearance of palpable tumors in any group, calipers are used to determine the volume in $mm^3 = L \times W \times H$, and the final volume adjusted by multiplying by 0.5236.
6. Ten days following inoculation of bacteria, mice may be given enrofloxacin (Bayer, 0.2 µg/mL drinking water) for a total of 2 wk, which increases the survival of mice.

3.8. Cloning and Expression of HSV-tK in Bacteria

Whereas the antitumor activity of tumor-specific *Salmonella* is a useful find-ing by itself, perhaps even more promising is the ability of these bacteria to be used as tumor-specific delivery agents. An implicit part of a targeting/prodrug conversion system is that the targeting ratio be able to be translated into an activation ratio, resulting in specific antitumor activity. A wide range of effector gene systems has been explored in viral, liposome, and antibody-conjugated therapies. We initiated our studies on a system capable of activat-ing drugs already approved for use in humans and known to be effective in the inhibition of melanoma tumor growth *(39)*, the *HSV-tK*.

Prodrug enzyme studies could employ cytoplasmically located enzyme, relying upon permeability of the activated drug or lysis of the bacteria to release the enzyme, or the use of secretion constructs generated by formation heterolo-gous fusions of signal sequence from a variety of sources (e.g., **Table 1**) or from commercially available sources. The trc promoter (Pharmacia, Uppsala, Sweden) resulting in cytoplasmic expression has been used for intratumoral expression of cytosine deaminase by tumor targeted *Salmonella (40)*. Secre-tion vectors such as pMAL (New England Biolabs, Beverly, MA) and pEZZ18 *(41)* (Pharmacia) are also available. We utilized HSV-TK *(42,43)* fused to the β-lactamase secretory sequence *(17)* (Clonetech, no longer available; *see* **Note 5**). Transformation protocols of *Salmonella* strains *(44)*, are similar to widely used protocols for *E. coli* transformation *(45)*. Strains such as LB5010 used by O'Callahan and Charbit *(44)* which are restriction minus and methyla-tion positive (r^-, m^+) greatly increase transformation efficiency, and serve as an intermediate host for plasmids being transferred from *E. coli* to *Salmonella*. A modified thymidine kinase assay *(46)* (P. Tung and W. Summers, personal com-munication) suitable for bacterial strains expressing *HSV-tK* is described below:

1. Bacterial lysates are prepared by pelleting 1 mL of log-phase bacterial culture for 30 s at 12,000g in a microfuge centrifuge. The pellet and supernatant are retained separately for determinations of secreted or lytically released activity, and the supernatant was further cleared by centrifugation for 10 min at 12,000g.
2. The pellet material, where both cytoplasmically expressed and periplasmically secreted activity are found, is further treated by resuspension in 100 μL of PBS containing 1 mg/mL lysozyme and 1% (v/v) Triton X-100 and subjected to three cycles of rapid freezing and thawing.
3. The viscosity of the resulting material can be reduced by several passages through a 27-ga needle using a syringe, and then clarified by centrifugation at 12,000g for 2 min.
4. Thymidine kinase activity is conveniently assayed using the false substrate 5-iodo-2'-deoxycytidine (IdC; Sigma) and its ^{125}I-labeled counterpart (New England Nuclear). Other substrates including ^{3}H-ganciclovir (Moravek) and

[3]H-acyclovir (Moravek) may also be used. Initial screening employs a negative control bacterium containing the plasmid without HSV-TK, and a single time-point for incubation of the control and each of the test samples. The assay mixture contains 0.2 mM IdC, 5 μCi [125]IdC, 10 mM ATP, 0.6 mg/mL bovine serum albumin, 10 mM MgCl$_2$, 25 mM NaF, and 100 mM sodium phosphate buffer pH 6.0. 5 μL of the enzyme extract are combined with 20 μL of the reaction mix and incubated at 37°C for 1 h and then bound to DE81 paper (Whatman), washed with distilled water three times, and once with 70% ethanol, dried, and the associated radioactivity determined in a gamma counter.

5. Verification of the enzyme activity requires determination kinetics, using time-points from 30 to 120 min, in the assay **step 4** above (*see* **Note 5**).

3.9. In Vivo Activity of Prodrug Activation Systems

Evaluation of the efficacy of *Salmonella* combined with a prodrug activation systems requires several important controls. We have found that the *Salmonella* carrying the effector gene plasmid exhibit less antitumor activity than their plasmid-free counterparts. Furthermore, although in theory, prodrugs such as ganciclovir are relatively non-toxic and have no inherent antitumor activity, effects on tumor growth and/or toxicity are sometimes measured by control experiments. Therefore, the following sets of groups are helpful in assessing antitumor activity in tumored animal experiments:

1. Control, no treatment.
2. GCV only.
3. *Salmonella* strain X.
4. *Salmonella* strain X, plus GCV.
5. *Salmonella* strain X, plus HSV-TK plasmid.
6. *Salmonella* strain X, plus HSV-TK plasmid, plus GCV.

Furthermore, varying amounts of GCV may be administered, causing considerable expansion of the size of the experiment. The experimental protocol is essentially that of the efficacy experiments described above, with the addition of the GCV.

1. C57BL6 mice are implanted sc with 5×10^5 B16F10 mouse melanoma cells, and staged between day 5 and day 12.
2. *Salmonella* are cultured on LB agar containing the appropriate antibiotic for maintenance of the plasmid overnight at 37°.
3. The following day the bacteria are transferred to LB broth without antibiotic, adjusted in concentration to OD$_{600}$ = 0.1 (~2×10^8 CFU/mL), and subjected to further growth at 37° on a rotator to OD$_{600}$ = 0.8, and placed on ice.
4. Following growth, they are diluted to a concentration of 10^4 to 10^8 CFU/mL (usually 10^7)in PBS on ice, warmed to room temperature, and 0.2 mL injected ip or iv into C57B6 mice (n = 5–10).

5. Three days postbacterial inoculation, the appropriate groups receive GCV ip under the following protocols:
   a. 330 mg/kg (2.5 mg day 11, 1.25 mg day 12; 2.5 mg day 18, 1.25 mg day 19);
   b. 220 mg/kg (2.5 mg day 11, 2.5 mg day 12);
   c. 165 mg/kg (2.5 mg day 11, 1.25 mg day 12);
   d. 110 mg/kg (1.25 mg day 11, 1.25 mg day 12);
   e. 55 mg/kg (1.25 mg day 11).
6. Ten days following inoculation of bacteria, mice are routinely given enrofloxacin (0.2 mg/mL drinking water) for a total of 2 wk.
7. After the appearance of palpable tumors in any group, calipers are used to determine the volume in $mm^3 = L \times W \times H$, and the final volume adjusted by multiplying by 0.5236 9 (*see* **Note 6**).

4. Notes

1. During the maintenance of tumor cell lines, the possibility of mycoplasma infection should be monitored using standard procedures (e.g., Boeringer Mannheim mycoplasma assay kit). Mycoplasma infections may go undetected but can affect cell growth and other properties, and may interfere with invasion assays.
2. Late log cultures corresponding to OD_{600} of 0.8, which are acidic and hypoxic, give maximal infection rates for wild-type *Salmonella*. We have isolated strains hyperinvasive at low population densities corresponding to OD_{600} of 0.3, which are well oxygenated, but retain maximal invasive capacity under acidic and hypoxic conditions).
3. To assess stability of the auxotrophic phenotypes, bacterial isolates can be replated on rich media, organized on a numbered grid, and replica plated onto minimal media agar supplemented with the appropriate nutritional additives to monitor for persistence of the auxotrophic mutations. Highly unstable or leaky auxotrophs are identified by weak growth and/or revertant colonies on the printed patches.
4. For microscopic analyses, portions of the tumor may be fixed prior to homogenization (a complete descripion of microscopic analysis is beyond the scope of this chapter). $1-2\ mm^3$ pieces of tissue are removed from representative tumors, fixed and embedded in paraffin. Sectioned material can be stained with hemotoxylin and eosin or tissue gram stain (Brown-Brenn stain). In samples where biodistribution analysis indicates levels of 10^9, the presence of bacteria is readily detected.
5. PCR has improved considerably in recent years, including the protocols for thermocycling and in the fidelity of the polymerases. In our study (**4**) where the HSV-TK was cloned using *Taq* polymerase (Perkin Elmer, Norwalk, CT), we found variable activity of the cloned genes. The possibility of incorporation of errors in cloning should always be evaluated, including sequencing of junctions or the entire construct if practical.
6. After 2 and 10 d of bacterial infection without antibiotic treatment, representative tumor-bearing animals may be sacrificed and their tumors and livers homogenized and quantitated for CFU of *Salmonella*/g tissue. In addition, individual

clones of bacteria can be isolated from the liver and tumor homogenates and tested for the genetic markers, e.g., *tet*^res (resistance to the antibiotic tetracycline) by plating to LB agar containing 10 µg/mL tetracycline in order to infer the presence of the plasmid, and may be further tested by the enzyme assay described above. In our experiments, the *HSV-tK* plasmid was found to be 100% retained after 42 h of infection in tumor-bearing mice, whereas 80% retained the plasmid after 10 d.

5. Summary

Isolation of *Salmonella* strains with mutations in readily identifiable metabolic pathways provides a rapid means to generate strains for evaluation as tumor-targeted vectors from pathogenic bacteria. Selection schemes for tumor-amplification or invasion can be interspersed with the mutation processed in order to insure desirable properties have not been lost during strain construction. Attenuated, tumor-targeting bacterial strains are suitable for use as expression vectors of effector gene systems such as prodrug-converting enzymes. Experiments in mice can be complicated by the fact that the bacteria alone are so potent in retarding tumor growth that further GCV effects are relatively small. In addition, the antitumor activity of *Salmonella HSV-tK* plasmid-bearing strains is less than their plasmid-free counterparts, even though they are able to target and amplify within tumors similarly to plasmid-free strains. Nevertheless, tumor-targeted *Salmonella* show a high degree of promise as gene therapeutic agents for the treatment of cancer.

Acknowledgments

We wish to thank Drs. Jean Bolognia, Terrence Doyle, Keith Joiner, Ivan King, Stanley Lin, Xiang Luo, Samuel Miller, William Summers, Peter Tung, and Li-mou Zheng for helpful discussions. This study was supported by a Grant from Vion Pharmaceuticals.

References

1. Jain, R. K. (1994) Barriers to drug delivery in solid tumors. *Scient. Am.* **271 (July),** 58–65.
2. Parker, R. C., Plummber, H. C., Siebenmann, C. O., and Chapman, M. G. (1947) Effect of histolyticus infection and toxin on transplantable mouse tumors. *Proc. Soc. Exp. Biol. Med.* **66,** 461–465.
3. Fox, M. E., Lemmon, M. J., Mauchline, M. L., Davis, T. O., Giaccia, A. J., Minton, N. P., and Brown, J. M. (1996) Anaerobic bacteria as a delivery system for cancer gene therapy: in vitro activation of 5-fluorocytosine by genetically engineered clostridia. *Gene Ther.* **3,** 173–178.
4. Pawelek, J. M., Low, K. B., and Bermudes, D. (1997) Tumor-targeted Salmonella as a novel anticancer vector. *Cancer Res.* **57,** 4537–4544.

5. Zheng, L. M., Luo, X., Fischer, J., Le, T., Bermudes, D., Low, B., et al. (1997) Attenuated *Salmonella typhimurium* inhibited tumor metastasis in vivo. *Proc. Amer. Asoc. Cancer Res.* (abstrt.) **38,** 9.

6. Bacon, G. A., Burrows, T. W., and Yates, M. (1950) The effects of biochemical mutation on the virulence of bacterium typhosum: the induction and isolation of mutants. *Br. J. Exp. Path.* **31,** 703–713.

7. Bacon, G. A., Burrows T. W., and Yates, M. (1951) The effects of biochemical mutation on the birulence of bacterium typhosum: the loss of virulence of certain mutants. *Br. J. Exp. Path.* **32,** 85–96.

8. Hoiseth, S. K. J. and Stocker, B. A. D. (1981) Aromatic-dependent *Salmonella typhimurium* are non-virulent and effective as live vaccines. *Nature* **291,** 238–239.

9. O'Callaghan, D., Maskell, D., Liew, F. Y., Easmon, C. S. F., and Dougan, G. (1988) Characterization of aromatic- and purine-dependent *Salmonella typhimurium*: attenuation, persistence, and ability induce protective immunity in BALB/c mice. *Infect. Immun.* **56,** 419–423.

10. Pidherney, M. S., Alizadeh, H., Steward, G. L., McCulley, J. P., and Niederkorn, J. Y. (1993) In vitro and in vivo tumorcidal properties of a pathogenic/free-living amoeba. *Cancer Lett.* **72,** 91–98.

11. Alizadeh, H., Pidherney, M. S., McCulley, J. P., and Niederkorn, J. Y. (1994) Apoptosis as a mechanism of cytolysis of tumor cells by a pathogenic free-living amoeba. *Infect. Immun.* **62,** 1298–1303.

12. Miller, J. H. (1992) *A Short Course in Bacterial Genetics.* Cold Spring Harbor Laboratory, Cold Spring Harbor.

13. Hutchinson, F. (1996) Mutagenesis, in *Escherichia coli and Salmonella typhimurium, Cellular and Molecular Biology* (Neidhardt, F. C., Curtiss III, R., Ingraham, J. L., Lin, E. C. C., Low, K. B., Magasanik, B., et al., eds.), Am. Soc. Microbiol., Washington, DC, pp. 2218–2235.

14. Cunningham, C. C., Gorlin, J. B., Kwiatkowski, D. J., Hartwig, H. J., Janmey, P. A., Byers, H. R., and Stossel, T. P. (1992) Actin-binding protein requirement for cortical stability and efficient locomotion. *Science* **255,** 325–327.

15. Vile, R. G. and Hart, I. R. (1993) Use of tissue-specific expression of the herpes simples virus thymidine kinase gene to inhibit growth of established murine melanomas following direct intratumoral injection of DNA. *Cancer Res.* **53,** 3860–3864.

16. Moolten, F. L. and Wells, J. M. (1990) Curability of tumors bearing herpes thymidine kinase genes transferred by retroviral vectors. *J. Natl. Cancer Inst.* **82,** 297–300.

17. Talmadge, K,. Stahl, S., and Gilbert, W. (1980) Eukaryotic signal sequence transports insulin antigen in *Escherchia coli. Proc. Natl. Acad. Sci. USA* **77,** 3369–3373.

18. Pugsley, A. P. (1988) Protein secretion across the outer membrane of gram-negative bacteria, in *Protein Transfer and Organelle Biogenesis* (Das, R. C. and Robbins, P. W., eds.), Academic, New York, pp. 607–652.

19. Holland, I. B., Wang, R., Seror, S. J., and Blight, M. (1989) Haemolysin secretion and other protein translocation mechanisms in gram-negative bacteria, in *Micro-*

bial Products, New Approaches (Baumberg, S., Hinster, I., and Rhodes, M., eds.), Cambridge University Press, Cambridge, pp. 219–254.

20. Wagner, W., Vogel, M. l., and Goebel, W. (1983) Transport of haemolysin across the outermembrane of *Escherichia coli* requires two functions. *J. Bacteriol.* **154,** 200–210.

21. Su, G-F., Brahmbhatt, H. N., deLorenzo, V., Wehland, J., and Timmis, K. N. (1992) Extracellular export of shiga toxin B-subunit/haemolysin A (C-terminus) fusion protein expressed in *Salmonella typhimurium aro*A-mutant and stimulation of B-subunit specific antibody responses in mice. *Microbial. Pathogenesis* **13,** 465–476.

22. Jones, J. D. G., Grady, K. L., Suslow, T. V., and Bedbrook, J. R. (1986) Isolation and characterization of genes encoding two chitinase enzymes from *Serratia marcescens. EMBO J.* **5,** 2377–2383.

23. Goebel, W., Hacker, J., Knapp, S., Then, J., Wagner, W., Hughes, C., and Juarez, A. (1984) Structure, function and regulation of the plasmid-encoded hemolysin determinant of *E. coli,* in *Plasmids in Bacteria* (Helinski, D. R., Cohen, S. N., Cloewell, D. B., Jackson, D. A., and Hollaender, A., eds.,) Plenum, New York, pp. 791–805.

24. Guzmán-Verduzco, L. M., Fonseca, R., and Kaperszotch-Portnoy, Y. M. (1983) Thermoactivation of a periplasmic heat-stable enterotoxin of *Escherichia coli. J. Bacteriol.* **154,** 146–151.

25. So, M. and McCarthy, B. T. (1980) Nucleotide sequence of the bacterial transposon Tn1681 encoding a heat-stable (ST) toxin and its identification in enterotoxigenic coli strains. *Proc. Natl. Acad. Sci. USA* **77,** 4011–4015.

26. Chapon, C. and Raibaud, O. (1985) Structure of two divergent promoters located in front of the gene encoding pullulanase in *Klebsiella pneumoniae* and positively reguylated by the *malT.* product. *J. Bacteriol.* **164,** 639–645.

27. d'Enfert, C., Ryter, A., and Pugsely, A. P. (1987) Cloning and expression in *Escherichia coli* of the *Klebsiella pneumoniue* genes for production, surface localization and secretion of the lipoprotein pullanase. *EMBO J.* **6,** 3531–3538.

28. Yanigida, N., Ouozumi, T., and Beppu, T. (1986) Specific excretion of *Serratia marcescens* protease through the outer membrane of *Escherichia coli. J. Bacteriol.* **166,** 937–944.

29. Collmer, A., Schoedel, C., Roeder, D. L., Ried, J. L., and Rissler, J. F. (1985) Molecular cloning in *Escherichia coli* of *Erwinia chrysanthemi* genes encoding multiple forms of pectate lyase. *J. Bacteriol.* **161,** 913–920.

30. Keen, N.T., Dahlbreck, D., Staskawicz, B., and Belser, W. (1984) Molecular cloning of pectate lyase genes from *Erwinia chrysanthemi* and their expression in *Escherichia coli. J. Bacteriol.* **159,** 825–831.

31. Lei, S.-P., Lin, H.-C., Hefferman, L., and Wilcox, G. (1985) Cloning of the pectate lyase genes from *Erwinia carotovora* and their expression in *Escherichia coli. Gene* **35,** 63–70.

32. Zink, R.T. and Chatterjee, A.K. (1985) Cloning and expression in *Escherichia*

coli of pectinase gene of *Erwinia carotovora* subsp. *carotovora*. *Appl. Environ. Microbiol.* **49,** 714–717.

33. Barras, F., Thurn, K. K., and Chatterjee, A. K. (1986) Export of *Erwinia chrysanthemi* (EC16) protease by *Escherichia coli*. *FEMS Microbiol. Lett.* **34,** 343–348.

34. Elsinghorst, E. A. (1994) Measurement of invasion by gentamycin resistance. *Meth. Enzymol.* **236,** 405–420.

35. Lee, C. A. and Falkow, S. (1994) Isolation of hyperinvasive mutants of Salmonella. *Meth. Enzymol.* **236,** 531–545.

36. Reed, L., J. and Muench, H. (1938) A simple method of estimating fifty percent endpoints. *Am. J. Hyg.* **27,** 493–497.

37. Welkos, S. and O'Brien, A. (1994) Determination of median lethal and infectious doses in animal model systems. *Meth. Enzymol.* **235,** 29–39.

38. Bonnekoh, B., Greenhalgh, D. A., Bundman, D. S., Ekhardt, J. N., Longley, M. A., Chen., S. H., et al. (1995) Inhibition of melanoma growth by adenoviral-mediated HSV thymidine kinase gene tranfer in vivo. *J. Invest. Derm.* **104,** 313–317.

39. King, I., Feng, M., Lou, X., Lin, S., Bermudes, D., and Zheng, L.-M. (1998) Tumor-targeted *Salmonella* expressing cytosine deaminase converted 5-fluorocytosine to 5-fluorouricil and inhibited tumor growth in vivo. Ann. Meet. Am. Assoc. Cancer Res., New Orleans, LA, March 28 to April 2, (abstr.).

40. Liljeqvist, S., Haddad, D., Berzins, K., Uhlén, M., and Ståhl, S. (1996) A novel expression system for *Salmonella typhimurium* allowing high production levels, product secretion and efficient recovery. *Biochem. Biophys. Res. Comm.* **218,** 356–359.

41. McKnight, S. L. (1980) The nucleotide sequence and transcript map of the herpes simplex virus thymidine kinase gene. *Nuc. Acids. Res.* **8,** 5949–5964.

42. Wagner, M..J., Sharp, J.A., and Summers, W.C. (1981) Nucleotide sequence of the thymidine kinase gene of herpes simplex virus type 1. *Proc. Natl. Acad. Sci. USA* **78,** 1441–1445.

43. O'Callaghan, D. and Charbit, A. (1990) High efficiency transformation of *Salmonella typhimurium* and *Salmonella typhi* by electroporation. *Mol. Gen. Genet.* **223,** 156–158.

44. Sambrook, J., Fritsch, E. F., and Maniatis, T. (1989) *Molecular Cloning: A Laboratory Manual*, 2nd Ed., Cold Spring Harbor, Cold Spring Harbor.

45. Summers, W. C. and Summers, W. P. (1977) [^{125}I]deoxycytidine used in a rapid, sensitive, and specific assay for herpes simplex virus type 1 thymidine kinase. *J. Virol.* **24,** 314–318.

II

CLINICAL PROTOCOLS FOR CANCER GENE THERAPY

A: Immunotherapy/Tumor Vaccination

27

Ex Vivo Cytokine Gene Transfer
in Melanomas by Using Particle Bombardment

Dirk Schadendorf

1. Introduction
1.1. Melanoma and Tumor Immunology

Melanoma is a malignant tumor of neuroectodermal origin with an increasing incidence and mortality. It needs to be detected and eliminated early, because melanoma is characterized by its high resistance to the conventional therapies, including surgery and chemotherapy *(1–3)*. On the other hand, melanoma is supposed to be one of the most immunogenic tumors which is demonstrated by tumor-infiltrating lymphocytes (TIL) destroying melanoma cells *(4–6)*. This may also be responsible for the occurrence of spontaneous partial or complete melanoma regression and for concomitant destruction of melanocytes in benign lesions, leading to clinical phenomena such as halo nevi, uveitis, and vitiligo in melanoma patients.

It is generally accepted that the spontaneous generation of cancer cells is a common event, and that the immune system assures a strict surveillance with the detection and elimination of these cells. In order to fight cancer, the idea to use the destructive power of immunologic reactions is easily visualized in autoimmune diseases and by the rejection of allografts in transplantation medicine. A number of clinical observations in human malignant melanoma suggest a particularly vigorous occurring immune response *(4–7)*. In the recent years, it has became more and more clear that T lymphocytes may play a critical role in antitumor immune responses and surveillance *(4,8)*. Furthermore, CD8+ T lymphocytes derived from melanoma lesions or the peripheral blood were shown to be capable to mediate impressive tumor regressions in vivo

From: *Methods in Molecular Medicine, Vol. 35: Gene Therapy: Methods and Protocols*
Edited by: W. Walther and U. Stein © Humana Press, Inc., Totowa, NJ

(9,10). The availability and further characterization of such tumor-specific T-cell clones in the recent years led to the identification of several melanoma-associated antigens [*see (8)*]. There are different approaches to utilize the host's immune system to fight the tumor, including the augmentation of the immunogeneity of tumor cells by cytokine gene transfer [*see (11,12)*].

1.2. The Rationale for a Cytokine Gene Transfer

In past decades, the identification and cloning of cytokines provided an important set of tools for the manipulation of immunologic responses. Systemic infusions of interleukin-2 (IL-2), originally named T-cell growth factor, into patients suffering from advanced melanoma were shown to achieve comparable clinical responses as conventional therapies, however, effects were associated with dramatic side effects *(13)*. Today, IL-2 and interferon alpha (IFN-α) are commonly used in combination with conventional chemotherapies (so-called chemoimmunotherapy) in order to improve response rates and survival *(3)*. Since 1989, a different immunotherapy approach using cytokines in a more physiological (paracrine) mode has been tested in various animal tumor models. Starting from the pioneering work of Tepper and coworkers *(14)*, who showed that tumor cells after transfection with the IL-4-gene were rejected and work by Fearon and colleagues *(15)* who demonstrated that paracrine-secreted IL-2 after gene transfer into a poorly immunogenic murine tumor can bypass T-helper function in the generation of antitumor response including protection against subsequent challenge with parental tumor cells, numerous cytokines have been tested in such tumor-bearing animal models *(12,16)*. Gene transfer of cytokine genes such as IL-2, IL-4, IL-7, IL-12, IFN-γ, TNF-α and GM-CSF were shown to be able to induce an systemic antitumor immune memory demonstrated by a subsequent challenge with wild-type tumor cells at a distance. This antitumor immunity required CD8+ T cells and in part CD4+ T cells *(12,16)*. Possibly, CD8+ and CD4+ T lymphocytes were activated directly by transfected tumor cells or more likely indirectly via antigen presenting cells (APC) *(17)*. Certain cytokines are active in some, but not in all, animal tumor models *(12,16)*.

Recently, the combination of cytokine-genes such as IL-7 and the costimulatory B7 molecule seemed to significantly enhance the antitumor effect *(18)*. In conclusion, experimental tumor models using gene-modified tumor cells demonstrated the antitumor effects of various cytokines and point to the need of CTL-induction for long-lived tumorimmunity. Although these results are encouraging, because they show the feasibility of the approach, a long way is still to go before one can imagine to treat patients tumor-specific leading to a *curative* T-cell response.

1.3. Ex Vivo Gene Transfer

The era of gene therapy has become a clinical reality. Since the first therapeutic experiments in 1970, more than 250 additional clinical gene trials were approved and more than 2000 patients treated worldwide at the end of 1996 *(19)*. Almost 25% of these studies have no therapeutic intent and are gene-marking trials. The majority (60%) of the trials are aimed to treat cancer. The great majority of investigators used immunization strategies with cytokine-gene modified tumor cells. Because melanoma is supposedly one of the most immunogenic tumors, it was therefore a favorable target for gene-modified cancer vaccines (summarized in **Table 1**). Based on the animal tumor models, a number of clinical protocols have been developed to treat cancer patients with cytokine gene-modified tumor cells.

1.4. Results of IL-7 and IL-12
Gene Transfer in Melanoma Treatment

Clinical phase I studies were initiated aiming at the induction of T-cell-mediated cytotoxicity and tumor immunity by immunizing melanoma patients *(21–24)*. Autologous melanoma cells were gene-modified by genetic manipulation in order to attract immunological competent cells to the tumor and to elicit a systemic antitumor immunity. Therefore, melanoma metastases from melanoma patients who have failed to respond to other therapies are surgically removed and melanoma cells are expanded in vitro (**Fig. 1**). Autologous melanoma cells were transfected either with both chains of the IL-12 gene *(24)* or with the IL-7 gene *(23)*. Patients are vaccinated sc with 5×10^{-6} to 5×10^{-7} autologous cells in week 1, week 2, week 3, and week 6. In parallel, DTH-reactivity and an extensive immunological monitoring including flow cytometry, NK-and LAK-activity as well as CTL analysis are performed. The cytokine gene transfer protocol uses a newly developed gene transfer technology that combines ballistic transfer of biological molecules and magnetic cell sorting *(22)*.

Evaluation of the first 10 patients immunized with autologous, IL-7 gene-modified melanoma cells demonstrated the safety, the lack of toxicity, and the feasibility of such an approach, however, no major clinical response was achieved *(23)*. Eight of ten patients completed the initial three sc vaccinations with IL-7 gene-modified cells and were eligible for immunological evaluation. Nonspecific cytotoxicity (NK- and LAK-activity) increased upon vaccination in 4/8 and 7/8 patients, respectively. Furthermore, peripheral blood lymphocytes were found to contain an increased number of tumor-reactive T cells after immunization. The number of tumor-reactive as well as cytolytic T-cell

Table 1
Clinical Trials Designed to Treat Melanoma Patients
by Cytokine Gene Transfer[a]

Gene	Cell target	Vector	Investigator	No. of Patients
IL-2	allogeneic tumor lines	RVV	Osanto/Schrier	35
IL-2	allogeneic tumor lines	RVV	Parmiani/Cascinelli/Foa	12
IL-2/B7	allogeneic tumor lines	RVV	Parmiani/Cascinelli/Foa	0
IL-4	allogeneic tumor lines	RVV	Parmiani/Cascinelli/Foa	12
IL-2	allogeneic tumor lines	RVV	Das Gupta	3
IL-2	allogeneic tumor lines	RVV	Ecomonu	0
IL-2	allogeneic tumor lines	RVV	Gänsbacher	12
IL-7	allogeneic tumor lines	RVV	Ecomonu	4
IL-2	fibroblasts + autol. tumor	lipofection	Mertelsmann/Lindemann	14
IL-4	fibroblasts + autol. tumor	RVV	Lotze	18
IL-12	fibroblasts + autol. tumor	RVV	Lotze	14
IL-2	autologous tumor	RVV	Gore/Collins	12
IL-2	autologous tumor	RMT	Stingl/Bröcker/Mertelsmann	12
IL-7	autologous tumor	ballistic	Schadendorf	10
IL-12	autologous tumor	ballistic	Schadendorf	6
GM-CSF	autologous tumor	RVV	Rankin	33
GM-CSF	autologous tumor	RVV	Ellem	10
GM-CSF	autologous tumor	RVV	Chang	3
GM-CSF	autologous tumor	ballistic	Mahvi	2
IFN-g	autologous tumor	RVV	Seigler	20

Abbreviations: RVV: Retroviral Vectors; RMT: receptor-mediated gene transfer; TF: Transfection
[a]Adapted from **ref. 19**.

lines was significantly higher after vaccination, as determined by a limited dilution analysis in seven patients. Furthermore, in 3/6 patients, the frequency of cytolytic microcultures increased from 2.6- to 28-fold. The magnitude of the T-cell reactivity was found to be highly associated with the patients' Karnofsky-index and recall antigen skin reactivity before vaccination. Nevertheless, only one mixed-clinical response could be observed during the treatment period. In a subsequent phase, six patients were immunized with autologous IL-12 gene-modified melanoma cells *(24)*. Clinically, there was no major toxicity except for mild fever. All patients completed more than four vaccinations and were eligible for immunological evaluation.

Postvaccination, the number of tumor-reactive proliferative as well as cytotoxic T cells was significantly increased in two patients (up to 15-fold). Two

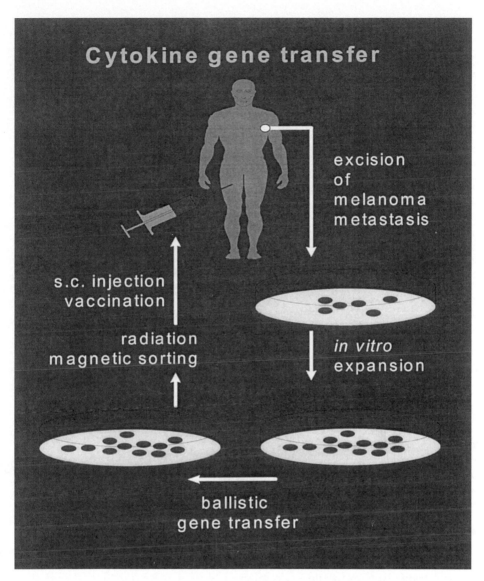

Fig. 1. Vaccination Procedure. Principle outline of vaccination preparation used for immunization of patients with advanced melanoma. Surgical excision of melanoma metastases, and subsequent expansion of tumor cells ex vivo, gene transfer using the magnetoballistic transfer technique, and irradiation is followed by sc injection of genetically modified, cytokine-secreting, autologous melanoma cells in weekly intervals (21–24).

patients developed DTH-reactivity against autologous melanoma cells and one had a minor clinical response. Biopsies taken from that patient's metastases revealed a heavy infiltration of CD4- and CD8-positive T lymphocytes. In conclusion, vaccination of patients with advanced melanoma using autologous gene-modified melanoma cells induced—even in far-advanced terminally ill patients—immunological changes that can be interpreted as an increased antitumor immune response *(23,24)*.

1.5. Cytokine Gene Transfer by Particle Bombardment

There are several nonviral methods of gene transfer that seem to be less risky in general, particularly in terms of integration into the host genome or potential infectiousness when compared to the viral vector systems. Transfer techniques in use are calcium phosphate precipitation, DEAE-dextrane transfection, electroporation, in vitro DNA-microinjection, receptor-mediated DNA transfection, liposomal DNA complexes, direct DNA-injection in vivo, and ballistic gene transfer [reviewed in *(20)*]. Most of the techniques have been known for years and are well established in small-scale approaches in the laboratory, however, are not useful for a clinical application because of low transfection efficacy or certain technical requirements, which cannot be fulfilled for clinical trials.

Naked DNA coated on gold microprojectiles that is directly propelled into in vivo target cells is an elegant method of gene transfer. This ballistic transfer is also applicable for an in vitro gene transfer allowing for a subsequent selection of transfected and nontransfected cells. This can be achieved by selection over several weeks for antibiotical resistance coexpressed with the gene of interest or by using the recently described ballisto-magnetic transfer system *(21,22)*. This gene transfer technology, which combines ballistic transfer of biological molecules and magnetic cell sorting, has originally been developed to study gene regulation on the chromatin level. It now opens the possibility to transfect large cell numbers for gene therapy protocols in a reasonable amount of time. Using this technique, more than 10^8 cells can be transfected each day, thus eliminating the need for viral vector systems, and is convenient when a cancer vaccine has to be quickly prepared from autologous tumor cells in short time (**Fig. 2**).

2. Materials

1. Ballistic gene transfer: Colloidal gold (0.5 mg, 1.6 mm), particle carrier membrane (purchased as macrocarrier) and the biolistic PDS-1000/He apparatus (1550 psi rupture disk, 500 mg Hg of vaccum) were all abtained from Bio-Rad, München, Germany. Colloidal supramagnetic particles (65-nm diameter) were used as purchased from Miltenyi GmbH, Bergisch Gladbach, Germany.

2. Cell enrichment by magnetic separation: high-gradient magnetic separation column (capacity 3×10^7 cells, type AS) was obtained from Miltenyi GmbH. Washing buffer: PBS +0.25 % human serum albumin.
3. Cytokine secretion and bioactivity after gene transfer: ELISA (IL-12, IFNγ) were purchased from R&D Systems (Minneapolis, MN); Ficoll-Hypaque, RPMI-1640, PBS from Seromed (Berlin, Germany); 24-well plates (Nunc, Wiesbaden, Germany); human IL-12 and IL-12 neutralizing antibodies (goat antihuman) (Sigma, Deisenhofen, Germany).

3. Methods

3.1. Ballistic Gene Transfer

1. A suspension of colloidal gold is pipeted onto each of seven particle carrier membranes and allowed to sediment.
2. After removal of the supernatant, the gold particles are resuspended in a mixture of three parts of an aqueous solution of DNA and two parts of a suspension of colloidal supraparamagnetic particles. The suspension was allowed to sediment, the supernatant was removed, and the particle carrier membranes were kept at room temperature until residual liquid had completely evaporated.
3. The accelerating system for ballistic transfer is based on the biolistic PDS-1000/ He apparatus. The biolistic unit was modified by a pressure-outlet manifold, a multiparticle carrier assembly, and an adjustable bearing to carry a 10-cm Petri dish. Cell-culture medium is removed from the Petri dish immediately prior to operating the ballistomagnetic vector system (*see* **Note 1**).

3.2. Cell Enrichment by Magnetic Separation

Subsequent enrichment of transduced cells by magnetic selection without need of in-vitro selection over months allows for fast, easy, and cost-effective vaccination of suitable patients.

1. A magnetic separation column is prepared according to the supplier's protocol. Following ballistomagnetic transfer, cells are immediately resuspended in 2 mL PBS, supplemented with 0.25% of serum albumin, and transferred onto the column. An aliquot of the cell suspension is kept for reference (unsorted fraction).
2. The cell suspension is passed through a high-gradient magnetic separation column, followed by a washing step with 3 mL PBS. The effluent is collected as negative or nonmagnetic fraction.
3. Following removal of the column from the magnetic separator, the retained cells are flushed back to the top of the column. The column is put back into the separator, washed with 3 mL PBS, and the effluent collected (wash fraction).
4. Finally, the column is again removed from the separator and eluted with 5 mL PBS (magnetic fraction). The fractions collected are further processed according to experimental conditions required for the subsequent assay (*see* **Note 2**).

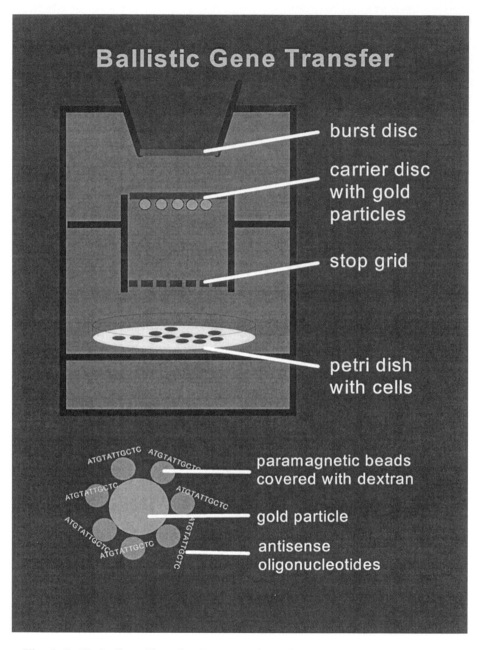

Fig. 2. Ballistic Gene Transfer. Pressure via Helium gas is applied onto a rupture membrane causing its rupturation and an acceleration of the carrier disk, which is coated with gold beads, paramagnetic particles, and plasmid DNA. The particle-carrying disk is abruptly stopped at a stopping grid causing a sudden release of the paramagnetic

3.3. Cytokine Secretion and Bioactivity After Gene Transfer

In order to test the cytokine secretion and activity, the following procedure was employed:

1. The following day, gene-modified melanoma cells were irradiated with 100 gy in 1–2 mL. Cells were subsequently detached from flasks by mechanical scraping into ice-cold, sterile PBS, washed three times, counted, and finally resuspended at 5×10^6 gene-modified melanoma cells per mL.
2. An aliquot of 10^6 cells was transferred to a single well of a 24-well plate (Nunc) for determining cytokine secretion after 24 h, using an IL-12 ELISA (*see* **Note 3**).
3. The bioactivity of IL-12-containing supernatant was analyzed and confirmed with a bioassay analyzing the release of IFN-γ from PBL upon contact to cell-culture supernatants (*see* **Note 4**).

3.4. Conclusion and Perspectives

Tumor immunology has made great progress in recent years. Recent animal studies have indicated that a potent protective immune response can be generated in vivo using cytokine gene-modified tumor cells. Locally secreted cytokines such as IL-2, IL-4, IL-7, IL-12, or GM-CSF and others from genetically modified tumor cells were shown to mediate tumor rejection and long-lived antitumor immunity. Based on these successful animal studies, various clinical protocols for the treatment of human cancer, predominantly using cytokine gene modifications, have been initiated in recent years.

In following years, the large number of ongoing first-clinical studies using gene-therapeutic strategies will provide the necessary scientific basis to proceed on this new avenue of medicine. At present, it seems safe to conclude that gene-therapeutic strategies involving cytokine gene-modified tumor cells can influence the immunological tumor–host relationship. In most cases, however, the response seems not to be strong enough to completely erradicate the tumor in patients with highly pretreated and far-metastatically advanced tumors. Although gene therapy is still in its infancy after five years of first-clinical practice, the potential of this new therapeutic opportunity has become already

Fig. 2. *(continued)* gold particles, which will subsequently hit the cells maintained in the Petri culture disk at the bottom of the apparatus. Gold particles coated with paramagnetic particles and the plasmid DNA encoding human recombinant IL-7 or IL-12 will hit the tumor cells and pass the nucleus packed with chromatin. Because of the charge of the nuclear chromatin the passing gold particles will lose most of their coated paramagnetic beads and plasmid DNA. Subsequently, cells hit are easily recovered by magnetic separation and selected for live cells, if necessary, by attachment to culture dishes.

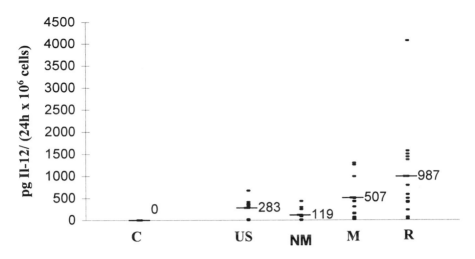

Fig. 3. Cytokine Release. Primary melanoma cell cultures from 15 metastases of patients were analyzed for the release of IL-12 from tumor cells after gene transfer. Gold particles coated with *p35* and *p40* encoding vector constructs were used for ballistic transfer. Cell fractions were magnetically separated and aliquots of all fractions were analyzed for IL-12 secretion after 24 h by ELISA. Nontransfected cells (**C**) did not secrete any IL-12. The whole cell mixture after ballistic transfer without separation (**US**) released a mean of 283 pg IL-12 (24h; 10^6 cells) which increased to 507 pg IL-12 (24 h; 10^6 cells), after magnetic separation (**M**) compared to 119 pg IL-12 (24 h; 10^6 cells) in the nonmagnetic cell fraction (**NM**). Irradiation (100 gy) of the magnetic fraction (**R**) further increased IL-12 secretion to 987 pg IL-12 (24 h; 10^6 cells).

visible. Even though enormous work, however, is currently put in the development of suitable vector systems and genetic tools, it is only a matter of time that gene therapy will be a standard treatment option in medicine and cancer therapy. One should keep in mind that standard therapy modalities, such as chemotherapy, needed decades before at least a few cancer entities could be cured. For patients with advanced malignant melanoma, however, no significant benefit was gained.

4. Notes

1. Ballistomagnetic transfer of biomolecules into 10^7–3×10^7 cells seeded onto 10 cm Petri dishes is achieved by simultaneous delivery of particles from seven-particle carrier membranes that are arranged in a way to cover the entire area of the Petri dish evenly.
2. Fractions are being tested for IL-12 detection by ELISA and for IFNγ-release. Examples of data obtained using the ballistomagnetic vector system to transfer both chains of the IL-12 gene are shown in **Fig. 3.**

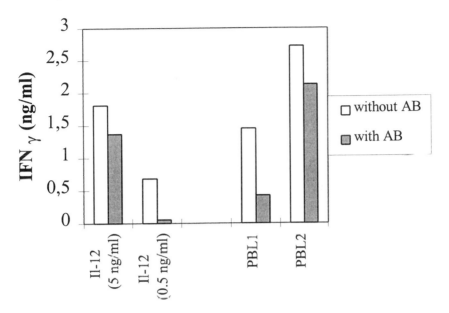

Fig. 4. Bioactivity. In order to test the bioactivity of the IL-12 secreted, IFN-γ release from PBL obtained from two healthy donors was analyzed. Both PBL preparations secreted IFN-γ in a dose-dependent fashion after addition of recombinant IL-12 (left panel), which could be blocked by a goat antihuman IL-12 antiserum (2 µg/mL—gray columns). Even higher release of IFN-γ was observed upon addition of cell-culture supernatant of IL-12 transfected melanoma cells (right panel). That effect could only partly to be blocked by antihuman IL-12 antiserum, however, supernatants of nontransfected cells had no effect on IFN-γ secretion (not shown). Proliferation kinetics of five human melanoma cell lines were not affected upon addition of recombinant IL-12 (1 pg/mL to 1 µg/mL) up to 7 d (not shown).

3. Detection range was between 10 to 200 pg/mL, according to the manufacturer's instructions.
4. PBMC were separated by Ficoll-Hypaque density gradient (Seromed) from two independent healthy donors. PBL were prepared from PBMC after partial depletion of monocytes by adherence to plastic surfaces (45 min, 37°C) and plated in U-bottom microtiter plates (10^6 cells/100 µL RPMI/10% FCS). 100 µL of IL-12-containing supernatant were added in duplicates to the PBL and incubated for 18 h (37°C, 5% CO_2). Controls included recombinant human IL-12 (Sigma) at 0.5 and 5.0 ng/mL. Furthermore, each sample was tested in parallel by the addition of IL-12-neutralizing goat antihuman antibodies (Sigma) at 2 µg/ml (=20 fold EC50 concentration) with PBL being preincubated with antiserum (30 min, 37°C, 5%CO_2) before the addition of the supernatants. Examples of data obtained analyzing IL-12 secretion and bioactivity after ballistic gene transfer of both chains are shown in **Fig. 4.**

Acknowledgments

This work was supported by the DFG and would not have possible without the contributions of Drs. B. Wittig, P. Möller, Y. Sun, B. Henz, K. Jurgovsky, and the excellent technical assistance of A. Sucker and T. Dorbic.

References

1. Ahmann, D. L., Creagan, E. T., Hahn, R. G., Edmonson, J. H., Bisel, H. F., and Schaid D. J. (1989) Complete responses and long-term survivals after systemic chemotherapy for patients with advanced malignant melanoma. *Cancer* **63,** 224–227.
2. Johnson, T. M., Smith, J. W., Nelson, B. R., and Chang A. (1995) Current therapy for cutaneous melanoma. *J. Am. Acad. Dermatol.* **32,** 689–707.
3. Garbe, C. (1993) Chemotherapy and chemoimmunotherapy in disseminated malignant melanoma. *Melanoma Res.* **3,** 291–299.
4. Oettgen, H. F. and Old, L. J. (1991) The history of cancer immunotherapy, in *Biologic Therapy of Cancer, Principles and Practice* (de Vita, V. T., Hellman, S., and Rosenberg, S. A., eds.), Lippincott, Philadelphia, PA, pp. 87–99.
5. Parkinson, D. R., Houghton, A. N., Hersey, P., and Borden, E. C. (1992) Biologic therapy for melanoma, in *Cutaneous Melanoma* (Balch, C. M., Houghton, A. N., Milton, G. W., Sober, A. J., and Soong, S. J., eds.), Lippincott, Philadelphia, PA, p. 522.
6. Dagleish, A. (1996) The case for therapeutic vaccines. *Melanoma Res* **6,** 5–10.
7. Mackensen, A., Carcelain, G., Viel, S., Raynal, M.-C., Michalaki, H., Triebel, F., et al. (1994) Direct evidence to support the immunosurveillance concept in a human regressive melanoma. *J. Clin. Invest.* **93,** 1391–1402.
8. Maeurer, M. J., Storkus, W. J., Kirkwood, J. M., and Lotze, M. T. (1996) New treatment options for patients with melanoma: review of melanoma-derived T-cell epitope-based peptide vaccines. *Melanoma Res.* **6,** 11–24.
9. Kawakami, Y., Eliyahu, S., Delgado, C. H., Robbins, P. F., Sakaguchi, K., Appella, E., et al. (1994) Identification of a human melanoma antigen recognized by tumor-infiltrating lymphocytes associated with in vivo tumor rejection. *Proc. Natl. Acad. Sci. USA* **91,** 6458–6462.
10. Robbins, P. F., El-Gamil, M., Kawakami, Y., and Rosenberg, S. A. (1994) Recognition of tyrosinase by tumor-infiltrating lymphocytes from a patient responding to immunotherapy. *Cancer Res* **54,** 3124–3126.
11. Möller, P. and Schadendorf, D. (1997) Somatic gene therapy and its implication for the treatment of malignant melanoma. *Arch. Dermatol. Res.* **289,** 71–77.
12. Schadendorf, D. (1997) Cytokines, autologous cell immunostimulatory and gene therapy for cancer treatment, in *Skin Immune System*, 2nd ed. (Bos, J. D., ed.), CRC, Boca Raton, FL, pp. 657–669.
13. Rosenberg, S. A., Lotze, M. T., Muul, L. M., Leitman, S., Chang, A. E., Ettinhhausen, S. E., et al. (1985) Observation on the systemic administration of autologous lymphokine-activated killer cells and recombinant interleukin-2 to patients with cancer. *N. Engl. J. Med.* **313,** 1485–1492.

14. Tepper, R. I., Pattengale, P. K., and Leder, P. (1989) Murine interleukin 4 displays potent anti-tumor activity in vivo. *Cell* **57**, 503–512.
15. Fearon, E. R., Pardoll, D. M., Itaya, T., Golumbek, P., Livitsky, H. I., Simons, J. W., et al. (1990) Interleukin-2 production by tumor cells bypasses T helper function in the generation of an antitumor response. *Cell* **60**, 397–403.
17. Pardoll, D. M. and Beckerleg, A. M. (1995) Exposing the immunology of naked DNA vaccines. *Immunity* **3**, 165–169.
18. Cayeux, S., Beck, C., Aicher, A., Dörken, B., and Blankenstein, T. (1995) Tumor cells cotransfected with interleukin-7 and B7.1 genes induce CD25 and CD28 on tumor-infiltrating T lymphocytes and are strong vaccines. *Eur. J. Immunol.* **25**, 2325 2331.
19. Marcel, T. and Grausz, J. D. (1997) The TMC worldwide gene therapy enrollment report, end 1996. *Hum. Gene Ther.* **8**, 775–800.
20. Ledley, F. D. (1995) Nonviral gene therapy: the promise of genes as pharmaceutical products. *Hum. Gene Ther.* **6**, 1129–1144.
21. Schadendorf, D., Czarnetzki, B. M., and Wittig, B. (1995) Clinical protocol-interleukin-7-, interleukin-12-, and GM-CSF gene transfer in patients with metastatic melanoma. *J. Mol. Med.* **73**, 473–477.
22. Schadendorf, D., Henz, B. M., and Wittig, B. (1996) Interleukin 7 trials for melanoma treatment. *Mol. Med. Today* **2**, 143–144.
23. Möller, P., Sun, Y. S., Dorbic, T, Möller H., Makki, A., Jurgovsky, K., et al. (1998) Vaccination with IL-7-gene modified autologous melanoma cells can enhances the anti-melanoma lytic activity in peripheral blood of advanced melanoma patients—a clinical phase I study. *Brit. J. Cancer*, **77**, 1907–1916.
24. Sun, Y., Jurgovsky, K., Möller, P., Alijagic, S., Dorbic, T., Georgieva, J., et al. (1998) Vaccination with Il-12-gene modified autologous melanoma cells—preclinical results and a first clinical phase I study. *Gene Ther.* **5**, 481–490.

28

Intratumoral Gene Transfer of the *HLA-B7* Gene Into Colon Carcinoma Metastases

Evanthia Galanis and Joseph Rubin

1. Introduction

Colorectal adenocarcinoma, with more than 150,000 new cases diagnosed in the United States yearly and approximately 50,000 deaths every year, is a significant public health problem. Despite the emergence of new agents, chemotherapeutic options are of limited efficacy, and novel therapeutic approaches are needed.

Colorectal adenocarcinoma has been one of the targets for cancer immunotherapy in the past. By using IL-2 and lymphokine activated killer (LAK) cells, Rosenberg and colleagues *(1)* achieved one complete regression (CR) and three partial regressions (PRs) out of 30 patients with advanced colorectal cancer.

Tumor-infiltrating lymphocytes (TILs) obtained from the MC-38 colorectal adenocarcinoma cell line were found specifically to lyse the tumor from which they are derived *(2)*. Specific cytokine release was demonstrated when these TILs came in contact with their autologous tumors *(3,4)* and the preliminary results of a clinical trial using genetically modified TILs have been reported *(5)*.

Tumor recognition by the cellular immune system requires tumor antigen presentation in the context of MHC class I or II molecules *(6)*. Presentation of antigen-derived peptide fragments by MHC class II molecules to the T-cell receptors, is considered to be the initiating event in T-cell mediated antitumor response. Histocompatibility molecules belonging to the class I major histocompatibility complex (MHC) (especially the *HLA-B7* family) provide a second signal resulting in the stabilization of messenger RNA for a number of T-cell-derived cytokines *(7,8)*. CD8$^+$ cytotoxic T lymphocytes (CTL) are activated by MHC class I bearing cells, whereas CD4$^+$ helper T cells are stimulated primarily by cells that express MHC class II molecules *(9)*.

From: *Methods in Molecular Medicine, Vol. 35: Gene Therapy: Methods and Protocols*
Edited by: W. Walther and U. Stein © Humana Press, Inc., Totowa, NJ

Total or selective loss of MHC class I antigens has been reported in up to 60% of colorectal carcinoma biopsy as well as in other solid tumors and hematologic malignancies *(10,11)*.

Transfer of an allogeneic MHC class I gene into murine tumor cells by Plautz et al. *(12)* resulted in immunologic rejection of transfected tumor cells. Additionally, intratumoral injection of allogeneic MHC genes into murine tumors resulted in induction of cytotoxic T lymphocytes against both nontransfected and modified tumor cells. Plautz et al. hypothesized that expression of the foreign histocompatibility protein triggered a cytokine cascade and stimulated an allogeneic antitumor response against tumor cells.

Nabel et al. *(13)* treated five patients with malignant melanoma with intratumoral injection of an *HLA-B7* gene/lipid complex. All the patients demonstrated evidence of gene transfer without treatment-related toxicity. In one of the patients, the injected lesion as well as distant metastases regressed, a response that appeared to be mediated by a CD8$^+$ lymphocytic infiltrate. The number of *HLA-B7* reactive cytotoxic lymphocytes increased after gene therapy in two patients, consistent with the generation of a specific immune response.

Further work on *HLA-B7* gene/lipid vector complex led to the creation of the plasmid VCL-1005 (Allovectin-7, Vical, Inc., San Diego, CA).

As will be described in the Materials and Methods sections, Allovectin-7 is a positively charged complex consisting of a cationic two-lipid cytofectin that is administered in combination with a double-stranded DNA plasmid that contains the *HLA-B7* and β2 microglobulin genes. The second gene was included to enhance the expression of the complex *HLA-B7* molecule and eliminate a possible tumor mechanism of immunologic escape. Deletion of β2 microglobulin gene has been described in human tumors, including colon cancer, and has been associated with decreased expression of MHC class I antigens *(14)*.

Preclinical animal studies showed that injection of the VCL-1005 plasmid into subcutaneous B16 melanoma tumors in mice significantly slowed tumor growth. The direct intratumoral injection of either the plasmid DNA encoding *HLA-B7* and β2 microglobulin alone or of the cationic lipid formulation alone had no significant effect on tumor growth. In mice that received direct intrahepatic injection of the same plasmid VCL-1005/lipid combination, no adverse effects were detected by histopathology or clinical biochemistry tests. In addition, repeated intravenous injection of the plasmid in monkeys and mice proved it safe, and allowed the study of its pharmacokinetics *(15)*.

These findings prompted us to evaluate the clinical applicability of VCL-1005 injection for treatment of colorectal liver metastases in an initial phase I and subsequent phase II trial looking for feasibility, toxicity, schedules, dosing, and therapeutic results.

The clinical protocol involving application of the *HLA-B7/β2* microglobulin gene transfer for treatment of colorectal liver metastases can be subdivided as follows:

1. Study drug.
2. Clinical trial; 2.1. Patient screening/eligibility criteria; 2.2. Treatment plan/study design; 2.3. Allovectin-7 administration; 2.4. Treatment assessment; 3. Laboratory evaluation of transfection and gene expression; 3.1. PCR analysis of tumor biopsies for plasmid DNA; 3.2. RT-PCR of tumor biopsies for plasmid mRNA; 3.3. FACS analysis of biopsy samples for *HLA-B7*; 3.4. Immunohistochemistry of biopsy samples for *HLA-B7* and infiltrating lymphocytes; 3.5. FACS analysis for circulating antibodies to *HLA-B7*; and 3.6. Limiting dilution assay (LDA) of peripheral blood monocular cells to evaluate alterations in the frequency of *HLA-B7* cytotoxic T lymphocytes (CTL), lymphocyte activated killer (LAK) and natural killer (NK) cells.

2. Treatment

2.1. Study Drug

2.1.1. Phase I

The drug, Allovectin-7 was supplied by Vical, Inc., in separate vials containing the following:

1. Plasmid DNA at a concentration of 1 mg/mL in 400 µL Lactated Ringer's solution. The plasmid, VCL-1005, contains the Rous Sarcoma Virus (RSV) promoter/enhancer that drives transcription of both the MHC class I human leukocyte antigen *B7* gene (*HLA-B7*), cloned from a human B-cell library, and the chimpanzee *β2* microglobulin gene (**Fig. 1**). An internal ribosomal entry site, designated as CITE, was used to enable coexpression of the two genes from a single promoter in eukaryotic cells *(16)*. To facilitate purification of the plasmid, the gene-encoding kanamycin resistance (aminoglycocide phosphotransferase) originally derived from the bacterial transposon *Tn903* *(17)* was also introduced. In addition, the plasmid contains transcript polyadenylation and termination signals from the bovine growth hormone polyadenylation sequence *(18)*. A pBR322-derived backbone was used for the construction of the plasmid, and the plasmid DNA was propagated in the *Escherichia coli* strain DH10B (Life Technologies, Baltimore, MD) *(19)*. Fermentation in complete TB medium containing 50 µg/mL kanamycin was performed in a 10-L Braun Biostat ED fermenter. Fermentation conditions were maintained as follows: temperature was controlled at 30°C, agitation at 600 rpm, airflow at 10 lt/min and pH at 7.0. The average fermentation yielded 4 mg of plasmid DNA/lt. Bacteria were harvested in late log phase (10–11 hours

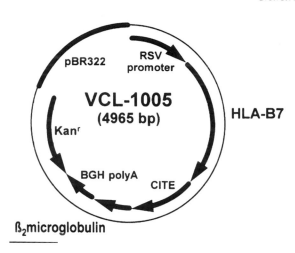

Fig. 1. Plasmid map of Allovectin 7. The RSV promoter drives expression of the HLA-B7 and β_2-microglobulin cDNAs. The two genes are separated by an internal chromosomal entry site (CITE) which allows coexpression of the two genes from a single promoter in eukaryotic cells; BGH poly A, bovine growth hormone transcription terminator and polyadenylation signal; kan[r] kanamycin resistance gene.

postinoculation), at a final OD_{600} of approx 30, in a Jouan Centrifuge at 3000g for 30 min and stored at –20°C. Fresh or frozen bacteria were lysed using a modification of the standard alkaline method *(19)*. Subsequent purification included precipitation with 2-propanol, resuspension and precipitation of impurities with ammonium acetate, precipitation with PEG-8000, Sephacryl S-1000 chromatography, precipitation with ethanol and sterilizing infiltration through a pyrogen-free 0.2 mg Acrodisc filter (Gelman, Ann Arbor, MI). All the steps for purification of pharmaceutical grade plasmid DNA for in vivo gene therapy have been described in detail by Horn et al. *(19)*.

All lots of plasmid DNA were qualified by the following criteria: appearance, concentration (UV absorbance A_{260}), size and integrity (agarose gel electrophoresis), DNA/protein ratio (UV absorbence, A_{260}/A_{280} of 1.75 to 2), total protein (BCA colormetric assay, less than 1 µg/mL), RNA (agarose gel electrophoresis, not visible by ethidium bromide stain), E. coli DNA (Southern blot, ≤0.01 µg/µg of plasmid DNA), endotoxin (LAL, <0.1 EU/µg of plasmid DNA), restriction enzyme analysis, pyrogenicity in rabbits, and sterility in fluid thioglycollate media.

2. The second vial contained the lipid mixture, which is a formulation of two compounds containing 77 mg of DMRIE (1,2 Dimyristyloxypropyl-3-dimethylhydroxyethyl ammonium bromide) and 90 µg of DOPE (dioleoyl-phosphatidyl-ethanolamine). The cationic lipid was prepared until GLP conditions as previously described *(20)*. All lots were qualified by migration on thin layer chromatography (TLC), lipid vesicle size (Time Resolved Laser Light Scatter, 500–900 nm), residual chloroform (GC-photoionization detection, <50 ppm),

sterility in fluid thioglycollate media, pyrogenicity in rabbits, and transfection potency in vitro with reporter genes.

3. Two vials of Lactated Ringer's solution.

The DNA lipid complexes were prepared immediately before administration. Each lipid vial (supplied as a dry film) was reconstituted with 400 µL Lactated Ringer's solution by vortexing until homogeneous. The content of the lipid vial was transferred into the DNA vial and mixed well by repeated inversion. The final concentration of the *HLA-B7* plasmid DNA was 500 µg/mL.

2.1.2. Phase II

Allovectin-7 (Vical, Inc.) was provided in sing-dose aliquots contained in sterile vials, each with 1.2 ml of a sterile solution of VCL-1005 plasmid DNA/ DMRIE/DOPE lipid complex in an injection vehicle composed of 0.9% NaCl with 1% glycerin and 0.01% Vitamin E. The concentration of the VCL-1005 plasmid DNA in the solution was 0.01 mg/mL. In addition, each vial contained a 4 µg/mL of the DMRIE/DOPE cytofectin.

Allovectin-7 vials were stored at –20°C. Thirty minutes prior to use, the vials were allowed to thaw at room temperature until injection.

2.2. Clinical Trial

2.2.1. Patient Screening/Eligibility Criteria

1. Histologically confirmed hepatic metastasis of primary colorectal adenocarcinoma beyond surgical cure. Patients had to have at least two liver metastases that were measurable in two dimensions on computer tomographic scans (CT). One lesion measured at least 2 cm in greatest diameter and was accessible for intralesional injection, whereas the second measurable lesion was to serve as a control for evaluation of possible distant responses. All patients had either prior standard chemotherapy for their disease and were unresponsive or had made the decision to delay or refuse standard chemotherapy.
2. Age older than 18 yrs.
3. Acceptable hematologic parameters (WBC higher than 3×10^9/L, and platelet count higher or equal to 100×10^9/L).
4. Adequate liver function (AST and alkaline phosphatase less or equal to three times above the upper limit of normal with normal serum direct bilirubin).
5. Adequate renal function as indicated by a creatinine less than 125% of upper limit of normal.
6. Efficient hemostasis: prothrombin time less or equal to 1 second above control;
7. Baseline Karnofsky performance score of at least 70 (ECOG 0,1).
8. Estimated life expectancy of at least 12 week.
9. For females of reproductive age: negative pregnancy test prior to the study and assurance of adequate contraception during the study.
10. HIV negative.

11. Hepatitis B surface antigen (HBsAg) negative.
12. Normal cellular immunity as indicated by a normal in vitro lymphocyte response to phytohemagglutinin (PHA).
13. *HLA-B7* negativity as shown by HLA typing performed prior to the study.

Contraindications for treatment were:

1. Active autoimmune disease.
2. Hepatitis.
3. Active infection.
4. Immunosuppressive therapy including use of steroids.
5. Surgery within the past 2 wk.
6. Radiation or chemotherapy within the past 3 wk.

The protocol was approved by the recombinant DNA advisory committee (RAC) of NIH. All patients gave informed consent prior to study entry.

2.2.2. Treatment Plan/Study Design

2.2.2.1. Phase I Study

Patients were divided into five groups each consisting of three patients:

1. Group A1: 10 μg of Allovectin-7 day 1.
2. Group A2: 50 μg of Allovectin-7 daily, day 1.
3. Group A3: 250 μg of Allovectin-7 on day 1.

All three patients at each escalation of schedule A were observed for toxicity and response for 30 d before patients received Allovectin-7 at the next planned higher dose. If responses were seen, patients were eligible for repeat treatment.

Schedule B was initiated after all three patients receiving 250 μg DNA were observed without toxicity.

4. Group B1: 10 μg of Allovectin-7 at weeks 0 and 2 (2 intratumoral biweekly injections).
5. Group B2: 10 μg of Allovectin-7 at weeks 0, 2, and 4 (3 intratumoral biweekly injections).

After a month of observation, responding patients were eligible for repeat treatment.

2.2.2.2. Phase II Study

10 μg of Allovectin-7 are administered biweekly at 0, 2, 6, and 8 wk, provided that tumor progression had not occurred in the interim.

2.2.3. Allovectin-7 Administration

1. A tumor biopsy was performed prior to injection of the study drug using an 18-gage needle.

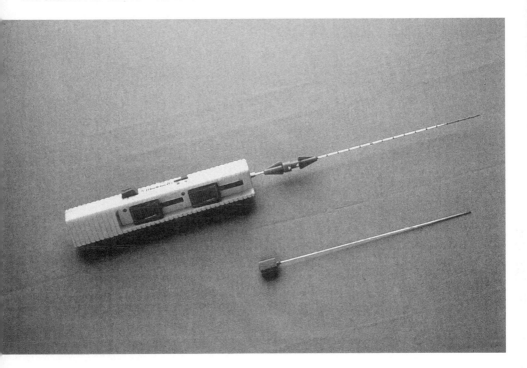

Fig. 2. Biopsy gun (18-gauge) and needle (22-gauge) used for tumor biopsies and Allovectin-7 injections, respectively.

2. Using a 22-gage spinal needle, the study drug was injected into multiple sites (up to 4) within the tumor under direct sonographic visualization (**Fig. 2**). Before injection and following the placement of the needle, gentle aspiration was applied to the syringe to assure that no material was injected intravenously.
3. Vital signs were measured before and every 15 min after the injection for at least 2 h or until the patiens were stable.
4. Postdrug administration observation.
    a. Phase I study: All patients were observed for 48 h after the injection in our General Clinical Research Center. Blood samples were obtained prior to dismissal to check serum enzymes, blood chemistry, and hematology values.
    b. Phase II study: Given the lack of any substantial toxicity related to injection in our phase I trial, patient observation was limited to 2 h postbiopsy and injection or until the patient was hemodynamically stable for the phase II study.

2.2.4. Treatment Assessment

1. Pretreatment evaluation included physical examination, chest x-ray, ECG, hematology and chemistry groups, delayed hypersensitivity skin test, and IV contrast-enhanced CT of the liver for measurement of the injected and control lesions.
2. Disease Status Assessment.

    a. Phase I: Evaluation by a study investigator for overall disease status and treatment response occurred every 2 wk for a total of 8 wk. Hematology and chemistry group were performed during those visits.

    b. Phase II: Patients were evaluated regarding disease status at weeks 2, 6, 8, and 16.

3. Biopsy of the injected lesion.

    a. Phase I: Biopsy of the injected lesion were performed at 2, 4, 6, and 8 weeks with follow-up CT scans being performed before the biopsy on the biopsy days. On the biopsy day, blood samples were collected to be screened for antibodies against *HLA-B7* DNA or protein.

    b. Phase II: Follow-up tumor biopsies were performed at weeks 6 and 16.

4. After the completion of the study, the patients were followed every 6 weeks until progression, and then every 8–12 wk.

2.2.5. Response Criteria

The definition of responses was as follows:

1. Complete regression (CR) was defined as a total disappearance of all evidence of tumor.
2. Partial regression (PR) was defined as >50% reduction of the product of the two perpendicular diameters of the indicator lesion as seen in the CT scan.
3. Progression was defined as an increase in size of the indicator lesion by at least 25% or as the appearance of new lesions.
4. Stable disease: Patients not meeting criteria for CR, PR, or progression were defined as stable.

3. Laboratory Evaluation of Transfection and Gene Expression

3.1. Materials

3.1.1. PCR Analysis of Tumor Biopsies for Plasmid DNA

1. TRIZOL (Life Technologies).
2. Oligonucleotide primers. The sense primer corresponds to the RSV promoter (sense 5′GGGAGGGGGAAATGTAGTCCTA3′). The antisense primer corresponds to the human *HLA-B7* sequence: bases 251–272 deposited in GenBank under accession number M6102 (5′TGTGTTCCGGTCCCAATACTC3′).
3. Standard PCR reagents.
4. Programmable thermal controller (MJ Research, Watertown, MA).
5. Standard reagents and apparatus for agarose gel electrophoresis.
6. Ethidium bromide.

3.1.2. RT-PRC Analysis of Tumor Biopsies for Plasmid mRNA

1. TRIZOL (Life Technologies, Gaithersburg, Maryland).
2. DNase I (Life Technologies).
3. cDNA Cycle Kit (Invitrogen, San Diego, CA).
4. Standard PCR reagents.

5. Thermocycler.
6. Oligonucleotide primers. The sense primer corresponds to bases 35–57 of the β2-microglobulin sequence deposited in the Gen Bank under accession number T00105 (5′TCCAGCGTACTCCAAAGATTCAG3′), while the antisense primer used corresponds to the bovine growth hormone (BGH) terminator region (5′GGGGAGGGGCAAACAACAGAT3′).
7. Standard reagents and apparatus for agarose gel electrophoresis.
8. Ethidium bromide.

3.1.3. FACS Analysis of Tumor Biopsy Samples for HLA-B7 (The Recombinant Gene Product)

1. Collagenase.
2. Trypan blue dye.
3. Monoclonal antibodies for the flow cytometric analysis;
   a. FITC-labeled antimouse IgG Ab (Sigma, St. Louis, MO).
   b. BB7.1 MAb (American Type Culture Collection) against human *HLA-B7*.
   c. biotin-labeled Ab against human MHC class I (HLA-A,B,C) (Becton Dickinson, San Jose, CA).
4. Becton Dickinson FACStar–plus flow cytometer.
5. 1% paraformaldehyde.

3.1.4. Imunohistochemical Staining of Biopsy Samples for HLA-B7 and Infiltrating Lymphocytes

1. Monoclonal antibodies against CD4 and CD8 (Becton Dickinson) and *HLA-B7* antigen (BB7.1 MAb, American Type Culture Collection).
2. Automated instrument for immunohistochemistry (Ventana Medical Systems, Tucson, AZ).

3.1.5. FACS Analysis for Circulating Antibodies to HLA-B7

1. FITC-labeled antihuman Ig (Sigma).
2. *HLA-B7* positive or negative peripheral blood mononuclear cells.
3. Becton Dickinson FACStar-plus flow cytometer.
4. 1% formaldehyde.

3.1.6. Limiting Dilution Assay of Peripheral Blood Mononuclear Cells to Evaluate Alterations of the Frequency of HLA-B7 Specific Cytotoxic T Lymphocytes (CTL), Lymphokine-Activated Killers (LAK), and Natural Killer (NK) Cells in the Peripheral Blood Following Gene Transfer

1. Patient's peripheral blood mononuclear cells (PBMC).
2. Phytohemagglutinin (PHA, 10 mg/mL).
3. IL-2 (30 mg/mL).

4. Allogeneic tumor cell line IM9; the IM9 cells are HLA class I positive, but *HLA-B7* negative.
5. PBMC from an *HLA-B7* positive donor to serve as *HLA-B7* positive cells.
6. *HLA-B7* positive target cell line JY to test for *HLA-B7* specific CTL activity.
7. K562 target cell line to test for NK cell activity.

3.2. Methods

3.2.1. PCR Analysis of Tumor Biopsies for Plasmid DNA

1. Genomic DNA was isolated from the core needle biopsy material using TRIZOL.
2. PCR was performed using 1–2000 ng of genomic DNA for 45 cycles of denaturation (94°C, 4 min), annealing (60°C, 30 s) and extension (75°C, 30s) in a programmable thermal controller using an in-sample probe.
3. Samples were analyzed by ethidium bromide staining on a 1.5% agagrose gel for the expected 549 bp PCR product.

3.2.2. RT-PCR Analysis of Tumor Biopsies for Plasmid mRNA

1. Total RNA was isolated from the core needle biopsy material using TRIZOL.
2. 0.1–1 µg of total RNA was treated with DNase I.
3. cDNA was synthesized using the cDNA Cycle Kit and primed with oligo-dT.
4. PCR analysis of the synthesized cDNA was performed using 45 cycles of denaturation (94°C, 4 min), annealing (58°, 30 s), and extension (75° 30 s).
5. Samples were analyzed by ethidium bromide staining on a 1.5% agarose gel for the expected 397 bp cDNA product.

3.2.3. FACS Analysis of Tumor Biopsy Samples for HLA-B7

1. Tumor biopsies were digested in collagenase at 37°C for 30 min or until a single cell suspension was achieved.
2. Cells were pelleted, washed, resuspended, and viability was determined by Trypan blue dye exclusion.
3. Cells were divided into three equal quantities for staining with
   a. FITC-labeled anti-mouse IgG;
   b. BB7.1 MAb directed against human *HLA-B7*, counterstained with FITC-labeled anti-mouse IgG, and
   c. biotin-labeled *HLA-A,B,C* antibody counterstained with avidin FITC.
4. Samples were fixed in 1% paraformaldehyde, and 20,000 events per histogram (when possible) were analyzed on the Becton Dickinson FACStar-plus cytometer.

3.2.4. Immunohistochemical Staining of the Biopsy Samples for HLA-B7 and Infiltrating Lymphocytes

1. Snap frozen tissue sections were stained for tumor infiltrating T cells and *HLA-B7* antigen by using the anti-CD4, anti-CD8, and anti-HLA-B7 Abs on the automated instrument.
2. Tumor infiltrating T cells were judged in a relative scale (0–4+).

3. HLA-B7 was judged as absent or present (1+ to 4+) based on signal presence or absence in the neoplastic cells.
4. Negative controls included isotype-matched irrelevant antibodies. Positive controls included:
   a. Normal tissue for CD4 and CD8 positivity,
   b. Cytospin concentration (Ficoll-Hypague separation) of known *HLA-B7* positive blood lymphocytes.

3.2.5. FACS Analysis for Circulating Antibodies to HLA-B7

1. Patient plasma was thawed, centrifuged at 1500*g* for 30 min, heat inactivated (56°C for 30 min), and diluted 1:2, 1:4, 1:8, 1:16, and 1:32.
2. The plasma was subsequently incubated with *HLA-B7* positive or negative peripheral blood mononuclear cells for 30 min before staining with FITC-labeled antihuman Ig. Hyperimmune anti-*HLA-B7* were used as positive controls.
3. Cells were washed, fixed in 1% formaldehyde, and analyzed on a Becton Dickinson FACStar-plus flow cytometer. The samples were considered positive if staining was ≥10% above background. Volunteer plasma, nonreactive against *HLA-B7* positive peripheral blood mononuclear cells and patient plasma at time 0 (prior to the first treatment) were used as negative controls.

3.2.6. Limiting Dilution Assay of PBMC to Evaluate Alterations of the Frequency of HLA-B7 specific Cytotoxic T Lymphocytes (CTL), Lymphokine-Activated Killers (LAK), and Natural Killer (NK) Cells in the Blood Following Gene Transfer

1. Cell dose titration was performed using 10^3, 10^4, 10^5, and 5×10^5 patient's PBMC in replicates of 12.
2. Each culture was stimulated with either
   a. Media (control).
   b. PHA + IL-2 (positive control).
   c. IM9 cells to assess general alloreactivity.
   d. *HLA-B7* positive cells. After 10–14 days of incubation, the cultures were assessed for lytic activity by split well analysis.
3. The cultures were retested for anti *HLA-B7* specific CTL activity using the JY target cell line, NK cell activity using the K562 target cell line and LAK cell activity using the IM9 cell line. A positive anti-*HLA-B7* CTL response required the following:
   a. The frequency of the *HLA-B7* CTLs posttreatment exceeded that of *HLA-B7* CTLs pretreatment,
   b. The frequency of the *HLA-B7* cells posttreatment exceeded that of general alloreactive CTLs posttreatment.

   Stimulated wells were considered positive for lytic activity if cytotoxicity levels were >3 standard deviations above the control lysis level for the target cells. Positive NK and LAK activity required lysis of the indicated cell lines >3 standard deviations above the control lysis.

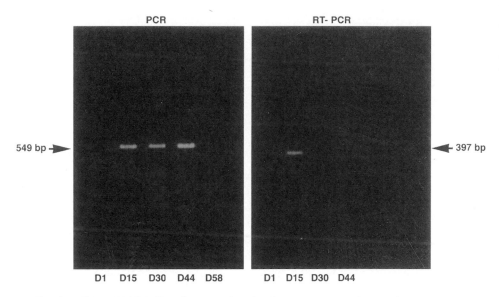

Fig. 3. PCR and RT-PCR of tumor biopsies from a study patient before (Day 1) and after treatment with a single dose of 250 µg of plasmid (Days 15, 30, 44, 58). In addition to the presence of the HLA-B7 plasmid through Day 44, there was transgene expression, as demonstrated by the 397 bp RT-PCR product on Day 15. (Photo courtesy of Dr. E. T. Akporiaye.)

4. Notes

1. Application of the dose escalation as described in the phase I in 15 patients resulted in transfection as indicated by detection of the plasmid DNA in 14/15 (**Fig. 3**) patients (93%). In 5/14 patients, the plasmid was detected until day 43 and in 9/14 until day 57. *HLA-B7* mRNA was detected in 5/15 patients (33%). The *HLA-B7* protein was detected by FACS in 7/14 patients (50%) (**Fig. 4**) and by immunohistochemistry in 4/7 patients (57%) *(21)*. The lower dose (10 µg of injected *HLA-B7*/plasmid/lipid complex) was roughly equivalent to the higher dose of 50 µg and 250 µg in terms of transfection and antigen expression. Consequently, the 10 µg dose in multiple biweekly injections was used as our phase II dose.

2. In the phase I trial, specific anti-*HLA-B7* cytotoxic lymphocytes were generated in 8/15 patients (53%). In addition, NK cells were detected in 14/15 patients (93%) and LAK cells in 9/15 patients (60%), indicating nonspecific immune-mediated killing. Again, the lower dose of 10 µg of injected *HLA-B7* plasmid/lipid complex was equivalent to higher doses in regards to generation of cellular immune response. CD8+ lymphocytes were infiltrating the biopsy site in 7/7 patients tested. No patient has developed circulating antibodies against *HLA-B7*.

3. There were no adverse events directly related to the study drug and in no instances did the administration of drugs have to be discontinued. Directed

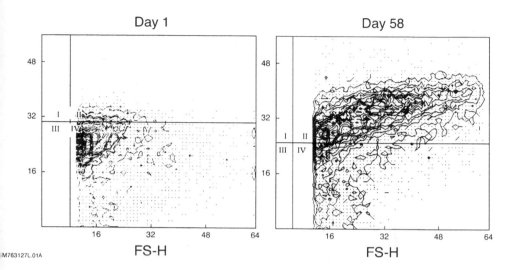

Fig. 4. FACS analysis of tumor biopsies from a study patient showing HLA-B7 expression on Day 58 post-treatment. The patient had received 10 µg of plasmid DNA on Day 1. x axis: forward scatter; y axis: fluorescence intensity. (Photo courtesy of Dr. D. T. Harris.)

ultrasound-guided biopsies of the liver as well as the injections of Allovectin-7 were well tolerated. After the drug administration, 3/15 phase I patients complained of soreness at the biopsy site and 1/15 experienced right shoulder pain. One patient had an episode of severe anxiety associated with the drug administration. In addition, 1/15 patients had an allergic reaction to contrast dye and developed hypotension during CT scanning performed during the study *(21)*. There were no deaths at the time of completion of the study, and five patients remained stable; however, there were no objective responses as part of the study *(21)*. Despite the lack of clinical responses, the expression of transgene in the majority of our patients proves that hepatic intratumoral injection of cytofectin-encoated genes represents an efficient means of gene transfer to liver metastases or primary hepatic tumors. Whether MHC class I gene transfer mediated immunotherapy will prove beneficial in patients with metastatic colorectal carcinoma remains to be determined. A possible future strategy may include combination gene transfer strategies, for example combination of MHC class I genes and cell cycle inhibitors such as p21 cyclin dependent kinase inhibitor *(22)*. Another approach could be the administration of generated TILs, as shown in patients with malignant melanoma in whom intratumoral injection of Allovectin-7 resulted in generated TILs that, when isolated and reinfused to the patients, were capable of inducing tumor response in two of the nine recipients *(23)*, proving the specificity of the *HLA-B7*-induced antitumor immunity.

References

1. Rosenberg, S. (1992) Immunotherapy and gene therapy of cancer. Karnofsky Memorial Lecture. *J. Clin. Oncol.* **10**, 180–199.
2. Barth, R. J. Jr., et al. (1990) Unique murine tumor associated antigens identified by tumor infiltrating lymphocytes. *J. Immunol.* **144**, 1531–1537.
3. Barth, R. J., et al. (1991) Interferon gamma and tumor necrosis factor have a role in tumor regressions mediated by murine CD8+ tumor infiltrating lymphocytes. *J. Exp. Med.* **173**, 647–658.
4. Barth, R. J., et al. (1991) Identification of unique murine tumor associated antigens by tumor infiltrating lymphocytes using tumor specific secretion of interferon-gamma and tumor necrosis factor. *J. Immunol. Meth.* **140**, 269–279.
5. Rosenberg, S. A., et al. (1992) Gene therapy of patients with advanced cancer using tumor infiltration lymphocytes transduced with the gene coding for tumor necrosis factor. *Hum. Gene Ther.* **3**, 57–73.
6. Lanzavecchia, A. (1993) Identifying strategies for immune intervention. *Science* **260**, 937–943.
7. Zier, K. S. and Gansbacher, B. (1996) IL-2 gene therapy of solid tumors: an approach for the prevention of signal transduction defects in T cells. *J. Mol. Med.* **74**, 127–134.
8. Lindsten, T., June, C. H., Ledbetter, J. A., Stella, G. T., and Thompson, C. B. (1989) Regulation of lymphokine messenger RNA stability by a surface-mediated T cell activation pathway. *Science* **244**, 339–343.
9. Germain R. N. and Margulies, D. H. (1993) The biochemistry and cell biology of antigen processing and presentation. *Annu. Rev. Immunol.* **11**, 403–450.
10. Garrido, F., Gabrera, T., Lopez-Nevok, M. A., and Ruiz-Cabello, F. (1995) HLA class I antigens in human tumors. *Adv. Cancer Res.* **67**, 155–195.
11. Schmidt, W., Leben, L., Atfield, G., and Festenstein, H. (1981) Variation of expression of histocompatibility antigens on tumor cells: absence of H-2Kk-gene products from a gross virus-induced leukemia in BALB.K. *Immunogenetics* **14**, 323–339.
12. Plautz, G. E., Yang, Z. Y., Wu, B. Y., et al. (1993) Immunotherapy of malignancy by in vivo gene transfer into tumors. *Proc. Natl. Acad. Sci. USA* **90**, 4645–4649.
13. Nabel, G. J., Nabel, E. G., Yang, Z. Y., et al. (1993) Direct gene transfer with DNA-liposome complexes in melanoma: expression, biologic activity, and lack of toxicity in humans. *Proc. Natl. Acad. Sci. USA* **90**, 11,307–11,311.
14. Funa, K., Gazdar, A. F., Minna, J. D., and Linnoila, R. I. (1986) Paucity of beta 2-microglobulin expression on small cell lung cancer, bronchial carcinoids and certain other neuroendocrine tumors. *Lab. Invest.* **55**, 186–193.
15. Parker, S. E., Vahlsing, H. L., Serfilippi, L. M., Franklin, C. L., Doh, S. G., Gromkowski, S. H., et al. (1995) Cancer gene therapy using plasmid DNA: safety evaluation in rodents and non-human primates. *Hum. Gene Ther.* **6**, 575–590.
16. Morgan, R. A., Couture, L., Elroy-Stein, O., Ragheb, J., Moss, B., and Anderson, W. F. (1992) Retroviral vectors containing putative internal ribosome entry sites:

development of a polycistronic gene transfer system and applications to human gene therapy. *Nucl. Acids Res.* **20,** 1293–1299.

17. Nomura, N., Yamagishi, H., and Oka, A. (1978) Isolation and characterization of transducing coliphage fd carrying a kanamycin resistance gene. *Gene* **3,** 39–51.

18. Gordon, D. F., Quick, D. P., Erwin, C. R., Donelson, J. E., and Maurer, R. A. (1983) Nucleotide sequence of the bovine growth hormone chromosomal gene. *Mol. Cell Endocrinol.* **33,** 81–95.

19. Horn, N. A., Meek, J. A., Budahazi, G., and Marquet, M. (1995) Cancer gene therapy using plasmid DNA: purification of DNA for human clinical trials. *Hum. Gene Ther.* **6,** 565–573.

20. Felgner, J. H., Kumar, R., Sridhar, C. N., Wheeler, C. J., Tsai, Y. J., Border, R., et al. (1994) Enhanced gene delivery and mechanism studies with a novel series of cationic lipid formulations. *J. Biol. Chem.* **269,** 2550–2561.

21. Rubin, J., Galanis, E., Pitot, H. C., Richardson, R. L., Burch, P. A., Charboneau, J. W., et al. (1997) Phase I study of immunotherapy of hepatic metastases of colorectal carcinoma by direct gene transfer of an allogeneic histocompatibility antigen, HLA-B7. *Gene Ther.* **4,** 419–425.

22. Ohno, T., Yang, Z., Ling, X., Jaffe, M., Nabel, E. G., Normolle, D., and Nabel, G. J. (1997) Combination gene transfer to potentiate tumor regression. *Gene Ther.* **4,** 361–366.

23. Nabel, G. J., Gordon, D., Bishop, D. K., Nickoloff, B. J., Yang, Z-Y., Aruga, A., et al. (1996) Immune response in human melanoma after transfer of an allogeneic class I major histocompatibility complex gene with DNA-liposome complexes. *Proc. Natl. Acad. Sci. USA* **93,** 15,388–15,393.

29

Hybrid Cell Vaccination
in Patients With Metastatic Melanoma

Uwe Trefzer, Guido Weingart, Wolfram Sterry, and Peter Walden

1. Introduction

Hybrid cell vaccination is a novel approach for immunotherapy of cancers by inducing specific antitumor immunity (*1,2*). The hybrid cells are generated by electrofusing autologous tumor cells with allogeneic MHC class II expressing cells such as B lymphocytes. The fused cells are irradiated and injected subcutaneously as a vaccine. This immune therapeutical approach aims at recruitment of T-cell help for the induction of tumor-specific cytolytic immunity. It is based on the observation that epitope linkage is a prerequisite for productive T–T cell collaboration, i.e., cytolytic precursor and helper T cells have to be activated by the same antigen presenting cell that displays epitopes for both T-cell types on the corresponding MHC class I and class II molecules (*3,4*). Neither of the two epitopes nor the corresponding T cells need to be related. The implications of this concept are, first, only MHC class I and II expressing cells can induce cytolytic T-cell responses (*5–7*), second, cognate antigens must be presented for both T-cell and MHC types (*4,8*) and, third, there must be T cells with the corresponding specificities in the T-cell receptor repertoire of the response-competent individual.

The hybrid cell vaccination approach to cancer immunotherapy was developed to meet the above requirements (*1*). In initial studies in patients with melanoma (*9*) or renal cell carcinoma (*10*) it could be shown that this vaccine therapy is well tolerated and can induce tumor regressions including complete remissions in some of the patients. The hybrid cells are usually not viable in long-term culture because of the genetic and physiologic differences between the fused partner cells. Therefore, the fusion protocol used to generate the

From: *Methods in Molecular Medicine, Vol. 35: Gene Therapy: Methods and Protocols*
Edited by: W. Walther and U. Stein © Humana Press, Inc., Totowa, NJ

hybrid cells must be designed to yield high numbers of hybridomas. The following protocol describes a high efficiency procedure. The principle of this protocol is that fusion partner cells are aligned in an inhomogenous electric field and fused with high voltage pulses.

2. Materials

2.1. Isolation of Autologous Melanoma Cells

1. Laminar flow hood.
2. Sterile flat-bottom glass dish (10 cm).
3. Scalpel, forceps, scissors.
4. Tissue sieve with metal grid, 50 mesh (#CD-1, Sigma, St. Louis, MO).
5. Sterile 1X PBS.
6. 37°C water bath with magnetic stirring.
7. Centrifuge for 15-mL conical tubes (Nunc, Naperville, IL).
8. 100-ml sterile glass bottle with screw cap and 2-cm magnetic stir bar.
9. 5 g collagenase type VIII (Sigma). Dissolve the enzyme in 40-mL TES buffer with stirring, fill to 50 mL, filter sterile and store in aliquots of 1.4 mL (= 140 mg) at –20°C.
10. Enzyme solution: 52 mg DNase II Type IV (Sigma) and 2 aliquots of collagenase type VIII are added to 500 mL of RPMI-1640, sterile filtered and stored at –20°C in aliquots of 50 mL.
11. Microscope, trypan blue.
12. Cryo medium: RPMI-1640, 30% FCS, 10% DMSO.

2.2. Isolation of Allogeneic B Lymphocytes

1. 50-ml conical tubes with screw cap.
2. Ficoll-Paque Plus (Pharmacia, Uppsala, Sweden).
3. Buffy coat of healthy donor.
4. rh IL-4 (Promega, Madison, WI), rh IL-6 (Promega), LPS from *Escherichia coli* serotype 055-B5 (Sigma).

2.3. Electrofusion

1. Electroporation chambers (0.4 cm, Bio-Rad, Munich, Germany).
2. Gene pulser (Bio-Rad).
3. Pasteur pipets (230 mm).
4. Nontoxic paraffin wax.
5. Relaxation buffer: 100 mM KCL, 3 mM NaCl, 1.25 mM EDTA, 10 mM PIPES, 0.5 mM ATP, adjusted to pH 6.8.

2.4. Cell Labeling

1. PKH26-GL (red) and PKH2-GL (green) fluorescent cell linker kit (Sigma).
2. Polypropylene conical centrifuge tubes.
3. Fluorescence microscope or flow cytometer for analysis.

3. Methods

3.1. Isolation of Autologous Melanoma Cells

1. Perform all work under sterile conditions.
2. After surgical removal, the tumor nodule is placed in sterile PBS.
3. Place the tumor nodule in a glass dish and remove all fibrous tissue and fat.
4. Transfer the tumor nodule to a new glass dish and cut in pieces of 2–3 mm.
5. Transfer the pieces into a glass bottle, add stir bar and 25 mL of enzyme solution at RT.
6. Place the bottle in a 1-L beaker filled with 100 cc water and let stir at 200 rpm at 37°C for 60 min.
7. Filter the cell suspension through the tissue sieve, place in a 50-mL conical tube, and wash 4X in glucose solution at 800g at RT.
8. Resuspend the pellet in 2 mL glucose solution, count tumor cells, and determine viability by trypan blue exclusion. Expect viability >90%.
9. If not used the same day, keep at –80°C in cryo medium.

3.2. Isolation and Activation of Allogeneic B Lymphocytes Containing PBMC

1. Dilute buffy coat 1:3 with PBS.
2. Pipet Ficoll-Paque (20 mL) into the centrifuge tube.
3. Carefully layer 30 mL diluted blood sample on the Ficoll-Paque. Do not mix Ficoll-Paque and blood sample.
4. Centrifuge at 1180g for 20 min at RT.
5. Aspirate off the upper layer using a clean Pasteur pipet, leaving the lymphocyte layer undisturbed at the interface.
6. Transfer the lymphocyte layer to a clean 50-mL centrifuge tube with a Pasteur pipet.
7. Fill the tube with PBS and centrifuge at 240g for 10 min. Wash twice.
8. Resuspend the pellet in 10 mL RPMI-1640 and count the cells.
9. Suspend the pellet in with RPMI-1640, 10% FCS, 1X antimycotic/antibiotic solution and place in 375-mL tissue-culture flask at 10^7 cells/mL. Add 200 U/mL rh IL-6, 200 U/mL rh IL-4, and 50 µg/mL LPS.
10. Incubate the cells for 3 d at 37°C in a 5% CO_2 atmosphere.
11. Pellet activated PBMC at 800g and wash with glucose solution at 800g for 5 min.
12. Resuspend the cells in 5 mL glucose solution and count.
13. If not used the same day, cryopreserve at –80°C.
14. Otherwise, dilute with glucose solution to 10^7 cells/mL.

3.3. Hybrid Cell Generation

1. Mix the tumor cells and the PBMC at a ratio between 1:1 and 1:3 and a total density of 2 × 10^7 cells/mL.
2. Apply nontoxic paraffin wax to a portion of one of the two aspects of the electroporation cuvet to obtain an inhomogenous electrical field for the alignment of the cells.

3. Carefully transfer 0.5 mL of the cell suspension to the electroporation chamber with a Pasteur pipet and let it rest for 5 min.
4. Electrophorectic alignment of cells is achieved by placing the electroporation chamber with the cell suspension for 15 s in the alignment field of 25 V/cm (*see* **Fig. 1**).
5. Apply three pulses of 1000 V/cm at a 25 μF setting of the gene pulser. The pulse times will be between 1 and 10 μs.
6. Let the cells rest for another 5 min and transfer them to 0.5 mL of relaxation buffer at RT in a 15-mL tube.
7. The same electroporation chambers can be used for further electrofusions.
8. Irradiate hybridized cells with 200 gy and then wash with PBS at 800g at RT.
9. Submit a sample for microbiological analyses (absence of pathogens and pyrogens).
10. Carefully resuspend pellet and aliquot in 2.5 mL glucose solution at a cell density of 2×10^7 cells/mL for immediate subcutaneous injection or add cryo medium and store at –80°C.

3.4. Assessment of the Fusion Efficiency with Membrane Dyes

1. Before the fusion, take an aliquot of 4×10^7 melanoma cells or PBMC, pellet them at 400g for 5 min and aspirate supernatant. Resuspend the cells in 2 mL diluent provided with the dyes.
2. Immediately prior to staining, dilute 1 μL of PKH26 or PKH2 dye in 1 mL of the respective diluent for the two cell types in a polypropylene tube. This is the 2X dye stock.
3. Rapidly add the cell suspension to the dye stocks, e.g., green for tumor cells and red for PBMC, and mix the sample gently.
4. Incubate at RT for 5 min. Periodically invert the tube.
5. Stop the reaction by adding an equal volume of serum. Incubate for 1 min.
6. Dilute the sample with an equal volume of medium and wash the cells four times at 400g for 10 min at RT with glucose solution.
7. Mix the tumor cells and PBMC at a ratio of 1 : 1 to 1 : 3 and subject them to the above described electrofusion.
8. Resuspend the cells in PBS and analyze for double positive cells using flow cytometry or fluorescence microscopy. As controls, use unstained cells and stained, but unfused cells.

3.5. Vaccination of Melanoma Patients and DTH Reaction

1. Perform complete staging examinations.
2. Prior to vaccination, determine the reactivity to common recall antigens (Mérieux-test) on the volar aspect of one lower arm. Patients who fail to mount a reactivity after 48 h are unlikely to benefit from vaccination therapy and are therefore excluded from hybrid cell vaccination.
3. For testing delayed-type hypersensitivity (DTH) to autologous tumor cells, inject 1 wk prior to vaccination 3×10^6 irradiated tumor cells in 100 μL glucose

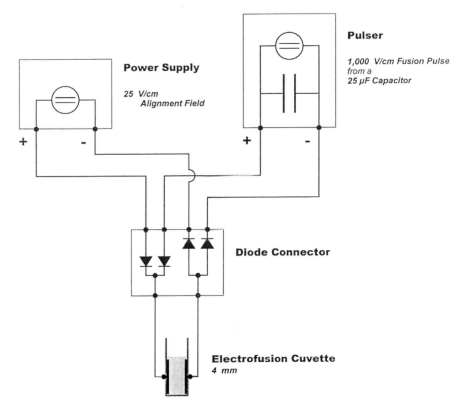

Fig. 1. Schematic diagram of the electrofusion apparatus.

solution intracutaneously on the upper arm. Use a 1-mL syringe with a 12-gauge needle. Check for reactivity after 48 hours and repeat 1 wk after the third injection.

4. For the vaccination therapy, take an aliquot (*see* **Subheading 3.3., step 10**) and gently transfer the cells to a 5-mL syringe with a 21-gage needle. If a cryopreserved aliquot is used, thaw and wash twice with glucose solution. Resuspend the cells in 2.5 mL glucose solution.

5. Divide the 2.5-mL vaccine between two separate sites distant from tumor lesions and slowly inject intracutaneously, e.g., at the lower abdomen and the upper thigh.

6. Use upper arms if lymph nodes in the inguinal area had been removed.

7. Repeat vaccination twice in intervals of 4 wk, followed by complete staging examinations another 4 wk thereafter.

8. Continue treatment in intervals of 4 wk if a clinical response is evident.

4. Notes

Electrofusion as compared to other cell-fusion techniques, such as polyethylene glycol fusion, offers the advantage of much higher fusion efficiency and better hybrid viability. Moreover, it is a highly reproducible approach. There is no need for fusogenic reagents as part of the procedure *(11)*. The fusion efficiency obtained with this protocol ranges from 15–25% for heterogenous fusion. The cell viability is usually >80%. The triple pulse protocol yielded the best fusion efficiency when compared to various single pulse settings. B lymphocytes as fusion partner for tumor cells are used because of their potent antigen presenting capacity *(12)* and, more importantly, because it is easy to obtain large numbers from buffy coats of healthy donors. However, over the past years the procedures to generate large numbers of activated dendritic cells were refined *(13)*. Because those dendritic cells are superior in antigen presentation and costimulation capacity, they are currently used for hybrid cell production. The protocol for electrofusion of tumor and dendritic cells is identical to the aforementioned.

1. Because of the relative small number of patients treated with this approach, the dose-response relationship has not yet been established. We generally use $5–10 \times 10^7$ hybrid cells for each vaccination. We have observed tumor regressions with as little as 4×10^7 hybrid cells.
2. Although some tumor cell types might be more fusogenic than others, it is of importance to refine the exact fusion conditions for every new tumor cell type.
3. With the high cell density used in this protocol, one will observe the formation of pearl chains in the fusion chamber at the time of cell alignment.
4. Clumping of cells is seen in some instances after electrofusion. This may be caused by cellular DNA released from damaged cells. If gently pipeting the cell suspension is not sufficient to resolve clumping, incubate for 10 min with DNase (100 U/mL) at RT and wash twice with PBS.
5. Applying three pulses will increase the fusion efficiency, although not significantly affect the cell viabilty.
6. Pulses above 1500 V/cm should be avoided. Fusion efficiency will be only slightly increased, but cell viability will decrease drastically.
7. Cell densities above 2×10^7 cells/mL will result in a lower yield of fused cells.

References

1. Stuhler, G. and Walden, P. (1994) Recruitment of helper T-cells for induction of tumour rejection by cytolytic T lymphocytes. *Cancer Immunol. Immunother.* **39**, 342–345.
2. Guo, Y., Wu, M., Chen, H., Wang, X., Liu, G., Li, G., et al. (1994) Effective tumour vaccine generated by fusion of hepatoma cells with activated B cells. *Science* **263**, 518–520.
3. Mitchison, N. A., Rajewski, K., and Taylor, R. B. (1970) Cooperation of antigenic determinants of cells in the induction of antibodies, in *Developmental Aspects of Antibody Formation and Structure* (Sterzl, J. and Riha, I., eds.), Academic, New York, pp. 547–547.

4. Mitchison, N. A. and O'Malley, C. (1987) Three-cell-type clusters of T cells with antigen-presenting cells best explain the epitope linkage and noncognate requirements of the in-vivo cytolytic response. *Eur. J. Immunol.* **17,** 1479–1483.

5. Borges, E., Wiesmüller, K. H., Jung, G., and Walden, P. (1994) Efficacy of synthetic vaccines in the induction of cytotoxic T lymphocyte responses. *J. Immunol. Meth.* **173,** 253–263.

6. Stuhler, G. and Walden, P. (1993) Collaboration of helper and cytotoxic T lymphocytes. *Eur. J. Immunol.* **23,** 2279–2286.

7. Grabbe, S., Beissert, S., Schwarz, T., and Granstein, R. (1995) Dendritic cells as initiators of tumour immune responses: a possible strategy for tumour immunotherapy? *Immunol. Today* **16,** 117–121.

8. Mitchison, N. A. (1990) An exact comparison between the efficiency of two-and three-cell-type clusters mediating helper activity. *Eur. J. Immunol.* **20,** 699–702.

9. Trefzer, U., Weingart, G., Chen, Y., Adrian, K., Audring, H., Winter, H., et al. (1998) A phase I trial with a hybrid cell vaccine in patients with metastatic melanoma, in *Proc. 3rd Europ. Conf. Gene Ther. 1997* (P. Walden, U. Trefzer, W. Sterry, and Farzaneh, F., eds.), Plenum, London, pp. 519–525.

10. Kugler, A., Seseke, F., Thelen, P., Kallerhoff, M., Müller, G. A., Stuhler, G., et al. (1998) Autologous and allogeneic hybrid cell vaccine in patients with metastatic renal cell carcinoma. *Brit. J. Urol.* **82,** 487–493.

11. Neil, G. A and Zimmermann, U. (1993) Electrofusion, in *Methods in Enzymology* (Moldave, K. and Grossman, L., eds.). Academic, New York, pp. 174–196.

12. Chesnut, R. W. and Grey, H. M. (1981) Studies on the capacity of B-cells to serve as antigen-presenting cells. *J. Immunol.* **126,** 1075–1079.

13. Wen, Y. J., Ling, M., Bailey-Wood, R., and Lim, S. H. (1998) Idiotypic protein-pulsed adherent peripheral blood mononuclear cell derived dendritic cells prime immune system in multiple myeloma. *Clin. Cancer Res.* **4,** 957–962.

II

CLINICAL PROTOCOLS FOR CANCER GENE THERAPY

B: Suicide Gene Therapy

30

Retroviral Transfer of the Herpes Simplex Virus-Thymidine Kinase (*HSV-tK*) Gene for the Treatment of Cancer

Rajagopal Ramesh, Anupama Munshi, Aizen J. Marrogi, and Scott M. Freeman

1. Introduction

1.1. Gene Therapy, Suicide Genes, and Suicide Cancer Gene Therapy

Gene therapy is defined as the alteration of the genetic material of a cell with resultant benefit to a patient. Gene transfer has two broad categories: one in which a therapeutic gene is delivered to the cells with the aim of treating a disease; and another where a marker gene is delivered to label a cell type to determine the fate of a cell or the marker gene. Gene therapy is now becoming a rapidly developing therapeutic modality for experimental treatment of some cancers and diseases that have no alternative treatment *(1,2)*.

Suicide gene therapy was originally developed as a safety measure to control the expression of a foreign gene introduced into a cell such that the gene-modified cell could be eliminated if gene expression was no longer desired, or if the gene-modified cells became transformed *(3)*. During the course of developing the suicide genes, it was realized that if the suicide gene can be delivered directly to a tumor, it could be used for cancer therapy. This concept forms the basis for suicide gene therapy.

The most common approach used in suicide gene therapy involves the delivery of a gene encoding an enzyme that will metabolize a nontoxic prodrug into a toxic metabolite, leading to killing of the cells expressing the gene. Early studies demonstrated that the activated prodrug interferes with the replication of the transfected cells, while not affecting the nearby normal nontransfected

From: *Methods in Molecular Medicine, Vol. 35: Gene Therapy: Methods and Protocols*
Edited by: W. Walther and U. Stein © Humana Press, Inc., Totowa, NJ

cells. However, as will be described below, the fundamental basis for thera-peutic suicide gene therapy trials is the ability of the gene-modified tumor cells to kill nearby unmodified tumor cells when exposed to the prodrug. Therefore, systemic toxicity is minimal making this approach attractive for cancer gene therapy or as a safety device in the use of live tumor cell vaccines. The most widely used suicide gene, that has progressed into clinical trials, is the herpes simplex virus thymidine kinase (*HSV-tK*) gene coupled with the prodrug ganciclovir (GCV) *(4)*.

1.2. HSV/tk *GCV System and the Bystander Effect*

The ability of the *HSV-tK* gene to sensitize *HSV-tK* gene-modified tumor cells to the antiviral drug GCV was first demonstrated both in vitro and in vivo by Moolten et al. *(5)*. The *HSV-tK* gene specifically monophosphorylates the guanosine analog GCV which is subsequently converted into the toxic GCV-triphosphate form by endogenous mammalian kinases. Cellular DNA poly-merase incorporate the GCV-triphosphate into replicating DNA, thereby arresting DNA replication and causing cell death *(6)*. The *HSV-tK* enzyme is almost 1000-fold more efficient at monophosphorylating GCV than the cellu-lar thymidine kinase *(7)*. Therefore, GCV is highly toxic to cells that express *HSV-tK*, but is minimally toxic to unmodified or uninfected cells at therapeutic concentrations of the drug (1–10 mmol/L). However, neutropenia can be a clinical manifestation as result of GCV administration *(6,8)*. The phosphoryla-tion of GCV curtails its movement across the cell membrane resulting in a longer half-life ($t1/2=18$–24 h) within the cells than unmodified GCV *(6)*. The increased half-life of GCV is an important feature in the antitumor effects of *HSV-tK* gene-modified tumors.

Because most cancers are clonal in origin, and that *HSV-tK* gene-modified tumor cells are sensitive to GCV, the initial strategy was to generate a mosa-icism within an individual such that cells become *HSV-tK* positive randomly *(9,10)*. Any tumor arising subsequently from one of the *HSV-tK* sensitized cells will result in all tumor cells carrying the sensitivity gene as a clonal property and thereby treatment with GCV will lead to elimination of the tumor *(10)*. Thus, if a cancer developed later from a cell carrying the *HSV-tK* gene, then treating with GCV can selectively eliminate those cells. Thus, normal nonma-lignant cells will be spared and thereby can repopulate.

Although the mosaic theory for cancer therapy using suicide genes is an attractive approach, several limitations in the available technology exists, which makes it less attractive for immediate application clinically. These diffi-culties include: 1) inefficient gene transfer into cells of an organ, in particular when retroviral vectors are used as a result of which only a small portion of an organ can be modified; 2) transient gene expression when adenoviral vectors are used as a result of which gene expression is lost in a rapidly dividing cell population (e.g., malignant growth); 3) silencing of the gene (e.g., methylation) resulting in loss of expression of the recombinant protein; and 4) incomplete tumor killing. Thus, modifications of the existing approach are required before suicide gene therapy can be applied as a prophylaxis for cancer.

The inability to genetically modify all tumor cells within an individual necessitates killing of the unmodified tumor cells for this approach to be therapeutically effective. Using the *HSV-tK*/GCV system, Freeman and colleagues *(4,11,12)* demonstrated that *HSV-tK* gene-modified tumor cells are toxic to nearby unmodified tumor cells when the mixed tumor population is exposed to GCV. This phenomenon where untransduced tumor cells not expressing the *HSV-tK* enzyme are killed by nearby *HSV-tK*-transduced tumor cells, has been termed the "bystander effect." The effectiveness of the "bystander effect" to kill tumor cells was initially demonstrated in in vitro mixing experiments *(11,12)* and was shown to be owing to the transfer of toxic GCV metabolites *(12–14)*. Based on these in vitro experiments, where *HSV-tK* gene-modified tumor cells were sensitive to GCV and could generate a bystander effect on adjacent TK negative tumor cells, in vivo studies were performed. Mice with sc tumors, comprised of TK positive and TK negative tumor cells rejected their tumors with GCV treatment thus indicating the occurrence of the bystander effect. Furthermore, the bystander effect occurs even when only a fraction (10%) of the tumor mass contains the *HSV-tK* gene-modified tumor cells *(12)*. In addition, the bystander effect was demonstrated when syngeneic, allogeneic, or xenogeneic *HSV-tK* gene-modified tumor cells were used, indicating that irrespective of the cell type, the gene-modified cells need to be in close proximity to the unmodified tumor cells for the antitumor effect to occur *(15)*. The occurrence of the bystander effect has subsequently been demonstrated in various experimental tumors expressing the *HSV-tK* gene *(16–19)*. Thus, the demonstration of the bystander effect has important implications in cancer therapy because it removes the need for delivery of the gene to 100% of the tumor cell population.

Another important observation from these in vivo experiments was the abrogation of bystander effect in immunodeficient mice indicating the requirement of an intact host immune system *(20–23)*. Thus in vivo, both the local effects of GCV and the systemic immunity, have been demonstrated to contribute toward tumor rejection.

Because the above findings were based on experiments where tumor cells are in close proximity in a relatively confined subcutaneous space; it was reasonable to question if a similar bystander effect would occur in an intraperitoneal (ip) tumor-bearing animal. Mice were injected with a mixed population of *HSV-tK* positive and negative tumor cells. The animals rejected the tumors with GCV treatment *(12,20)*.

Although mice with an ip tumor comprising a mixture of TK positive and TK negative tumor cells rejected their tumors when treated with GCV, it may not be feasible in a clinical setting where a patient has a preexisting tumor. To model this clinical setting, animals with an ip *HSV-tK* negative tumor showed a prolonged survival when treated with *HSV-tK* gene-modified tumor cells and GCV *(12)*. Thus a preexisting tumor within a large enclosed body cavity could be treated resulting in prolonged survival. This observation formed the basis for the development of *HSV-tK*-based clinical trial for the treatment of ovarian cancer, which is mainly confined to the peritoneal cavity. In addition, the use of *HSV-tK*/GCV system in the treatment of cancer offers several advantages: 1) rapidly replicating tumor cells are more susceptible to impairment of DNA synthesis; 2) chemotherapy-resistant tumors, such as ovarian cancer, can be made sensitive when genetically modified with the *HSV-tK* gene; and 3) *HSV-tK*/GCV-treated tumor cells have the ability to kill neighboring tumor cells through the bystander effect.

1.3. Ovarian Cancer

Cancer of the ovary is the fifth most common malignant condition among women in the United States with an annual incidence of 22,000 new cases *(24)*. The disease predominantly affects postmenopausal women in their sixth decade, accounting for approx 13,300 deaths each year and for more than half of all deaths from genital cancer. The average lifetime risk for the development of ovarian cancer in women in the United States is 1 in 70. The highly lethal nature of this tumor is related to the absence of symptoms in the majority of women with early stages of the disease. Seventy percent of women present with advanced disease stages in which the tumor has spread to the peritoneal surfaces of the upper abdomen. Extensive intraabdominal disease is difficult to eradicate completely by surgery and many patients only have a partial response to adjuvant chemotherapy. Ovarian cancer is staged into four categories: Stage I tumors are limited to the ovaries; Stage II includes tumors with pelvic extension; Stage III includes tumors with peritoneal implants outside the pelvis and retroperitoneal or inguinal nodes and also tumors with extension to the small bowel or omentum; and Stage IV includes tumors with distant metastasis including parenchymal liver metastasis. Each of the first three stages (I–III) of ovarian cancer can be further divided into substages of more progressive disease (a-b-c) based on the involvement of the contralateral ovary.

Patient survival can be evaluated based on the stage of the disease at diagnosis. Higher stage disease correlates with a worse prognosis. Treatment of ovarian cancer is based on the stage of the disease with the higher stage of disease being treated more aggressively. Stage I disease can be treated with either surgery or a combination of surgery and chemotherapy. Stage II, III, and IV patients are initially surgically debulked of tumor before receiving chemotherapy and /or radiotherapy. The treatment is based on the ability to surgically remove the tumor and the location of the remaining tumor. The initial chemotherapy usually includes the drug cisplatin and taxol in the regimen, as it is highly active against this tumor. The present protocol requires that patients previously receive either cisplatin or carboplatin and taxol treatment, and following the initial chemotherapy patients may be treated with ip chemotherapy. Therefore, the technology allowing the insertion of fluid into the peritoneal cavity for treatment of ovarian cancer is established and these methods are used during this investigation.

The follow up 5-yr disease-free survival in various stages of ovarian cancer are 80–100% (Stage I), 30–40% (Stage II to IIIa), 20% (Stage IIIb), and 5–10% (Stage IIIc–IV). Prognosis of an ovarian cancer patient is also dependent on 1) size of the largest tumor lesion at the time of diagnosis or 2) diameter of the largest remaining metastatic lesion after surgical reduction. Patients presenting with a >10-cm tumor mass exhibited a 0% 3-yr survival and a 9-mo mean survival. In addition, patients who relapse following the initial chemotherapy only have a 10–20% response to second-line therapy that has not been shown to prolong patient survival.

CA125 is a tumor marker identified for ovarian cancer and is present on the surface of malignant ovarian cells, normal ovary, pleura, mesothelium, peritoneum, and gut. It is a cell-surface glycoprotein shed by malignant cells and is detectable in the serum. Detection of CA125 is, therefore, useful in determining microscopic disease recurrence if the patient presented with a possible titer that decreased with treatment. In a patient with ovarian cancer, a CA125 titer of 35 IU/mL is almost always associated with disease. A negative titer is a poor indicator for lack of disease. Changes in the CA125 titer provide a good indication of the tumor's response to treatment and can be used to follow the success or failure of treatment. Thus, persistently elevated titers during treatment usually indicate treatment failure.

Based on the encouraging results obtained from preclinical experimental animal studies and with limited treatment availability for ovarian cancer patients, the first *HSV-tK* suicide gene therapy Phase I clinical trial for the treatment of human ovarian cancer was approved by the FDA and the Recombinant DNA Advisory Committee (RAC) *(4,20)*. The methods involved in the development of a clinical protocol for ovarian cancer include: 1) developing an allogeneic ovarian cancer cell line expressing the *HSV-tK* gene, which primarily involves transduction with a retroviral vector carrying the *HSV-tK* gene;

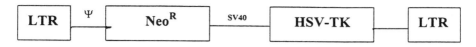

Fig. 1. The retroviral vector carrying the *HSV-tK* gene.

2) selection and testing of the *HSV-tK* transduced cell line for drug (GCV) sensitivity; 3) testing for recombinant retrovirus production; 4) testing for endotoxin production; 5) evaluation for mycoplasma contamination; and 6) preparation of the cells for infusion into the patient. The aforementioned procedures, along with the criteria for inclusion and patient selection, will be discussed in detail in the following sections.

2. Materials

2.1. Cell Lines

The human ovarian tumor cell line (PA1), the amphotropic packaging cell line (PA 317), and the 3T3 cell line (mouse fibroblast) were obtained from the American Type Culture Collection (ATCC, Rockville, MD). The cells were maintained in Dulbecco's modified Eagle's medium (DMEM) supplemented with 10% fetal bovine serum (FBS) at 37°C in a 5% CO_2 incubator. The cells were passaged by trypsinization when they were 80–90% confluent.

2.2. Retroviral Vectors

The retroviral vector carrying the *HSV-tK* gene used for transduction of PA-1 ovarian carcinoma cells is shown in **Fig. 1** *(10)*. The vector used is a type C Moloney murine leukemia virus (MoMuLV) based retrovirus carrying the neomycin resistance gene (*Neo*^R) and the *HSV-tK* gene under the control of the viral long-terminal repeats (LTR). The viral packaging sequence (Ψ) is included and is upstream of the *neo*^R gene. The SV40 promoter drives expression of *HSV-tK*.

2.3. 6X Bromophenol Blue

Bromophenol blue – (0.25%), sucrose – (40% (w/v) in water) solution stored at 4°C is stable for very long periods of time. Use of bromophenol blue as a gel-loading dye serves to 1) increase the density of the sample ensuring that the sample drops evenly into the agarose wells; 2) add color to the sample thereby simplifying the loading process; and 3) they contain dyes that in an electric field move toward the anode at predictable rates. The migration of bromophenol blue in 0.5X TBE buffer is approximately the same as linear double-stranded DNA 300 base pair (bp) in length.

2.4. 5X Tris-Borate Buffer (TBE): Tris base–(54 g), boric acid–(27.5 g), 0.5 M EDTA (pH 8.0)–(20 mL)

A precipitate forms when concentrated solutions of TBE are stored for long periods of time. To avoid this, autoclaving the 5X solution at 15 lbs/15 min and storage at room temperature is recommended. For agarose gel electrophoresis, dilution of TBE to 1X (1:5 dilution) in water is recommended.

2.5. 1% Methylene Blue

Prepare 1% methylene blue (Sigma Chemicals, St. Louis, MO) by dissolving 1 g in 100 mL of methanol. Store solution at room temperature. Solution stored for more than 1 mo is not recommended for use. Prepare fresh solution at regular intervals.

2.6. Ethidium Bromide

Dissolve 1 g of ethidium bromide (Et.Br) in 100 mL of water by mixing for several hours. Cover the container with aluminum foil or transfer the solution to a dark bottle to protect from light. Store the stock solution (1 mg/mL) at room temperature. Care should be taken when handling Et.Br. or solutions containing it, because it is a powerful mutagen and is moderately toxic. Use of gloves is strongly recommended.

2.7. Geneticin (G418 Sulfate)

Stock solution of G418 is prepared by dissolving the powder in water. However, the microbiological potency of G418 varies and is usually between 50–75% of the actual concentration. For example, if G418 is 50% active, then 1 mg of G418 dissolved in water will give 500 µg/mL of active solution. G418 is stable as a clear colorless solution when stored at 4°C. Solution is prepared under sterile conditions inside a laminar flow hood.

2.8. Protamine

Protamine sulfate is obtained commercially at 10 mg/mL concentration. Store solution at 4°C and handle inside a laminar flow hood.

2.9. Ganciclovir (GCV)

GCV is prepared by dissolving the lyophilized powder (500 mg) in 10 mL of sterile water to a final concentration of 50 mg/mL. The solution is sterilized by filtration through syringe filter (0.22 µ) and stored at 4°C. Storing GCV at 4°C for long periods of time results in formation of crystals. Incubation at 37°C for 30–60 min prior to use is recommended. Solution is prepared under sterile conditions inside a laminar flow hood. GCV should be prepared fresh every couple of weeks.

3. Methods

3.1. Retrovirus Supernatant

The amphotropic packaging/producer cell line (PA317), which has been previously transfected with the plasmid carrying the *HSV-tK* gene, is grown to confluence in DMEM supplemented with 10% FBS. Fresh medium is added to the cells 24 h before the virus supernatant is harvested. The media (viral supernatant) is then filtered through a 0.45-μm syringe filter, aliquoted, and stored at −80°C until use. Freezing the viral supernatant prevents inactivation and decay of retroviral particles present in the supernatant (*see* **Note 1**).

3.2. Retroviral Transduction

Tumor cells (PA-1) are seeded at 30–40% confluency in 60-mm^2 tissue-culture plates (Corning, NY) prior to transduction with viral supernatant. Protamine sulfate (positively charged) is added to the retroviral supernatant (50 μg/mL) to increase the retroviral transduction efficiency by modulating the natural charge repulsion barrier *(25)*. Cells are incubated with the viral supernatant at 37°C for 2 h following which the supernatant is replaced with fresh supernatant and incubation continued overnight at 37°C. The next day, viral supernatant is removed, cells are washed twice with PBS to remove any unbound virus, and fresh medium is added. Cells are allowed to grow for 24 h before the cultures are assayed for transduction efficiency by G418 selection.

3.3. G418 Selection

Geneticin, also known as G418 sulfate, is an aminoglycoside related to Gentamicin that is commonly used as a selective agent in molecular genetics experiments. It is commonly known as neomycin and is toxic to both prokaryotic and eukaryotic cells. The resistance genes (*neo^R*) are dominant and are located on bacterial transposons (Tn 601 and Tn 5) that can also be expressed in eukaryotic cells. Efficient expression is achieved when the *neo* DNA sequence is linked to the eukaryotic DNA sequence thereby permitting transcription and processing of the Neo coding sequence into mRNA. Introduction of this gene into cells can confer resistance to Geneticin-enabling cells to grow in media containing Geneticin.

3.3.1. Principle

PA-1 cells transduced with retroviral vector carrying the neomycin resistance (*neo^R*) when exposed to G418 will grow, whereas cells not transduced will be killed. Thus transduced cells can be selectively grown, expanded, and used for all experimental purposes.

3.3.2. Procedure

The PA-1 cells transduced with the retroviral vector carrying the neomycin resistance gene and the *HSV-tK* gene are plated in 60-mm^2 6-well tissue-culture plates (Corning, NY) and incubated at 37°C in a 5% CO_2 incubator. The following day, the cells are exposed to G418 (800 μg/mL) in duplicate for 14 d (*see* **Note 2**). Cells unexposed to G418 serve as a control. On day 14, the culture medium is aspirated and fresh culture medium without G418 is added and the cells are allowed to grow. Cells growing at this point of time carry the *neo*R gene. Two rounds of G418 selection are performed. When the cells are at 70–80% confluency, the cells are trypsinized and replated in 100-mm^2 culture plates (Corning, NY). When the cells are close to confluency, the cells are again trypsinized and an aliquot is frozen and stored in liquid nitrogen. The cells are frozen at regular intervals in liquid nitrogen for future use. It is recommended that freshly thawed cells be selected for G418 resistance before using for any other purpose. This is because cells may lose the gene over a period of time resulting in the loss of G418 resistance.

3.4. In Vitro Testing for GCV Sensitivity

Evaluation of the TK retrovirus transduced PA-1 cells for GCV sensitivity is essential if cells have to be used for therapeutic purposes. Determining the sensitivity is essential because it indicates the concentration at which maximal killing can be obtained.

3.4.1. Principle

PA-1 cells transduced with the retroviral vector carrying the *HSV-tK* gene and subsequently selected for G418 resistance by the procedure mentioned above are next tested for GCV sensitivity. The rationale is that cells resistant to G418 need not necessarily express the thymidine kinase (*TK*) gene. Failure to express *HSV-tK*, because of methylation or gene loss, will result in the inability to convert GCV to its monophosphate form that is a crucial step in the tumoricidal effect. Testing for expression of *TK* will also indicate the sensitivity range of the cells to GCV. Hence, exposing these cells to GCV at regular intervals is recommended.

3.4.2. Protocol

The PA-1 cells transduced with retroviral vector carrying both the neomycin resistance gene and the *HSV-tK* gene are plated in 60-mm^2 6-well tissue-culture plates (Corning, NY) and incubated at 37°C in a 5% CO_2 incubator. The following day, the cells are exposed to varying concentrations of GCV

(0–100 μM) in duplicates for 10 d. Cells unexposed to GCV serve as a control. On day 14, the culture medium is aspirated and 2 mL of 1% methylene blue are added to each well. Following incubation for 5 min at room temperature, the plates are thoroughly washed in running tap water, air-dried, and the number of blue-staining colonies counted. The number of colonies present in each well exposed to varying concentrations of GCV serves as an indicator of sensitivity.

3.5. Stock Culture Preparation of HSV-tK Gene-Modified PA-1STK Cells

Following transduction and selection, the allogeneic gene-modified cell line PA-1STK is initially grown as a primary (1°) seed lot in AIM-V medium containing 1% calf serum. The cells are trypsinized when about 70% confluency is attained and stored in 30–40 vials at 10^7 cells/vial in a freezing medium (20% calf serum and 7.5% DMSO in M199) at –80°C overnight in an insulated container and then stored in liquid nitrogen.

From the primary seed lot, a vial of cells is thawed, washed, and used to grow a similarly sized secondary (2°) seed lot (from which the cells for patient treatment will be grown), which are also frozen away as above. Single lot numbers of medium, serum, and other reagents used for growing cells are obtained in sufficient quantity to be used for the production of all cells for patient treatment from the 2° seed lot.

3.6. Replication Competent Retrovirus (RCR) Assay

Detection of RCR in tissue culture is performed as a preventive measure to protect humans from developing cancer as a consequence of injecting these DNA vectors. The method used is known as the Helper-Rescue Assay.

3.6.1. Principle

The ability of retroviral vectors to undergo recombination events to produce replication competent virus can be detected by S+/L– assay, which has been established over the past decade (26). Recently, a more rapid and sensitive assay, the Helper-Rescue Assay, has been developed that is widely used for detecting ecotropic, amphotropic, and xenotropic viruses. If a recombination event occurs, it will almost always occur in the producer cell as producer cell line (PA-317) contains both, a helper virus and the retrovirus vector. The producer cell line generates the viral particles used for transduction. Therefore, the producer cell lines need to be continually monitored for the presence of RCR. Cells (PA-1) transduced with replication incompetent viral stock as measured by the above assay are very unlikely to generate replication competent virus themselves. However, as described in the protocol below, transduced cells (PA-1STK) can be monitored for a few weeks after transduction, a period sufficient to detect replication competent virus by the above assays. Thus monitoring the *HSV-tK*-transduced cells for a few weeks in vitro before infusion into a patient will greatly reduce the risk of generating replication competent retrovirus (RCR's).

3.6.2. Protocol

1. Plate PA-1 cells and NIH3T3 cells in 60-mm^2 tissue-culture plates at 40–50% confluency and incubate the plates at 37°C overnight in 5% CO_2 incubator.
2. The following day, collect the supernatant from PA-1STK cells that are to be used for the clinical trial purpose.
3. Add the supernatant from PA-1STK cells onto plates growing PA-1 and NIH3T3 cells in duplicates and incubate at 37°C in a 5% CO_2 incubator for 1 wk.
4. Following incubation for 1 wk, discard the supernatant and replenish with fresh culture medium. Add G418 (50 mg/mL stock) to a final concentration of 800 µg/mL. Incubate the cells for 1 wk.
5. On day 7, remove the plates from the incubator and check for G418 resistant colonies.
6. It is expected that PA-1 and NIH3T3 cells exposed to PA-1STK supernatant will not be resistant to G418. However, appearance of G418 resistant colonies is an indication of RCR production.

3.7. Mycoplasma Detection by PCR

Presence or association of mycoplasma with the PA-1STK tissue-culture cells to be injected into humans is not favorable and can be detected by the use of a polymerase chain reaction (PCR)-based assay.

3.7.1. Principle

The PCR is a rapid technique for the in vitro amplification of a specific sequences from genomic DNA (or from RNA) between a 5' and 3' primer each complementary to one of the strands of the DNA and flanking target sequence. The sequence-specific oligonucleotide primers used in the PCR are extended in the presence of DNA polymerase enzyme (e.g., *Taq* polymerase) with repeated cycles of heat denaturation, annealing, and extension resulting in the exponential amplification of the target DNA. This method is very sensitive to amplify a single copy of DNA present in a sample to approximately a millionfold that can be detected by running an agarose-gel electrophoresis.

The mycoplasma PCR primer kit (Stratagene, CA) can detect most mycoplasma infections from 100 µL of cell-culture supernatant. Cell growth-inhibiting or weak mycoplasma infections can also be detected by harvesting and testing culture cells. The assay is performed 24 h before preparing the cells for injecting into the patient. The protocol described below detects almost all cases of mycoplasma infection.

3.7.2. Protocol

3.7.2.1. TEMPLATE PREPARATION

Collect 100 µL of culture supernatant into a sterile microcentrifuge tube and boil for 5 min. Spin the tube briefly for 5 s in a microcentifuge.

Add 10 µL of resuspended StrataClean™ resin (provided in the kit) to the supernatant and mix briefly (gentle flicking is sufficient). Spin the tubes for 10 s in a microcentrifuge to pellet the resin.

Take 10 µL of the treated supernatant to a fresh sterile tube and dilute 1:10 with sterile water (10 µL of the diluted template is required per PCR). The diluted supernatant serves as the template for detection of mycoplasma. Care must be taken to avoid aspirating the resin into the aliquot.

3.7.2.2. PCR REACTION CONDITIONS.

The optimal reaction conditions for a standard 50 µL reaction mixture to detect mycoplasma are as follows:

$10mM$ Tris-HCl (pH 8.3–8.8)
50 mM KCl   *Taq* Buffer (*see* **Notes 3** and **4**)
1.5–2.5 mM MgCl2
200 µM of each deoxynucleotide triphosphates (dATP, dCTP, dGTP, and dTTP) and 1 U of *Taq* DNA polymerase/reaction tube.

The recipe described below is for one reaction and can be adjusted accordingly for the number of samples to be tested.

1. In a 0.5-mL microcentrifuge tube, add 5 µL of 10X *Taq* reaction buffer to 29 µL of sterile water.
2. To the above mixture, add 1 µL of 200 µM dNTP mixture followed by 2 µL of primer mix (stock primer mix is 5 mM for each primer) and 1 µL of *Taq* DNA polymerase (2.5 U/µL stock).
3. Add either 2 µL of internal control template or, if the template is not used, add 2 µL of water instead. The total volume of the PCR reaction mixture should be 40 µL.
4. Add 10 µL of the diluted sample to the appropriate reaction tube. Add 10 µL of the negative control (water or negative extract) to the appropriate reaction tube.
5. Add 10 µL of the positive control template (provided in the kit) to the appropriate reaction tube.
6. Briefly mix the reaction components by vortexing and centrifuge in an Eppendorf tube. Overlay the reaction mixture with 50 µL of light mineral oil (Sigma Chemicals) and subject to 45 amplification cycles in a thermocycler (Thermolyne-Barnstead). The cycling parameters are shown in **Table 1** (*see* **Note 5**).

Table 1
Cycling Parameters for Detection of Mycoplasma
by Polymerase Chain Reaction (PCR)

Cycle #	Temperature parameters		Number of Cycles
1	94°C	5 min	1
	55°C	1 min, 45 s	
2	72°C	3 min	3
	94°C	45 s	
	55°C	1 min, 45 s	
3	72°C	3 min	40
	94°C	45 s	
	55°C	45 s	
4	72°C	10 min	1

7. After completion of the PCR amplification, 15 µL of the amplified PCR product is mixed with 4 µL of 6X gel-loading buffer (bromophenol blue) and analyzed on a 2% agarose gel.
8. The sample is electrophoresed in 1X TBE buffer containing 0.5 µg/mL ethidium bromide (10 mg/mL stock) at 60 V/cm^2 for 2 h at room temperature to ensure separation between PCR products associated with the internal control template and those owing to mycoplasma.
9. Following electrophoresis, the gel is visualized under a UV transilluminator and the results are recorded using a Polaroid photograph system.

3.8. Endotoxin Assay (Limulus Amebocyte Lysate)

This assay is a quantitative test and is used to test for the presence of endotoxin that are produced by gram negative bacteria in the tissue-culture supernatant. Presence of endotoxin in the culture supernatant of PA-1STK cells is not suitable for use as a cancer vaccine. The assay is performed 24–48 hours before preparing the cells for treatment using the commercially available endotoxin assay kit (BioWhitaker, Walkersville, MD).

3.8.1 Principle

Gram-negative bacterial endotoxin catalyzes the activation of proenzyme in the Limulus Amebocyte Lysate (LAL). The initial rate of activation is determined by the concentration of endotoxin present. The activated enzyme catalyzes the splitting of *p*-nitroaniline (pNA) from the colorless substrate Ac-Ile-Glu-Ala-Arg-pNA. The pNA release is measured photometrically at 405–410 nm after the reaction is stopped with stop reagent. The correlation between the absorbance and the endotoxin concentration is linear in the 0.1–1.0 eu/mL range. The concentration of endotoxin in a sample is calculated from the absorbance values of solutions containing known amounts of endotoxin standard.

3.8.2. Procedure

To test the presence of endotoxin, 50 µL of culture supernatant is mixed with 50 µL of LAL reagent in a 96-well flat-bottomed ELISA plate (Corning, NY) and incubated at 37°C for 30 min. Following incubation, 100 µL of substrate solution is added and incubation continued for 6 min at 37°C. The reaction is stopped by the addition of 50 µL of stop reagent (25% acetic acid v/v in water). Development of yellow color in the sample indicates the presence of endotoxin and the absorbance is determined spectrophotometrically at 405–410 nm. Because the absorbance is in direct proportion to the amount of endotoxin present, the concentration of endotoxin can be calculated from a standard curve (*see* **Notes 6–9**).

3.9. Treatment of Ovarian Cancer with Gene-Modified Cancer Vaccine

1. Eligiblity criteria
   a. Stage I, II, or III ovarian cancer patients.
   b. Patients who have completed surgery and chemotherapy.
   c. Evidence of residual disease by tumor marker or imaging must be present.
2. Patient selection
   a. A diagnosis of epithelial ovarian carcinoma must be established histologically.
   b. Patients may initially have been Stage I, II, or III. Stage IV patients initially or at present are not eligible.
   c. Patients must have completed the initial surgery and chemotherapy and have been off treatment for at least 6 wk. Previous chemotherapy must have included cisplatin or carboplatin containing regimens.
   d. Patients must have clinical evidence of recurrent, progressive, or residual disease by laparscopy, laparotomy, imaging, surgery, or successive elevation of the CA 125 marker. If possible, resistance or progression should be documented by histology/cytology. If CA 125 is used as evidence of residual disease, then the level must be greater than 35 IU/mL and increasing on two successive determinations, greater than 1 mo apart, and the patient must not have had a laparotomy within the preceding 3 mo.
   e. The patient's performance status must be 0 or 1 by ECOG standards.
   f. Any tumor masses found by imaging must be 2.0 cm or less to be eligible for this study.

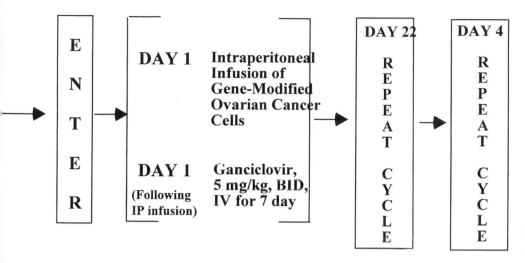

Fig. 2. Schematic representation of treatment schedule for ovarian cancer using the *HSV-tK* gene-modified cancer vaccine.

    g. Adequate bone marrow, kidney, and liver function must be shown by: Hct > 30, WBC > 4000, platelets > 100,000, creatinine < 1.5 mg%, Creat. Cl > 50, normal bilirubin, SGOT and alkaline phosphatase < 1.5 × normal.

    h. Patients must not have a significant history of heart disease (frequent angina, MI within the past 6 mo, congestive heart failure requiring daily treatment).

    i. A patient is not eligible if there is a history of a previous malignancy, other than squamous or basal cell carcinoma of the skin. Patients with childbearing potential are not eligible.

    j. Patients with extensive abdominal adhesions and lack of free flow of fluid within the peritoneal cavity are not eligible.

    k. Patients with evidence of moderate to severe pulmonary disease (COPD) will not be eligible.

    l. Patients requiring steroid treatment are not eligible.

    m. Patients with a negative Epstein Barr antibody test are not eligible.

3.10. Preparation and Administration of HSV-tK Gene-Modified Cancer Vaccine

1. Treatment Plan
   a. The patients will be admitted to the hospital for the first 8 d of each cycle.
   b. The vaccine is given on day 1 and GCV is given for 7 d, beginning on day 1 (**Fig. 2**).
   c. The treatment is repeated at 3-wk intervals for a total of three cycles of treatment.

   d. At the completion of treatment, patients will be followed regularly until there is progression of disease.
2. Preparation of cancer vaccine
   a. A few days before a patient's treatment is scheduled, a vial of cells from the 2° seed lot is thawed and seeded in the requisite number of flasks needed for the vaccine treatment.
   b. The cell-culture supernatant is tested for mycoplasma, bacterial and fungal contamination, and endotoxin production 24 h prior to harvesting the cells as mentioned above.
   c. On the day of use, the cells are harvested, washed twice with normal saline, counted, and irradiated at 10,000 rads from a cesium source. Following irradiation, the cells are washed 3X with normal saline and resuspended in 1000 mL normal saline for administration of the vaccine.
3. Administration of the cancer vaccine
   a. Patients are assigned, in order of entrance on study, to one of the four treatment schedules as shown in **Table 2**. The dose escalates with each treatment unless any toxicity of Grade II or higher level has occurred. For Grade II toxicity (except for neutropenia or thrombocytopenia), the dose is repeated, but physician discretion could lower the dose if overall toxicity is of concern. For Grade III or IV toxicity, the dose is lowered one level. If these Grade III/IV toxicities do not resolve within 1 wk, the patient will be taken off the study.

      The patient is admitted to the hospital the day before the treatment or on the same day of treatment and the vaccine is administered through a small ip catheter. The catheter is placed on the day of treatment and removed at the conclusion of treatment.
   b. The vaccine is administered in 1000 mL of normal saline through the catheter over a 2-h time period. GCV treatment is started within 24 h following ip infusion of the cells and is given 5 mg/kg, 2×/d for 7 d. GCV is reconstituted in sterile water and is not compatible with bacteriostatic water (*see* **Notes 10–15**). For iv administration, GCV is prepared in 100 mL of normal saline or 5% Dextrose and water and infused over a 1-h time period.

3.11. Vaccine Side Effects

1. Irradiated tumor cells have been administered as vaccines at intradermal sites in previous studies. At intradermal sites, the local side effects are usually only a transient nontender bump and even this side effect is largely determined by the adjuvant used rather than the tumor cells. The side effects from ip vaccine administration are largely unknown. The GCV activation of the tumoricidal effect could lead to some local inflammatory response, which may be a beneficial antitumor effect. However, whether symptoms will occur is unknown. For this reason, the study is designed with an escalating dose plan and the patients will be hospitalized and monitored daily for side effects.
2. Grading of side effects and toxicity will be determined by the NCI's "Common toxicity criteria."

Table 2

Patients	First Dose	Second Dose	Third Dose
1–4	1×10^7	1×10^8	3×10^8
5–8	1×10^8	3×10^8	1×10^9
9–12	3×10^8	1×10^9	3×10^9
13–16	1×10^9	3×10^9	1×10^{10}

3. To document the patient reported incidence and severity of side effects, each diary lists 23 possible side effects and includes space for patients to write in additional side effects. Patients also rate the efficacy of self-care activities in alleviating treatment side effects. In addition, patients are asked to give an overall rating of the degree of discomfort resulting from the side effects. The diary takes approximately 15 min to complete. The diary has been shown to have adequate variance and is acceptable to patients. The diary will be completed daily for the 8-d hospital stay for each treatment and at 1 wk and 2 wk following discharge.

4. Conclusions

The *HSV-tK* gene has been identified to function as a suicide gene when exposed to the prodrug, ganciclovir (GCV). Based on its ability to generate a "bystander effect," a number of clinical protocols, including ours (ovarian cancer), have been initiated for the treatment of cancer. The success of this technology has relied on the bystander effect and is currently limited to the treatment of localized solid tumors, such as ovarian and brain. The efficacies of this treatment protocol using the *HSV-tK* gene will be evaluated from the reports of several Phase I trials and a Phase III trial that is currently being carried out. However, preliminary reports indicate that delivery of *HSV-tK* gene in cancer gene therapy is nontoxic with some patients achieving either partial or complete clinical remission. Furthermore, advances made in the existing protocols will lead to the application of *HSV-tK* suicide gene therapy for metastatic cancers.

5. Notes

1. The half-life of retrovirus at 37°C is 5–8 h. Viral titer can be increased (10–100-fold) by growing the packaging cell line at 32°C. This change in temperature prolongs the extracellular half-life of the retroviral particles.
2. The amount of G418 to be added in culture to select for resistant cells varies for different cell type. Hence, the optimal concentration required to maintain and select cells must be determined for each type of cells that has to be transduced.
3. In our experience, 10X *Taq* buffer and MgCl$_2$ (25 m*M*) provided by Promega (Madison, WI) in the *Taq* DNA polymerase kit gives good amplification and circumvents the need to prepare individual reagents.

4. It is recommended that cells be cultured in the absence of antibiotics for several days in order to maximize the strength of the signal, which is observed in PCR. Test supernatants to be used in PCR should be derived from cells that are at or near confluence.

5. The cycling parameters shown in **Table 1** are applicable to most thermocyclers. However, thermalcyclers whose transition times are long will inadvertently add time to the PCR program and may result in excessive signals in both the test samples and controls. In such a situation, one can attempt to reduce the signal by elimination of segment 2 in the PCR program. If a problem still persists, changing the parameters is suggested.

6. When using 25% acetic acid as stop reagent, samples such as tissue-culture medium may turn yellow because of acid environment.

7. All material coming in contact with the sample or test material should be pyrogen-free (sterile Eppendorf tubes are suitable).

8. Samples (e.g., tissue-culture medium) should be stored at 2–8°C if they are to be used within 24 h; samples to be tested later than 24 h should be frozen.

9. Prewarming the microtiter plate at 37°C prior to starting the experiments gives better results.

10. GCV is a nucleoside analog that is supplied as a sterile powder. The original sterile powder supplied in 10-mL sterile vials, 25 in a carton, should be stored at room temperature avoiding heat above 40°C (104°F). Reconstituted solution in the vial should be stored at room temperature. It should not be refrigerated. When stored accordingly, it will be stable for 12 h. Final diluted infusion solution (admixture preparation) should be refrigerated, but freezing is not recommended. The solution must be used within 24 h of dilution to reduce the risk of bacterial contamination.

11. Mild cytopenias may occur during the 7-d GCV administration. Pain and phlebitis at the site of administration may occur. Anemia, fever, rash, and abnormal liver enzymes can also occur.

12. Administration of GCV should be stopped if absolute granulocyte count falls below 750 or the platelets are less than 50,000.

13. GCV solution used for injection into patients is stored separately from one that is used for testing GCV sensitivity following transduction of cells in culture.

14. The PA1STK cells to be injected into the patient are handled in a separate tissue-culture laminar hood isolated from that which is used for transducing cells with retroviral vector. This avoids any contamination that might otherwise take place.

15. Tissue-culture incubators have to be dedicated exclusively for growing cells for clinical trials.

References

1. Anderson, W. F. (1992) Human gene therapy. *Science* **256**, 808–813.
2. Friedman, T. and Roblin, R. (1972) Gene therapy for human genetic diseases. *Science* **175**, 949–955.

3. Blaese, R. M. (1992) Gene therapy using suicide genes, in *Biologic Therapy of Cancer* (DeVita Jr., V. T., Hellman, S., and Rosenberg, S. A., eds.), J. B. Lippincot, Philadelphia, PA, pp. 746–750.
4. Freeman, S. M., McCune, C. S., Abboud, C. N., and Abraham G. N. (1992) Treatment of ovarian cancer using *HSV-tK* gene-modified cells. *Hum. Gene Ther.* **3,** 342–349.
5. Moolten, F. L. (1986) Tumor chemosensitivity conferred by inserted herpes thymidine kinase genes: paradigm for a prospective cancer control strategy. *Cancer Res.* **46,** 5276–5281.
6. Elion, G. B. (1980) The chemotherapeutic exploitation of virus specified enzymes. *Adv. Enzyme Regul.* **18,** 53–60.
7. Elion, G. B., Furman, P. A., Fyfe, J. A., deMiranda, P., Beauchamp, L., and Schaeffer, H. J. (1977) Selectivity of action of an antiherpetic agent, 9-(2-hydroxyethoxymethyl) guanine. *Proc. Natl. Acad. Sci. USA* **74,** 5716–5720.
8. Shepp, D. H., Dandliker, P., deMiranda, P., Burnette, T. C., Cederberg, D. M., Kirk, L. E., and Meyer, J. D. (1985). Activity of 9-[2-hydroxymethyl) ethoxymethyl} guanine in the treatment of cytomegalovirus penumonia. *Ann. Intern. Med.* **103,** 368–373.
9. Moolten, F. L. (1990a) Mosaicism induced by gene insertion as a means of improving chemotherapeutic selectivity. *Crit. Rev. Immunol.* **10,** 203–233.
10. Moolten, F. and Wells, J. M. (1990b) Curability of tumors bearing herpes thymidine kinase genes transferred by retroviral vectors. *J. Natl. Cancer Inst.* **82,** 297–300.
11. Freeman, S. M., Whartenby, K. A., Koeplin, D. S., Moolten, F. L., Abboud, C. N., and Abraham, G. N. (1992b) Tumor regression when a fraction of the tumor mass contains the *HSV-tK* gene. *J. Cell Biochem.* **16F** (abstr. 47).
12. Freeman, S. M., Abboud, C. N., Whartenby, K. A., Packman, C. H., Koeplin, D. S., Moolten, F. L., and Abraham, G. N. (1993) The Bystander effect: tumor regression when a fraction of the tumor mass is genetically modified. *Cancer Res.* **53,** 5274–5283.
13. Bi, W. L., Parysek, L. M., Warnick, R., and Stambrook, P. J. (1993) In vitro evidence that metabolic cooperation is responsible for the Bystander Effect observed with *HSV-tK* retroviral gene therapy. *Hum. Gene Ther.* **4,** 725–731.
14. Mesnil, M., Piccoli, C., Tiraby, G., Willecke, K., and Yamasaki, H. (1996) Bystander killing of cancer cells by herpes simplex virus thymidine kinase gene is mediated by connexins. *Proc. Natl. Acad. Sci. USA* **93,** 1831–1835.
15. Freeman, S. M., Ramesh, R., Shastri, M., Munshi, A., Jensen, A., and Marrogi, A. J. (1995) The role of cytokines in mediating the bystander effect using *HSV-tK* xenogeneic cells. *Cancer Lett.* **92,** 167–174.
16. Barba, D., Hardin, J., Ray, J., and Gage, F. H. (1993) Thymidine kinase mediated killing of rat brain tumors. *J. Neurosurg.* **79,** 729–735.
17. Culver, K. W., Ram, Z., Oldfield, E. H., and Blaese, M. (1992) Regression of brain tumors using gene-modified cells. *Science* **256,** 1550–1552.

18. Ram, Z., Culver, K. W., Walbridge, S. W., Blaese, R. M., and Oldfield, E. H. (1993) In situ retroviral-mediated gene transfer for the treatment of brain tumors. *Cancer Res.* **53,** 83–88.

19. Ezzedine, Z. D., Martuza, R. L., Platika, D., Short, M. P., Malick, T., Choi, B., et al. (1991) Selective killing of glioma cells in culture and in vivo by retrovirus transfer of the Herpes Simplex thymidine kinase gene. *New Biol.* **3,** 608–614.

20. Freeman, S. M., McCune, C., Robinson, W., Abboud, C. N., Angel, C., Abraham G. N., et al. (1995) Treatment of ovarian cancer using a gene-modified vaccine. *Hum. Gene Ther.* **6,** 927–939.

21. Freeman, S. M., Ramesh, R., Munshi, A., Abboud, C. N., and Marrogi, A. J. (1995) Enhanced tumor recognition and killing using the HSV-tK suicide gene. *Cancer Gene Ther.* **2,** 240–241.

22. Ramesh, R., Marrogi, A. J., Munshi, A., Abboud, C. N., and Freeman, S. M. (1996) In-vivo analysis of the "Bystander effect": a cytokine cascade. *Exp. Hematol.* **24,** 829–838.

23. Gagandeep, S., Brew, R., Green, B., Christmas, S. E., Klatzman, D., Poston, G. J., and Kinsella, A. R. (1996) Prodrug activated gene therapy. Involvement of an immunological component in the bystander effect. *Cancer Gene Ther.* **3,** 83–88.

24. Boring, C. C., Squires, T. S., and Tong, T. (1993) Cancer statistics, 1993. *CA Cancer J. Clin.* **43,** 7–26.

25. Cornetta, K. and Anderson, W. F. (xxxx) Protamine sulfate as an effective alternative to polybrene in retroviral-mediated gene-transfer: implications for human gene therapy. *J. Virol.* **23,** 187–194.

26. Aaronson, S. A., Bassin, R. H., and Weaver, C. (1972) Comparison of the murine sarcoma viruses in non-producer and S+/L– transformed cells. *J. Virol.* **9,** 701–704.

31

Gene Therapy for Treatment of Brain Tumors (*HSV-tK* In Vivo Gene Transfer)

A Case Study

Friedrich Weber, Frank Floeth, and Hans Bojar

1. Introduction

Despite a high effort in the research of malignant brain tumors, the clinical results in treatment of malignant brain tumors are still very poor. Brain tumors are a major cause of morbidity and mortality in the population. New primary brain tumors develop in 2–4 of 100,000 adults each year (*1*). Recent evidence indicates that the prevalence of primary brain tumors is increasing, especially in the elderly (*2*). The astroglial brain tumors, including the highly malignant glioblastoma multiforme (GBM), are the most common primary brain tumors. For these tumors, the first line of treatment is surgery and almost always radiotherapy as an adjuvant. A variety of patient-management strategies are currently used for GBM, from supportive care to aggressive multimodality approaches. The principal reason for this wide spectrum of approaches is that, despite aggressive therapy, which includes surgical removal of the tumor, postoperative high-dose radiation (60 gy), chemotherapy, and other adjuvant treatments, the prognosis of patients with GBM is very poor (*3–6*). In a series of NCOG protocols on glioblastoma multiforme patients with Karnofsky performance scores of 60 or higher, who were treated with postsurgical radiation therapy and adjuvant chemotherapy with nitrosourea-based drug combinations, the median survival and time of tumor progression were consistently above 50 and 34 wk, respectively (*7–9*). The nitrosoureas (BCNU and CCNU), alone and in combination, are the most active cytotoxic drugs for recurrent and progressive tumors, although most of these responses are transient and in patients

From: *Methods in Molecular Medicine, Vol. 35: Gene Therapy: Methods and Protocols*
Edited by: W. Walther and U. Stein © Humana Press, Inc., Totowa, NJ

with well-differentiated gliomas. When glioblastoma multiforme recurs, which happens in nearly 100% of all cases, however, the median survival from the start of treatment is about 6 mo, with only 22% of patients surviving longer than 1 yr *(11)*. Therefore, there is a great interest in local treatment modalities. A wafer impregnated with carmustine, for use as an implant after surgical removal of recurrent GBM showed a prolongation in the median survival time of only 2 mo, from 20 to 28 wk in a study with a total of 222 patients. In another study, a median survival of 9 mo was found in a selected group of patients with recurrent GBM who underwent a second operation, but a reasonable quality of life in those patients was limited to 10 wk *(12)*.

Advances in molecular biology and immunology have induced the development of modern immuno- and genetherapeutical strategies. Within different gene therapy strategies is the suicide gene therapy using the herpes simplex thymidine kinase gene. The enzyme thymidine kinase (*tk*) from herpes simplex virus (HSV) are normally not present in human cells,

The *HSV-tK* gene not normally present in human cells, sensitizes transduced cells to ganciclovir (GCV) by adding phosphate to the drug molecule, which is then transformed into GCV triphosphate, which is mistaken by DNA polymerase for deoxyguanosine triphosphate, thus causing chain termination leading to cell destruction. The *HSV-tK* enzyme phosphorylates GCV to a monophosphate form and further phosphorylation by cellular kinases leads to GCV triphosphate compounds that are potent inhibitors of DNA synthesis *(13–15)*. Retroviral vectors encoding the *HSV-tK* suicide gene can be delivered to tumors either by direct injection of viral particles *(16)* or by implantation into the target tissue of cells that continuously produce the virus *(17)*. In this project, living mouse-derived cells that produce large amounts of retroviral vectors carrying the *HSV-tK* gene are injected into brain tumors. New vectors are continuously produced in the tumor for as long as the producer cells survive, therefore, more transduction of tumor cells is expected than with the injection of retroviral vectors alone. For retroviral-mediated in vivo gene transfer, the central nervous system has several advantages of safety and efficacy. Retroviral vectors integrate and, therefore, express vector genes only in proliferating cells. In the brain, the cancer is the most mitotically active tissue and includes the malignant cells and tumor-associated blood vessels, while macrophage-derived cells, blood cells, and endothelial cells have minimal mitotic activity and healthy brain tissue has none. In addition, the brain is a partially immunologically privileged site, which should allow xenogeneic vector-producer cells to survive longer than in other sites and to transduce a very large population of the dividing tumor cells. This immunological "privilege" is further increased because human gliomas are known to depress local immunity

(18). The period of survival of these cells remains however limited—recognized as xenogeneic, they are eliminated by the immune system, alternatively they would be destroyed by GCV treatment.

2. Materials
2.1. The Retroviral Vector and the Vector-Producing Cell Line

GLI 328 is a retroviral vector-producer cell line containing the *herpes simplex* virus type 1 thymidine kinase gene (*HSV-tK*) and the bacterial neomycin resistance gene (*neo'* from Stratagene, La Jolla, CA) in GTI's patented G1 vector backbone. The *HSV-tK* gene is transcribed from the viral Long Terminal Repeat (LTR), the *neo'* gene, encoding for the enzyme neomycin phosphotransferase is transcribed from an internal SV40 (simian virus 40) early promoter (LTR-*HSV-tK*-SV40–*neo'*-LTR). The *HSV-tK* gene confers sensitivity to the nucleotide analog GCV whereas the *neo'* gene product serves as a marker gene and confers resistance to the neomycin analog G418. In these retroviral vector-producer cells, the structural genes of the retrovirus were introduced using the plasmid pPAM3. pPAM3 is a derivative of the Moloney murine leukemia virus (MoMLV) and contains the *gag* gene from MoMLV and a hybrid pol gene from MoMLV and 4070A. The envelope gene in pPAM3 is a hybrid: 82% from the murine amphotrophic 4070A retrovirus, 18% from an ecotrophic laboratory virus, AM-MLV. To provide the structural proteins without generating wild-type retrovirus, further changes were made in the structure of pPAM3, so that two recombination events are required to regenerate a wild-type virus. In addition to deleting the packaging signal, the 3' LTR from MoMLV was replaced with the SV40 polyadenylation signal and part of the 5' LTR was removed. There is also a mutation in the start codon for the *gag* gene. A producer cell line is made from vector plasmid and packaging cells; GLI 328 is a eukaryotic producer cell line and contains the vector plasmid pG1Tk1SvNa stably integrated into PA317 packaging cells. The plasmid DNA was extracted from a culture of transformed *Escherichia coli* DH5-a. The vector plasmid DNA was transfected into an ecotropic packaging cell. Supernatant from the PE501 transfected cells was then used to transduce the 3T3 fibroblast-derived amphotropic packaging cell line PA317. Clones of the transduced producer cells were then grown in G418 medium to select clones that contain the *neo'* gene. The clones were then tested for resistance to G418.

It has been discovered that a low percentage of the GLI 328 VPCs contain a spliced form of the G1Tk1SvNa provirus. Semiquantitative (polymerase chain reaction) PCR assays performed using primers that specifically amplify the spliced form have established that the percentage of producer cells exhibiting the spliced form is about 1.9%. This level of splice is well below the detection limit of a Southern blot analysis. DNA sequencing shows the spliced form to be a 227 bp sequence bordered by consensus splice donor and acceptor sequences that is deleted from the *HSV-tK* gene. Any truncated protein derived from this spliced *HSV-tK* gene could not phosphorylate GCV.

3. Methods

3.1. Ethics and Good Clinical Practice

Clinical studies have to be performed under standard operating procedures that correspond to GCP conditions. Within Europe, the Rules Governing Medicinal Products in the European Community (directive 91/507/EEC.) and additionally, the U.S. Code of Federal Regulations dealing with clinical studies have to be considered.

3.2. Study Synopsis

Patients suffering from a recurrence of a GBM or showing clinical and radiological evidence of a recurrence of a previously operated malignant glioma, were chosen as a target population (*see* **Notes**).

Primary and secondary study objectives were defined. First, the safety of intracerebral administration of GLI328 followed by GCV treatment should be investigated. Second, evidence of any antitumor efficacy should be assessed by survival as well as time to progression.

3.3. Overall Study Design

This was an open, single group, multicenter, prospective study investigating in a pilot manner the value of *HSV-tK/GCV* gene therapy as an adjuvant to the surgical resection of recurrent glioblastoma in adult patients. The target population was patients with recurrence of a previously resected GBM or a presumption of GBM according to the clinical and radiological characteristics after prior resection of a malignant glioma. In addition, patients were required to meet the selection criteria (*see* **Notes**).

3.4. Shipment of the PA317/G1Tk1SvNa.7 Producer Cells to the Clinical Sites and Handling of the Frozen Material

Dry ice shipments are sent with indicators to monitor the temperature of the container during shipment. If the indicators show that the correct temperature was not maintained during shipment, the product must be destroyed. Upon receipt in the clinical site, the cell bags/cassettes have to be quickly transferred from the shipper to a liquid nitrogen vapor freezer.

3.5. Preparation of PA317/G1Tk1SvNa.7 Producer Cells for Administration to Patients

The product from the freezer bag is processed in a 3-bag wash system (Baxter Healthcare Corporation, Muskegon, MI, Fenwal Division, FTX-1058). Working in a certified laminar flow biological safety cabinet (LFBSC), one spike of the 3-bag wash set is inserted into the spike port of a Ringer's Lactate (RL) bag. After opening the appropriate clamps, 150 mL of RL by weight is transferred into one of the bags of the 3-bag wash system. All clamps are closed and the tubing of the spike port is heat-sealed using a hand-held tube sealer (SEBRA® Model 2380). The tubing is then cut off, leaving the spike in the RL bag.

If it is verified by the surgeon that the patient is ready for surgery, a preselected product lot bag/cassette is retrieved from the liquid nitrogen storage tank. If it has to be transported to the laboratory it has to be placed under dry ice in an insulated box. The bag is removed from the cassette and rapidly thawed by immersing in a $37 \pm 1°C$ water bath (calibrated, filled with sterile water, without additives) to above the frozen content level. Thawing takes approx 2 min. During this step semifrozen material must not be massaged to avoid cell damage. The bag must be kept immersed until the cells are completely thawed. Once the cells are thawed, they must be administered within 4 h. As soon as the bag is thawed it is removed from the water bath and has to be sprayed with 70–85% ethanol prior to transfer to the LFBSC. After gently mixing of the thawed cell bag, the product is processed in a 3-bag wash system. Using a spike port of the 3-bag wash set, the entire cell suspension of the product lot bag is transferred into one of the empty bags, making sure that no cells remain in the tubing. After closure of all clamps on the wash set, the tubing is heat-sealed just below the Y and the empty product lot bag is discarded. The clamps of the cell bag and the RL bag are then opened and 40 mL of RL by weight are transferred to the cell bag over 45 s while mixing. All clamps are closed. The cells are pelleted by placing the 3-bag wash set into a precooled centrifuge (Beckman J-6B, rotor JS 4.2, Fullerton, CA) and spinning at 1100 rpm for 5 min at $4 \pm 2°C$. The wash supernatant is then expressed from the cell bag into the waste bag of the 3-bag system by use of a plasma extractor (Baxter Healthcare Corporation, Fenwal Division), taking care that no cells go into the waste bag. After closure of the clamps of the cell bag and waste bag, the pelleted cells are resuspended by gently massaging the cell bag. The clamps of the cell bag and RL bag are then opened and 40–50 mL of RL are transferred to the cell bag by weight. After closure of all clamps, the cells are mixed by massaging and the described steps are repeated for a second and third wash. After the final waste expression using the plasma extractor, cells are left in approx

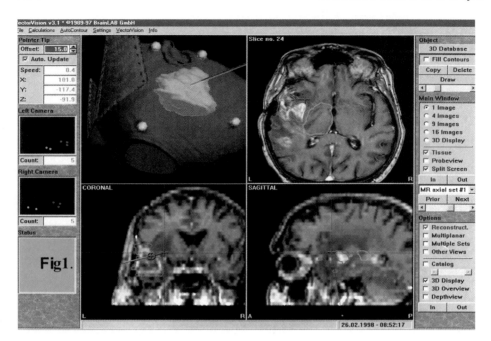

Fig. 1. Resection area and installation area was carefully planned using three-dimensional reconstructions of CT/MRI scans.This procedure provides the surgeon with more safety during the surgical procedure. The VPC can be administered with higher accuracy.

10 mL. After closure of the clamp on the cell bag, the cells are resuspended by massaging. After appropriate heat-sealing, the cell bag is cut off from the 3-bag wash set. Working in the LFBSC, a sampling site coupler is inserted into the cell bag. The total volume of washed cell suspension is determined by weighing. An aliquot of the cell suspension is removed for cell counts. The cell bag has to be kept on ice while counting cells. For cell count, 0.1 mL of cell suspension is added to 49.9 mL of diluted Trypan blue (0.4%, Sigma, St. Louis, MO). Using brightfield optics, viable and nonviable cells are counted in a hemacytometer (Neubauer improved). The cells should appear spherical with neither swelling nor shrinkage.

If the requirements for yield ($\geq 0.9 \times 10^9$ cells in a total volume of about 9 mL) and viability ($\geq 75\%$) are met, the cell bag is placed into an isolated ice container for transport to the operating room.

3.6. Experimental Treatment

The therapy was initiated by a gross total resection (**Fig. 1**), whereby the opening of the ventricles should be avoided. After resection, the cavity wall

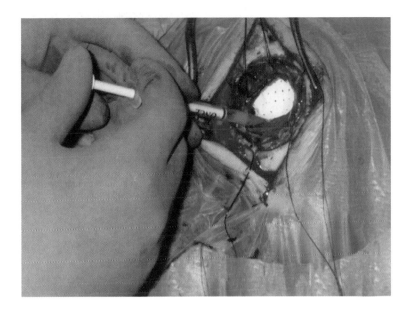

Fig. 2. Procedure of application of VPC after tumor debulking into the tissue adjacent to the recection border.

was infiltrated by 50 single injections (**Fig. 2**) in a depth of 1.5 cm (*see* **Notes**). The injections were homogenously distributed over the whole surface. The tumor tissue was histopathological examined during the surgical procedure. Only when the assumed diagnosis was histologically verified, the administration of the vector producer cells was performed. Preoperatively, the tumor was neuroradiologally evaluated by MRI scan. In order to get a good discrimination between residual tumor and unspecific contrast enhancing owing to breakdown of the blood-brain barrier, the first postoperative control was performed within 24 h. GCV treatment was started 14 d after surgery over a period of 14 d (5 mg/kg twice a day):

DAYS

0 1 2 3 4 5 6 7 8 9 10 11 12 13 14 15 16 17 18 19 20 21 22 23 24 25 26 27 28 29 30 31 32 33 34 35 36

↑   ↑ ↑ ↑ ↑ ↑ ↑ ↑ ↑ ↑ ↑ ↑ ↑ ↑ ↑   ↑

Application   Ganciclovir   End of cycle

of vector producer

cells (VPC)

Tumoral tissue taken at surgery underwent central histopathological examination. Ganciclovir, was given twice daily as an iv perfusion between days 14–27. MRI scans were carried out immediately before surgery within 48 h after resection, on day 35, every second month until month 12, and thereafter every 3 mo. Clinical and routine blood examinations were repeated at weekly intervals until day 35, at month 2, every 2 mo until month 12, and thereafter every 3 mo. Blood samples for biosafety monitoring were taken at baseline, day 14 (for the first 10 patients only), day 35, every 2 mo until month 12, and then annually for life. Brain tissue samples were to be obtained at subsequent resection or at autopsy and CSF and other tissue samples whenever possible. The biosafety testing was aimed at detecting the presence of transduced normal cells, the presence of recombination events leading to the formation of replication competent retrovirus, as well as the presence of antibodies to either the vector-producer cell or the retroviral vector core protein. The samples were frozen immediately after being obtained, shipped and stored in liquid nitrogen. A central neuroradiologist reviewed the MR scans of all patients in a sequential manner.

3.7. Posttreatment

Patients were to be seen as out-patients at months 2, 4, 6, 8, 10, and 12 after the cell injection, then every 3 mo for the second year, and then at least annually until they terminated the study or died. Each of these evaluations was to include the following evaluations, unless stated otherwise.

1. Complete physical examination.
2. Karnofsky assessment.
3. MRI or CT scan of the brain.
4. Laboratory assays: hematology, chemistry, urinalysis.
5. Collection of samples for biosafety monitoring: whole blood (uncoagulated for the isolation of PBLs at the central laboratory), frozen serum, and autopsy samples where possible.
6. Annual visits after 24 mo of follow-up to include collection of biosafety samples for study specific evaluations.
7. If, at any time, the patient underwent reresection of the tumor, tissue was to be obtained for biosafety analysis.

3.8. Efficacy Variables

Survival time was estimated by measuring the time interval from surgery and administration of GLI 328 to death. The response of the tumor was to be based on the quantification of the tumor-enhancement volume observed on either MRI or CT scans. Response was to be estimated according to the following criteria: complete response (disappearance of all detectable malignant disease); partial response (>50% decrease in volume); minor response (25–49% decrease in volume); stable disease (<25% decrease 8 <25% increase in volume); locally progressive disease (>50% increase in volume or development of new lesion locally); and nonlocally progressive disease (development of a new tumor or >50% increase in volume of a tumor which is noncontiguous with the treated tumor).

Quality of survival was estimated by monitoring the Karnofsky performance score (KPS). This was defined as the time since surgery and GLI 328 injection until the sustained fall in the KPS to below 40. The same analysis was done for a KPS threshold of 60.

3.9. Biosafety Monitoring

3.9.1. Detection of Vector in Peripheral Blood Leucocytes (PBL) by PCR

1. PBL DNA was tested for vector-specific proviral sequences using a PCR assay with primers specific to the *NeoR* gene or *HSV-tK* gene.
   a. The assay sensitivity was validated to detect one copy per 500,000 cells. At a set detection limit of 10 copies, the assay was capable of detecting 10 or more copies of proviral vector DNA with a confidence of 99.99%.
   b. To distinguish between transduced lymphocytes and VPCs, all positive results were tested for the presence of *env* helper sequences, which are only present in VPCs.
2. Detection of replication-competent retrovirus (RCR) DNA sequences by PCR: PBL DNA was tested for the presence of RCR-specific proviral sequences using a PCR assay with primers selected to detect recombinant RCR, but not vector proviral DNA or producer-cell DNA.
   a. The assay sensitivity was validated to dectect one copy per 500,000 cells. At a set detection limit of 10 copies, the assay was capable of detecting 10 or more copies of proviral vector DNA with a confidence of 99.99%.
3. Cocultivation for detection of RCR. Peripheral blood mononuclear cells (PBMC) were cocultured with *Mus dunni*, a murine cell line permissive for a range of viruses. If PBMCs produced RCR, the *Mus dunni* cells would become infected from RCR virions shed from the patients' PBMCs leading to cell death that could be observed in culture.
   a. The assay sensitivity was validated to detect 50 RCR positive cells per 10,000,000.

4. Notes

1. Before starting therapy, the patients were carefully evaluted regarding tumor localization and extension. If the lesion involved both hemispheres, the corpus callosum, the brainstem, or was in close approximity of the ventricular system, the patient was excluded from the study.

2. If the ventricular system was opened during surgery, no vector-producing cells were administered because of the occurrence of some neurotoxic events when VPC had been administered intrathecally. With respect to feasibility, multiple injections of small volumes of VPC suspension into the resection cavity wall were technically complicated by the need to ensure that the injection tracks were evenly distributed and as perpendicular as possible to the cavity wall. Inevitably, with the irregular nature of the cavity some overlapping of the tracks occurred whereas other zones were nearly inaccessible. Although the aim was to inject the maximum volume, injection varied depending on the size of the cavity.

3. The greatest problem, however, was that of reflux, which was extremely variable. The declared injected volume is likely to be an overestimate of the actual amount retained in the brain tissue because of the reflux of suspension up and out of the injection track in many cases.

4. Additionally, the penetration of VPCs beyond the injection site is limited to several mm and presents a major problem regarding in vivo transduction efficacy. As primary safety concerns treatment-related CNS events, brain lesions or hemorrhage because of mechanical stresses of multiple injections of VPCs have to be considered. Inflammatory reactions resulting from the application of xenogenic cells have not occured.

References

1. Radhakrishan, K., Bohnen, N. I., and Kurland, L. T. (1994) Epidemiology of brain tumors, in *Brain Tumors, A Comprehensive Text* (Morantz, R. A. and Walsh, J. W., eds.), New York, pp. 1–18.
2. Salcman, M. (1990) Epidemiology and factors affecting survival, in *Malignant Cerebral Glioma* (Apuzzo, M. L. J., ed.), Am. Assoc. Neurolog. Surg. Park Ridge, IL, pp. xx.
3. Werner, M. H., Phuphanich, S., and Lyman, G. H. (1995) The increasing incidence of malignant gliomas and primary central nervous system lymphoma in the elderly. *Cancer* **76** 1634–1642.
4. Black, P. (1991) Brain tumors. *N. Engl. J. Med.* **324,** 1471–1476.
5. Bauman, G. S., Gaspar, L. E., Fisher, B. J., et al. (1994) A prospective study of short-course radiotherapy in poor prognosis glioblastoma multiforme. *Int. J. Radiat. Oncol. Biol. Phy.* **29,** 835–839.
6. Färkkilä, M., Jääskeläinen, J., Kallio, M., et al. (1994) Randomised, controlled study of intratumoral recombinant y-interferon treatment in newly diagnosed glioblastoma. *Br. J. Cancer* **70,** 138–141.
7. Hildebrand, J., Sahmoud, T., Mignolet, F., et al. EORTC Brain Tumor Group. (1994) Adjuvent therapy with dibromodulcitol and BCNU increases survival of adults with malignant gliomas. *Neurology* **44,** 1479–1483.
8. Levin, V. A., Silver, P., Hannigan, J., et al. (1990) Superiority of post-radiotherapy adjuvant chemotherapy with CCNU, procarbazine, and vincristine (PCV) over BCNU for anaplastic gliomas: NCOG 6G61 Final Report. *Int. J. Radiat. Oncol. Biol. Phys.* **18,** 321–324.

9. Levin, V. A., Wara, W. M., Davis, R. L., et al. (1986) NCOG protocol 6G91: Response to treatment with radiation therapy and seven-drug chemotherapy in patients with glioblastoma multiforme. *Cancer Treat. Rep.* **70,** 739–743.

10. Phillips, T. L., Levin, V. A., Ahn, D. K., et al. (1991) Evaluation of bromodeoxyuridine in glioblastoma multiforme: a Northern California Cancer Center phase II study. *Int. J. Radiat. Oncol. Biol. Phys.* **21,** 709–714.

11. Ammirati, M., Galicich, J. H., and Arbit, E., et al. (1987) Reoperation in the treatment of recurrent intracranial malignant gliomas. *Neurosurgery* **21,** 607–614.

12. Rajan, B., Ross, G., Lim, C. C., et al. (1994) Survival in patients with recurrent glioma as a measure of treatment efficacy: prognostic factors following nitrosourea chemotherapy. *Eur. J. Cancer* **30A,** 1809–1815.

13. Moolten, F. L. (1986) Tumor chemosensitivity conferred by inserted herpes thymidine kinase genes: paradigm for a prospective cancer control strategy. *Cancer Res.* **46,** 5276–5281.

14. Plautz, G., Nabel, E. G., and Nabel, G. J. (1991) Selective elimination of recombinant genes in vivo with a suicide retroviral vector. *New Biologist* **3,** 709–715.

15. Borrelli, E, Heyman, R., Hsi, M., et al. (1988) Targeting of an inducible toxic phenotype in animal cells. *Proc. Natl. Acad. Sci. USA* **85,** 7572–7576.

16. Ezzedine, Z. D., Martuza, R. L., Platika, D., et al. (1991) Selective kitling of glioma cells in culture and in vivo by retrovirus transfer of the herpes simplex thymidine kinase gene. *New Biologist* **3,** 608–614.

17. Moolten, F. L. and Wells, J. M. (1990) Curability of tumors bearing herpes thymidine kinase genes transferred by retroviral vectors. *J. Natl. Cancer Inst.* **B2,** 297–300.

18. Gilboa, E., Eglitis, M. A., Kantoff, P. W., et al. (1986) Transfer and expression of cloned genes using retrpyjpg vectors. *BioTechniques* **4,** 504–512.

32

Gene Therapy of Glioblastoma Multiforme with a Bicistronic Retroviral Vector Expressing Human IL-2 and *HSV-tK*

Giorgio Palù, Massimo Pizzato, Roberta Bonaguro, and Federico Colombo

1. Introduction

Gene therapy of cancer includes strategies for augmentation of immuno-therapeutic and chemoterapeutic approaches. These strategies mainly involve ex vivo and in vivo cytokine gene transfer, drug sensitization with genes for prodrug delivery, and the use of drug-resistance genes for protecting bone marrow from high-dose chemotherapy *(1)*. Vector development remains the primary focus for any future research in the field. Retroviral vectors, especially those derived from Moloney murine leukemia virus (MoMLV), remain among the most widely utilized vectors in gene therapy trials.

Their efficiency relies upon the unique biological feature of retroviruses, i.e., the stable integration of the viral genome, generally at a low copy number, into the host chromosomes. This property guarantees that the transferred genes become constitutively acquired as new genetic elements in the transduced cells as well as in their progeny.

Retroviral vectors are engineered to be replication-defective by replacing part of the genome, the *gag-pol-env* genes, with the desired therapeutic genes. Infectious particles can still be generated in a single cycle of replication, if the deleted functions are provided *in trans*. This is normally achieved by introducing the defective virus (retroviral vector) into packaging cell lines containing a helper virus genome.

From: *Methods in Molecular Medicine, Vol. 35: Gene Therapy: Methods and Protocols*
Edited by: W. Walther and U. Stein © Humana Press, Inc., Totowa, NJ

Genetic integration, at least for some members of the Oncornavirinae, the prototype being represented by MoMLV, requires an active state of cell proliferation *(2)*. This aspect is a limitation for purposes of genetic transfer into resting cells, but turns into a clear advantage when a selective expression is to be achieved in actively proliferating neoplastic cells.

The main obstacles to the practical use of retroviral vectors in some clinical trials are represented by the limited size of genetic sequences that can be accommodated in their backbone, and by the almost exclusive ex vivo employment. When a combined therapeutic approach is conceived for gene therapy of cancer, the simultaneous expression of more than one antitumor gene, possibly with a synergistic effect, should ideally be achieved by the same vector *(3)*. Additionally, a gene for positive selection needs to be present in the vector. This basic design can saturate the vector expression capacity, which depends on the foreign genes complexity and promoter utilization.

The present session reports on the design and functional assay of a novel bicistronic, triple gene MoMLV-based vector (pLIL-2TKSN). Human interleukin 2 (IL-2) and herpesvirus thymidine kinase (TK) are produced from a long transcript driven by the 5' LTR, through a cap-dependent and an internal ribosome entry site (IRES)-regulated translation, respectively. The selectable marker, neomycin phosphotransferase, is expressed from a shorter transcript under control of an internal SV40 promoter *(4–6)*. This construct has the potential for allowing combination of cytokine and suicide gene therapy to be employed in areas, such as the brain, where normal cells are in a post-mitotic state, and thus refractory to transduction by retroviral vectors *(7–17)*.

The methods described will deal with vector construction, production from packaging lines, identification of clones yielding higher viral titer, cell cultures and recombinant retrovirus infections, helper-virus detection, efficiency of transgene expression, and functional assays.

A pilot study has been conducted in vivo. pLIL-2TKSN vector was used to treat four patients affected by recurrent glioblastoma multiforme (GBM), with evidence of disease progression after craniotomy removal plus fractionated radiotherapy *(18)*. These patients underwent stereotactic implantation of vector-producing cells (RVPC) into the tumor masses. Stereotactic GBM biopsies were taken at the time of RVPC implantation and before ganciclovir (GCV) administration (10–14 d after RVPC implantation) to evaluate presence and extent of tumor transduction, along with transcriptional activity of the vector and host reaction to the treatment. Clinical data, reported in **Table 1**, have shown that gene therapy of GBM, combining effects of TK/GCV with those mediated by IL-2, is safe and able to produce a significant reduction of the tumor mass or tumor necrosis around injection site. Antitumor activity may result both from metabolic suicide of malignant and endothelial cells, and from

Table 1
Brain Stereotactic Gene Therapy of GBM Patients: Main Clinical Features

Patient (age)	Previous treatment	Recurrence (volume)	KPS (*)	Inoculated RVPC n. × 10⁸ (vol.)	Number of targets	Pre-GCV biopsy	Clinical follow-up	Imaging follow-up
1. male (22)	MR FRT Stereotactic Curietherapy (^{125}I)	150 mL	70	1.5 (6 mL)	4	NT	5 mo survival	Tumor necrosis around injection site (2 mL/site)
2. male (50)	MR FRT MR	180 mL	75	2 (3 mL) 2.5 (3 mL)	3	T	12 mo survival	Tumor necrosis around injection site (2 mL/site)
3. female (58)	MR FRT	80 mL	90	2 (2 mL)	4	T	Clinical improvement 11 mo surviving	Decreased tumor volume (40 mL)
4. female (50)	MR FRT Chemotherapy Radioimmuno-Therapy	60 mL	70	3 (3 mL)	1	NT	Still surviving at 10 months	Stabilized

MR, microsurgical removal; FRT, fractionated radiotherapy. * KPS, Karnofsky score (*see* (**21**)); T, taken; NT, not taken an immune-inflammatory rejection. Bystander effects elicited by TK and IL-2 can explain tumor regression, notwithstanding the low transduction efficiency *(18)*. These findings give a new perspective on the genetic treatment of malignant brain tumors that exploits the immune system.

2. Materials

2.1. Materials for Method 1

1. Plasmids. pLIL-2 and pLIL-2TKSN were derived from the Moloney prototype vector LXSN, containing the selectable marker gene *neo* (neomycin phosphotransferase) driven by the simian virus 40 (SV40) early promoter. The 1.7-kb DNA containing the IRES-TK cassette was derived from pSXLC-TK (kindly provided by Pastan, I.) *(6)*.
2. Restriction enzymes, buffers, and reagents (New England Biolabs, Boehringer Mannheim) were employed following the manufacturer's protocol.
3. *Escherichia coli* cc118 for plasmid DNA large-scale preparations. Purification of plasmid DNA by equilibrium centrifugation in CsCl-ethidium bromide gradients.

2.2. Materials for Method 2

1. Helper cell lines. Amphotropic packaging cells PA317(ATCC CRL-9078) have been used, but other more recent packaging cells could be utilized as well. Before use, all cell lines should be tested for mycoplasma infection, a condition which would otherwise compromise all the experimental setting.
2. Culture media. Dulbecco's modified Eagle's medium (DMEM), supplemented with 10% (v/v) fetal calf serum (FCS), penicillin (P, 100 U/mL) and streptomycin (S, 100 µg/mL) (growth medium). Antibiotic for selection of transductants: G418 800 µg/mL in culture medium (selection medium). All antibiotics are resuspended in water at the desired concentration, filter-sterilized (0.22-µm filters, Millipore, Bedford, MA) and stored in aliquots at –20°C.
3. NIH3T3 murine fibroblast cell line (ATCC CRL-1658), A172 human glioblastoma cell line (ATCC CRL-1620), and AoU373 human astrocytoma cell line (ATCC HTB 17).
4. Calcium Phosphate Transfection System (Life Technologies, Gaithersburg, MD).
5. Polybrene (8 µg/mL) (Sigma, St. Louis, MO) in water, filter-sterilized (0.22-µm filters, Millipore), stored at –20°C.
6. Staining solution for CFU (colony forming units): 2% methylene blue, 50% ethanol.
7. 0.45-µm filters (Costar, Cambridge, MA), 10 cm diameter Petri dishes (Costar), 96-well tissue-culture plates (flat-bottom wells) (Costar).

2.3. Materials for Method 3

1. NIH3T3-LacZ, a cell line harboring a LacZ-containing retroviral vector (MFGnlsLacZ) (kindly provided by Y. Takeuchi).

2. DMEM + 10% FCS + P/S culture medium (growth medium).
3. Polybrene (8 µg/mL) (Sigma) in water, filter-sterilized.
4. Phosphate-buffered saline (PBS): 120 m*M* NaCl, 25 m*M* Na-phosphate, pH 7.3.
5. X-gal (5-bromo-4-chloro-3-indolyl-β-D-galactopyranoside) Staining Reagent: a) staining solution: 0.01% (w/v) sodium deoxycholic acid sodium salt, 0.02% NP40, 2 m*M* MgCl$_2$ (Sigma), 5 m*M* potassium ferricyanide (Sigma), 5 m*M* potassium ferrocyanide (Sigma), in PBS; b) X-gal 1 mg/mL (Sigma). The staining solution is light-sensitive, stable at room temperature. X-gal aliquots [40 mg/mL in DMSO (dimethylsulfoxid)] are stored at –20°C; X-gal is added to the staining solution just before use.
6. Six-well tissue culture plates (flat-bottom wells) (Costar).

2.4. Materials for Method 4

1. RNAzol™ B Kit reagents (Tel-Test, Inc., Friendswood, TX), chloroform, isopropanol and 70% ethanol. RNAzol is light-sensitive; stable at 4°C up to 9 mo; contains irritant (guanidinium thiocyanate) and poison (phenol).
2. Bovine pancreatic DNAse 10 U/µL (Boehringer Mannheim, Mannheim, Germany).
3. Sterile water containing 0.1% diethylpyrocarbonate (DEPC).
4. Reverse PCR. MuLV reverse transcriptase 50 U/µL (Perkin-Elmer, Norwalk, CT), RNase inhibitor 20 U/µL (Perkin-Elmer), 10X PCR buffer (Perkin-Elmer), 25 m*M* MgCl$_2$ (Perkin-Elmer), 10 m*M* dNTPs (Perkin-Elmer), 15 µ*M* reverse primer.
5. PCR. AmpliTaq DNA polymerase 5 U/µL (Perkin-Elmer), 10X PCR buffer (Perkin-Elmer), 25 m*M* MgCl$_2$ (Perkin-Elmer), 10 m*M* dNTPs (Perkin-Elmer), 15 µM sense and antisense primers.
6. Primers for IL-2: forward primer 5'GTA CAG GAT GCA ACT CCT GTC TTG 3'; reverse primer 5'AGA GGA CGA TAG AAG GCG ATG 3'.
7. Primers for TK: forward primer 5'CTG CGG GTT TAT ATA GAC GG 3'; reverse primer 5'CAT TGT TAT CTG GGC GCT 3'.
8. Agarose (Seakem LE, FMC), 1X Tris-borate/EDTA electrophoresis buffer, ethidium bromide (stock solution 10 mg/mL; stored at room temperature, in dark bottle).

2.5. Method 5

1. CTLL mouse cell line culture (kindly provided by Dr. K. Smith); murine tumor-specific cytotoxic T lymphocytes.
2. RPMI-1640 medium.
3. RPMI-1640 medium containing 10% FCS.
4. Trypan-blue solution 0.4% (w/v) (Sigma).
5. Human recombinant IL-2 (Eurocetus, Amsterdam, The Netherlands).
6. ^{3}H-thymidine (S.A. 25 Ci/mMol) (Amersham, Arlington Heights, IL).
7. 96-well microtitre plates (Costar).

8. Filter mats (GF/C filters, Whatman, Clifton, NJ).
9. Liquid scintillation counter system.

2.6. Method 6

1. Ganciclovir (Sigma) diluted in sterile water.
2. Cell proliferation Kit (MTT) (Boehringer Mannheim); light sensitive; stable at –20°C. After thawing, the MTT labeling reagents may be stored at +4°C for up to 4 wk, protected from light.
3. 96-well tissue-culture plates (flat-bottom wells) (Costar).

3. Methods

3.1. Method 1: Plasmid Construction

1. The Moloney prototype vector LXSN was used to construct pLIL-2SN (3.2 kb), as described by Melani, C., et al. *(19)*. pLIL-2TKSN vector (4.9 kb) was derived from pLIL-2SN using standard recombinant DNA techniques *(20)*. The 1.7-kb DNA fragment containing IRES-TK was derived from pSXLC-TK following digestion with *Bam*HI and *Xho*I restriction enzymes. IRES-TK cassette was then inserted into the *Bam*HI site of pLIL-2SN by blunt-end ligation with T4 DNA ligase after fill-in of DNA ends using Klenow polymerase (**Fig. 1**).
2. The correct insertion was confirmed by restriction endonuclease mapping and sequencing on the resulting 8.1-kb plasmid pLIL-2TKSN.

3.2. Method 2: Cell Culture and Recombinant Retrovirus Infections

3.2.1. Generation of Producer Cells

1. Grow and maintain PA 317 amphotropic packaging cell line in DMEM + 10% FCS + P/S at 37°C in a humidified, 5% CO_2 incubator (*see* **Note 1**).
2. 24 h prior to transfection, remove the medium, rinse cells with PBS. Trypsinize and count cells. Plate 1×10^6 cells on 10-cm Petri dishes in a final volume of 10 mL DMEM + 10% FCS + P/S.
3. Four h prior to transfection, replace the culture medium with 8 mL fresh medium.
4. Day 1. Resuspend 20 µg retroviral vector DNA in sterile water to be used for transfection. Transfect cells with Calcium Phosphate Transfection System (Life Technologies) reagents, following the manufacturer's protocol.
5. Day 2. Aspirate medium and replace with 10 mL fresh medium. Incubate for two more days.
6. Selection for stable lines. On day 4, aspirate medium and replace with fresh medium supplemented with G418 at 800 µg/mL final concentration (selection medium).
7. Incubate under standard conditions, feeding with fresh selective medium every 2–3 d until resistant colonies appear (generally after 2 wk).

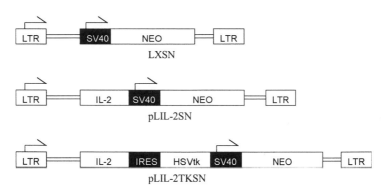

Fig. 1. Schematic representation of LXSN, pLIL-2SN, and pLIL-2TKSN vectors. The Moloney prototype vector LXSN was used to construct pLIL-2SN, as previously described *(19)*. pLIL-2TKSN was derived from pLIL-2SN using standard recombinant DNA techniques *(20)*. The DNA fragment containing IRES-TK cassette was derived from pSXLC-TK, kindly provided by I. Pastan *(6)*, following digestion with *Bam*HI and *Xho*I restriction enzymes. IRES-TK cassette was then inserted into the *Bam*HI site of pLIL-2SN by blunt-end litigation with T4 DNA polymerase, after fill-in of DNA ends using Klenow polymerase.

3.2.2. Isolation of Single Cell-Derived Clones

1. Trypsinize the resistant colonies and seed the obtained cells at limiting dilution in 96-well tissue-culture plates (flat bottom) in 100 µl selection medium.
2. Incubate until cells at the final dilution reach confluence.
3. Trypsinize each single cell-derived clone and seed in 25-cm^2 flasks in 10 mL selection medium.
4. Incubate until a confluent monolayer forms.

3.2.3. Determination of Viral Titer

1. Grow NIH3T3 cells in growth medium in 25-cm^2 flasks, until confluence is reached.
2. Trypsinize and count cells. Seed 6×10^5 cells per Petri dish.
3. Incubate for 24 h at 37°C (a semiconfluent monolayer is reached).
4. Trypsinize and dilute packaging cells to obtain an equivalent number of cells per mL from each clone, and plate in 10-cm Petri dishes (10 mL final volume).
5. Incubate in selection medium at 37°C until confluence is reached.
6. Incubate at 32°C for 3 d, feeding cells with fresh medium every day.
7. 24 h before collecting the supernatants, replace medium with 8 mL growth medium.
8. Collect virus-containing supernatants and filter through 0.45-µm filters to remove cells and debris.

9. Place serially diluted or undiluted virus-containing supernatants onto NIH3T3 cells in the presence or in the absense of Polybrene (8 µg/mL).
10. Incubate at 37°C for 4 h to allow virus to absorb to cells.
11. Rinse cells with 5 mL sterile saline solution. Add 10 mL growth medium and incubate for an additional 48 h.
12. Trypsinize cells and seed serial dilutions, from 1:10 to 1:10.000, in 10-cm Petri dishes. Add selection medium to 10 mL final volume.
13. Incubate under standard conditions, feeding with fresh selection medium every 2–3 d, until resistant colonies appear.
14. Remove medium. Visualize resistant colonies by adding methylene blue staining solution, leaving at room temperature for 2 h. Express the viral titer, for every single clone, as CFU per milliliter of supernatant (CFU/mL).

3.2.4. Transduction of Human Glioma Cells

1. Grow A172 human glioblastoma cells and AoU373 human astrocytoma cells in growth medium at 37°C, in a humidified, 5% CO_2 incubator (as previously described for PA317 cells).
2. Seed 6×10^5 cells per Petri dish. Incubate overnight.
3. Add undiluted or serially diluted virus-containing supernatant of PA317 producer cells, in the presence or in the absence of Polybrene (8 µg/mL). Incubate at 37°C for 4 h.
4. Remove the viral solution, rinse with saline, and replace with fresh growth medium.
5. After 48 h incubation, add G418 (800 µg/ml) to the culture medium for production of stable transfectants (as previously described for NIH3T3 cells).

3.3. Helper-Virus Detection. LacZ Provirus Mobilization Assay

1. Transduce NIH3T3-LacZ (as previously described) with supernatant from: PA317; PA317/LXSN; PA317/LIL-2SN; PA317/LIL-2TKSN and Mv1-Lu (cells producing wild-type MLV A, positive control) cultures.
2. Incubate for 14 d, feeding with fresh medium every 2–3 d.
3. Collect supernatants, filter through 0.45-µm filters, and use to infect NIH3T3 cells (indicator), as previously described.
4. Incubate for 48 h.
5. Fix cells with 95% ethanol for 15 min. Wash twice in PBS.
6. Expose cultures to X-gal staining reagent (3 mL each), at 37°C for 3–5 h.
7. Examine cultures for presence of X-gal stained cells.

3.4. Monitoring Efficiency of Transgene Expression from PA317 Cell Clones. RT PCR for neo, IL-2, and TK

3.4.1. Isolation of RNA

1. Extract RNA from 1.5×10^6 cells of each clone using the RNAzol™ B method, following manufacturer's protocol (*see* **Note 2**).

2. Resuspend RNA in 43 µL of sterile water, add 5 µL 10X DNase Buffer and 2 µL DNase (20 U). Incubate at 37°C for 60 min.
3. Extract with phenol/chloroform and precipitate in ethanol/sodium acetate. Resuspend in 25 µL of deionized water (DI) containing 0.1% DEPC (*see* **Note 3**).
4. Quantitate the amount of RNA obtained by spectrophotometric readings at 260-nm wavelength. Adjust the final volume in order to have equal concentrations of RNA in each sample.

3.4.2. Reverse PCR

1. To synthesize cDNA for *neo*, IL-2, and TK, use ~1µg of template RNA. Reaction components: 50 U MuLV reverse transcriptase, 20 U RNase inhibitor, 0.6 μM specific reverse primer, 1.6 mM dNTPs, 1X PCR buffer, 3.5 mM MgCl$_2$, 0.001% (w/v) gelatin, and DEPC-treated DI to 25 µL final volume.
2. Incubate at 42°C for 50 min and denaturate at 95°C for 5 min.

3.4.3. Direct PCR

1. Reaction components: 1X PCR Buffer (adjust to 100 µL final volume), 2 mM MgCl$_2$, 1 U AmpliTaq DNA polymerase, 0.5 μM specific forward and reverse primers.
2. Submit reaction samples to 40 cycles of PCR. PCR conditions include similar denaturation (94°C for 1 min) and extension (72°C for 1 min) steps for *neo*, IL-2, and TK. Perform the annealing step (1 min) at 60°C, 66°C, and 53°C for *neo*, IL-2, and TK respectively. Terminate all reactions by a final 10 min extension at 72°C.
3. Controls. Exclude presence of contaminating DNA in the samples by performing a direct PCR for β-globin. Confirm competence of extracted RNA by performing a reverse PCR for β actin.
4. Visualize amplicons by electrophoresis in 1.5% agarose gel (Seakem LE, FMC) with 0.5 µg/mL ethidium bromide staining.

3.5. Bioassay of IL-2 Using CTLL Cell Line

3.5.1. Maintenance of CTLL Cell Line

1. Culture CTLL in RPMI-1640 medium containing 10% FCS, supplemented with partially purified rat splenocyte conditioned medium (or recombinant IL-2) in upright 25-cm^2 flasks.
2. Maintain the cultures using a 3-d feeding schedule. Seed the cells at approximately 2×10^4 cells/mL and feed with 1–5% purified conditioned medium (this corresponds to a concentration of approx 15–20 IL-2 international units—IU/mL). After 3 d, when the cell density is approximately 2×10^5 cells/mL, cultures are split to 2×10^4 cells/mL and refed with IL-2.

3.5.2. IL-2 Bioassay

1. Wash CTLL cells (3 days after feeding) three times with RPMI-1640 by centrifuging the cells at 250 g for 10 min.

2. Determine viability of the cells, e.g., by trypan blue dye exclusion (cells should be >80% viable) and resuspend them to a final concentration of 1×10^5 cells/mL in RPMI-1640 containing 10% FCS.
3. Titrate the IL-2 standard in triplicate in 96-well microtitre plates. Prepare dilutions of the samples in triplicate. Include a negative control, i.e., culture medium alone. Each well should contain a volume of 50 µL.
4. Add 50 µL of cell suspension to each well and incubate the plates for 18 h at 37°C in a humidified CO_2 incubator.
5. Add 0.5 µCi of tritiated thymidine to each well and return the plates to the incubator for 3–4 h.
6. Harvest the contents of each well onto filter mats and determine the radioactivity incorporated into DNA by liquid scintillation counting.
7. Plot a standard curve of cycles per minute vs concentration of IL-2. For quantitation of activity in unknown samples, compare test results with standard curve.

3.6. GCV Sensitivity Assay

1. Plate cells from resistant bulk populations of AoU373 and A172 infected with the recombinant retrovirus and selected as previously described, at a concentration of 5×10^3 cells/well in 96-well flat-bottom plates.
2. Incubate for 24 h in growth medium at 37°C.
3. Aspirate medium and replace with medium containing GCV at different concentrations, ranging from 0.01–100 µ*M*.
4. Incubate for 5 d under the same conditions.
5. Measure cytotoxicity by the MTT (tetrazolium salt) Kit I colorimetric assay (Boehringer Mannheim), following manufacturer's protocol.
6. Measure spectrophotometrical absorbance of the formazan product, formed in the samples, using a microtiter plate (ELISA) reader at 550–600 nm, according to the filters (available for the ELISA reader) used.
7. Express results as percentage of infected, drug-free controls. Calculate IC_{50} as the concentration of drug that inhibits cell growth by 50%, by plotting percentage of surviving cells (ordinate) versus $\log_{10}$ GCV concentration (abscissa).

4. Notes

1. PA 317 cells grow rapidly. To maintain the line in culture cells must be split (1:10) every 3 d.
2. To extract RNA from cells, resuspension with RNazol must be performed very gently, otherwise DNA will be extracted as well.
3. After extraction and precipitation, RNA has to be kept in ice (or stored at –80°C), in order to prevent its degradation.

References

1. Roth, J. A. and Cristiano, R. J. (1997) Gene therapy for cancer: what have we done and where are we going? *J. Natl. Cancer Inst.* **89,** 21–39.

2. Miller, D. G., Adam, M. A., and Miller, A. D. (1990) Gene transfer by retrovirus vectors occurs only in cells that are actively replicating at the time of infection (published erratum appears in *Mol. Cell. Biol.* 1992, **12**, 433). *Mol. Cell. Biol.* **10**, 4239–4242.

3. Chen S. H., Kosai K., Xu B., et al. (1996) Combination suicide and cytokine gene therapy for hepatic metastases of colon carcinoma: sustained antitumor immunity prolongs animal survival. *Cancer Res.* **56**, 3758–3762.

4. Saleh, M. (1997) A retroviral vector that allows efficient co-expression of two genes and the versatility of alternate selection markers. *Hum. Gene Ther.* **8**, 979–983.

5. Hsieh, C. I., Chen, B. F., Wang, C. C., Liu, H. H., Chen, D. S., and Hwang L. H. (1995) Improved gene expression by a modified bicistronic retroviral vector. *Biochem. Biophys. Res. Commun.* **214**, 910–917.

6. Sugimoto Y., Aksentijevich I., Gottesman M. M., and Pastan I. (1994) Efficient expression of drug-selectable genes in retroviral vectors under control of an internal ribosome entry site. *Biotechnology* **12**, 694–698.

7. Freeman, S. M., Ramesh, R., Shastri, M., Munshi, A., Jensen, A. K., and Marrogi, A. J. (1995) The role of cytokines in mediating the bystander effect using *HSV-tK* xenogeneic cells. *Cancer Lett.* **92**, 167–174.

8. Culver, K. W. (1996) Gene therapy for malignant neoplasms of the CNS. *Bone Marrow Transplant* **18**, S6–9.

9. Gagandeep, S., Brew, R., Green, B., et al. (1996) Prodrug-activated gene therapy: involvement of an immunological component in the "bystander effect." *Cancer Gene Ther.* **3**, 83–88.

10. Yamamoto, S., Suzuki, S., Hoshino, A., Akimoto, M., and Shimada, T. (1997) Herpes simplex virus thymidine kinase/ganciclovir-mediated killing of tumor cell induces tumor-specific cytotoxic T cells in mice. *Cancer Gene Ther.* **4**, 91–96.

11. Meazza, R., Marciano, S., Sforzini, S., et al. (1996) Analysis of IL-2 receptor expression and of the biological effects of IL-2 gene transfection in small-cell lung cancer. *Br. J. Cancer* **74**, 788–795.

12. Corrias, M. V., Basso, S., Meazza, R., Musiani, P., Occhino, M., Ferrini, S., and Pistoia, V. (1998) Characterization and tumorigeniticy of human neuroblastoma cells transfected with the IL-2 gene. *Cancer Gene Ther.* **5**, 38–44.

13. Tjuvajev, J., Gansbacher, B., Desai, R., et al. (1995) RG-2 glioma growth attenuation and severe brain edema caused by local production of interleukin-2 and interferon-gamma. *Cancer Res.* **55**, 1902–1910.

14. Bi, W. L., Parysek, L. M., Warnick, R., and Stambrook, P. J. (1993) In vitro evidence that metabolic cooperation is responsible for the bystander effect observed with HSV tk retroviral gene therapy. *Hum. Gene Ther.* **4**, 725–731.

15. Freeman, S. M., Abboud, C. N., Whartenby, K. A., et al. (1993) The "bystander effect": tumor regression when a fraction of the tumor mass is genetically modified. *Cancer Res.* **53**, 5274–5283.

16. Elshami, A. A., Saavedra, A., Zhang, H., et al. (1996) Gap junctions play a role in the "bystander effect" of the herpes simplex virus thymidine kinase/ganciclovir system in vitro. *Gene Ther.* **3**, 85–92.

17. Hamel, W., Magnelli, L., Chiarugi, V. P., and Israel, M. A. (1996) Herpes simplex virus thymidine kinase/ganciclovir-mediated apoptotic death of bystander cells. *Cancer Res.* **56,** 2697–2702.

18. Palù, G., Cavaggioni, A., Calvi, P., Franchin, E., Pizzato, M., Boschetto, R., et al. (1999) Gene therapy of glioblastoma multiforme via combined expression of suicide and cytokine genes: a pilot study in humans. *Gene Ther.* **6,** 330–337.

19. Melani, C., Chiodoni, C., Arienti, F., et al. (1994) Cytokine gene transduction in tumor cells: interleukin (IL)-2 or IL-4 gene transfer in human melanoma cells. *Nat. Immun.* **13,** 76–84.

20. Sambrook, J., Fritsch, E. F., and Maniatis, T. (1989) *Molecular Cloning: A Laboratory Manual.* Cold Spring Harbor Laboratory, Cold Spring Harbor, NY, pp. 1–110.

21. Karnofsky, D. A. and Burchenal, J. H. (1945) The clinical evaluation of chemiotherapeutic agents in cancer, in *Evaluation of Chemiotherapeutic Agents* (McLeod, C. M., ed.), Columbia University Press, New York.

33

Intratumoral Gene Transfer of the Cytosine Deaminase Gene for the Treatment of Breast Cancer

Hardev S. Pandha and Nicholas R. Lemoine

1. Introduction

One of the major limitations of conventional cancer chemotherapy is its lack of selectivity; there is cytotoxicity to both tumor cells and normal cells. Genetic prodrug activation therapy (GPAT) uses transcriptional differences between normal and neoplastic cells to drive the selective expression of a metabolic suicide gene able to convert a nontoxic prodrug into its toxic metabolite. Genetically modified cells that express the nonmammalian enzyme cytosine deaminase (CD) gene are able to convert the nontoxic prodrug 5-fluorocytosine (5-FC) to the toxic metabolite 5-fluorouracil (5-FU), which inhibits RNA and DNA synthesis during S-phase of the cell cycle (1,2). We have devised a transcriptionally targeted GPAT strategy in which expression of CD is restricted to ERBB2-expressing tumor cells. Exposure of CD-expressing cells to 5-FC should result in tumor-selective cell kill thereby sparing normal breast cells.

ERBB2 protein plays a crucial role in the pathogenesis of many human cancers such as breast, pancreas, lung, and ovarian carcinomas. Overexpression of ERBB2 in 25–30% of breast carcinomas is associated with reduced relapse-free and overall patient survival (3). High ERBB2 receptor levels has been shown to correlate with poor prognosis in node-positive patients (4,5), in a subset of node-negative patients (6,7) and in entire cohorts irrespective of nodal involvement (8). ERBB2 status has also been predictive of resistance to endocrine and cytotoxic therapies (9–11). Overexpression of ERBB2 is owing both to increased gene transcription and gene amplification. The activity of the ERBB2 promoter is enhanced in overexpressing cells through binding of

From: *Methods in Molecular Medicine, Vol. 35: Gene Therapy: Methods and Protocols*
Edited by: W. Walther and U. Stein © Humana Press, Inc., Totowa, NJ

members of the AP-2 family of transcription factors to a response element in the proximal part of the promoter. We have previously shown that a 500 base-pair fragment of the proximal promoter (containing the AP-2 binding site) driving the CD gene transduced into a panel of breast and pancreatic tumor cell lines, resulted in levels of CD expression and cell death (upon exposure to 5-FC) directly proportional to the ERBB2 status of the cells *(12)*. The recent availability of a monoclonal antibody (16D8F2) to bacterial cytosine deaminase has allowed direct examination of *Escherichia coli* CD protein expression in clinical biopsy tissue by immunohistochemistry *(13)*. In previous in vitro and murine studies, it has only been possible to monitor CD expression indirectly by cell killing or enzymatic assays *(14,15)*.

1.1. Clinical Protocol

The aim of the clinical study is:

1. To establish a safe and effective dose of a recombinant ERBB2-CD chimaeric gene to sc breast cancer metastases.
2. To confirm the expression of CD in injected ERBB2-positive sc breast cancer metastases.
3. To determine the ability of metastases expressing CD to activate 5-fluorocytosine to 5-fluorouracil.
4. To examine the effects of the local release of 5-fluorouracil on tumor growth in subcutaneous nodules.

1.1.1. Inclusion Criteria

Patients require:

1. At least three well demarcated, nonulcerating skin metastases less than 2 cm diameter.
2. Histologically proven cutaneous relapse of breast cancer.
3. Good performance status (WHO 0, 1, or 2).
4. Normal renal and haematological parameters.
5. Life expectancy of at least 3 mo.
6. Failure on conventional treatment (radiotherapy, endocrine therapy and at least one systemic form of chemotherapy) with an interval of at least 4 wk since previous chemotherapy.
7. Positive ERBB2 status established by immunohistochemistry using two antibodies to the human ERBB2 receptor, which should give concordant results. Only membrane-associated (and not cytoplasmic) staining is considered significant. A positive result to qualify for trial entry is taken as membrane immunoreactivity in at least 30% of tumor cells *(16)*. Previous studies have shown that membrane immunoreactivity correlates with at least threefold overexpression compared to normal breast. The degree of overexpression of ERBB2 by immunohistochemis-

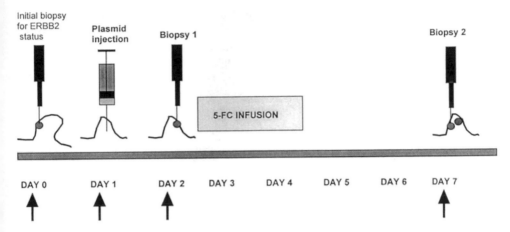

Fig. 1. Schematic representation of the clinical schedule. Three discrete well-demarcated nonulcerating skin lesions are selected, measured, marked, and photographed. After an initial biopsy for ERBB2 status lesions, two of the three lesions are injected with pERCY or polyNeo plasmid in 0.2 mL of sterile water. This is directed into the centre of the tumor nodules using a 22-gage needle. The third lesion selected is the uninjected control. A biopsy is taken from the injected nodules after 24 h and the 2-d 5-FC infusion commenced after 48 h (for the first eight patients only). Further biopsies, measurements, and photographs are taken 7 d after initial intralesional injections.

try was designated according to the proportion of tumor cells expressing the oncoprotein: moderate(+) staining indicated up to 30% of all tumor cells positive, intermediate(++) 30%–70%, high degree of positive staining (+++) over 70%.

1.1.2. Exclusion Criteria

1. Systemic progression of disease.
2. Active autoimmune disease.
3. Concomitant infection with hepatitis virus or HIV.
4. History of psychiatric illness that could influence compliance.
5. Documented presence of cerebral metastases.
6. If chemotherapy given within previous 4 wk.
7. Anaemia or leucopenia as a result of recent chemotherapy.

1.1.3. Clinical Schedule

The clinical schedule is shown in **Fig. 1**.

1. Three similar-sized discrete lesions are marked, measured, and photographed.
2. One lesion is injected with pERCY plasmid containing the proximal ERBB2/CD chimera, the second with the control plasmid polyNeo, which has the same plasmid backbone as pERCY with the ERBB2 promoter/CD chimera removed. The

third lesion is not injected and served as a further control. All injections were in 0.2 mL of sterile water and directed into the center of the tumor nodules using a 22-gauge needle.

3. A biopsy is taken from the injected nodules at 24 h.
4. Infusion of 200 mg/kg/24 hr 5-FC (Alcobon, Roche) prodrug is commenced after 48 h, and given for a total of 48 h duration.
5. Further biopsies, measurements, and photographs are taken 7 d after initial injection.

Responses to GPAT are evaluated clinically (e.g., changes in shape of nodules), by two perpendicular measurements of the tumor nodule diameters and by clinical photography. Complete tumor response is defined as the complete disappearance of the injected cutaneous tumor nodule; partial response is defined as 50% or greater reduction of the sum of the products of perpendicular diameters. Biopsies are taken posttreatment on day 2 and day 7 using a 3-mm punch biopsy. The tissue is orientated and divided longitudinally using a sterile scalpel. One half was snap frozen in liquid nitrogen, the other fixed in formalin and paraffin-embedded the same day.

2. Materials
2.1. The Plasmids Used

For this clinical study, a 544 bp DNA fragment of the proximal 5′ flanking region of ERBB2 (containing the promoter response element) was isolated as described by Hollywood and Hurst *(17)* and cloned into pBluescript II SK+ (Strategen Ltd., Cambridge, UK). A 1522 bp DNA fragment encoding *E. coli* cytosine deaminase was cloned downstream of the 544 bp DNA fragment of ERBB2 to produce and intermediate plasmid pERBB2. The plasmids used for patient injection were based on the commercially available vector pcDNA3. The 2.1-kb chimaeric minigene comprising the ERBB2 promoter response element and the CD gene was subcloned into pcDNA3 into the *Bam*HI restriction site after the CMV promoter/enhancer had been removed, and was designated pERCY. The control plasmid polyNeo was created by *Bgl*I and *Bam*HI digestion of pcDNA3 to remove the CMV promoter/enhancer and religation of the free ends which destroyed the *Bam*H I restriction site. The plasmid constructs used in clinical trial are shown in **Fig. 2**.

3. Methods
3.1. Immunocytochemistry to Establish ERBB2 Status

This may be performed on fresh biopsy tissue or paraffin-embedded archival tissue. Two antibodies to the human ERBB2 receptor should be used such as those supplied by Dako (High Wycombe, U.K.) or Signet (Cambridge,

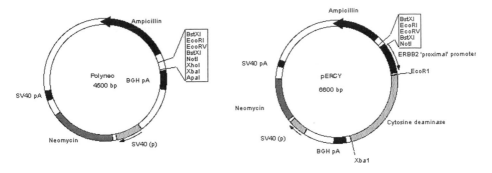

Fig. 2. Plasmid maps of the constructs used in the clinical trial.

U.K.), and should give concordant results. A positive result to qualify for trial entry is taken as membrane immunoreactivity in at least 30% of tumor cells.

1. Mount biopsy tissue onto polysine-coated or Vectabond-coated (not polylysine) slides.
2. Block endogenous peroxidases by incubating slides in 0.3% H_2O_2 for 15 min.
3. Reduce nonspecific binding of ERBB2 antibody by blocking in normal goat serum at 1/20 dilution for 30 min.
4. Incubate in primary antibodies diluted according to the manufacturer's recommendation at 4°C overnight; Dako 1:3000 and Signet 1:100.
5. Incubate for 30 min at room temperature with the appropriate biotinylated secondary antibody (for Dako swine antirabbit, for Signet goat antimouse).
6. Label with peroxidase-streptavidin at 1:500 dilution for 30 min at room temperature.
7. Incubate slides in diaminobenzidine (DAB) chromogen for 10 min. Positive immunoreactivity is visible as brown staining.

3.2. Immunocytochemistry to Detect Cytosine Deaminase in Cells and Tissues

This is performed initially on cell lines (to provide positive and negative controls) before evaluating cryostat cut sections of snap-frozen tissue from clinical biopsies.

1. Fixed and permeabilize both cultured cells grown on sterile glass slides and tissue sections.
2. Incubate slides/sections in 3% paraformaldehyde/PBS for 5 min and then in 0.05M NH4Cl/PBS both at room temperature.
3. Incubation in cold absolute methanol at –20°C for 10 min, followed by permeabilization in 0.1% Triton-X-100/PBS at room temperature for 5 min.
4. Incubate in primary monoclonal antibody 16D8F2[18] diluted 10 µg/mL for 30 min at room temperature.

5. Incubate in secondary antibody (biotinylated goat antimouse).
6. Label with peroxidase-streptavidin at 1/500 dilution for 30 min at room temperature.
7. Incubate slides in DAB chromogen for 10 min. Positive immunoreactivity is visible as brown staining.

It is recommended that the antibody is initially tested on cells transfected with the CD gene as well as the nontransfected line (negative for CD). The biopsy samples the degree of CD expression by immunohistochemistry is designated according to the proportion of tumor cells expressing the CD protein: (+++) indicated over 70% of tumour cells positive, (++) 50–70% positive, and (+) less than 50% positive.

3.3. In Situ *Hybridisation for Cytosine Deaminase mRNA Detection*

Cytosine deaminase mRNA expression in paraffin-embedded clinical trial biopsy tissue may be determined by an *in situ* hybridization technique (based on Senior et al. 1990) *(18)*.

3.3.1. Preparation of Slides

1. Wash microscope slides held in a metal slide rack and coverslips overnight in 10% Decon-90, then in hot running tap water for 60 min, and finally rinse in milli-Q water prior to baking slides covered in aluminium foil at 180°C for 4 h.
2. Immerse slides for 10 s in freshly prepared 3-aminopropylethoxysilane (TESPA, Sigma) 2% (v/v) in acetone, then rinse twice in acetone and twice in DEPC-treated water prior to drying in an oven at 40°C. Discard remaining TESPA as only freshly prepared solution should be used.
3. Cut 4 μm sections from paraffin-embedded biopsies using a microtome and float on DEPC-treated milli-Q water. Use disposable microtome blades or ensure rigorous cleaning of the blade with alcohol prior to use. Collect sections onto TESPA-coated slides and oven-dry overnight at 40°C. Coverslips are washed in 70% alcohol in a metal rack and oven-baked at 180°C for 4 h.
4. De-wax sections in fresh xylene and 0.1% DEPC for 8 min, and then rehydrate through 100%, 80%, 60%, and 30% ethanol containing 0.1% DEPC.
5. Permeabilize tissues with proteinase K (final concentration 20 μg/mL) in PBS 37°C for 10 min, and rinse in 2X PBS containing 0.2% (w/v) glycine for 5 min.
6. After two further rinses in PBS, fix sections in 4% paraformaldehyde in PBS for 20 min (*see* **Note 1**).
7. Rinse in PBS twice.
8. Acetylate sections with 500 mL 0.1*M* triethanolamine and 1.25 mL of acetic anhydride. Mix well for 10 min.
9. Wash slides in PBS 3 more times for 5 min, and dehydrate through graded alcohol from 30% to 100% containing 0.1% DEPC.
10. Air-dry sections prior to hybridization.

3.3.2. Preparation of ^{35}S-labeled Riboprobes

1. Add 1 µg of each restriction digest template to the in vitro transcription mix: (1X transcription buffer (Promega, Madison, WI), 1.5 U/mL RNAsin (Promega), DTT (5.6 mM plus 5.6 mM from ^{35}S-UTP), ATP, GTP, CTP mix (each 6.25 µM), 10 U/µg template of RNA polymerase plus 3.5 µL (800 Ci/mmol) ^{35}S-UTP (Amersham, Arlington Heights, IL).
2. Incubate this mixture plus templates at 37°C for 60 min.
3. Destroy the template by adding 1 µL of DNase I (RNase free) to the reaction tube and incubating for 15 min.
4. Dilute the reaction mix in 25 µL of 10 mM DTT and 1.5 µL of ribosomal RNA (10 µg/mL used as a carrier).
5. Take 1 µL into 50 µL of water and 3 mL scintillant to assess total ^{35}S present.
6. Equlibrate a Chromospin-30 column (Clontech, Palo Alto, CA).
7. Add the bulk of the reaction mix to the column, spin at 700g for 3 min at 15°C and collect eluate.
7. Add 4 µL of 100 mM DTT, mix well then count 1 µL in 50 µL water and 3 mL scintillant: calculate the percentage incorporation of ^{35}S (should be 40–80%)
8. The riboprobe eluate is assessed for quality on a 6% polyacrylamide sequencing gel and, if satisfactory, stored at –20°C until required (*see* **Note 2**).

3.3.3. Hybridization

The hybridization buffer consists of 10% 10X salts mix in Denhart's solution, 50% formamide, 3% rRNA, 20% dextran sulphate, 1% 1M DTT, and the remaining 16% of the total volume of the probe is made up with DEPC-treated milli-Q water.

1. Heat the hybridization buffer containing the probe to 80°C for 1 min.
2. Pipet 20 µL of hybridization buffer onto each slide.
3. Place slides in a humidified box containing blotting paper saturated with 1X salts and 50% formamide. Seal box with tape and incubate overnight at 55°C.
4. After hybridization, place slides in 50% formamide at 55°C for 4 h, then wash slides for 5 min 10 times using TNE buffer.
5. Incubate slides in 100 µg/mL RNase A in TNE buffer solution at 37°C for 1 h.
6. Wash slides in 2X SSC and 0.5X SSC each for 30 min at 65°C.
7. Finally, to ensure that the labeled hybrids remain in place, pass the slides through graded ethanols increasing from 30% to absolute ethanol all containing 0.3M ammonium acetate.
8. Air-dry slides overnight prior to autoradiography.

3.3.4. Autoradiography and Slide Developing

For the autoradiography process, melt 25 mL of Ilford K5 emulsion in 2.4 mL of 5M ammonium acetate, and dilute with 25 mL of milli-Q water warmed to 45°C.

1. Dip slides into the emulsion to cover the tissue, then cool and dry in total darkness by placing slides on a metal plate overlying ice.
2. Once dry, place slides in a plastic rack, sealed in a light-tight bag and expose for 15 d at 4°C.
3. Develop slides in Kodak D-19 developer at 18°C for 4 min and fix in 30% sodium thiosulphate.

3.3.5. Counterstaining

The Giemsa stain discriminates individual cell structures. Giemsa staining of slides in parallel to those used for *in situ* hybridization are prepared by immersing slides in dilute stock Giemsa solution (1 in 100 with distilled water) for 60 s. Excess stain is washed off with tap water and the slides air drying prior to examination.

The CD gene required for preparation of the riboprobes for this *in situ* work was directionally cloned into pGEM-4 vector using the *Eco*RI and *Hind*III sites. Linearized pGEM-4 containing a 428 base pair CD insert was used for in vitro transcription of the riboprobe with:

1. *Eco*RI for production of sense strand (negative control) under control of the T7 promoter.
2. *Hind*III for production of antisense strand under the control of the SP6 promoter.
3. Linearized pBluescript containing β-actin cDNA with *Dra*I, also under the control of the SP6 promoter.

The digestion products were phenol/chloroform extracted and ethanol precipitated. The activity of radiolabelled probes eluted from Chromaspin-30 columns were assessed in a scintillation counter and were between 3.0×10^6 cpm and 3.65×10^6 cpm. All sections should be examined with CD sense, CD antisense, and β-actin antisense probes.

3.4. Quantitative Assay for Cytosine Deaminase Activity In Vitro

To detect cytosine deaminase activity in either cell lines expressing CD or in clinical biopsies, a thin layer chromatography method (TLC) was developed. The method relies on the enzyme's ability to convert cytosine to uracil; a reaction which merely converts the amine group to a ketone group. The two compounds have different mobilities through a liquid phase (in this case a mixture of butanol and water). These compounds can be radioactively labeled and separated by TLC. The method was modified from that described by Andersen and co-workers *(19)* (*see* **Note 3**).

1. A minimum of 1×10^6 cells are washed in Hanks Balanced Salt Solution and resuspended in 200 μL of lysis buffer (100 m*M* Tris-Cl pH 7.8, 1 m*M* EDTA, 1 m*M* dithiothreitol).

2. Freeze/thaw lysates by immersion in liquid nitrogen, and centifuge at 15,800*g* for 10 min.
3. Take 10-µL aliquots of cleared lysates and mix with 10 µL of "cytosine label mix" (consisting of 0.97 mCi, 12.2 Ci/mmol [³H]-cytosine in 100m*M* Tris-Cl, pH 7.8).
4. Incubate lysates in the presence of [³H]-radiolabeled cytosine for 1 h at 37°C, then spot 5–10 µL onto fluorescent TLC sheets (Merk, plates 1.05735).
5. Spot nonradioactive standard samples of cytosine and uracil (0.4 mg/mL) at either ends of the TLC plate. Because these absorb UV light, their positions on the TLC plate can be estimated using a hand-held UV source (λ^2 240 nm).
6. Place the TLC sheets in a chromatography chamber containing butan-1-ol and water (86 : 14 v/v), seal the chamber with clingfilm and allow to run for 4 h (*see* **Note 4**).
7. To calculate rate of uracil formation, cut out bands corresponding to the radioactive products (i.e., at the level of the nonradioactive uracil control) and place in scintillation tubes containing 5 mL of liquid scintillation analyzer (TriCarb 1500). Measure radioactivity by scintillation counter.
8. The amount of radioactivity recovered from the cytosine and uracil bands should account for all of the label introduced. This is confirmed by assaying activity of the same amount of label not separated by chromatography. The percentage conversion of cytosine to uracil over the time period is calculated as the amount of uracil produced divided by the amount of cytosine substrate introduced into the reaction. Each time-point gives a value in radioactivity, which is converted to the amount of uracil produced at each time point and the results plotted on a graph. The gradient of the resulting line is the rate of deamination, i.e., the enzyme activity, because this may be expressed as product/amount of cells/time period. A typical result of TLC using CD-expressing cells lines HPAF CD500 and control HPAF cells is shown in **Fig. 3**; deamination of radiolabeled cytosine results in cytosine to uracil conversion by the CD-expressing cell line only.

The conversion of cytosine to uracil expressed as a percentage is calculated as:

$$\text{\% conversion to uracil} = \frac{\text{dpm uracil band}}{\text{total dpm in uracil and cytosine bands}} \times 100\%$$

(dpm = decay per minute)

4. Notes

1. The paraformaldehyde should be made up fresh for each experiment. In order to ensure the 4% solution dissolves completely, the paraformaldehyde is added to PBS that has just boiled, then the 4% solution is allowed to cool gently at room temperature.
2. For 100% incorporation, total incorporated counts will be 3.2×10^8, equivalent to 243 ng RNA. Expect 10 million dpm (decay per minute)/mL. One million dpm is approximately 0.7 ng RNA probe. Specific activity of RNA transcript will be $1.3–1.7 \times 10^9$ dpm/µg RNA using the ³⁵S as the only source of UTP.

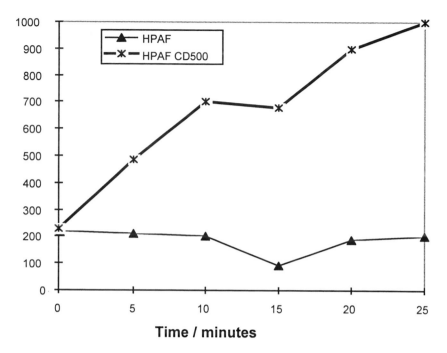

Fig. 3. Example of a quantitative assay for cytosine deaminase activity in vitro by conversion of cytosine to uracil in HPAF CD500 cell line compared to HPAF parental cells.

3. It is recommended that determination of CD activity is performed initially on CD-transduced and control cell lines to determine the sensitivity of the technique.It will be possible to evaluate the minimum number cells required for detection of converted uracil before committing clinical tissue. In our experience this technique requires a minimum of 1 million cells.

4. The TLC should be run in a fume cupboard as butan-1-ol fumes are irritant. To ensure uniform movement of all bands it is important to ensure that the TLC plate is surrounded by a butan-1-ol atmosphere within the chromatography chamber. This is best achieved by sealing the chamber using either a heavy glass lid with Vaseline smeared onto the rim of the chamber, or several layers of clingfilm.

References

1. Huber, B., Austin, E., Good, S., Knick, V., and Richards, C. (1993) In vivo antitumour activity of 5-fluorocytosine on human colorectal carcinoma cell lines genetically modified to express CD. *Cancer Res.* **53,** 4619–4626.
2. Mullen, C. A., Coale, M. M., Lowe, R. M., and Blaese, R. M. (1994) Tumors expressing the cytosine deaminase suicide gene can be eliminated in vivo with

5-fluorocytosine and induce protective immunity to wild type tumor. *Cancer Res.* **54,** 1503–1506.

3. Lovekin, C., Ellis, I., Locker, A., et al. (1991) c-erbB2 oncoprotein expression in primary and advanced breast cancer. *Br. J. Cancer* **63,** 439–443.

4. Gustrson, B. A., et al. (1992) prognostic importance of c-erbB2 expression in breast cancer. *J. Clin. Oncol.* **10,** 1049–1056.

5. Borg, A., Tandon, A., and Sigurdsson, H. (1990) HER-2/neu amplification predicts poor survival in node-positive breast cancer. *Cancer Res.* **50,** 4332–4337.

6. Richner, J., Gerber, H., and Locher, G. (1990) c-erbB2 protein expression in node negative breast cancer. *Ann. Oncol.* **1,** 263–268.

7. Alfred, D., Clark, G., and Tandon, A. (1992) HER-2/neu in node-negative breast cancer: prognostic significance of overexpression influenced by the presence of in situ carcinoma. *J. Clin. Oncol.* **10,** 599–605.

8. Gullick, W., Love, S., and Wright, C. (1991) c-erbB2 protein overexpression in breast cancer is a risk in patients with involved and uninvolved lymph nodes. *Br. J. Cancer* **63,** 434–438.

9. Borg, A., Baldertorp, B., Ferno, M., Killander, D., Olsson, H., and Sigurdsson, H. (1994) ERBB2 amplification is associated with tamoxifen resistance in steroid receptor-positive breast cancer. *Cancer Lett.* **81,** 137–144.

10. Tetu, B. and Brisson, J. (1994) Prognostic significance of HER-2/neu oncoprotein expression in node-positive breast cancer. *Cancer* **73,** 2359–2365.

11. Slamon, D., Clark, G., Wong, S., Levin, W., and Ullrich, A. (1987) Human breast cancer: Correlation of relapse and survival with amplification of the Her-2/neu oncogene. *Science* **235,** 177–182.

12. Harris, J. D., Gutierrez, A. A., Hurst, H. C., Sikora, K., and Lemoine, N. R. (1994) Gene therapy for cancer using tumour-specific prodrug activation. *Gene Ther.* **1,** 170–175.

13. Haak, K., Moebius, U., Knebel Docbcritz, M., and Gebert, J. (1997) Detection of cytosine deaminase in genetically modified tumour cells by specific antibodies. *Hum. Gene Ther.* **8,** 1395–1401.

14. Mullen, C. A., Kilstrup, M., and Blaese, R. M. (1992) Transfer of the bacterial gene for cytosine deaminasc to mammalian cells confers lethal sensitivity to 5-fluorocytosine: A negative selection system. *Proc. Nat. Acad. Sci. USA* **89,** 33–37.

15. Austin, E. A. and Huber, B. E. (1993) A first step in the development of gene therapy for colorectal carcinoma: Cloning, sequencing and expression *Escherichia coli* cytosine deaminase. *Mol. Pharmacol.* **43,** 380–387.

16. Slamon, D. J., Godolphin, W., Jones, I., Holt, J., Wong, S., Keith, D., and Press, M. (1989) Studies of the HER-2/neu proto-oncogene in human breast and ovarian cancer. *Science* **244,** 707–711.

17. Hollywood, D. P. and Hurst, H. C. (1993) A novel transcription factor, OB2-1, is required for overexpression of the proto-oncogene c-erbB2 in mammary tumour cell lines. *EMBO J.* **2,** 2369–2375.

18. Senior, P. V., Byrne, S., Brammar, W. J., and Beck, F. (1990) Expression of the IGF-II/ mannose-6-phosphate receptor mRNA and protein in the developing rat. *Development* **109,** 67–73.

19. Anderson, L., Kilstrup, M., and Neuhard, J. (1989) Pyrimidine, purine and nitrogen control of cytosine deaminase synthesis in E coli. *Arch. Microbiol.* **153,** 115–118.

II

CLINICAL PROTOCOLS FOR CANCER GENE THERAPY

C: Anti-Oncogene and Suppressor Gene Therapy

34

Adenovirus-Mediated Wild-Type *p53* Gene Transfer into Head and Neck Cancers

Gary L. Clayman, Douglas K. Frank, and Patricia A. Bruso

1. Introduction

Mutation of the *p53* tumor-suppressor gene is recognized as one of the most common genetic alterations in human malignancy to date *(1)*. Approximately 60% of human tumors are thought to possess mutation at the *p53* locus. Transient overexpression of the wild-type *p53* gene in various malignancies has been considered a potential molecular intervention strategy *(2–7)*. This strategy is based on the role that wild-type *p53* plays as a tumor-suppressor gene and inducer of cell-cycle arrest and apoptosis *(1,8–11)*.

Previous work in our laboratory has focused upon the potential of wild-type *p53* gene transfer as a strategy for the selective induction of apoptosis in human head and neck squamous cell carcinoma of the upper-aerodigestive tract (SCCHN). The recombinant adenovirus, Ad-p53, has been used as the gene delivery tool in all of our preclinical and clinical studies. This replication-defective vector has been described in detail elsewhere *(4)*. The tropism of adenovirus for tissues of the upper-aerodigestive tract make it an ideal gene-delivery vehicle for our purposes. It is important to point out that the genetic material introduced into mammalian cells via Ad-p53 remains episomal (not integrated into the DNA) and is overexpressed. Gene expression is transient as the episomal DNA is not passed on to daughter cells.

Our interest in new treatment strategies for SCCHN is generated by the humbling survival rates (50%) for these tumors, which have not changed over the last several decades with current standard treatment modalities (radiation, surgery, chemotherapy) *(12)*. Furthermore, after undergoing standard therapy (including radiotherapy), the SCCHN patient with recurrent disease has a

From: *Methods in Molecular Medicine, Vol. 35: Gene Therapy: Methods and Protocols*
Edited by: W. Walther and U. Stein © Humana Press, Inc., Totowa, NJ

particularly dismal prognosis and has few meaningful treatment options. The principal cause of death in SCCHN is local-regional recurrence *(13,14)*. Clearly, new treatment strategies need to be developed and investigated. Thus, the study of novel molecular therapies involving genes such as wild-type *p53* seemed appropriate. The fact that local-regionally recurrent SCCHN is readily accessible, even in the most advanced cases, enhanced its candidacy for investigation as a target for wild-type *p53* molecular intervention.

Our preclinical laboratory investigations demonstrated that introduction of the wild-type *p53* gene via Ad-p53 into SCCHN cell lines and established tumor nodules in nude mice suppressed in vitro and in vivo tumor growth, respectively *(4)*. Further studies demonstrated that this suppression of cell growth was via cell death, and that the mechanism of cell death was apoptosis *(3)*. Our group was able to demonstrate that the apoptotic process occurred in malignant cells regardless of their *p53* status, albeit at different rates. Furthermore, normal fibroblasts were not sensitive to these effects, suggesting that the induced apoptotic process was selective for malignant cells *(2)*.

The results of the preliminary data regarding wild-type *p53* molecular therapy in our laboratory led to investigating its utility in a residual SCCHN murine model *(2)*. Such a model was developed secondary to the high incidence of locoregional failure in this disease, presumably secondary to microscopic residual disease following initial standard therapy. Introduction of Ad-p53 locally into sites of SCCHN tumor cell inoculation in nude mice prevented the establishment of tumors. This study (and its precursors) laid the groundwork for the current adenovirus-mediated wild-type *p53* human gene therapy trial at the Department of Head and Neck Surgery, University of Texas M.D. Anderson Cancer Center, for patients with advanced local-regionally recurrent head and neck squamous cell carcinoma of the upper-aerodigestive tract that has failed other standard therapeutic modalities. The first phase of this trial has been completed, and an international phase II trial has been initiated.

As aforementioned, patients with local-regionally advanced, recurrent SCCHN that have failed initial standard therapy have a dismal prognosis. If radiation was included in the treatment regimen for such patients, they are furthermore left with few therapeutic options. Patients with these characteristics formed the study population for our Ad-p53 clinical trial. Thus, we present our materials and methodology for the administration of Ad-p53 molecular therapy in the management of SCCHN within the context of our phase I clinical trial.

Patients in phase I were randomized into two treatment arms. The first arm consisted of inoperable patients. The second arm consisted of patients who were deemed operable but incurable. The patients in the second arm received Ad-p53 preoperatively in six doses over 2 wk and then intraoperatively and postoperatively as an adjuvant approach to the surgical extirpation of their recurrence. For simplicity, we will discuss the administration of Ad-p53 molecular therapy in the management of SCCHN in the context of the patients in this second treatment arm.

2. Materials

The replication-defective recombinant adenovirus, Ad-p53 was utilized for all wild-type *p53* gene transfers. This vector contains the cytomegalovirus (CMV) promoter, and wild-type *p53* cDNA in a minigene cassette inserted into the E1-deleted region of human adenovirus, type 5. Details regarding the preparation of recombinant adenovirus can be found in the publication Zhang et al. *(15)* Ad-p53 is a BL-2 agent and should be handled with the appropriate level of biological containment. After production, Ad-p53 was stored at –80°C at concentrations of 2–3.5 × 10^{10} particle forming units (pfu) per mL in phosphate-buffered saline (PBS) supplemented with 10% glycerol in the hospital pharmacy. Ad-p53 was thawed and diluted in PBS at 4°C within 2 hours of use.

All staff wore glasses, gowns, and gloves at the time of administration of Ad-p53. Hepa masks (3M Corp., St. Paul, MN), fit tested and 99% efficient respirators, were also worn at the time of vector delivery to patients (*see* **Note 1**). Technol 2010 masks (Technol Inc., Fort Worth, TX), not fit tested and 95% efficient respirator, were worn while in the room with patients subsequent to vector delivery for the purposes of patient monitoring and blood draws. Ad-p53 administration was carried out with sterile 5–10 mL syringes and 27-gauge needles. The vector was drawn out of the stock vials (containing 2–3.5 × 10^{10} pfu per mL) using 18-gage needles for the purposes of dilution.

3. Methods

In phase 1 of the clinical trial, all Ad-p53 administration was performed on an inpatient basis. The first cycle consisted of treatments (direct tumor injections) given three times weekly for 2 wk, excluding weekends (six treatments overall). Seventy-two hours following the last treatment in the first cycle, patients had surgery. At the time of surgery and just prior to closure, an administration of a single dose of Ad-p53 was delivered to the surgical bed and left in contact for 60 min. Seventy-two hours after surgery, a retrograde instillation of Ad-p53 was administered through wound catheters, which had been placed intraoperatively.

3.1. Administration of Ad-p53

The clinical trial was designed in a dose escalation manner in order to determine a maximum tolerated dose per treatment. Whereas patients early in the study received 1 × 10^6 pfu total to the tumor (or tumor bed) during each treatment (including each of the six treatments of the first cycle), doses were increased in log increments until 1×10^9 pfu was reached, and then in one-half log increments until 1×10^{11} pfu was reached.

1. After acquiring the Ad-p53 stock vial(s) from the pharmacy for a given patient treatment, the sample was thawed. The pharmacy stock vials were prepared as 2×10^{10} pfu in 0.1 mL to 1 mL PBS.
2. Under aseptic conditions, the appropriate amount of vector was withdrawn from the stock vial(s) for a given patient treatment. As stated, this ranged from 1×10^6 pfu to 1×10^{11} pfu per treatment. The amount of vector administered to a given patient from treatment to treatment never varied.
3. After withdrawing the necessary amount of Ad-p53 from the stock vial(s), dilution in PBS for the purposes of administration, under sterile conditions, was performed (*see* **Subheadings 3.1.1.** and **3.1.2.**). **Step 4** of the protocol varied depending upon whether direct tumor injection or surgical bed administration of vector was performed. This is clarified below as the procedure for Ad-p53 administration for each delivery scenario is described.

3.1.1. Direct Tumor Injection of Ad-p53

For direct intratumoral administrations, Ad-p53 was diluted to a volume of PBS concordant with the number of tumor injections to be performed. Generally, we injected about 0.5 mL of vector solution at 1 cm (surface area) tumor increments. Thus, a very large tumor required the appropriate amount of vector to be diluted in a larger volume of PBS.

4. Injections were carried out by first passing the injection needle as far into the tumor as possible and injecting the vector solution slowly (*see* **Note 2**) as the needle and syringe were withdrawn. For the purposes of the first cycle, a tumor map was made so that subsequent Ad-p53 administrations during the cycle occurred in the exact locations as prior injections (**Fig. 1**). Hypopharyngeal, laryngeal, and cervical lesions were injected transcutaneously (*see* **Notes 3** and **4**). Oral cavity and oropharyngeal tumors were injected directly (*see* **Note 4**).

3.1.2. Intraoperative and Retrograde Catheter Administrations of Ad-p53 to the Tumor Bed

For these administrations, the appropriate amount of vector was always diluted to 10 mL in PBS.

5. At the completion of tumor extirpation, Ad-p53 was administered liberally (a "vector wash") to the tumor bed via a syringe and left in contact for 60 min prior to wound closure. Injections were performed along the margins of the resected neoplasms as well (**Fig. 2**). For the retrograde catheter administrations performed 72 h after surgery, the appropriate amount of Ad-p53 was also always diluted to 10 mL in PBS.

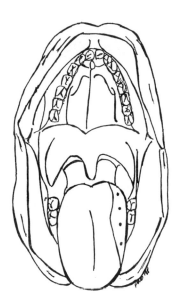

Fig. 1. Example of a typical tumor map for a left tongue carcinoma. Note incremental markings along left tongue lesion, indicating sites where Ad-p53 is injected.

6. Vector was administered via a syringe through the drains into the wound bed with clamps utilized to prevent efflux of the Ad-p53 for 1 h. The drains were subsequently removed in 24–48 h.

3.2. Patient Monitoring During Ad-p53 Administration

Because the treatment of SCCHN patients with Ad-p53 was within the context of a phase I clinical trial, patient monitoring for the detection of untoward effects and toxicities was quite stringent (*see* **Note 5**). All patients had vital signs, hematology, chest X-ray, blood chemistry, and performance status evaluated at the start of each treatment cycle. Patients were closely observed for a 2-h period following each treatment.

4. Notes

1. The healthcare workers with the greatest risk of Ad-p53 exposure had their serum and urine tested for the presence of infectious Ad-p53 and/or Ad-p53 DNA. All tests were negative. Low levels of anti-Ad-p53 antibody were detected in some serum samples, suggesting that no significant exposures to the adenovirus vector occurred.
2. To date, our clinical experience with the administration of Ad-p53 has been limited to patients with advanced recurrent SCCHN that had failed standard treatment modalities, including radiotherapy. This experience has been in the form of

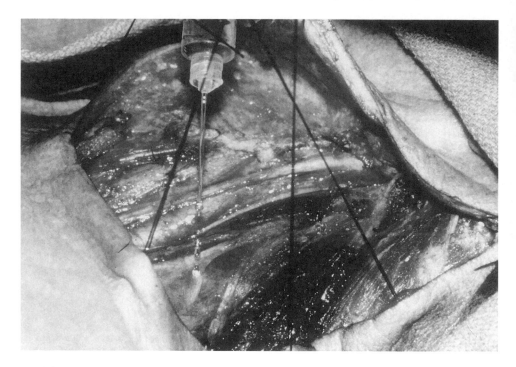

Fig. 2. Intraoperative delivery of Ad-p53 to tumor bed. Ad-p53 is being injected into the tumor margins subsequent to a "vector wash" of the tumor bed.

the clinical trial described. A consistent observation that has been made in the delivery of Ad-p53 to patients during the first cycle has been pain at the site of injection. It has been determined that this is secondary to the cold temperature of the recently thawed and diluted vector. It was initially thought that the Ad-p53 needed to be kept cold in order to preserve its infection ability. Stability studies suggest that the vector can be warmed to room temperature prior to patient injection. We anticipate that this may significantly diminish patient discomfort during administration.

3. Erythema at the site of injection was noted among several patients following transcutaneous injection of Ad-p53. This effect was never dose-limiting.

4. During the first cycle, it was not unusual for patients receiving higher viral doses per treatment ($1 \times 10^{9.5}$–1×10^{11}) to experience mild flu-like symtoms following Ad-p53 injections. These symptoms often extended through or recurred after the second treatment. Symptoms usually did not last into or beyond the third treatment of the first cycle. Flu-like symptoms could include all or only some of the following: Fever (as high as 39.4°C in one patient), sinus congestion, headache, and sore throat. Flu-like symptoms were never dose-limiting in our phase I experience.

5. Determining the patient biological distribution of Ad-p53 after administration was an important aspect of the phase I clinical trial. Patient blood, urine, and upper-aerodigestive tract secretions were assayed for the presence of Ad-p53 by a cytopathic effect assay (CPE) and Ad-p53 specific PCR. Although the technical details of the performance of these assays is beyond the scope of this chapter, it is important to point out that Ad-p53 was detected in blood and urine at higher vector concentrations. Vector quickly disappeared from blood within 24 h after a treatment. At high doses, vector could be detected in the urine of patients throughout treatment. The presence of vector in the urine ultimately disappeared within 3–17 d after the last Ad-p53 administration. As with blood and urine, Ad-p53 could also be detected in the sputum of patients after treatment at the higher doses, and would be present throughout a cycle. Ad-p53 would usually be cleared from the sputum within a week.

Acknowledgments

This work was supported in part by an American Cancer Society Career Development Award, National Institute of Dental Research 1-P50-DE11906 (93-9) (GLC), National Institute of Health First Investigator Award R29 DE11689-01A1 (GLC), and Training of the Academic Surgical Oncologist Grant T32 CA60374-03 (GLC), and a sponsored research agreement from Introgen Therapeutics, Inc. (Austin, TX 78701).

References

1. Levine, A. J., Momand, J., and Finlay, C. A. (1991) The p53 tumor suppressor gene. *Nature* **351,** 453–456.
2. Clayman, G. L., El-Naggar, A. K., Roth, J. A., Zhang, W. W., Goepfert, H., Taylor, D. L., and Liu, T. J. (1995) In vivo molecular therapy with p53 adenovirus for microscopic residual head and neck squamous carcinoma. *Cancer. Res.* **55,** 1–6.
3. Liu, T. J., El-Naggar, A. K., McDonnell, T. J., Steck, K. D., Wang, M., Taylor, D. L., and Clayman, G. L. (1995) Apoptosis induction mediated by wild-type p53 adenoviral gene transfer in squamous cell carcinoma of the head and neck. *Cancer Res.* **55,** 3117–3122.
4. Liu, T. J., Zhang, W. W., Taylor, D. L., Roth, J. A., Goepfert, H., and Clayman, G. L.. (1994) Growth suppression of human head and neck cancer cells by the introduction of a wild-type p53 gene via a recombinant adenovirus. *Cancer Res.* **54,** 3662–3667.
5. Fujiwara, T., Grimm, E. A., Mukhopadhyay, T., Cai, D. W., Owen-Schaub, L. B., and Roth, J. A. (1993) A retroviralwild-type p53 expression vector penetrates human lung spheroids and inhibits growth by inducing apoptosis. *Cancer Res.* **53,** 4129–4133.
6. Mercer, W. E., Shields, M. T., Amin, M., Sauve, G. J., Appella, E., Romano, J. W., and Ullrich, S. J. (1990) Negative growth regulation in a glioblastoma cell line that conditionally expresses human wild-type p53. *Proc. Natl. Acad. Sci. USA* **87,** 6166–6170.

7. Shaw, P., Bovey, R., Tardy, S., Sahli, R., Sordat, B., and Costa, J. (1992) Induction of apoptosis by wild-type p53 in a human colon tumor-derived cell line. *Proc. Natl. Acad. Sci. USA* **89,** 4495–4499.

8. Martinez, J., Georgoff, I., Martinez, J., and Levine, A. J. (1991) Cellular localization and cell cycle regulation by a temperature-sensitive p53 protein. *Genes Dev.* **5,** 151–159.

9. Diller, L., Kassel, J., Nelson, C. E., Gryka, M. A., Litwak, G., Gebhardt, M., et al. (1990) p53 functions as a cell cycle control protein in osteosarcomas. *Mol. Cell Biol.* **10,** 5772–5781.

10. Baker, S. J., Markowitz, S., Fearon, E. R., Willson, J. K., and Vogelstein, B. (1990) Suppression of human colorectal carcinoma cell growth by wild-type p53. *Science* **249,** 912–915.

11. Yonish-Rouach, E., Resnitzky, D., Lotem, J., Sachs, L., Kimchi, A., and Oren, M. (1991) Wild-type p53 induces apoptosis of myeloid leukemic cells that is inhibited by interleukin-6. *Nature* **352,** 345–347.

12. Publ. No. 93-400. (1993) *American Cancer Society Facts and Figures.* American Cancer Society, Washington, DC.

13. Day, G. L., Blot, R. E., Shore, R. E., et al. (1994) Second cancers following oral and pharyngeal cancers: role of tobacco and alcohol. *J. Natl. Cancer Inst.* **86,** 131–137.

14. Vokes, E. E., Weichselbaum, R. R., Lippman, S. M., et al. (1993) Head and neck cancer. *N. Engl. J. Med.* **328,** 184–194.

15. Zhang, W. W., Fang, X., Branch, C. D., et al. (1993) Generation and identification of recombinant adenovirus by liposome-mediated transfection and PCR analysis. *Biotechniques* **15,** 869–872.

35

Direct DNA Injection (*p53*) into HCC Tumors

Ragai R. Mitry and Nagy A. Habib

1. Introduction

Liver tumors, specially HCC, are among the most common malignancies in the world, and their annual world incidence is about 250,000 cases, with a male to female ratio 4 : 1 *(1)*. HCC is one of the most important neoplasms in tropical and subtropical regions, particularly among the sub-Saharan African black population and ethnic Chinese *(2)*. The prognosis is very poor, and patients with advanced tumors are unlikely to survive 3 mo *(3)*. Most HCC cases are beyond radical resection when detected. All other forms of the currently available therapies are rarely beneficial *(2)*.

Methods for modern molecular genetics have been developed to allow transfer and expression of foreign DNA sequences in human somatic cells and make human gene therapy possible *(4)*. In fact, gene therapy has altered the conventional path for cancer research. It offers the potential for developing innovative treatments for both inherited monogenic diseases like cystic fibrosis, and polygenic disorders such as cancer *(5)*. Various gene delivery systems are available including nonviral "naked" DNA or liposome/DNA complexes and viral retroviruses and adenoviruses.

Direct injection of naked DNA is a method that involves the direct injection of pure plasmid DNA into the desired tissue *(6)*. It is inexpensive and considered as one of the safest gene transfer techniques. The mechanism of naked DNA uptake by cells/tissues in vivo is not very clear, but the possible mechanisms involved are pinocytosis and endocytosis. In 1990, Wolff et al. injected β-galactosidase (*lacZ*) reporter gene DNA constructs into mouse skeletal muscles and showed that the *lacZ* expression was at significant levels *(7)*.

From: *Methods in Molecular Medicine, Vol. 35: Gene Therapy: Methods and Protocols*
Edited by: W. Walther and U. Stein © Humana Press, Inc., Totowa, NJ

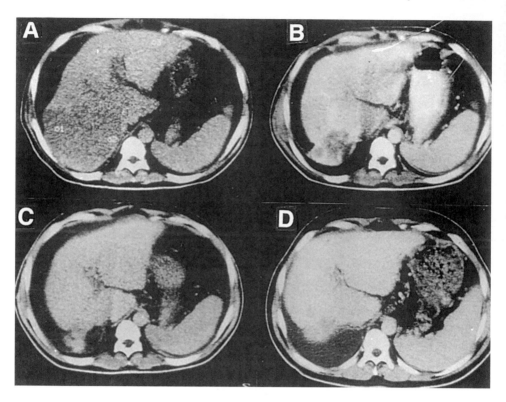

Fig. 1. CT scans of one of the HCC patients that have undergone wt-*p53* gene therapy. (**A**) Unenhanced CT scan case 4 prior to therapy. A 12-cm diameter tumor is seen in the posterior position of the right lobe of liver (AFP 1900 IU/L). (**B**) Contrast-enhanced CT scan of the same patient 3 mo later after two intratumoral injections of wt-*p53* shows a considerable reduction in size of the tumor, which now measures 5 cm in diameter (normal AFP). (**C**) Contrast-enhanced CT scan of same patient 6 mo after the commencement of therapy. The tumor now measures 2 cm in diameter (normal AFP). (**D**) Contrast-enhanced CT scan of the same patient 19 mo after the commencement of therapy. No tumor is seen (normal AFP).

In 1996, Habib and colleagues published the results of a pilot study carried out on five HCC patients, to assess the therapeutic potential of percutaneous injection of naked wild-type *p53* plasmid DNA, pC53-SN3 (wt-*p53*). The results showed objective tumor response in three of the five patients with reduction of the tumor volume (75, 90, and 95%) on computed tomographic (CT) scan measurements (**Fig. 1**) as well as a significant fall of serum α-fetoprotein (AFP). No mortality or morbidity owing to the injections *(8)*. The procedures used in that study are explained in details in the methods section.

2. Materials

1. Bacterial resuspension buffer: 50 mM glucose, 25 mM Tris-HCl (pH 8.0), 10 mM EDTA (pH 8.0) and autoclave.
2. Bacterial lysis buffer: 0.2 N NaOH, 1% SDS.
3. Bacterial neutralisation buffer: 60 mL of 5M potassium acetate, 11.5 mL glacial acetic acid, 28.5 mL ddH$_2$O.
4. Lauria-Bertani (LB) broth: 10 g NaCl, 5 g Bacto-yeast extract, 10 g Bacto tryptone, 2 mL 1M NaOH, add distilled H$_2$O to make up 1000 mL and autoclave.
5. LB agar plates: 0.7% agar in LB broth (w/v), then autoclave.
6. Ampicillin: 50 mg/mL dissolved in sterile ddH$_2$O and filtered through a 0.2-µm filter; stored as small aliquots.
7. *Escherichia coli* (XL-1 Blue) purchased from Stratagene (La Jolla, CA) and processed according to the manufacturer's instructions. The bacteria is then stored at –80°C as 100-µL aliquots in sterile 0.5-mL microfuge tubes.
8. Tris-EDTA buffer (TE): 10 mM Tris base, pH 7.5, 1 mM EDTA (disodium salt).
9. Phosphate-buffered saline (PBS): 2.3 g anhydrous Na$_2$HPO$_4$, 0.59 g NaH$_2$PO$_4$.2H$_2$O, 18 g NaCl. Add distilled H$_2$O to make 2000 mL. pH should be ~7.3.
10. Lysis buffer: 0.32M sucrose, 10 mM Tris base, pH 7.5, 5 mM MgCl$_2$, 1% (w/v) Triton-x100.
11. 10% SDS in ddH$_2$O.
12. Proteinase K solution: proteinase K dissolved in autoclaved 0.075M NaCl, 0.024M EDTA, pH 7.5 at a concentration of 10 mg/mL.
13. Sodium acetate (NaAc): 3M, pH7.0.
14. Phenol/Chloroform mixture: 1:1 ready mixed (purchased from Sigma-Aldrich). This mixture is TOXIC and should be handled with gloves in fume cupboard.
15. Choloroform.
16. Absolute alcohol (ethanol).
17. 70% ethanol: diluted in ddH$_2$O.
18. DNA *Taq* polymerase enzyme.
19. KCl, 10X *Taq* polymerase buffer (supplied with the DNA *Taq* polymerase enzyme).
20. Deoxynucleotide triphosphates mixture (dNTP's): 1.25 mM dATP, 1.25 mM dCTP, 1.25 mM dGTP, 1.25 mM dTTP.
21. Loading buffer: 40% sucrose, 0.025% w/v bromophenol blue, 0.025% w/v xylene cyanol.
22. Ethidium bromide (EtBr) solution: 10 mg dissolved in distilled H$_2$O. HIGHLY TOXIC, handle with care. Store in a dark bottle at 4°C.
23. 10X TBE running buffer: 890 mM Tris-HCl, pH 8.0, 890 mM boric acid, 200 mM EDTA (disodium salt).
24. Fixation solution: 2% formaldehyde, 0.2% glutaraldehyde, in PBS.
25. X-gal substrate solution: 5 mM potassium ferricyanide, 5 mM potassium ferrocyanide, 2 mM magnesium chloride, in PBS.

Store SDS, NaAc solutions, chloroform, absolute alcohol, and bacterial lysis buffer at room temperature (RT). Store DNA template(s), loading buffer, lysis buffer, LB broth, LB agar plates, bacterial resuspension buffer, and bacterial neutralization buffer, in a refrigerator or cold room (4°C). Other solutions should be stored at –20°C.

3. Methods

3.1. Preparation of Plasmid DNA

3.1.1. E. coli Cultures Transformation and Glycerol Stock Preparation

Plasmids are introduced into *E. coli* by a process know as transformation. This process can be used for any plasmid. The transformed bacteria are then selected twice on Lauria-Bertani agar plates containing the appropriate antibiotic. For example, in the following procedure, the antibiotic used is ampicillin. Small LB liquid cultures are then prepared and used for preparation of glycerol stocks of the transformed bacteria. Note that all the following steps should be carried out close to a flame.

1. Defrost a 100-µL *E. coli* aliquot on ice.
2. Flame mouth of the tube containing the bacteria then using a sterile loop and close to the flame, introduce a small quantity of the plasmid (dissolved in TE) onto the bacteria by dipping the loop into the *E. coli* aliquot. Recap the tube and mix contents by gentle shaking. Centrifuge tube briefly (pulse centrifugation) in a microfuge then place on ice for 30 min.
3. Close to the flame and using a sterile tip, transfer the bacterial aliquot onto an LB agar plate containing ampicillin. Using a sterile loop or glass spreader, spread the bacteria on the surface of the agar.
4. Incubate the plate overnight at 37°C. The next day, using a sterile loop, pick a single well isolated colony and spread it on another fresh LB agar plate/ampicillin. Incubate plate overnight at 37°C. Seal the first plate using "para-film" and place in the refrigerator for up to 1 mo.
5. The following day, in two sterile universal tubes (10-mL sample tubes), place 5 mL LB broth in each. Add 5 µL of ampicillin stock solution and using a sterile loop, transfer a well isolated colony from the plate to each of the two tubes. Recap tubes and mix the contents by vigorous shaking, then place in a shaking incubator, overnight at 37°C. Seal the plate and store in fridge.
6. The following cultures should be turbid because of bacterial growth. Label two "cryo-tubes" with the name of the plasmid and date. Close to a flame, place 1.5 mL of culture in corresponding cryo-tube, then add 300 µL glycerol. Recap the cryo-tubes and mix contents by inversion (6–7 times). Store tubes in –80°C. Part of the remaining 3.5 mL of the culture will be used in confirmatory tests (**Subheadings 3.1.2.** and **3.2.5.**).

3.1.2. Confirmation of Successful Transformation

Subheading 3.1.1., steps 3 and **4**, confirm that transformation was successful because the *E. coli* was able to grow on plates containing an antibiotic, i.e., the bacteria became resistant. A more reliable way for confirmation of successful transformation would be restriction enzyme (endonuclease) digestion. The supplier of the plasmid(s) should provide a schematic map for the plasmid, which would show the insertion site (cloning site) of the gene of interest, e.g., wt-*p53*. Also, this map would show the restriction enzyme sites that could be used to confirm the "structure" of the plasmid. For example, *Bam*HI (**Fig. 2**) could be used to digest the wt-*p53* plasmid (8.4 kb in length) resulting in two DNA fragments of 1.8 kb of wt-*p53* gene and 6.6 kb of vector.

1. Transfer 1.5 mL of each LB culture into a microfuge tube (1.5-mL or 2-mL tube), and centrifuge tubes at high speed for 1.5 min.
2. Carefully remove supernatant and centrifuge tubes for few seconds, then remove any remaining traces of supernatant.
3. Using a vortex, resuspend pellet in 150 μL of bacterial resuspension buffer.
4. Add 150 μL bacterial lysis buffer and mix contents by gently inverting the tube (6–7 times). Do not vortex.
5. Add 150 μL neutralisztion buffer and mix contents by inverting the tube (about 10 times), followed by centrifugation at a high speed and 4°C for 5 min.
6. Carefully and without disturbing the pellet, transfer the supernatant into a fresh microfuge tube. Precipitate the plasmid DNA by adding 1.0 mL ice-cold absolute alcohol. Mix by inverting the tubes about 10 times.
7. Centrifuge tube at high speed and 4°C for 5 min. Then remove supernatant and remove all traces of the supernatant.
8. Let air-dry for about 2 min, then resuspend pellet in 40 μL TE by gentle tapping.
9. Transfer 20 μL plasmid solution into a fresh microfuge tube, then digest the sample with the appropriate restriction enzyme(s), (*see* **Subheading 3.2.5.**).
10. Prepare 0.8% agarose gel (*see* **Note 11**) and run samples of the undigested and digested plasmid, alongside a DNA marker ladder. Check for the presence of bands at the expected lengths. One band should appear in the lane of undigested plasmid and more than one band in the lane of digested plasmid depending on the enzyme(s) used (*see* **Fig. 2**) and number of sites.

3.1.3. Plasmid Extraction and Sterilization

3.1.3.1. PLASMID EXTRACTION

Commercially available plasmid extraction kits are reliable and easy to use. The kits used in the pilot study carried out by Habib et al. *(8)*, were purchased from Qiagen Ltd., Chatsworth, CA. The following steps will explain the preparation of large cultures required for use with any plasmid extraction kit or protocol.

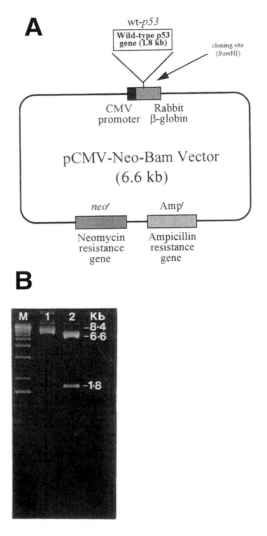

Fig. 2. **(A)** A schematic of pC53-SN3 plasmid, and **(B)** *Bam*HI restriction (endonuclease) enzyme digestion of pC53-SN3 plasmid. Lane M: 1 kb DNA markers ladder; lane 2: plasmid before digestion, and lane 3: plasmid after digestion.

1. In sterile universal tubes, place 10 mL LB broth per tube, then add 10 µL ampicillin stock solution. Using a sterile loop, transfer a "pinch" of the bacterial glycerol stock into each of the tubes. Recap tubes and mix contents by vigorous shaking, then place in a shaking incubator overnight, at 37°C. The contents of each tube will be used to seed 250–500 mL LB broth.
2. The following day, use 2 L sterile conical glass flasks to prepare large cultures. The number of flasks used will depend on the amount of plasmid to be prepared

and kit used. Use 500 mL LB broth per flask. Add 500 µL ampicillin stock solution, followed by a single 10-mL culture from **step 1**. Recap the flasks and incubate flasks in a shaking incubator (200–250 throws per min) overnight, at 37°C.

3. Pellet the bacterial cells in large centrifuge bottles. The speed of centrifugation will depend on the bottles type and the plasmid extraction protocol used. Follow the instructions supplied with the extraction kit.
4. Dissolve the plasmid in TE. The volume depends on the expected amount of extracted plasmid. The final plasmid concentration should be ≥ 1 µg/µL.
5. The final product can be analysed using the restriction enzyme digestion technique (**Subheading 3.2.5.**).

3.1.3.2. PLASMID STERILIZATION

The following procedure must be carried out in a class II laminar flow cabinet.

1. Determine the exact plasmid DNA concentration using a spectrophotometer set for UV absorption at 260 nm. For example, dilute 10 µL concentrated plasmid in TE to a total volume of 1 mL. A reading of 1 corresponds to 50 µg of DNA (plasmid or genomic). Work out the original concentration of the undiluted solution.
2. In the laminar flow cabinet, dilute the plasmid using sterile TE to give a final concentration of about 1 µg/mL. Using a sterile disposable syringe, filter the solution through a sterile 0.2-µm filter in a sterile universal tube. Repeat the filtration step. At this point, the sterilized solution can be stored at 4°C until use.
3. Samples of the sterilised plasmid should be tested for bacterial, viral, and mycoplasma contamination.

3.2. Patients and Treatment with wt-p53 Naked Plasmid DNA

3.2.1. Patients

1. Confirm malignancy histologically.
2. Perform CT scan before and after treatment. Monitoring of tumor size is always reported on the injected lesion. Also monitor the appearance and progress of other untreated lesion(s), if present.
3. Check the level of one of the appropriate tumor markers before and after treatment. For example in case of HCC patients, use serum AFP.
4. Prior to and following the wt-*p53* injections, all patients should have: full blood count, serum electrolytes, urea, creatinine, liver function, and coagulation profiles.
5. On the day of treatment, specially postinjection, all patients should be monitored for pulse, blood pressure, central venous pressure, urine output, and body temperature.
6. Patients should sign a consent form. This form should explain the nature of the procedures, the risks involved, and the unproven results of this therapeutic approach.

7. Most of the patients would be discharged on the same day of the procedure. The complications that may be observed include transient fever, hypotension, or hypertension. These side effects are expected to last for about 2 h and usually cease without treatment. Some patients might require hospitalization for 24 h.

3.2.2. Therapeutic Protocol

1. The first injection would be a single injection of 2 mg naked wt-*p53* plasmid DNA.
2. Inject plasmid percutaneously and intratumorally under CT scan.
3. Consider 50% reduction in serum AFP level and 50% diminution of tumor volume post-treatment, as a positive response. When estimating the volume of tumor, always use the greater diameter measured on CT scan.
4. Patients showing positive response or stable disease could be offered further injections at monthly intervals.
5. Two core biopsies of the treated lesion ~36 h postinjection could be analyzed for gene transfer and expression. Immediately place each biopsy in a labeled cryotube and snap-freeze in liquid nitrogen. At this point, the biopsies could be stored in a –80°C freezer or processed for DNA and/or RNA extraction. Make use of the marker gene(s) of the plasmid, e.g., *neo*[r] or *lacZ*.

3.2.3. Use of lacZ as a Marker Gene and β-galactosidase Activity Analysis

The genes of interest (e.g., *p53*) could be obtained already cloned in vectors that express *lacZ* marker gene, other than the antibiotic resistance genes. Well-established molecular biology laboratories could be asked to clone the gene of interest into a vector that expresses the *lacZ* gene.

1. Thirty-six h postinjection, a core biopsy of the treated lesion is obtained and split into two halves. One half is placed in a cryo-tube and immediately snap-frozen in liquid nitrogen. This sample could be analyzed biochemically for β-galactosidase activity using a commercially available β-galactosidase assay kits or published protocols. The other half is immediately processed for histochemical analysis (*see* **steps 4–8**).
2. Cut 5-μm frozen sections in the specimens. These sections are then stained using the chromogenic substrate X-gal (*9*).
3. On each tissue section, place 100 μL of fixation solution and incubate for 10 min at RT.
4. Remove fixation solution, then wash sections by placing 300 μL PBS, for 2 min at RT, then discard PBS. Repeat the washing step twice.
5. Remove traces of PBS around the sections using a filter paper.
6. Place the slides on 3–4 layers of water-moistened filter paper inside a "lunch box." Place 100 μL X-gal staining solution on each section and cover the box with the lid. Gently place the box in an incubator at 37°C for 4–5 h.

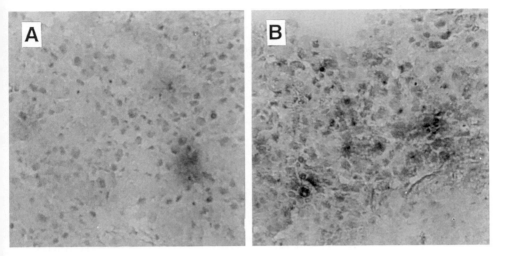

Fig. 3. Histochemical detection of β-galactosidase activity in 5-μm frozen sections in HCC tumors grown subcutaneously in nude mice. Thirty-six h posttreatment **(A)** control tumors injected with buffer and **(B)** tumors injected with a single dose of 50 μg of naked β-gal plasmid DNA. The sections were counter-stained with light haematoxylin and eosin.

7. Remove the staining solution. Gently and briefly, dip sections in PBS (in a beaker).
8. The sections are ready to be counter-stained with light haematoxylin/eosin. Then examine the sections under a light microscope (×100 or ×200 magnification). The cells showing high activity of β-galactosidase activity will stain blue (**Fig. 3**). The percentage of blue-stained cells can be worked out. In fact, if nontumor biopsies are processed/stained in the same way, you might not see any blue-stained cells in the section because all the cells should have low enzymatic activity.

3.2.4. DNA Extraction

1. Crush the frozen tissue specimen inside the cryo-tube using a sterile glass rod. Split the crushed tissue into two equal parts and store one part at –80°C which will be used in RNA extraction. Process the other part as follows.
2. Add 0.5 mL lysis buffer (containing 0.5% SDS per mL). Add 100 μg proteinase K per mL and recap the tubes. Place tubes in a shaking incubator (gentle shaking, about 70–80 throws per minute) at 37°C overnight.
3. Transfer the digested sample into a fresh sterile 1.5-mL microfuge tube. Add equal volume of phenol:chloroform and 1/10 volume NaAc and mix contents using a roller or gyratory shaker for 15 min, at RT.
4. Centrifuge tubes at 7000*g* and RT for 10 min, then carefully, without disturbing interface layer, transfer the top aqueous layer into a fresh microfuge tube.
5. Add equal volume of phenol:chloroform and mix on a shaker for 15 min at RT.

6. Repeat **steps 4** and **5** until no interface layer is visible. Finally, transfer the aqueous layer into a fresh microfuge tube.

7. Precipitate DNA by adding an equal volume of ice-cold absolute alcohol and mix by inversion (about 10 times), then place in –20°C freezer overnight. At this point, tubes can be stored in freezer for several months.

8. If DNA is required, then centrifuge tubes at 7000g and 4°C for 10 min. Discard supernatant, then resuspend DNA pellet in 0.5 mL 70% alcohol.

9. Transfer the suspension into a sterile 1.5-mL microfuge tube and centrifuge at 7,000g and RT for 10 min.

10. Discard supernatant and let pellets air-dry for 2–3 min, then resuspend each pellet in 0.5 mL TE. Resuspension could be done by gentle tapping. Place tubes in the refrigerator to allow DNA to dissolve slowly.

3.2.5. Restriction Enzyme Digestion of DNA

1. Place ~5 μg DNA sample (plasmid DNA, genomic DNA, and PCR product) in a microfuge, then add: 4 μL 10X buffer (supplied with enzyme), 20 U restriction enzyme. Add ddH$_2$O to make up total volume to 40 μL, then mix contents by gentle tapping.

2. Centrifuge tube for 1 s (pulse centrifugation), then place the tubes at the appropriate optimal temperature for the enzyme used for about 4 h. Sometimes a longer period of incubation is required. In fact, to ensure that digestion is complete, the tubes could be incubated overnight.

3. Analyze samples of undigested and digested DNA agarose gel electrophoresis alongside a DNA marker ladder. Prepare agarose gel of appropriate percentage, depending on the length of the DNA fragments.

3.2.6. Use of neo ^{r} as a Marker Gene

Tumor biopsies can be analyzed for exogenous gene transfer and expression by using the neomycin resistance gene as a marker gene.

3.2.6.1. DETECTION OF GENE TRANSFER USING PCR TECHNIQUE

Ensure that all diposable tips, tubes and plasticware, and solutions used are sterile. Use fresh tips when pipeting the various solutions and samples. The following protocol is used with a thermocycler (PCR machine) that does not require mineral oil to be placed on top of reaction mixture. If mineral oil is required, then carefully and gently place a drop of the oil on the surface of reaction mixture in each tube.

1. Dilute each DNA sample in sterile ddH$_2$O to a final concentration of ~25 ng/μL. Place 10 μL sample in the reaction tube.

2. In a sterile 1.5-mL microfuge tube, prepare sufficient "master mix" solution for the samples to be analyzed. For example: 5 μL 10X reaction buffer, 8 μL dNTP's mixture, 1 μL primer1, 1 μL primer2, ~24.5 μL sterile ddH$_2$O, ~2 U *Taq* poly-

merase (~0.5 µL, depending on the concentration of the polymerase). Mix contents of tube by gentle tapping, followed by brief centrifugation.

3. Add 40 µL master mix to each DNA sample. A negative control tube can be included in which 10 µL sterile ddH$_2$O are used instead of DNA. Gently triturate samples (mixing sample by up/down pipeting). Cap the tubes and place in PCR machine and start the run. For example, to detect a 791 bp fragment of *neo^r* (**Fig. 4**), the following primers (*10*) and PCR cycles could be used:

primer1 (forward): 5′ CAA GAT GGA TTG CAC GCA GG 3′
primer2 (reverse): 5′ CCC GCT CAG AAG AAC TCG TC 3′

PCR cycles: 1X cycle   5 min at 94°C
             30X cycles   1 min at 94°C (denaturing)
                          2 min at 64°C (annealing)
                          3 min at 72°C (extension)
            1X cycle   7 min at 72°C

4. The final product can be stored at 4°C until analyzed, or samples of the PCR products and their *Pst*I restriction enzyme digestion products could be analyzed on a 1% agarose gel (**Fig. 5**).

3.2.6.2. DETECTION OF GENE EXPRESSION USING RT-PCR TECHNIQUE

Reverse transcriptase polymerase chain reaction (RT-PCR) can be used to find out if a gene has been expressed or not. Many commercially available kits could be used to carry out RT-PCR. Most of these kits are easy to use and reliable. This technique involves the extraction of messenger RNA (mRNA) from cells/tissue using, e.g., Micro-FastTrack mRNA Isolation Kit (Invitrogen, San Diego, CA) and reverse transcribe it into complementary DNA (cDNA) using, e.g., cDNA Cycle Kit (Invitrogen).

1. Extract mRNA from treated and control tissues.
2. Reverse transcribe the mRNA into cDNA.
3. Analyze samples of the cDNA using the *neo^r* PCR primers (**Subheading 3.2.6.1.**).
4. Digest samples of the PCR products using *Pst*I restriction enzyme.
5. Analyze the PCR and digestion products on agarose gel (**Fig. 5**).
6. The results should show if there is gene expression or not.

4. Notes

1. All buffers/solutions are prepared in deionised distilled water (ddH$_2$O) and autoclaved wherever appropriate.
2. Dissolve SDS by slow mixing in order to avoid foaming. Do not attempt to autoclave SDS solution, as autoclaving leads to foaming. SDS precipitates at low temperature or if placed in fridge by mistake. If precipitate is formed, warm up the solution under running hot water or by brief microwaving.
3. All tubes and disposables must be sterilized by autoclaving wherever appropriate or purchased ready sterile.

Fig. 4. The neomycin resistance gene sequence. Obtained from the database at European Molecular Biology Laboratory (EMBL) through the World Wide Web. P1: sequence of forward primer, Primer1; P2: complementary sequence to reverse primer, Primer2.

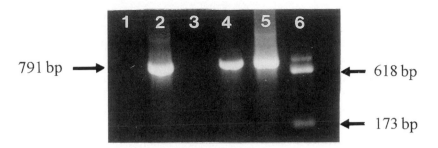

Fig. 5. An example for PCR amplification products of *neo*[r] gene, analyzed on 1% agarose gel. Control samples (lane 1: DNA and lane 3: cDNA) and treatment samples (lane 2: DNA and lane 4: cDNA). Lane 5: pC53-SN3 DNA sample as positive control for *neo*[r]. Lane 6: *Pst*I digestion products.

4. Defrost all solutions/mixtures required for PCR reactions at RT. During use, place defrosted solutions/mixtures on ice until ready to place back in freezer. Always keep the *Taq* polymerase in the freezer until it is required to be added to PCR reaction, then immediately place back in freezer.

5. Preparation of agar plates: place 100 mL LB broth in an autoclavable glass bottle, then add 0.7 g agar and sterilize by autoclaving. Allow to cool to ~45°C, then add the appropriate amount of antibiotic and mix contents by gentle shaking. Close to a flame pour about 20–25 mL molten agar/LB into each 10-cm Petri dish. Allow plates to set (cool to RT), then place dishes upside down in an incubator overnight at 37°C. The following day, label the dishes on the bottom surface with the antibiotic's name. Seal dishes with parafilm and store in the refrigerator until use.

6. Bacterial plates should be clearly labeled on bottom surface with the full name of the plasmid and date because you may need to use them again, if the small cultures (5 mL) were not successful.

7. X-gal stock solution is colorless. Discard solution if it shows a light pink coloration.

8. Always keep a bottle of absolute alcohol (about 200 mL) in –20°C freezer, required for the DNA precipitation.

9. Formalin-fixed tumor biopsies pre- and posttreatment could also be analyzed immunohistochemically for *p53* activity.

10. The endotoxin (lipopolysaccharides) level in the final plasmid product obtained using Qiagen kits is usually less than the level set by the FDA. Endotoxin-free plasmid extraction kits are commercially available, e.g., from Qiagen.

11. Preparation of agarose gel: place the appropriate volume of 1X TBE in a conical flask and add the agarose (weight depends on % required). Microwave for about 1–2 min and let stand until temperature is about 50°C. Add 0.5 µL of EtBr per 10 mL of prepared gel. Gently swirl the mixture. Pour mixture into the casting "boat," insert comb and let stand at RT for ~45 min. Place sample(s) in fresh microfuge tube(s), add half volume of loading buffer and mix by gentle tapping. Carefully, remove comb and place gel in the electrophoresis tank. Pour 1X TBE

on gel until its level about 2–3 mm above surface of gel, ensuring that there are no air bubbles trapped in wells. Place samples in the wells. The amount of sample depends on tooth width of comb used. Load 1 µL sample (PCR or digestion products) per mm of tooth width.

12. Change gloves often and use freshly sterilized microfuge tubes, disposables, and solutions/ddH$_2$O as contamination is possible especially with PCR/RT-PCR work.

13. Disposing EtBr and cleaning contaminated/spillage areas are carried out according the regulations and rules set by the senior staff in charge of the laboratory.

14. If dark bottles are not available, wrap the tube or bottle in alimunium foil. Do not forget to label both the bottle and the wrapper.

Acknowledgments

We thank Dr. Bert Vogelstein for kindly providing the wt-*p53* plasmid.

References

1. Lotze, M. T., Flickinger, J. C., and Carr, B. I. (1993) Hepatobiliary neoplasm in *Cancer: Principles and Practice of Oncology,* 4th ed. (DeVita, V. T. Jr., Hellman, S., and Rosenberg, S. A., eds.), J. B. Lippincott, Philadelphia, PA, pp. 883–914.

2. Okuda, K. and Okuda, H. (1991) Primary liver cell carcinoma, in *Oxford Textbook of Clinical Hepatology* (McIntyre, N., Benhamou, J.-P., Bircher, J., Rizzetto, M., and Rodes, J., eds.). Oxford University Press, Oxford, England, pp. 1019–1053.

3. Sherlock, S. and Dooley, J. (1993) *Diseases of the Liver and Biliary System.* 9th ed. Blackwell Scientific, Oxford, England.

4. Anderson, W. F. (1984) Prospects for human gene therapy. *Science* **226,** 401–409.

5. Miler, A. D. (1992) Human gene therapy comes of age. *Nature* **357,** 455–460.

6. Schofield, J. P. and Caskey, C. T. (1995) Non-viral approaches to gene therapy. *Br. Med. Bulletin.* **5,** 56–71.

7. Wolff, J. A., Malone, R. W., Williams, P., Chong, W., Acsadi, G., Jani, A., and Felgner, P. L. (1990) Direct gene transfer into mouse muscle in vivo. *Science* **247,** 1465–1468.

8. Habib, N. A., Ding, S.-F., El-Masry, R., Mitry, R. R., Honda, K., Michail, N. E., et al. (1996) Preliminary report: the short-term effects of direct p53 DNA injection in primary hepatocellular carinomas. *Cancer Detect. Preven.* **20,** 103–107.

9. Rols, M.-P., Dahhou, F., and Teissié, J. (1994) Pulse-first heterofusion of cells by electric field pulses and associated loading of macromolecules into mammalian cells. *BioTechniques* **17,** 762–769.

10. Rill, D. R., Moen, R. C., Buschle, M., Bartholomew, C., Foreman, N. K., Mirro, J., et al. (1992) An approach for the analysis of relapse and marrow reconstitution after autologous marrow transplantation using retrovirus-mediated gene transfer. *Blood* **79,** 2694–2700.

Further Reading

Sambrook, J., Fritsch, E. F., and Maniatis, T. (1989) *Molecular Cloning: A Laboratory Manual.* Cold Spring Harbor Laboratory, New York.

36

A Phase II Trial of Intratumoral Injection with a Selectively Replicating Adenovirus (ONYX-015) in Patients with Recurrent, Refractory Squamous Cell Carcinoma of the Head and Neck

David H. Kirn

1. Introduction

Selectively replicating viruses may offer a new approach to cancer treatment. If successful in clinical trials, these agents will constitute a new category in the antitumoral armamentarium. Many viruses are currently being studied, and an adenovirus (ONYX-015) first entered clinical trials in 1996; herpesvirus agents are scheduled to enter clinical trials in 1998. Critical issues need to be addressed if the utility of these agents is to be optimized. For each virus, the effect of antiviral immunity on antitumoral efficacy must be better understood. For all viruses, physical barriers to spread within tumors (e.g., fibrosis, pressure gradients) must be overcome. Although proof-of-concept experiments with chemotherapy and ONYX-015 have been encouraging, further studies are required to determine optimal treatment-regimen sequencing. Combination studies with radiation therapy are also underway with ONYX-015. Finally, these agents may require modification (e.g., coat modification) in order to maximize effectiveness against systemic metastases following intravenous administration.

1.1. Preclinical Development of ONYX-015

p53 is mutated in roughly 50% of all human cancers, including nonsmall cell lung (60%), colon (50%), breast (40%), head and neck (60%), and ovarian (60%), cancers in the advanced stages. Loss of *p53* function is associated with

From: *Methods in Molecular Medicine, Vol. 35: Gene Therapy: Methods and Protocols*
Edited by: W. Walther and U. Stein © Humana Press, Inc., Totowa, NJ

resistance to chemotherapy and/or decreased survival in numerous tumor types, including breast, colon, bladder, ovarian, and nonsmall cell lung cancers. Therefore, effective therapies for tumors that lack functional *p53* are clearly needed.

p53 mediates cell cycle arrest and/or apoptosis in response to DNA damage (e.g., owing to chemotherapy or radiation) or foreign DNA synthesis (e.g., during virus replication). Consequently, DNA tumor viruses such as adenovirus, SV40, and human papilloma virus encode for proteins that inactivate *p53* and thereby allow efficient viral replication. For example, the adenovirus E1B-region 55 kD protein binds and inactivates *p53*, in complex with the E4orf6 protein. Because *p53* function must be blocked in order to allow efficient virus replication, Dr. Frank McCormick hypothesized that an adenovirus lacking E1B, 55 kDa gene expression might be severely limited in its ability to replicate in normal cells; however, cancer cells that lack *p53* function should support virus replication and resultant cell destruction. ONYX-015 (ONYX Pharmaceuticals, Richmond, CA) is an attenuated adenovirus type 2/5 chimera (dl1520) with two mutations in the early region E1B, 55 kDa gene; this virus was created in the laboratory of Dr. Arnie Berk *(1)*. The cytopathic effects of wild-type adenovirus and ONYX-015 were studied on a pair of cell lines that are identical except for *p53* function: the RKO human colon cancer cell line with normal *p53* function (the parent line), and an RKO subclone transfected with dominant-negative *p53* (courtesy of Dr. Michael Kastan) *(2)*. As predicted, ONYX-015 induced cytopathic effects identical to wild-type adenovirus in the subclone lacking functional *p53*, whereas cytopathic effects with ONYX-015 were reduced by approximately two orders of magnitude in the parental tumor line harboring normal *p53*. Subsequently, a tumor cell line that was resistant to ONYX-015 because of normal *p53* function (U2OS), became sensitive to ONYX-015 following transfection and expression of the E1B, 55 kDa gene. Therefore, ONYX-015 is able to replicate selectively in *p53*-deficient cancer cells resulting from a deletion in the E1B, 55 kDa gene.

Subsequent experiments demonstrated that primary (nonimmortalized) human endothelial cells, fibroblasts, small airway cells, and mammary epithelial cells highly resistant to ONYX-015 replication and cytolysis, in contrast to effects seen with wild-type adenovirus *(3)*. Replication-dependent cytopathic effects were demonstrated in human tumor cell lines of many different histologies following infection with ONYX-015. Tumor cells that lack *p53* function through different mechanisms (*p53* gene mutation and/or deletion, or *p53* degradation by human papilloma virus E6 protein) were shown to be destroyed by ONYX-015. In addition, several carcinoma lines with normal *p53* gene sequence, including two chemotherapy-resistant ovarian cancer subclones, were efficiently lysed. ONYX-015 had significant in vivo antitumoral activity against subcutaneous (sc) human tumor xenografts in nude mice following intratumoral or intravenous injection. The in vivo efficacy against each tumor type correlated with the in vitro sensitivity of the cell line to ONYX-015. Efficacy against intraperitoneal (ip) carcinoma was documented following ip virus administration (C. Heise and D. Kirn, publication pending). Because of the lack of efficient replication in rodent cells, however, immunocompetent (syngeneic) tumor models have not been useful for studying replication-dependent effects. Therefore, the role of the antiviral and antitumoral immune responses may only be determined in cancer patients until a novel model is developed.

2. Clinical Development of ONYX-015

ONYX-015 is a novel agent with a novel mechanism of action *(3)*. We predicted that both toxicity and efficacy would be dependent on the intrinsic ability of a given tumor to replicate the virus, to the location of the tumor to be treated (e.g., intracranial vs peripheral), and to the route of administration of the virus. In addition, data on viral replication, antiviral immune responses, and their relationship to antitumoral efficacy were critical in the early stages of development. We, therefore, elected to treat patients with recurrent head and neck carcinomas initially.

2.1. Phase I Trial: Head and Neck Cancer

The rationale for targeting this population as follows. These tumors are frequently amenable to direct injection and biopsy in the outpatient clinic setting. *p53* abnormalities are very common; gene mutations or deletions are present in up to 70% of recurrent tumors *(4,5)*, and other *p53*-inactivating mechanisms such as mdm-2 overexpression and HPV E6 expression appear to be present in another 15–20% of these tumors. Finally, most patients suffer severe morbidity, and even mortality, from the local/regional progression of these tumors. Up to two-thirds of these patients die because of local complications. Therefore, a local therapy might lead to significant palliation and even survival prolongation.

Patients enrolled onto the phase I trial had recurrent squamous cell carcinoma of the head and neck that was not surgically curable and had failed either prior to radiation or chemotherapy *(6)*. *p53* gene sequence and immunohistochemical staining were determined on all tumors, but were not used as entry criteria. Other baseline tests included lymphocyte subsets (CD3, 4, 8), delayed-type hypersensitivity skin testing (including mumps and candida), and neutralizing antibodies to ONYX-015. This was a standard phase I dose escalation trial in which at least three patients are treated per dose level prior to escalation to the next cohort; intrapatient dose escalation was not allowed. Six patient cohorts received single intratumoral injections of ONYX-015 every 4 wk (until progression) at doses from 10^7 to 10^{11} PFU per dose. Two additional cohorts received five consecutive daily doses of 10^9 or 10^{10} per day (total dose 5×10^9 or 5×10^{10}) every 4 wk. Following treatment, patients were observed for toxicity and for target (injected) tumor response. Additional biological end points included changes in neutralizing antibodies, the presence of virus in the blood (PCR days 3, 8), viral replication within the injected tumor (in tumor biopsies on days 8 and 22), and associated immune cell infiltration.

No significant toxicity was seen in any of the 32 patients treated. Eleven patients received repeat treatments (2–7 total). Grade 3 tumor site pain was noted on a single occasion in one patient. Otherwise, tumor-injection site pain was either nonexistent or mild. Flu-like symptoms were noted in approximately one-third of patients on the single-dose regimen and two-thirds of patients on the daily X 5 regimen. Symptoms included low grade fevers (less than 38.5°C), grade 1–2 myalgias and grade 1 nausea. Symptoms typically started within 12 to 24 h of injection and lasted for 1–5 d. Following ONYX-015-induced tumor necrosis, nonbleeding ulcerations developed over several injected tumors. However, no significant local complications occurred.

Neutralizing antibodies were positive in approximately 70% of the cases prior to treatment. Following treatment, all patients had positive antibody titers, and all patients had an increase in antibody titer. Replication was identified infrequently on day 8 tumor biopsies in patients on the single injection protocol, whereas day 8 biopsies were almost uniformly positive in tumors from patients on the multidose regimen. Day 22 biopsies were negative for viral replication.

Three of the 23 patients on the single-dose regimen had formal partial responses (PR) of the injected tumor and nine had tumor stabilization (8+–16+ wk). In addition, three patients with stable disease had ≥50% necrosis of the injected tumor. In contrast, three of nine patients on the multidose regimen had PR's and an additional three had stabilization with significant necrosis; only two patients had progressive disease. One patient received seven treatments over 7 mo while maintaining a partial remission. These results are consistent with experiments comparing these two regimens in nude mouse human tumor xenograft models (D. Kirn, publication pending). Responding patients included some with positive baseline neutralizing antibodies and tumors with a normal *p53* gene sequence. However, definitive correlations between these variables and the degree of tumor response cannot be made until larger phase II trials are completed.

2.2. Phase II trial: Head and Neck Cancer

Based on these results, two phase II trials in head and neck cancer patients were initiated. In a study using ONYX-015 treatment alone, approximately 30 patients refractory to chemotherapy or radiotherapy following recurrence are being treated with ONYX-015 alone; final data are pending. This clinical trial protocol is the subject of this chapter. In a second phase II trial, patients are treated simultaneously over 5 d with ONYX-015 intratumorally and cisplatin (day 1 bolus) and continuous infusion 5-fluorouracil (days 1–5) intravenously. These patients are all chemotherapy-naive in the setting of recurrent disease.

3. Material and Methods

3.1. ONYX-015 Viral Therapeutic Construct and Production

ONYX-015 is an E1B-55 kDa gene-deleted adenovirus that selectively replicates in and lyses *p53*-deficient tumor cells. The virus contains a deletion between nucleotides 2496 and 3323 in the E1B region encoding the 55 kDa protein. In addition, a C to T transition at position 2022 in E1B generates a stop codon at the third codon position of the protein. These alterations eliminate expression of the E1B 55 kDa gene in ONYX-015 infected cells. Viruses were grown in the human embryonic kidney cell line HEK293 and purified by CsCl gradient ultracentrifugation as previously described.

3.2. Study

3.2.1. Objectives

1. Primary End Points
   - Objective response rate of injected target tumors: Percent of patients with PRs or complete responses (CRs).
   - Pain response rate: Percent of patients with a 50% reduction in pain or pain medication usage ($\geq$4 wk): pain assessment by visual analog pain scale.
   - Safety of intratumoral injections of ONYX-015: assessment of local, systemic toxicities
2. Secondary End Points
   - Progression-free survival
   - Survival
   - Quality of life (assessed by EORTC global QLQ-C30 and EORTC disease specific QLQ -H&N35)
   - Performance status response: Percent of patients with a $\geq$20 point increase in Karnofsky performance status ($\geq$ 4 wk).
   - Immune response: neutralizing antibody response

3.2.2. Study Design

This phase II study is designed to evaluate the efficacy and safety of Onyx's attenuated adenovirus, ONYX-015, when administered intratumorally to patients with recurrent and refractory head and neck cancer. Patients eligible for study participation will have unresectable disease, which is refractory to at least one prior chemotherapeutic regimen and/or radiation therapy. The efficacy of ONYX-015 treatment will be evaluated based on the injected tumor(s) response. The clinical benefit of ONYX-015 will be evaluated through quality-of-life assessment (EORTC instrument), Karnofsky performance score, and pain assessment. Survival and progression-free survival intervals will also be recorded. The humoral (antibody-mediated) immune response will be evaluated to determine its potential for affecting efficacy or safety.

3.2.2.1. ONYX-015 DOSAGES AND DOSING RATIONALE

Eligible patients will be treated with ONYX-015 administered daily for 5 d at a dose of 10^{10} pfu per day. This was the highest dose administered daily for 5 d in the phase I study and was shown to be safe (i.e., no dose-limiting toxicities).

3.2.2.2. TREATMENT WITH ONYX-015

a. Dosing Regimen: For administration of each dose of ONYX-015, patients will be treated and observed in a properly equipped outpatient clinic. The target tumor will be injected with 10^{10} PFU of ONYX-015 daily over 5 d (i.e., a total dose 5×10^{10} PFU) (with day 1 being the first day of ONYX-015 injection (*see* **Note 1**). Nontarget tumor(s) (where applicable) may be injected with either diluent or ONYX-015 on the same days in identical fashion to the target tumor following the guidelines detailed in **steps 2c** and **3** below.

b. Target Tumor Masses: The dominant, symptom-causing tumor (if symptoms are present) should be identified as the target tumor and should be the only tumor injected with ONYX-015 during the first two treatment cycles. The identification of the most symptomatic, problematic lesion is based on the judgement of the Principal Investigator. Multinodular, but contiguous tumors can be treated and evaluated as a single lesion.

c. Secondary, Nontarget Tumor Masses: If additional, smaller, accessible lesions are present, these lesions may be injected with diluent for the first two treatment cycles as described in **step 3** below. Thereafter, treatments may be divided between up to three separate lesions (i.e., the initial two cycles must be concentrated within the dominant lesion; thereafter, 6 wk after treatment initiation, two additional secondary lesions may be injected). However, the total dose to the patient will remain the same (i.e., the same total dose will be divided up between the tumors to be treated); the total volume in which the ONYX-015 is suspended will be increased based on the total tumor volume of the tumors to be treated. If a

CR occurs in a treated lesion, injections can be continued as outlined above with newly defined dominant and secondary lesions.

d. Immediate Posttreatment Monitoring of Patients: The patient's vital signs will be taken ≤15 min before each ONYX-015 injection. After each injection is completed, the patient will be observed in the clinic for a minimum of 30 min. Vital signs will be taken after 30 min ± 5 min. If vital sign(s) have changed by >15%, vital signs will be repeated every 30 min until returning to within baseline 15% of baseline values. Following the observation period, the patient will be sent home or hospitalized overnight at the discretion of the investigator.

3.2.2.3. REPEAT TREATMENT

At the discretion of the Principal Investigator, patients will be eligible for repeat treatment cycles of ONYX-015 at the same dosage every 3 wk (counting from the day 1 of the previous treatment cycle) if they meet the following criteria:

- No grade 4 toxicity with the prior treatment cycle of ONYX-015. Patients experiencing grade 4 toxicity will be eligible for repeat dosing at 10^8–10^9 PFU per day for 5 d at the discretion of the Principal Investigator after consultation with the Onyx Medical Director.
- No evidence of progressive disease at the target tumor site following at least two treatment cycles with ONYX-015.
- No interim development of any withdrawal criteria (**Subheading 3.2.3.**).

3.2.3. Study Population

3.2.3.1. SQUAMOUS CELL CARCINOMA OF THE HEAD AND NECK

Squamous cell carcinoma of the head and neck afflicts an estimated 125,000 patients annually in developed countries in Europe, North America, and the Far East. In the U.S., the annual incidence is estimated at 45,000 cases with 15,000 associated deaths. Head and neck tumors have been reported to harbor *p53* mutations in 45–70% of cases; both alcohol and tobacco use are associated with these mutations. Primary therapy for localized disease is surgery and adjuvant radiotherapy.

Tumors recur in approximately one-third of patients following surgery. In the majority of cases, they recur in the region of the original primary tumor and lead to severe morbidity because of pain and to oropharyngeal and laryngeal obstruction and the resultant difficulties in swallowing and speech. Once the cancer has recurred and/or metastasized, the patient is considered incurable. Palliative surgery is difficult and disfiguring, and further radiation therapy is not generally beneficial for more than a few months. Several chemotherapeutic agents have been used in recurrent squamous cell carcinoma of the head and neck. Combination regimens have been shown to induce responses in 30–40% of patients, but the therapy can be toxic and there is no clear impact on survival. Once a patient's tumor is refractory to chemotherapy and/or radiation therapy, the median life expectancy is 3 mo and tumor response rates to second or third-line chemotherapeutic agents are 15%. There remains an urgent need for more effective therapies for these terminally ill patients.

3.2.2.2. INCLUSION CRITERIA

For inclusion in this study, a patient must satisfy the following criteria:

Tumor status
- Histologically confirmed squamous cell carcinoma of the head and neck, including the oral cavity, pharynx, and larynx
- Recurrent disease, which is refractory to radiotherapy and/or chemotherapy. Recurrent disease refers to tumor that progresses following primary therapy (surgery and/or radiation and/or chemotherapy) and therefore may include locally advanced tumors which progress following primary treatment with surgery and/or radiation and/or chemotherapy.
- The entire tumor is amenable to direct injection in the clinic as described in the protocol
- Tumor amenable to measurement clinically and/or radiographically
- Tumor is unresectable (as defined by attending surgeon)

General
- Karnofsky Performance Status of ≥70% (**Subheading 3.2.6.**).
- Life expectancy of ≥3 mo.
- ≥18 yr of age (or the age of majority if different than 18 yr of age)
- Consent for study participation given before screening and treatment, as evidenced by patient's dated signature (or signature of legally acceptable representative, if patient unable to give informed consent).

3.2.3.3. EXCLUSION CRITERIA

Patients with any of the following will be excluded from the study:

- Ongoing active infection, including human immunodeficiency virus
- Viral syndrome diagnosed within the last 2 wk.
- Chemotherapy within the last 3 wk.
- Radiotherapy to the target tumor site within the last 4 wk.
- Concomitant hematological malignancy (e.g., chronic lymphocytic leukemia, non-Hodgkin's lymphoma).
- Impending airway obstruction or other condition requiring urgent (predicted within 2 wk) tumor debulking.
- Pregnant or lactating females.
- Prior participation in any research protocol, which involved administration of adenovirus vectors.

- Treatment with any other investigational therapy within the last 6 wk.
- Any condition that compromises compliance with the objectives and procedures of this protocol, as judged by the investigator.

3.2.3.4. WITHDRAWAL OF PATIENTS FROM STUDY

Patients may be withdrawn from the study, in terms of no further treatment with ONYX-015, for any of the reasons listed below. The day on which this occurs will be referenced as the "day withdrawn from study treatment." The last day on which the patient is seen will be considered the "day off study." In some case(s) these dates may be the same.

- Patient's decision to discontinue study participation.
- Intolerable adverse reaction(s) (judged to be either physically or psychologically detrimental to the patient).
- Intercurrent illness that may compromise the patient's safety or interfere with the evaluation of study treatment (e.g., chronic lymphocytic leukemia, non-Hodgkin's lymphoma).
- Impending airway obstruction or other condition requiring urgent tumor debulking.
- Requirement for urgent a) radiotherapy or b) chemotherapy (for the **target** tumor site).

  Note: For any ONYX-015 treated tumor showing stable disease or objective response, such tumor may continue to be treated with ONYX-015 even if the target tumor requires radiotherapy—at the Investigators discretion.
- Requirement for concomitant medication that may interfere with the evaluation of study treatment, including chronic immunosuppressive medication, e.g., glucocorticoid or cyclosporine, unless investigator and Onyx Medical Director or project manager mutually determine that patient's status warrants continuation on study treatment (*see* **Note 2**).

Pregnancy
- Clinical evidence of progressive disease at the *target* tumor site after a *minimum of 2 cycles of treatment.*
- Failure to comply with study procedures.
- Loss of patient to follow-up.

3.2.3.5. SAMPLE SIZE

Staged accrual will be used such that the study will be terminated after specific numbers of patients have been enrolled if a minimum number of responses have not been seen; the lowest significant response rate to be ruled out will be 20% (at alpha = 0.10; beta 0.10). If at least the minimum number of objective responses are seen to allow completion of accrual, a total of 30 evaluable patients will be accrued. For example, if no responses (symptomatic or shrinkage) are seen in any of the first 12 patients treated, or only 1 out of the first

20, the study would be terminated at that time. The estimated confidence interval on the response rate is ≤ (±)20 %.

Evaluable Patients: An evaluable patient is any patient who meets the enrollment criteria, receives at least two cycles of treatment, and has follow-up through the end of the second cycle with radiographic imaging (following the radiographic imaging guidelines) and/or adequate measurement by physical exam before and after treatment.

Correlations: An additional 10–20 evaluable patients may be enrolled (optional) in order to gain statistical power to allow meaningful comparisons between different subgroups of patients, should these appear critical to the planning of a pivotal trial with ONYX-015. These analyses might compare patients with 1) large vs small tumors (> or <10 cm^2), 2) differing *p53* status as defined by immunohistochemistry or sequenceing for *p53* (+/– normal), 3) the presence or absence of pre-treatment neutralizing antibodies (+/–).

3.2.4. Conduct of the Study—Schedule of Activities and Evaluations

3.2.4.1. SCREENING AND PRETREATMENT

A checklist of screening and pretreatment evaluations follows.

- Signed IRB- or LREC-approved informed consent
- Testing of tumor biopsy by immunohistochemistry (IHC) and *p53* gene sequencing for *p53* status (results not required prior to patient's treatment with ONYX-015). Biopsy material must have been obtained from the *target* tumor after becoming refractory to chemotherapy and/or radiation therapy.
- Complete medical history
- Complete physical examination, including vital signs, weight, and height
- Karnofsky performance score
- Hematological tests, including prothrombin time (PT) and INR, and partial thromboplastin time (PTT)
- CD3, CD4, CD8, and total lymphocyte counts
- Serum chemistry tests
- Serum antibody to type 5 adenovirus (neutralizing)
- Plasma sample for PCR testing for the presence of adenovirus, ONYX-015 DNA
- Archival plasma sample
- Urinalysis
- Urine or serum pregnancy test, if applicable
- Electrocardiogram (12-lead)
- Chest X-ray (PA and lateral)
- Delayed-type hypersensitivity skin testing
- Secondary diagnoses
- Baseline medical events, including signs, symptoms, and illnesses
- Medications within the last 2 mo
- EORTC quality-of-life assessment

- Pain evaluation: visual analog pain scale, pain medication usage
- Tumor size assessment by CT or MRI scan (excluding tumors evaluable by physical exam, but *not* by radiography):
  — cross-sectional area (computer-assisted measurement)
  — cross-sectional area (classical measurement)
  — non-necrotic volume (computer-assisted measurement)
- Clinical assessment of the tumor (size, consistency, color)
- Photography of tumor (if externally visible)

3.2.4.2. ENROLLMENT

Upon completion of the above screening procedures, each eligible patient will be enrolled. Each patient will be assigned a unique patient identification number. The patient number will be sequentially assigned to correspond with the order of enrollment into the study. This number along with the patient's initials will be documented on each page of the CRF. For patients who are screened for study participation, but who are not enrolled, CRFs recording the screening data collected, including reason not enrolled, will be completed.

3.2.4.3. OUT-PATIENT FOLLOW-UP DURING ONYX-015 TREATMENT PERIOD

The same schedule and visit requirements (except where differences are specified below) will be followed for each treatment cycle, including the initial ONYX-015 treatment cycle and any repeat treatment cycles (where later applicable). Any deviation from stated schedules must be approved by Onyx's Medical Director or either of the project managers.

3.2.4.4. POST-TREATMENT MONITORING OF PATIENTS

The patient's vital signs will be taken ≤15 min before each ONYX-015 injection. After each injection is completed, the patient will be observed in the clinic for a minimum of 30 min. Vital signs will be taken after 30 min ± 5 min. If vital sign(s) have changed by >15%, vital signs will be repeated every 30 min ± 5 min until returning to within 15% of baseline values < +/– 15%. Following the observation period, the patient will be sent home or hospitalized overnight at the discretion of the investigator.

Day 5 (± 2) Prior to the tumor injection on that day blood will be drawn for
- Hematological tests, including prothrombin time (PT), INR and partial thromboplastin time (PTT)
- Tumor bandage evaluation/changing, as required; assessment of drainage
- Photography of target tumor (optional)
- Serum chemistry tests
- Adenovirus DNA in blood by PCR
  Day 15 (± 2)
- Aspiration and measurement of necrotic tumor tissue/fluid (if present)

- Brief physical examination directed to relevant signs and symptoms, including vital signs and weight.
- Tumor bandage evaluation/changing, as required; assessment of drainage
- Photography of target tumor (optional)
- Hematological tests, including PT, INR, and PTT
- Serum chemistry tests
- Adenovirus DNA in blood by PCR (test to be performed if PCR positive on day 5 specimen)
- Changes in concomitant medications
- Reporting of adverse events
- Patients to be given visual pain scales, to be completed daily (one per day upon returning) until Day 22 visit

Days 22 (± 2)

- Clinical assessment of the treated tumors (size, consistency, color, etc.)
- Tumor size assessment by CT scan, MRI, or physical exam
- Complete physical examination, including vital signs and weight
- Karnofsky performance score
- Tumor bandage evaluation/changing, as required; assessment of drainage
- Photography of target tumor
- Hematological tests, including PT, INR, and PTT
- Serum chemistry tests
- Serum antibody to Ad5/ONYX-015 (neutralizing)
- Adenovirus DNA in blood by PCR (test to be performed if PCR positive on day 15 specimen)
- Archival plasma sample
- Urinalysis
- Pain evaluation: pain medication usage, visual analogue pain scales to be collected from patients
- EORTC quality of life assessment
- Changes in concomitant medications

3.2.4.5. LONG-TERM FOLLOW-UP AFTER COMPLETION OF ONYX-015 TREATMENT

Once patients have completed treatment with ONYX-015, they will be followed until target tumor progression as follows: every 4 wk for 6 mo, and every 3 mo thereafter for 6 mo (for a total of 12 mo from the end of the last ONYX-015 treatment cycle). (For the purposes of this study, 1 mo equals 4 wk, or 28 d). The date of death, if applicable, will be determined for all patients. The checklist below details procedures to be performed at each of these follow-up visits. The visits occurring every 4 wk may occur ± 1 wk, and all quarterly visits (after 6 mo) may occur ± 2 wk. The investigator may order other procedures as needed, based on the patient's clinical status. It is to be noted that the quarterly follow-up visits after the 3-mo visit may be performed at the study center or, if a patient is unable to return to the study center, the patient's primary oncologist may perform the assessments and provide the data to the study center using worksheets specially developed for this purpose.

- Brief physical examination directed to relevant signs and symptoms, including vital signs and weight
- Karnofsky performance score
- Tumor size assessment by CT scan, MRI, or physical exam
- Clinical assessment of the tumor (size, color, consistency, etc.)
- Tumor bandage evaluation/changing (if required), assessment of drainage
- Photography of target tumor
- EORTC quality of life assessments
- Pain evaluation: visual analog pain scale, pain medication usage
- Changes in concomitant medications (*see* **Note 3**)
- Reporting of adverse events (*see* **Note 4**)

3.2.5. Tumor and Patient Assessments

3.2.5.1. TUMOR RESPONSE CRITERIA

Using the following standard criteria, response is to be assessed separately on the injected target tumor, injected nontarget tumor(s) (including those injected with diluent) and noninjected tumor foci according to the schedule outlined above in **Subheading 3.2.4.** for "tumor size assessment." Duration of response and progression-free survival will be determined. *Classical/standard* cross-sectional tumor measurements used to assess response should be the following: (maximal tumor diameter × perpendicular diameter).

Complete response (CR): complete disappearance of tumor
Partial response (PR): regression of the tumor(s) by ≥50% but <100%
Minor response (MR): regression of the tumor(s) by ≤25% but <50%
Stable disease (SD) tumor decrease or increase in size by <25%
Progressive disease (PD): ≥25% increase in tumor size

3.2.5.2. CLINICAL BENEFIT RESPONSE CRITERIA (PAIN, PERFORMANCE STATUS)

- Pain response: A ≥50% reduction in pain and/or pain medication usage lasting ≤ 4 wk. Patients must have a baseline visual analogue pain score ≥20 in order to be evaluable for pain response.
- Performance status response: A ≥20-point increase in KPS lasting ≥4 wk. Patients must have a baseline ≥ KPS of 70 to be evaluable for performance status response.
- Weight changes of patients will be recorded during time on study.

3.2.6. Statistical Methods and Data Analysis

The primary objectives of this study are to estimate the objective response rate (tumor size and pain) and toxicity associated with ONYX-015 when administered into solid squamous cell carcinoma of the head and neck.

Secondary objectives are: 1) to estimate response rates using classical maximal cross-sectional measurements; 2) to estimate survival and time to disease progression; 3) to assess the quality of life benefit of ONYX-015; 4) to evaluate the performance status response, and 5) to determine the local and systemic immune response to ONYX-015.

3.2.6.1. SAMPLE SIZE CONSIDERATIONS

A staged accrual design will be used for this study. In the first stage, 12 patients will be enrolled and treated with ONYX-015. If none of the patients respond to treatment, then enrollment into the study will be terminated. If at least one patient responds to treatment, then enrollment may be continued. If, after the enrollment of 20 patients at least two patients respond to treatment, then enrollment will be continued until a total of 30 "evaluable" patients have completed two cycles of treatment (*see* **Subheading 3.2.3**).

Assuming the study goes to completion of all 30 evaluable patients in planned enrollment, then the 90% confidence interval for the estimated response rate will be (±) 12%, assuming 20% responders. Sufficient evidence to indicate that the true response rate is greater than 20% would be provided if the lower limit of the confidence interval is greater than 0.20 ($\alpha = 0.05$, 1-tailed test).

3.2.6.2. PRIMARY EFFICACY ANALYSIS

Because this is an uncontrolled study enrolling a small number of patients, formal hypothesis testing is not planned. However, comparisons of different subgroups may lead to the generation of hypotheses which will be studied prospectively in subsequent clinical trials.

The primary statistical analysis will be the estimation of the 95% confidence interval of the probability of response, defined as partial or complete response in injected target tumors using computer-assisted cross-sectional measurements (*see* **Subheading 3.2.5.**). The confidence interval will be determined using the binomial distribution. The proportion of patients with partial or complete response using computer-assisted non-necrotic volume measurements and the proportion of patients with a ≥50% reduction in pain as determined using Visual Analog Scales or pain medication usage will be estimated similarly.

The definition of response requires two observations a least 4 wk apart. The primary analysis, therefore, will be done on the following two groups of patients:

Evaluable: Patients who meet the enrollment criteria and receive at least two cycles of treatment, and have follow-up data through the end of the second cycle with radiographic imaging and/or adequate measurement by physical exam before and after treatment.

Intent to Treat: Patients who received at least one administration of study medication.

3.2.6.3. SECONDARY EFFICACY ANALYSIS

Secondary analyses will include the following:

- The proportion of patients with stable disease at the target tumor site using computer-assisted cross-sectional measurements (defined in **Subheading 3.2.5.**)
- The proportion of patients with partial or complete responses (defined in **Subheading 3.2.5.**) using classical maximal cross-sectional measurements
- Time to disease progression estimated by the method of Kaplan and Meier
- Survival evaluated with Kaplan Meier estimation
- Quality of life as assessed by EORTC global QLQ-C30 and EORTC disease specific QLQ-H&N35
- The proportion of patients with a $\geq$20-point increase in Karnofsky performance status ($\geq$4 wk)

  Relationships with the following variables will be examined as appropriate (these comparisons might generate hypotheses which could be addressed subsequently in prospectively designed trials):

- Baseline immunological status: CD3, CD4, and CD8 counts plus delayed-type hypersensitivity skin response
- Neutralizing antibody titer at baseline and end of treatment cycle
- Baseline tumor size (> or <10 cm^2)
- *p53* gene sequence, *p53* immunohistochemical test results

3.2.6.4. DEMOGRAPHICS AND BASELINE CHARACTERISTICS

Subject age, weight, and height will be summarized with descriptive statistics (mean standard deviation, minimum and maximum), whereas gender and race will be summarized with frequency tabulations. Individual patient listings will be produced. Medical history data will be summarized with frequency tabulations.

3.2.6.5. SAFETY DATA

Patients who receive at least one treatment with study medication (*evaluable for safety*) will be included in the safety analysis. Safety data including adverse events, laboratory results, toxicity, vital signs, and withdrawal information will be summarized over time. Individual patient listings will be produced. Data will also be listed by patient for physical examinations, electrocardiograms, and chest X-rays.

Adverse events will be coded with the COSTART coding thesaurus and tabulated using the COSTART body system classification scheme. The number and percent of subjects with adverse events will be tabulated; in addition, the data will be stratified by adverse event intensity and investigator-specified relationship to ONYX-015.

3.2.6.6. CONCOMITANT MEDICATIONS

All concomitant medication usage documented during the study period will be summarized in frequency tabulations. The Anatomical Therapeutical Chemical (ATC) coding scheme will be used to group medications into relevant categories for these tabulations.

4. Notes

1. Intratumoral injection technique: the most common problem encountered with the intratumoral injection treatments described in the protocol is suboptimal intratumoral distribution of the virus. The injection needle should be passed to its greatest depth initially, and the virus-containing solution should be injected as the needle is being withdrawn. This technique ensures distribution of the virus along the entire needle tract. In addition, injection should be out to and 0.2–0.5 cm. beyond the palpable edge of the tumor. This is to ensure that microscopic tumor deposits beyond the palpable tumor edge can be targeted with the viral therapy.
2. Limited courses of glucocorticoid therapy are allowable (e.g., for nausea control).
3. After the 1-mo follow-up visit, the only concomitant medications that will be recorded are those, if any, that are relevant to an adverse event (ongoing or delayed in onset) judged to be potentially causally related to ONYX-015 and antitumor therapy(ies).
4. After the 1-mo follow-up visit, only those adverse events (ongoing or delayed in onset) judged to be potentially causally related to ONYX-015 will be recorded.

References

1. Barker, D. D. and Berk, A. J. (1987) Adenovirus proteins from both E1B reading frames are required for transformation of rodent cells by viral infection and DNA transfection. *Virology* **156,** 107–121.
2. Bischoff, J. R., et al. (1996) An adenovirus mutant that replicates selectively in p53-deficient human tumor cells. *Science* **274,** 373–376.
3. Heise, C., et al. (1997) ONYX-015, an E1B gene-attenuated adenovirus, causes tumor-specific cytolysis and antitumoral efficacy that can be augmented by standard chemotherapeutic agents [see comments]. *Nat. Med.* **3,** 639–645.
4. Boyle, J. O., et al. (1993) The incidence of p53 mutations increases with progression of head and neck cancer. *Cancer Res.* **53,** 4477–4480.
5. Brennan, J. A., et al. (1995) Association between cigarette smoking and mutation of the p53 gene in squamous-cell carcinoma of the head and neck. *N. Engl. J. Med.* **332,** 712–717.
6. Ganly, I., Kirn, D., Rodriguez, G., et al., (1997) Phase I trial of intratumoral injection with an E1B-deleted adenovirus, ONYX-015, in patients with recurrent head and neck cancer. *Proc. Am. Soc. Clinic. Oncol.*

II

CLINICAL PROTOCOLS
FOR CANCER GENE THERAPY

D: Antisense Gene Therapy

37

c-*myb* Antisense Oligonucleotide Therapeutics for Hematologic Malignancies

Selina Luger

1. Introduction

Although improved significantly, conventional treatment of hematologic malignancy remains inadequate for many patients. Novel treatment approaches could be useful if they would be more efficacious and less toxic. One such approach could involve the manipulation of genes critical for leukemic cell growth and survival.

The usual way to determine the biological significance of a particular gene's function is to perturb its normal pattern of expression and observe the consequences on a cell's (organism's) growth or behavior. In the past several years, a number of strategies have been developed to accomplish such an objective at both the single cell and intact organism levels. One widely used approach has been to transfect a target cell with a genetically engineered construct, which transiently or inducibly overexpresses the gene of interest. Another has been to create transgenic animals, which overexpress the gene of interest in the living animal. A wealth of information has been gathered using these approaches, but whereas simple in theory, they have been hampered to some degree by technical difficulties relating to efficiency of transformation, choice of usable target cell systems, and particularly in the case of transgenic animals, expense. Another strategy for elucidating gene function has been through its disruption. Two main approaches have been developed to accomplish this end. One is carried out in an intact animal and involves microinjecting into the animal embryonic stem (ES) cells a genetically engineered construct containing a mutated, nonfunctional form of the targeted gene that inserts itself into the target gene by the natural process of homologous recombination (*1*). The effect

From: *Methods in Molecular Medicine, Vol. 35: Gene Therapy: Methods and Protocols*
Edited by: W. Walther and U. Stein © Humana Press, Inc., Totowa, NJ

of expressing the mutated dysfunctional gene in a developing animal may then be discerned. This method, though quite effective at generating heterozygous or homozygous loss of function mutants is hampered by that fact that it is nonetheless very inefficient, time consuming, and expensive. It is also unlikely that this approach will be appropriate for therapeutic applications anytime in the near future *(1)*. A far simpler and much less expensive approach has been to employ an "antisense" strategy *(2)*. Antisense (AS) oligodeoxynucleotides (ODN), traditionally 13–30 nucleotides in length are synthesized complementary to the mRNA, or sense sequence. The technique relies on either introducing, or expressing, antisense DNA or RNA in a target cell *(3,4)*. This allows formation of an mRNA-DNA or mRNA-RNA duplex, which ultimately inhibits the targeted gene's function. Additionally, oligonucleotides can also be used to disrupt gene function through triplex formation with the double -helical DNA or by mimicking the action of ribozymes, naturally occurring RNAs capable of degrading RNAs in the same manner that enzymes degrade proteins.

The mechanism whereby AS ODN inhibit gene expression is not straightforward and several possible explanations have been devised (numbers in text correspond to numbers in **Fig. 1**). The antisense sequence may work in the nucleus to prevent: **1** transcription, **2** hnRNA processing; or **3** transport of the message out of the nucleus. In the cytoplasm, the interaction of the antisense transcript or ODN and the protein synthesizing machinery may interfere with translation of mRNA. This may be brought about by inhibiting the association of the **4** mRNA and the ribosome, or **5** the ability of the ribosomal-tRNA complex to "read" and assemble nascent proteins as the complex moves along the mRNA. Finally, **6** an antisense DNA mRNA complex can be used as substrate by the enzyme RNaseH, which degrades the mRNA while the antisense DNA is left intact to hybridize with another message *(2,5)*. Regardless, the function of the gene in question is thereby either inhibited or totally abrogated. The effect seems to be efficient as well, as antisense oligonucleotides appear to disrupt their target in a very high percentage of cells exposed *(6)*.

The use of antisense oligodeoxynucleotides for disrupting gene function avoids potential complications arising from the use of viral vectors *(7)*. This methodology may then prove to be safer *vis a vis* the induction of malignancies and insertional mutagenesis. Second, the efficiency of cellular delivery appears to be much higher than what is usually observed with retroviral vectors *(7)*. The latter appears to have a target cell infection efficiency of only a few percent, whereas AS ODN appear to disrupt their target in a very high percentage of cells exposed *(6,7)*. Finally, from a drug manufacturing point of view, it is likely that it will be easier to produce consistent lots of antisense DNA than the components of viral-based delivery systems.

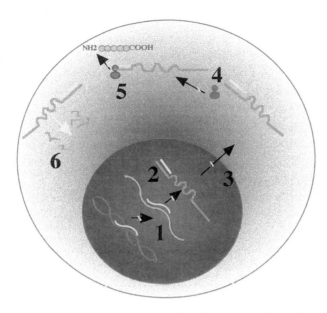

Fig. 1. Mechanism of antisense ODN action. Representation of potential sites for antisense oligodeoxynucleotide activity. See text for details.

The hematopoietic system has served a model to study potential therapies for hematologic malignancies as well as solid tumors. The accessibility of blood cells and bone marrow has allowed us to learn much about the molecular mechanisms involved in normal cell growth and development. By examining normal hematopoiesis we hope to better understand the changes that result in malignant transformation. The study of leukemia has provided much of the knowledge that we have about cancer genes and oncogenic mechanisms. Protooncogenes are the normal cellular homologs of oncogenes found in transforming retroviruses. They are highly conserved genes, often found through the *phyla*-from yeast to man. Investigations into the function have provided evidence that many play a role in the regulation of normal cell growth and development (*8*). Their encoded protein products have been postulated to effect cell growth by several mechanisms (*8*). These include production of growth factors (c-*sis*, PDGF), growth factor receptors (c-*kit*, c-*fms*), signal transduction proteins (*ras*), and transcription factors (c-*jun*, c-*fos*). Normal and malignant cells manifest differential sensitivity to the effect of disrupting the function of certain genes or protooncogenes, which are critical for cell growth. Perturbations in regulation of these genes is felt to contribute to or result in neoplastic growth. Synthetic antisense oligodeoxynucleotides may be employed to disrupt the function of specific genes in hematopoietic cells and thereby understand, in a more direct manner, their function.

In studying normal and malignant hematopoiesis, one gene we have chosen as a target is the c-*myb* protooncogene. c-*myb* is the normal cellular homolog of v-*myb*, the transforming gene of avian myeloblastosis and avian leukemia E26. v-*myb* has been found to preferentially transform hematopoietic cells. Its specificity for hematopoietic tissue is demonstrated by the fact that it does not, unlike most other oncogenes, transform fibroblasts *(9)*. v-*myb* has been detected in two replication defective avian acute leukemia viruses; AMV *(10,11)* and E 26 *(12)*.

Though a number of alternatively spliced c-*myb* products have been identified *(13)*, the major product appears to be a 74 kDa nuclear binding protein that recognizes a specific nucleotide consensus sequence *(14)*. Several functional domains have been identified in this protein (**Fig. 1**). It has three imperfect tandem repeat regions, which encode the DNA binding domain *(15)*. DNA binding in turn appears to be dependent on the phosphorylation state of this portion of the MYB protein *(16)*.

The protooncogene c-*myb* has been postulated to play an important role in regulating hematopoietic cell proliferation, and perhaps differentiation as well *(17–19)*. Evidence to support this hypothesis includes the observations that: 1) c-*myb* is preferentially expressed in primitive hematopoietic cell tissues and hematopoietic tumor cell lines of several species *(20)*; 2) increasing degree of cell maturation is associated with a significant decline in c-*myb* expression *(21)*; and 3) constitutive expression of exogenously introduced c-*myb* inhibits the ability of a murine erythroleukemia cell line (MEL) to undergo erythroid differentiation in response to known inducing agents *(22,23)*. Although data clearly implicate the c-*myb* gene product as a potentially important regulator of hematopoietic cell development, the evidence provided by these experiments is largely of an indirect nature. Accordingly, the function of the c-*myb* protooncogene as it related to normal hematopoiesis remained speculative until its function was definitively disrupted. This has been done using the antisense approach, and the results obtained have largely been confirmed by the technique of homologous recombination *(24)*.

In order to investigate the role of c-*myb* in normal human hematopoiesis, an 18-bp ODN based on either sense or antisense strands of the c-*myb* mRNA transcript from codons 2–7 was synthesized. Mononuclear cells (MNC) obtained from normal human bone marrow depleted of adherent cells and T lymphocytes were exposed to the ODN and colony formation was assayed in cultures with appropriate inducing agents *(25)*. Exposure of the MNC to the c-*myb* antisense ODN resulted in a decrease in the number of colonies formed. This was true for granulocyte-macrophage colony-forming units (CFU), as well as for erythroid and megakaryocyte progenitor cell growth. The colonies in the antisense-treated cultures were also found to be uniformly smaller, and composed of smaller numbers of individual cells There was a dose-dependent inhibition of colony formation for all lineages examined upon exposure to antisense ODN. No effect was noted upon exposure to c-*myb* sense ODN. Furthermore, it was demonstrated that if c-*myb* antisense ODN were added after 5 d of incubation, only slight decrease in colony formation was noted, suggesting that the c-*myb* protein was most critical during the early stages of colony formation. This hypothesis was subsequently confirmed by exposing populations of "early" and "late" progenitors to antisense ODN *(26)*. These data provide evidence that c-*myb* is required for proliferation of intermediate or late erythroid and myeloid progenitors and is less important for early progenitor amplification and lineage commitment.

With the above data suggesting a major role for c-*myb* in normal human hematopoiesis and considering the evidence that c-*myb* expression is increased in leukemias, further antisense experiments were carried out in leukemic cell lines to try and elucidate the role of c-*myb* in leukemic hematopoiesis *(27)*. Cells from four human myeloid leukemic cell lines, HL-60, K562, KG-1, and KG-1a, distinguished by their differing stages of arrest, were exposed to c-*myb* ODN and colony assays were performed after 5 d in culture. After exposure to c-*myb* antisense ODN, the proliferation of each leukemia cell line was inhibited as compared to the control. This effect was, however, most pronounced in the HL-60 cell line, which is the most mature and least significant in the KG-1a cell line, which is blocked at the most immature myeloid stage.

The possibility that normal and leukemic hematopoietic cells might manifest differential sensitivity to loss of c-*myb* function was then explored *(6,28)*. Cells used for these studies were normal bone marrow MNCs, CCRF-CEM cells (a human T-cell leukemia cell line), AML blast cells obtained from AML patient, and CML blast cells.

When untreated, or in the presence of sense ODN, leukemic cell colonies were too numerous to count. At a similar antisense dose, normal bone marrow MNC were unaffected and CEM cell growth was reduced by >90%. When normal BM MNC were mixed 1:1 with CEM and exposed to antisense ODN, the response to antisense ODN was found to be dose dependent. At a dose of <6 μmg/mL only leukemic colonies could be identified by morphologic, histochemical, and immunochemical analysis. When the dose was doubled, leukemia cell colony formation was decreased and normal colony formation was noted. With even higher doses of the ODN (>25 μg/mL), only normal colony formation could be identified (**Table 1**).

When primary patient material was utilized, at equivalent antisense DNA doses, AML blasts from 18 of 23 patients exhibited a 75% decrease in colony

Table 1
**Effect of c-*myb* Oligomer Exposure on Colony/Cluster Formation
by T-Cell Leukemia and Normal Bone Marrow Progenitor Cells (MNC)[a]**

Cells Plated	No. Added	Oligomer/Amt. Added[b]		Colony/Cluster
MNC	5×10^4/mL	NONE		24±4
		MYB S	(20; 5.0)	31±4
		MYB AS	(20; 5.0)	30±6
T leukemia	5×10^4/mL	NONE		TNTC[c]
		MYB S	(20; 5.0)	TNTC
		MYB AS	(20; 5.0)	1±1
MNC + leukemia	5×10^4/mL	NONE		TNTC
	of each	MYB S	(20; 5.0)	TNTC
		MYB AS	(2; 0.5)	TNTC
		MYB AS	(5; 1.0)	TNTC
		MYB AS	(10; 2.5)	41±5
		MYB AS	(20; 5.0)	34±1

[a]Cells were exposed to oligomers at indicated doses (mg/mL) for 4 d in suspension cultures, and then transferred to semisolid media. After 12 d in culture, colonies and clusters were counted in paired dishes with an inverted microscope. Colony/cluster counts are presented as mean ± SD. Reprinted from *(28)*.
[b]μg/mL added to the culture medium at time 0, and +18 h respectively
[c]Too numerous to count (> 1000 colonies)

and cluster formation compared to untreated or sense-treated controls. Similar experiments with blast cells from CML patients exhibited a similar decrease in colony formation in 12/16 patients. This effect was dose dependent and sequence specific (**Fig. 2**). At equivalent doses of c-*myb* AS, normal MNC colonies were inhibited by no more than 50%. Examination of the residual colonies for *bcr-abl* mRNA expression, using a reverse transcriptase-polymerase chain reaction (RT-PCR), revealed that although easily detectable in control and sense treated colonies, in each case where c-*myb* AS ODN inhibited growth, *bcr-abl* expression was either greatly decreased or nondetectable. No residual leukemic CFU were demonstrable on replating of treated cells *(6)*.

These studies suggest that ODN have the potential to become an important new therapeutic agent for the treatment of solid tumors as well as leukemias. There are several obstacles to antisense therapy *(29,30)*. If AS ODN are to be employed for in vivo therapy, the question of stability must first be addressed. DNA with unmodified phosphodiester bonds is susceptible to 3′, and 5′ exonuclease attack. Such exonucleases are common in plasma and are found intracellularly *(31)*. Capping or derivatizing the 5′ and 3′ ends of ODN have been used to prevent exonuclease attack as has changing the base glycosidic linkage

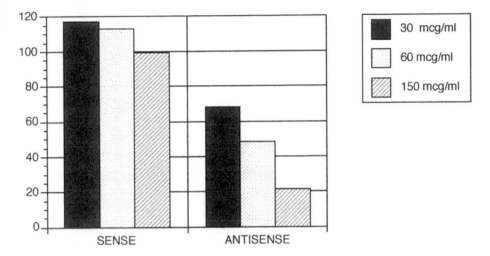

Fig. 2. Dose and sequence dependent effect of c-myb ODN on CML CFU-GM colony formation. Cells were exposed to oligodeoxynucleotides at indicated doses (µg/mL) for 24 hours in suspension cultures, and then transferred to semi-solid media. After ten days in culture, colonies and clusters were counted in paired dishes with an inverted microscope. CFU-GM Colony/cluster counts are presented as the percent Cells were exposed to oligomers at indicated doses (µg/mL) for four days in suspension cultures, and then transferred to semi-solid media. After twelves days in culture, colonies and clusters were counted in paired dishes with an inverted microscope. Colony/cluster counts are presented as the percent of colonies (mean ± SD) present in control dishes (no ODN added).

from *b* to *a* anomeric form. Modification of the phosphodiester bonds between the bases also renders the molecules less sensitive to nuclease attack and, therefore, increase their survival significantly.

Though many such modifications have been synthesized *(4,32)*, perhaps the two most widely employed are the methylphosphonates (CH_3–O–P–) and the phosphorothioates (S–O–P–). Methylphosphonates are highly nuclease resistant and tend to form RNA-DNA hybrids with high melting points *(33)*. Nevertheless, the lack of an ionizable hydrogen renders them relatively water insoluble. Furthermore, they are incapable of binding RNaseH thereby eliminating a potentially important mechanism for disrupting gene expression. Phosphorothioates are also quite stable to nuclease attack, but in contrast to the methylphosphonates retain their charge and thus their water solubility *(33,34)*. They also bind RNaseH. Some investigators have reported that the phosphorothioates may manifest significant nonsequence specific toxicity because of charge-related protein binding *(35)*. In our hands this has not proven to be a problem.

In order to evaluate the in vivo efficacy of c-*myb* AS phosphorothioate ODN (P-ODN), we established a human leukemia-SCID mouse chimeras with K562 cells and treated diseased animals with phosphorothioate modified antisense oligodeoxynucleotides *(36)*. K562 cells express the c-*myb* protooncogene, which served as the target for the antisense DNA. They also express the tumor specific *bcr/abl* fusion gene present in CML, which was utilized to track the human cells in the mouse host. The c-*myb* AS P-ODN was administered continuously for single-treatment periods of either 7 or 14 d by means of a subcutaneously implanted, constant infusion osmotic (Alzet™) pump. Once animals had detectable circulating leukemic blast cells the mean (±SD) survival of untreated control mice was 6 ± 3 d. The survival of animals treated for 7 or 14 d with either sense or scrambled sequence c-*myb* oligodeoxynucleotides was not statistically different from the control animals. In distinct contrast, animals treated for similar lengths of time with c-*myb* antisense oligodeoxy- nucleotides survived 3–8 times longer than the various control animals (untreated, sense, or scrambled sequence ODN).

In addition, animals receiving c-*myb* AS DNA had significantly less disease at the two sites most frequently manifesting leukemic cell infiltration, the cen- tral nervous system, and the ovary. These results suggest that phosphorothioate modified AS DNA may be efficacious for the treatment of human leukemia in vivo, and by analogy, for the treatment of other human neoplasias as well.

These studies employed a human c-*myb* sequence in a murine host. Because the human and murine sequences differ by at least five bases in the targeted regions, this system did not allow us to examine the toxicities attributable to c-*myb* AS P-ODN in particular, but does allow us to say that no systemic tox- icities attributable to the presence of extraneous short stranded phosphorothioate DNA were noted. In order to address this issue Balb-C mice received infusions of murine *myb* oligodeoxynucleotides in doses up to 10 times those used in the in vivo experiments. Effects of murine c-*myb* AS P-ODN on body weight and blood cell counts at doses up to 10 times those used therapeutically were assessed. Weight, leukocyte count, and hematocrit were unaffected. No apparent toxicities were noted other than local toxicity to the skin and thrombocytopenia, which appeared to be nonsequence specific.

Based on the preclinical data that has been obtained in the laboratory, we have begun several clinical studies to evaluate the clinical utility of c-*myb* AS P-ODN. CML is a clonal neoplasm arising from the malignant transformation of a pluripotent hematopoietic stem cell. Patients typically present with symp- toms related to leukocytosis, thrombocytosis, or splenomegaly. The disease is characterized by a 3–4-yr indolent phase that eventually accelerates and trans- forms into a blast crisis, which is rapidly fatal. Although symptoms can be controlled during the indolent or "chronic" phase with intermittent or continuous therapy with hydroxyurea or busulfan, the mean duration of the chronic phase of 3–4 yr cannot be prolonged with conventional chemotherapy. Allogeneic bone marrow transplantation is the only known cure for CML. As most patients do not have a suitable donor, autologous bone marrow transplantation (ABMT) has provided an alternative to allogeneic transplantation in a variety of hematologic malignancies. The major concern with ABMT is tumor contamination of the autograft. Several approaches have been attempted to purge Ph+ cells from bone marrow *(37–39)*. Studies have suggested that normal early progenitors or stem cells persist in the marrow of CML patients *(40,41)*.

We have initiated a pilot study to evaluate the effectiveness of c-*myb* AS P-ODN as ex vivo bone marrow purging agents for patients with CML in chronic or accelerated phase. We hope to, in this way eliminate the malignant clone from the autograft. Purging was performed for 24 h on CD34+ marrow cells. Patients received busulfan and cytoxan followed by reinfusion of previously cryopreserved ODN purged cells. Initially, 7 chronic phase and 1 accelerated phase CML patients have been treated. Seven of eight engrafted. In 4 of 6 evaluable chronic phase patients, metaphases were 85–100% normal 3 m after engraftment, suggesting that a significant purge had taken place. Sustained hematologic improvement and normalization of blood counts was maintained in five patients with follow-up ranging from 6 mo to 4 yr *(42)*.

In addition to our ex vivo purging study, we have initiated a phase I study of infusional c-*myb* AS P-ODN in patients with hematologic malignancies. Twenty courses of therapy were administered to 18 patients with refractory CML or acute leukemia (two patients were treated at two different dose levels). *myb* AS P-ODN was administered by continuous infusion over 7 d at dose levels ranging from 0.3 mg/kg/d to 2.0 mg/kg/d. No dose-related toxicity has been noted, although two idiosyncratic toxicities (transient renal insufficiency and pericarditis), not clearly drug related were observed in one patient each. One blast-crisis patient survived approximately 14 mo with transient restoration of chronic phase disease *(42)*.

Although clinical benefit is difficult to determine at this point, our preliminary results demonstrate that AS P-ODN can be administered safely to leukemic patients. Additional clinical studies are ongoing in leukemic and other patients using AS ODN directed against various gene targets. Further work needs to be done to allow us to understand the mechanism of action of these agents. Much remains to be understood about the kinetics of oligomer uptake and the fate of intracellular ODN. Determination of appropriate AS ODN target, delivery of ODN into cells, and the feasibility of large-scale synthesis continue to be addressed. The therapeutic utility of these agents is promising.

2. Materials

2.1. Plasticware

1. 5-mL polypropylene tubes (Fisher Scientific, Pittsburgh, PA).
2. Cell-culture dishes (Corning, Corning, NY).
3. Suspension culture tubes.
4. 50-mL centrifuge tubes.
5. 1.4-mL Eppendorf tubes.
6. 0.8-mL Eppendorf tubes.

2.2. Growth Factors

1. Diluted, Aliquoted (100–200 µL/aliquot) stored at –70°C long term and at –20°C after opening. Keep on ice while using.
2. IL-3 (R & D Systems, Minneapolis, MN).
3. Stem cell factor or kit ligand (SCF).
4. Granulocyte macrophage-colony stimulating factor (GM-CSF).
5. Erythropoietin (Epo).

2.3. Media

1. Methylcellulose (Terry Fox Laboratories, Vancouver, BC) light sensitive, store at 4°C.
2. Ficoll.
3. Iscove's modified Dulbecco's medium (IMDM), RPMI, or Minimal Essential Medium (MEM).
4. Bovine calf serum (Hyclone, Logan, UT).
5. HEPES buffer, pH 7.0

3. Methods

3.1. Adherent Cell Depletion of Bone Marrow and Peripheral Blood

1. Dilute peripheral blood/ bone marrow 1:1 with medium (RPMI, Iscove, MEM) (*see* **Note 1**).
2. Add to each 50-cc centrifuge tube (*see* **Note 2**) 15 cc of Ficoll; 35 cc of blood or bone marrrow.
3. Spin at 21°C, 1500g, 30 min.
4. Aspirate off 5–10 cc medium. Using 5 or 10 cc pipet remove layer of MNC into new 50-cc centrifuge tube (*see* **Note 3**).
5. Wash cells by adding medium and spin for 10 min, at 4°C, 200g.
6. Aspirate off medium and resuspend pellet in fresh medium.
7. Count cells.
8. Add medium to cells to concentration of $2–3 \times 10^6$mL.
9. Add 5% BCS.
10. Put 5–10 cc cell suspension in each Corning dish (untreated plates).

11. Incubate overnight for adherent cell depletion.
12. In AM, collect cells from Corning dishes (**Note 4**).
13. Spin cells for 10 min at 4°C, 200g.
14. Count cells—These are adherent depleted mononuclear cells (A⁻MNC).

3.2. T-Cell Depletion

1. Resuspend A⁻MNC cells to a concentration of $4–6 \times 10^6$/mL supplemented medium (*see* **Note 5**). Aliquot 4.5-cc cell suspension into each 15-mL centrifuge tube.
2. Add 0.5-mL prepared sheep red blood cells to each tube.
3. Spin cells for 5 min at 4°C, 200g.
4. Leave cells at 4°C for 55 min.
5. Mix cells and rosettes by inversion (*see* **Note 6**).
6. Underlayer with Ficoll, 6 mL of Ficoll per tube (*see* **Note 7**).
7. Spin at 21°C, 1500g, 30 min.
8. Using 5- or 10-cc pipet remove layer of mononuclear cells (MNC) into new 50-cc centrifuge tube (*see* **Notes 3** and **8**).
9. Wash cells by adding medium and spin for 10 min, at 4°C, 200g (*see* **Note 9**).

3.3. Oligodeoxynucleotide Exposure (for Cell Culture)

1. Prepare 0.4-mL suspension that contains 2×10^5 A⁻T–MNC; BCS 8 μL; HEPES 4 μL; Iscove to a total of 400 μL (*see* **Notes 10** and **11**).
2. Add oligonucleotides to tube and then add 50% of original dose at 18 h—Cells are incubated at 37°C overnight (*see* **Note 12**).
3. Twenty-four hours after the original dose, cells are cultured in methylcellulose with lineage specific growth factors added at this time (*see* **Note 13** and **14**).
   For CFU-GM: IL-3 20 U/mL, GM-CSF 5 ng/mL
   For BFU-E: IL-3 20 U/mL, Epo 5 U/mL, SCF 100 ng/mL
   For CFU-E: Epo 5 U/mL
4. Prepare culture dishes. Put 2 covered and 1 uncovered small dish in each large culture dish.
5. For each tube do the following (*see* **Note 15**): Add 1.8 cc methycellulose to each tube using glass pipet. Mix cells together with methylcellulose. When adequately mixed draw up all 2–2.2-mL cell suspension and plate half of suspension in each of two small dishes. Cover small and large dish and shake large dish to spread out cell suspension and remove all air bubbles.
6. Repeat as stated above for each tube.
7. When all tubes have been plated, add 3–5 cc water to each uncovered small dish.
8. Incubate at 37°C with 5% CO_2 (*see* **Note 16**).
9. Incubate until lineage-specific colonies are ready to be counted (*see* **Note 17**).

3.4. Oligodeoxynucleotide Exposure (For RNA Extraction)

1. Prepare 0.4-mL suspension containing $5–10 \times 10^6$ A–T–MNC; BCS 20 μL; IL-3 20 U/mL; GM-CSF 5 ng/mL; Iscove to a total of 400 μL (*see* **Notes 11** and **18**).

2. Add ODN to tubes and then add 50% of original dose at 18 h. Cells are incubated at 37°C overnight (*see* **Note 19**).
3. After 36-h total incubation, spin down cells and extract RNA.

3.5. RNA Extraction From Blood or Bone Marrow (For Patient Samples Before and After Treatment)

1. Dilute peripheral blood/ bone marrow 1:1 with medium (RPMI, Iscove, MEM).
2. To each 50-cc centrifuge tube add 15 cc Ficoll and 35 cc blood or bone marrrow. Pipet slowly downside of tube over Ficoll (*see* **Note 2**).
3. Spin at 21°C, 500*g*, 30 min.
4. Aspirate off 5–10 cc medium. Using 5- or 10-cc pipet, remove layer of MNC into new 50-cc centrifuge tube (*see* **Note 3**).
5. Wash cells by adding medium and spin for 10 min at 4°C, 200*g*.
6. Aspirate off medium and resuspend pellet in fresh medium.
7. Count cells.
8. Spin down $\leq 10 \times 10^6$ cells per 1.4-mL Eppendorf tube.
9. Aspirate off medium.
10. Proceed with RNA extraction.

4. Notes

1. 15–30 cc of aspirated bone marrow is obtained from consenting normal donors and patients with leukemia. If bone marrow aspiration is not possible, and patient has circulating leukemia, peripheral blood can be used.
2. Put Ficoll in tube first. Layer blood slowly over Ficoll, or the two will mix.
3. Cells of interest (MNC) are in the layer between medium and Ficoll. Be very careful not to remove cells when aspirating medium. Dense red blood cells will be at the bottom of the tube. Do not stir them while pipeting.
4. Wash plates 2–3 times with fresh medium to collect all cells.
5. For T-cell depletion, cells are aliquoted at $2–3 \times 10^7$ cells/4.5 mL medium (MEM or RPMI or Iscove) supplemented with 10% BCS.
6. Mix very gently so as not to break up rosettes.
7. Gently put pipet with 6-mL Ficoll under the rosettes. Slowly release Ficoll from pipet so as not to disturb rosettes.
8. Rosetted T cells should have pelleted to the bottom.
9. These are A⁻T⁻ MNC.
10. For ODN exposure for cell culture, ODN are typically added to 2×10^5 cells in 0.4-mL Iscove medium supplemented with 2% BCS.
11. Calculate the number of tubes that will be used in the experiment (*n*) and prepare cells in suspension for *n* + 1 tubes. Aliquot 400 µL into each culture tube.
12. Unmodified, 18-base ODN sequences were based on the human c-*myb* cDNA sequence and were as follows: 5′-GCC-CGA-AGA-CCC-CGG-CAC-3′ (sense); 5′ GTG-CCG-GGG-TCT-TCG-GGC-3′ (antisense). Typically we set up the experiment as in **Table 2**.

Table 2
Experiment

	Oligonucleotide	Concentration (mg/mL) 0 h–18 h	μL/400 μL–0 h–18 h
A	Control	—	—
B1	Sense	40–20	16 μL–8 μL
B2	Sense	100–50	40 μL–20 μL
B3	Antisense	40–20	16 μL–8 μL
B4	Antisense	100–50	40 μL–20 μL
B5	Scrambled	40–20	16 μL–8 μL
B6	Scrambled	100–50	40 μL–20 μL

13. Growth factors are diluted when they arrive and aliquoted into 100–200-μL portions to be stored at –70°C. New batches are evaluated so that growth factor doses result in optimal colony growth. After activity assay is done, dilutions are made so that growth factors can be added to suspension culture as follows: IL-3 20 U/mL = 5 μL; Erythropoietin. 5 U/mL = 2.5 μL; GM-CSF 5 ng/mL = 2.5 μL; SCF 100 ng/mL = 1 μL.
14. If we were plating CFU-GM would prepare enough growth factors for $n + 1$ tubes and mix together 80 μL IL-3 and 40 μL GM-CSF and aliquot 15 μL of the mixture to each tube.
15. Use glass pipets for methylcellulose as it will stick to the side of plastic pipettes. Add methycelullose and mix cells together slowly so as not to get any air bubbles.
16. Maintain incubator so as to minimize bacterial and fungal contamination.
17. Dishes remain in incubator until colonies are ready to be counted ; CFU-GM 7–10 d; BFU E 14 d; CFU-E 5 d.
18. For RNA extraction following ODN exposure, ODN are typically added to $5–10 \times 10^6$ cells in 0.4-mL Iscove medium supplemented with 5% BCS and growth factors.
19. Typically, experiment is set up with four tubes, control, sense, antisense, and scrambled. Only one dose of ODN is used 100 mg/mL at time 0, 50 mg/mL at 18 h.

References

1. Colman, A. (1990) Antisense strategies in cell and developmental biology. *J. Cell Sci.* **97,** 399–409.
2. Gewirtz, A., Sokol, D. L., and Ratajczak, M. (1998) Nucleic acid therapeutics: state of the art and future prospects. *Blood* **92,** 712–736.
3. Helene, C. and Toulme, J. (1990) Specific regulation of gene expression by antisense, sense and antigene nucleic acids. *Biochim. Biophys. Acta* **1049,** 99–125.

4. van der Krol, A. R., Mol, J. N. M., and Sruitje, A. R. (1988) Modulation of eukaryotic gene expression by complementary RNA or DNA sequences. *Bio-Techniques* **6,** 958–976.

5. Holt, J. T., Redner, R. L., and Nienhuis, A. W. (1988) An oligomer complementary to c-myc mRNA inhibits its proliferation of HL-60 cells and induces differentiation. *Mol. Cell Biol.* **8,** 963–973.

6. Ratajczak, M. Z., Hijiya, N., Catani, L., deRiel, K., Luger, S. M., McGlave, P., and Gewirtz, A. M. (1992) Acute- and chronic-phase chronic myelogenous leukemia colony-forming units are highly sensitive to the growth inhibitory effects of c-*myb* antisense oligodeoxynucleotides. *Blood* **80,** 1956–1961.

7. Miller, A. D. (1992) Human gene therapy come of age. *Nature* **357,** 455–460.

8. Bishop, J. M. (1991) Molecular themes in oncogenesis. *Cell* **64,** 235–248.

9. Shen-Ong, G. L. C. (1990) The *myb* oncogene. *Biochim. Biophys. Acta* **1032,** 39–52.

10. Baluda, M. A. and Goetz, I. E. (1961) Morphological conversion of cell cultures by avian myeloblastosis virus. *Virology* **15,** 185–199.

11. Moscovici, C. and Gazzolo, L. (1982) Transformation of hemopoietic cells and avian leukemia viruses, in *Advances in Viral Oncology*, vol. 1 (Oncogene Studies), Raven, New York, pp. 83–106.

12. Radka, K., Beug, H., Kornfeld, S., and Graf, T. (1982) Transformation of both erythroid and myeloid cells by E26, an avian leukemia virus that contains the *myb* gene. *Cell* **31,** 643–653.

13. Westin, E. H., Gorse, K. M., and Clarke, M. F. (1990) Alternative splicing of the human c-*myb* gene. *Oncogene* **5,** 117–124.

14. Luscher, B. and Eisenman, R. N. (1990) New light on *myc* and *myb*. Part II. *myb*. *Genes Dev.* **4,** 2235–2241.

15. Sakura, H. C., Kanei-Ishii, T., Nakagoshi, H., Gonda, T. J., and Ishii, S. (1989) Delineation of three functional domains of the transcriptional activator encoded by the c-*myb* protooncogene. *Proc. Natl. Acad. Sci. USA* **86,** 5758–5762.

16. Luscher, B., Christenson, E., Litchfield, D. W., Krebs, E. G., and Eisenman, R. N. (1990) *Myb* DNA binding inhibited by phosphorylation at a site deleted during oncogenic activation. *Nature* **344,** 517–522.

17. Thompson, C. B., Challoner, P. B., Neiman, P. E., and Groudine, M. (1986) Expression of the c-*myb* proto-oncogene during cellular proliferation. *Nature* **319,** 374–380.

18. Slamon, D. J., Boone, T. C., Murdock, D. C., Keith, D. F., Press, M. F., Larson, R. A., and Souza, L. M. (1986) Studies of the human c-*myb* gene and its product in human acute leuemias. *Science* **232,** 347–350.

19. Duprey, S. P. and Boettiger, D. (1985) Developmental regulation of c-*myb* in normal myeloid progenitor cells. *Proc. Natl. Acad. Sci. USA* **82,** 6937–6941.

20. Doolite, R. F., Hunkapiller, M. W., Hood, L. E., DeVare, S. G., Robbins, K. C., Aaronson, S. A., and Antonaides, H. N. (1983) Simian sarcoma onc gene, v-sis, is derived from the gene (or genes) encodding a platelet derived growth factor. *Science* **221,** 275–277.

21. Sherr, C. J., Rettenmier, C. W., Sacca, R., Roussel, M. F., Liook, A. T., and Stanley, R. F. (1985) The c-fms proto-oncogene product is related to the receptor for the mononuclear phagocyte growth factor, CSF-1. *Cell* **41,** 665–676.

22. Majumder, S., Brown, K., Qui, F. H., and Besmer, P. (1988) c-kit protein, a transmembrane kinase: identification in tissues and characterization. *Mol. Cell Biol.* **8,** 4896–4903.

23. Todokoro, K., Watson, R. J., Higo, H., Amanuma, H., Kuramochi, S., Yanagisawa, H., and Ikawa, Y. (1988) Down-regulation of c-*myb* gene expression is a prerequisite for erythropoietin-induced erythroid differentiation. *Proc. Natl. Acad. Sci. USA* **85,** 8900–8904.

24. Mucenski, M. L., McLain, K., Kier, A. B., Swerdlow, S. H., Schreiner, C. M., Miller, T. A., et al. (1991) A functional c-*myb* is required for normal murine fetal hepatic hematopoiesis. *Cell* **65,** 677–689.

25. Gewirtz, A. M. and Calabretta, B. (1988) A *c-myb* antisense oligodeoxynucleotide inhibits normal human hemaopoiesis in vitro. *Science* **242,** 1303–1306.

26. Caracciolo, D., Venturelli, D., Valtieri, M., Peschle, C., Gewirtz, A. M., and Calabretta, B. (1990) Stage-related proliferative activity determines c-*myb* functional requirements during normal human hematopoiesis. *J. Clin. Invest.* **85,** 55–61.

27. Anfossi, G., Gewirtz, A. M., and Calbretta, B. (1989) An oligomer complementary to c-*myb* encoded mRNA inhibits proliferation of human myeloid leukemia cell lines. *Proc. Natl. Acad. Sci. USA* **86,** 3379–3383.

28. Calabretta, B., Sims, R. B., Valtieri, M., Caracciolo, D., Szczylik, C., Venturelli, D., et al. (1991) Normal and leukemic hematopoietic cells manifest differential sensitivity to inhibitory effects of *c-myb* antisense oligodeoxynucleotides: An in vitro study relevant to bone marrow purging. *Proc. Natl. Acad. Sci. USA* **88,** 2351–2355.

29. Uhlmann, E. and Peyman, A. (1990) Antisense oligonucleotides: a new therapeutic principle. *Chem. Rev.* **90,** 543–584.

30. Zon, G. and Stec, W. J. (1991) Oligofdeoxynucleotides: pharmacological considerations, in *Oligonucleotides and Analogues: A Practical Approach* (Eckstein, F., ed.), Oxford Univ. Press, Oxford, pp. 87–108.

31. Eder, P. S., DeVine, R. J., Dagle, J. M., and Walder, J. A. (1991) Substrate specificity and kinetics of degradation of antisense oligonucleotides by a 3′ exonuclease in plasms. *Antisense Res. Dev.* **1,** 141–151.

32. Howe, K. M., Reakes, C. F., and Watson, R. J. (1990) Characterization of the sequence-specific interaction of mouse c-*myb* protein with DNA. *EMBO J* **9,** 161–169.

33. Miller, P. S. (1989) Non-ionic antisense oligonucleotides, in *Oligodeoxynucleotides:Antisense Inhibitors of Gene Expression* (Cohen, J. S., ed.), CRC, Boca Raton, FL, pp. 79–95.

34. Stein, C. A. and Cohen, J. S. (1988) Oligodeoxynucleotides as inhibitors of gene expression: a review. *Cancer Res.* **48,** 2959–2668.

35. Motoji, T., Takanashi, M., Fuchinour, M., Masuda, M., Oshimi, K., and Mizoguchi, H. (1989) Effect of recombinant GM-CSF and recombinant G-CSF on colony formation of blast progenitors ina cutew myeloblastic leukemia. *Exp. Hematol.* **17,** 56–60.

36. Ratajczak, M. Z., Kant, J. A., Luger, S. M., Hijiya, N., Zhang, J., Zon, G., and Gewirtz, A. M. (1992) In vivo treatment of human leukemia in a scid mouse model with c-myb antisense oligodeoxynucleotides. *Proc. Natl. Acad. Sci. USA* **89,** 11,823–11,827.

37. Rizzoli, V. and Mangoni, L. (1990) Pharmacological-mediated purging with mafosfamide in acute and chronic myeloid leukemias. The Italian Study Group. *Prog. Clin. Biol. Res.* **333,** 21–36.

38. McGlave, P. (1990) Bone marrow transplants in chronic myelogenous leukemia: an overview of determinants of survival. *Semin. Hematol.* **27,** 23–30.

39. Barnett, M. J., Eaves, A. C., and Phillips, G. L. (1990) An overview of bone marrow transplantation for chronic myeloid leukemia. *CMAJ* **143,** 187–193.

40. Dunbar, C. E. and Stewart, F. M. (1992) Separating the wheat from the chaff: selection of benign hematopoietic cells in chronic myeloid leukemia. *Blood* **79,** 1107–1110.

41. Verfaillie, C. M., Miller, W. J., Boylan, K., and McGlave, P. B. (1992) Selection of benign primitive hematopoietic progenitors in chronic myelogenous leukemia on the basis of HLA-DR antigen expression. *Blood* **79,** 1003–1007.

42. Gewirtz, A. M., Luger, S., Sokol, D., Gowdin, B., Stadtmauer, E., Recio, A., and Ratajczak, M. (1996) Oligodeoxynucleotide therapeutics for human myelogenous leukemia: interim results (abstr.). *Blood* **88,** 270a.

38

Ovarian Cancer Gene Therapy with *BRCA1*—An Overview

Patrice S. Obermiller and Jeffrey T. Holt

1. Introduction
1.1. BRCA1 *and Breast and Ovarian Cancer*

The human breast and ovarian cancer susceptibility gene *BRCA1* is a tumor-suppressor gene which is mutated and lost in hereditary breast and ovarian cancer, and has both alleles mutated in approximately 10–15% of cases of sporadic ovarian cancer. Studies of chromosome loss in ovarian cancer show that at least one allele of the *BRCA1* gene is lost or mutated in up to 70% of sporadic ovarian cancers. Although no sporadic breast cancers contain *BRCA1* mutations, our published study shows that expression of the mRNA is decreased suggesting that the *BRCA1* gene is altered quantitatively in sporadic cancer and qualitatively in hereditary cancer. Decreased expression of the *BRCA1* gene may also be important in cases of sporadic ovarian cancer that do not have *BRCA1* mutations. The majority of mutant alleles are nonsense and should produce truncated proteins, which are predicted to vary in length from 5% to 99% of full-length protein. A relatively small number of missense mutations have also been identified, most commonly in the predicted ring finger domain in the N-terminus. Patients with mutations in *BRCA1* differ clinically from nonfamilial breast cancer because the breast cancer is earlier in onset and more highly associated with ovarian cancer. We have recently obtained data indicating that families with *BRCA1* mutations in the 3′ portion of the gene develop early-onset breast cancer, but do not develop ovarian cancer, suggesting that expression of a truncated *BRCA1* protein may suppress ovarian tumors, but not breast tumors (*1*).

From: *Methods in Molecular Medicine, Vol. 35: Gene Therapy: Methods and Protocols*
Edited by: W. Walther and U. Stein © Humana Press, Inc., Totowa, NJ

Sporadic breast cancer in humans is clearly associated with early age of first pregnancy and this confers about a 50% reduction in the incidence of breast cancer. Thus, first pregnancy marks a key period of breast development involving proliferation, differentiation, and involution, which involve apoptosis.The demonstration that pregnancy induces *BRCA1* mRNA in mouse mammary gland supports a potential role for this gene product in breast development and differentiation. The primary function of the breast is lactation, a secretory process in which milk proteins are released in response to hormonal stimulation. This is characteristic of the regulated secretory pathway in which proteins accumulate intracellularly in secretory granules and are released only when the cells are stimulated with a secretogog. The granin family of proteins are regulated secretory proteins which colocalize in secretory granules with a number of peptide hormones such as parathyroid hormone, insulin, and prolactin. Granins contain a 10-amino acid motif, have a high percentage of acidic amino acids, are posttranslationally modified by glysocylation, phosphoryation, or sulfation and undergo proteolytic cleavage leading to peptides such as the chromogranin A-derived pancreastatin. This literature has been recently reviewed *(2)*. As an initial step in the biochemical characterization of the *BRCA1* gene product, we developed antibodies and studied the expression, localization, and function of *BRCA1* protein. These studies demonstrate that *BRCA1* is a growth inhibitory molecule that is released from cells, and represents a new member of the granin gene family *(3)*.

1.2. Retroviral Gene Therapy in Peritoneal and Pleural Effusions

Our preclinical data in mice and initial human data with a different retroviral vector suggest that malignant effusions may represent an ideal site for in vivo gene therapy approaches. The model system of metastatic ovarian cancer growing within peritoneal fluid has several advantages of safety and efficacy for retroviral-mediated gene transfer into solid tumors. First, the pathology of metastasis into mesothelial-lined spaces consists of relatively thin tumor plaques with extravasation of cancer cells into the fluid; potentially allowing a reservoir for delivering retroviral vectors to malignant cells. This spreading pattern is in contrast to primary tumors and more solid metastatic sites where cancer grows as a large three-dimensional mass, which could prevent delivery of retroviral vectors or other agents into the majority of tumor cells. In addition, infusion of retroviral vectors into these fluids should produce a greater effect on the growing cells within the fluid (predominantly cancer cells) than on proliferating host cells in regions of the body which do not directly connect to the mesothelial-lined spaces. Second, ovarian cancer provides a model system in which regional therapy could be curative in a high percentage of cases. This is true because ovarian cancer is confined to the peritoneal cavity at patient presentation in 60% of cases. The uptake and expression of the viral vectors can be readily assessed in these model systems because these fluids are readily accessible for cytologic, biochemical, and molecular analysis.

1.3. Scientific Rationale and Specific Objectives

To apply gene therapy to ovarian cancer we propose a method for in vivo gene replacement of the *BRCA1* gene regulated by the Moloney leukemia virus long terminal repeat (LTR): the vector is called LXSN-*BRCA1*sv (*4*). We have demonstrated that transduction of MCF-7 human cancer cells with LXSN-*BRCA1*sv inhibits their growth and their tumorigenesis in nude mice. MCF-7 cells were used in these experiments because they have a defect in the *BRCA1* gene that results in low levels of *BRCA1* protein, mimicking the genetic defect found in hereditary ovarian cancer. A control retroviral vector that does not produce *BRCA1* did not inhibit tumor formation, providing evidence that the antitumor effect is specifically mediated through expression of the transferred gene and not a nonspecific effect of retroviral transduction.

Our studies characterizing *BRCA1* expression have demonstrated that only certain tissues express *BRCA1*, and transfection studies demonstrate that *BRCA1* inhibits the growth of epithelial cancer cells, but not cultured fibroblasts. This suggests that the *BRCA1* protein may be a tissue-specific growth inhibitor, which could limit toxic effects of the vector in noncancer tissue. Our previous gene therapy protocols use tissue-selective gene regulation to limit toxicity, this vector expresses a tissue-selective growth inhibitor. This may contribute to the limited toxicity that we have observed in toxicity studies in nude mice. Transduction with the LXSN-*BRCA1*sv retroviral vector results in marked tumor inhibition or even cure of some experimental animals with no clearcut toxicity in nude mice. Therefore, we propose to apply this method for the treatment of human ovarian cancer.

The clinical trial will focus on maximizing the delivery of retroviral vector to the tumor cells within the malignant fluid space, along with repeated administration in an attempt to maximize the antitumor effect. Patients will undergo a fluid examination prior to infusion of retroviral vector (paracentesis for malignant ascites). Cytologic, biochemical, and molecular studies will be performed on aspirations of fluid to follow the extent of viral vector uptake by tumor cells. The clinical extent of tumor spread will be measured before and after retroviral vector infusion by clinical exam, conventional radiologic studies, and determination of *CA125* and secreted *BRCA1* levels (if detectable).

1.4. Preclinical Data

The specific retroviral vectors to be employed in these studies have been shown to produce a 90% inhibition in the growth and spread of established

MCF-7 peritoneal tumors in mice ($N = 6$ in each treatment group). Although our studies indicate that the retrovirus transduces no more than 40–70% of the cancer cells, it produces a 90% or greater reduction in the size of the tumors. Other gene therapy studies have shown a similar phenomenon (greater efficacy than can be explained by infection rates), which has been termed the bystander phenomenon. The bystander effect in our studies appears to be caused by secretion of *BRCA1*, because conditioned media from transfected cells also inhibits the growth of cancer cells. Published studies of flank tumors demonstrate that unselected cells transduced with LXSN-BRCA1sv have slow-growing tumors, whereas cells that were slected with *G418* to assure 100% transduction of the population have no tumor growth. This indicates that the dose of the viral vector will be important despite the presence of secretion. We have also seen no toxicity in nude mice that have been followed for at least 8 wk after treatment with the *BRCA1* retroviral vector. The retroviral vector for the patient trial has only been shown to be free of contaminating viruses including replication-competent retroviruses. This preclinical data has been published *(1,3)*.

1.5. Clinical Data

Two types of clinical data are available concerning this Phase I trial:

1. Stability of a different retroviral vector (XM6:antifos) in pleural and peritoneal effusions in vitro and in vivo in one patient;
2. Studies of expression, secretion, and growth inhibitory function of human cells expressing endogenous or transfected *BRCA1*.

Data presented show that retroviral vectors are stable in peritoneal fluid and that cells within this fluid can be transduced in vitro at high efficiency. (Some of this data is published *(5)*). In addition to this in vitro data, we have treated two patients with the starting dose of XM6:antifos and we have been able to show that the vector is stable in the pleural effusion for 24 h, such that samples aspirated from the pleural catheter 24 h after infusion can transduce target cells in in vitro transduction assays. This vector can be detected in the pleural effusion cell pellet and in supernatant, and a small amount of vector DNA can be detected in the blood for up to 24 h after infusion. Antibodies directed against the amphotropic envelope protein were detected in blood samples from the patient 4 wk after infusion, but were not detected in prior samples. One patient died 6 wk after treatment following talc pleurodesis. Extensive autopsy performed by the author (Dr. Holt) and pathology colleagues at Vanderbilt demonstrated that there was extensive lymphangitic spread of tumor within the lung. The cause of death was respiratory failure owing to the combination of lymphangitic tumor and pleurodesis, which together destroyed either mechanism of fluid removal from pulmonary parenchyma. PCR analysis of 24 tissues showed no detectable retroviral vector at autopsy including injection site (our detection sensitivity of PCR-southern is 1–5 mol/ sample). RCR studies on blood and tissue samples (including injection site) were negative for PG4 foci following amplification on Mus Dunni permissive cells.

Expression analysis of ovarian cancer cells by Western blot and immunohistochemistry indicates that more than 80% of ovarian cancer samples from patients have significantly decreased *BRCA1* protein expression compared to normal. This occurs in both hereditary and sporadic cases of ovarian cancer. Functional data showing growth inhibition of ovarian cancer cells have been published *(1,6)*.

1.6. Overall Aims and Objectives

Based on preclinical data (see preliminary studies) we hypothesize that *BRCA1* retroviral therapy may be effective in the treatment of metastatic ovarian cancer. The study is designed to test this hypothesis and specifically provide information on the following aspects of this therapy:

1. Is there effective uptake and expression of retroviral vector into malignant ovarian cancer cells that are growing within peritoneal fluid? What dose of retroviral vector is required to produce expression in a significant proportion of cancer cells?
2. Do peritoneal cells and other nonsecretory cells express the transduced *BRCA1* gene?
3. Does the viral vector enter the systemic circulation? Is there toxicity associated with infusion of viral vector in patients with ovarian cancer?

2. Material
2.1. Chemistry, Manufacturing, and Control

The LXSN-BRCA1sv clinical grade retroviral vector was produced under cGMP conditions in our dedicated facility (*see* **Notes 1** and **2**). This basically involves using AIM V media from Life Technologies (Bethesda, MD) as a perfusate for the PA317 producer line growing in a closed perfusion-based system (Corning Costar Cell Cube) at 37°C. We have adapted the producer cell line to serum-free growth in the Cell Cube at 37°C.

2.1.1. Construction of the Vector

The vector was constructed by cloning the *Sal*I linkered *BRCA1* cDNA into the *Xho*I site of LXSN, as we have described *(1)*. The LXSN vector was obtained from Dusty Miller at the University of Washington. The structure of the vector was confirmed by two methods: restriction mapping and DNA sequencing.

Summary of Evidence that the Presumed Vector Sequences are Correct:

1. Detailed strategy for plasmid construction with careful mapping of all cloning intermediates.
2. Restriction mapping, supported by DNA sequencing.
3. Western blots showing full-length protein is produced and retains growth suppression capacity.
4. Southern blot of *Pst*I-restricted transferred DNA showing integration of unrearranged vector into target cells.
5. PCR using primers derived from published *Neo* gene sequence.

2.1.2. Master Cell Bank: Generation and Characterization

The PA317 master cell bank was produced by transducing PA317 cells with virus stock from Bosc 23 cells, which were transfected with twice-cesium banded LXSN-BRCA1sv plasmid DNA. Following transfection, the PA317 cells were split and then treated with G418 until individual clones could be identified and expanded. Each clone was then screened for its titer by analyzing its ability to transfer G418 resistance (because the retroviral vector contains a *Neomycin* resistance gene). The clones that had the highest titer were then frozen in numerous aliquots and tested for sterility, presence of replication-competent retrovirus, and presence of mycoplasm. A single-cloned PA317 cell line has been used for all of the activity and toxicity studies, and for the published studies *(1)*.

Whenever cells are thawed from the master cell bank their viability will be tested by analyzing doubling time and by Trypan blue exclusion, and their function will be tested by repeating the titer of virus produced. We presently have 20 frozen vials of the master cell bank, which are derived from a single early passage and have been shown to be bacteria, fungus, and mycoplasm-free. Tests for RCR (replication-competent retrovirus) are negative by S+L– assay and by RCR tests using 3T3 amplification prior to PG4 S+L– testing. Tests for RCR were performed on both the master cell bank and on a single patient dose (highest dose) of vector preparation.

2.2. Control and Testing

2.2.1. Summary of Completed Testing for RCR

To perform these tests we incubated 100 mL of viral stock from the LXSN-BRCA1sv master cell bank with 10^7 Mus Dunni cells for 7 d followed by assay on PG4 S+L– cells as we have described in Arteaga and Holt *(5)*. We also cocultured 10^7 PA317 producer cells with Mus Dunni cells for 4 d and then added this media to Mus Dunni cells for 7 d, followed by asay on PG4 S+L–. Tests were also performed on each a 1-mL aliquot of clinical grade vector from each day of production, and from 50 mL of media that was incubated with the postproduction cells in the Cell Cube device (*see* **Note 2**).The following

Table 1

Virus stock	Amphotropic control virus	1 wk 3T3 amplification
None	None	–
None	10^{-5}	+
LXSN-BRCA1sv (stock)	None	–
LXSN-BRCA1sv (stock)	10^{-5}	+
LXSN-BRCA1sv (coculture)	None	–
LXSN-BRCA1sv (Feb 1)	None	–
LXSN-BRCA1sv (Feb 2)	None	–
LXSN-BRCA1sv (Feb 3)	None	–
LXSN-BRCA1sv (Feb 4)	None	–
LXSN-BRCA1sv (Feb 5)	None	–
LXSN-BRCA1sv (Feb 6)	None	–
LXSN-BRCA1sv (Feb 7)	None	–
LXSN-BRCA1sv (Feb 8)	None	–
LXSN-BRCA1sv (Feb 9)	None	–
LXSN-BRCA1sv (postproduction)	None	–

results (**Table 1**) demonstrate the absence of RCR in our master cell bank and viral vector stocks.

2.2.2. Other Tests on Master Cell Bank

We have completed all microbiologic testing on the master cell bank: including bacterial culture, mycoplasm testing by Hoescht and MAP testing (monoclonal antibody production) has been completed by Microbiological Associates (Rockville, MD). In vitro assays for cells from the master cell bank were innoculated into monolayer cultures of the following cell types and were negative for cytopathic effect or for hemabsorption:

1. NIH 3T3 cells.
2. WI38 (human diploid fibroblasts).
3. CV-1 cells (monkey kidney cells).

2.2.3. Lot Release Criteria

We will release lots that pass the following criteria;

1. Negative for RCR by PG4S+L– assay after Mus Dunni amplification.
2. Negative for bacteria and fungi and culture and Gram stain.
3. Negative for mycoplasm by Hoescht and PCR.
4. Vector prep produces greater than 80% inhibition of G418 resistant colonies compared to control vector.
5. Negative for pyrogens by limulus amebocyte lysate testing. We will reject any if the result of this test exceeds 0.5 U/mL.

3. Methods

3.1. Protocol Design

Patients with ovarian cancer who meet the study criteria will be treated with retroviral gene therapy by infusion of the retroviral vector into the peritoneal tumor site. Retroviral vectors will be manufactured in the Cancer Center Vector Production Facility from viral producer cells using serum free and phenol-red free conditions and will be tested for sterility, absence of specific pathogens, and an absence of RCR by standard assays (the FDA has specific requirements for biologic therapies of this type and we comply with their standards in our GMP virus production facility, *see* **Notes**). Retrovirus will be stored frozen in large aliquots that have been tested according to FDA standards.

Patients will first undergo surgical placement of a peritoneal catheter as an outpatient procedure performed by Dr. David Tait (surgical procedure, *see* **Note 3**). Patients will be admitted to the Clinical Research Center where they will have a complete physical exam, blood, and urine tests to determine overall health. They will also have a chest X-ray, electrocardiogram, and appropriate radiologic procedures to assess tumor stage (*see* Study Parameters in **Table 2**). Patients will spend 4 d in the Clinical Research Center for the initial infusions of retroviral vector. Peritoneal washings will be taken through the catheter prior to each treatment. Blood samples will also be drawn prior to each treatment and tested for the presence of retroviral vector by sensitive polymcrase chain reaction (PCR)-based assays. The fluids that are removed will be analyzed to determine:

1. The percentage of cancer cells taking up the vector/gene combination: by PCR and by *in situ* hybridization.

Table 2
Study Parameters for Clinical Trial

Routine Studies	Pre-Treatment (Rx)[5]	Daily during Rx	2 wk post-Rx	4 wk post-Rx	Monthly × 11	q 6 mo
History and Physical	X	X	X	X	X	X
Tumor Status	X	As clinically indicated(ACI)			ACI	
ACI						
(CT scan)						
Performance Status	X	X	X	X	X	X
Toxicity Assessment	X	X	X	X	X	X
Weight	X	X	X	X	X	X
Complete Blood Count[1]	X	X	X	X	X	X
PT, PTT	X	X	X	X	X	X
Urinalysis	X	X	X	X	X	X
BUN and Creatinine	X	X	X	X	X	X
Liver Function Tests[2]	X	X	X	X	X	X
Serum Chemistries[3]	X	X	X	X	X	X
Chest X-ray	X	ACI	ACI	X	X	X
EKG	X	ACI	ACI	ACI	ACI	ACI
Ascites Studies[4]	X	X	ACI	ACI	ACI	ACI
Circulating antibodies[6]	Control	X	X	X	X	X

ACI = As Clinically Indicated
[1] To include: hematocrit, hemoglobin, differential, and platelets.
[2] To include: alkaline phosphatase, serum transaminases, bilirubin, protein, LDH, and albumin. Ca125 will also be followed.
[3] To include: Na, K, Ca, PO4, Cl, Magnesium, C02, and glucose
[4] To include: cytology, cell count, differential, LDH, protein, glucose, bacterial cultures as clinically indicated.
[5] Lab tests within 5 d of treatment.
[6] Measurement of antibodies to amphotropic envelope.

2. The number of cancer cells present in the fluid.
3. *BRCA1* expression level of the cells.
4. Quantity of secreted *BRCA1* protein in the peritoneal effusion.

Patients will be continuously monitored while in the CRC. After the 4-d period in the Clinical Research Center they will be discharged, but will be asked to return at day 7 for a blood sample and a fluid sample. After completion of the viral vector infusion series, patients will proceed with chemotherapy options as clinically indicated to temporarily control their disease.

3.2. Research Design

This study will determine the maximally tolerated dose (MTD) of LXSN-BRCA1sv when administered in transcellular spaces. Primary end points will be:

1. The rate of transduction in tumor and/or nontumor cells in peritoneal ascites.
2. The presence and stability of this vector in the systemic circulation and in the peritoneal (tumor cell-containing) space.
3. The nature of the systemic (fever, myalgias) and local (peritonitis, pain) toxicities induced by this vector. A secondary end point will be the clinical efficacy of LXSN-BRCA1sv.

3.2.1. Protocol Inclusion Criteria

1. Patients with biopsy-proven recurrent epithelial ovarian cancer measurable in two dimensions radiographically or on physical exam.
2. Patients age $\geq$17 and $\leq$75 and who have signed informed consent.
3. GOG performance status (PS) $\leq$2.
4. Life expectancy of greater than 3 mo.
5. Recovery for at least 4 wk from previous surgery and/or other cancer therapies.
6. Adequate hematological (WBCs $\geq$4000/mm^3, platelet count $\geq$100,000/mm^3), hepatic (bilirubin $\leq$2 mg/dL, SGOT $\leq$2 × normal), and renal (creatinine $\leq$1.5 mg/dL) functions.
7. Patients using an acceptable form of birth control if hysterectomy was not performed at original ovarian cancer surgery.

3.2.2. Exclusion Criteria

1. All medical students (Vanderbilt policy) and pregnant patients.
2. Active bacterial infections.
3. Patients on concomitant experimental or other alternative therapies.
4. Patients with heart failure (NYHA class 4), recent myocardial infarction, respiratory insufficiency, or hematological, hepatic, or renal dysfunction.
5. Concomitant anticoagulant or antiplatelet drugs.

Effusion material that is not required for diagnostic purposes will be collected for molecular studies. A 0.1–2-L serum-free volume of retroviral vector (containing 10^9–10^{10} viral particles) will be administered four times daily into the peritoneal space under bedside ultrasonic guidance. Volume will be determined by the clinical PI (principal investigator) based on the presence or absence of ascites. A half-log dose escalation will be performed in patients duringthe Phase I trial. Ascitic fluid will be drawn daily before LXSN-BRCA1sv infusion.

3.2.3. Toxicity Evaluation

Patient evaluation will include history and physical examination prior to initiation of therapy and daily during the 4-d period of vector infusion. Toxicity grading will be done using the GOG Common Toxicity Criteria. CBC, SMA-20, urinalysis, as well as cytology and conventional studies in the effusates will be performed daily during this period (see **Table 2**, Study Parameters).

Although the LXSN-BRCA1sv vector is replication-incompetent, long-term toxicity from it is unknown. Hence, follow-up studies will be done at 2 and 4 wk and then every month during the first year with special attention to the persistence of retroviral vector in the systemic circulation. Patients will be then followed every 6 mo for the rest of their lives. We do not intend prospectively to retreat patients unless they experience a documented complete clinical or partial response to LXSN BRCA1sv. An autopsy will be requested for every patient (patient and families will be informed of the importance of autopsy and long-term follow-up for gene therapy studies at the time of initial interview and informed consent).

3.3. Protocol Parameters

3.3.1. Determination of Starting Dose

The doses of LXSN-BRCA1sv to be used in the Phase I Clinical Trial are based on our prior preclinical animal studies. Because our current titers of clinical grade vector are 4–7×10^7 per mL, a small volume of vector will be required for the initial dose.

Although our toxicology studies of intraperitoneal infusion of LXSN-BRCA1sv into immunocompetent mice are in progress, we have experience with ip infusion of the similar XM6:antifos. There was no clinical toxicity attributable to the XM6:antifos vector in any of the treated animals to date. PCR analysis of tissue distribution of ip infusion into nude mice showed vector DNA in peritoneum (also positive by Southern blot) and in serum during the first 48 h after infusion. Studies of tissue distribution following ip infusion into immunocompetent mice and intrapleural infusion into immunocompetent rats are in progress. Intraperitoneal infusion into mice in the absence of inflammation results in no detectable vector DNA even when tissues are analyzed as early as 4 h after the final infusion. Intraperitoneal infusion into mice treated with intraperitoneal oyster glycogen shows vector present in the kidney at 4 h (4/4 animals tested to date) and in certain other organs, but only at the 4×10^7 dose and not at the 4×10^6 dose *(7)*.

From these studies we obviously do not have a nude mouse (or immunocompetent mouse or rat) LD10. Therefore, we have selected 10% of the largest (safe) dose injected into mice as our initial dose in humans. Note that this dose does not show any tissue distribution by PCR analysis in mice, even when treated with oyster glycogen.

Considering the surface area of a 25-g mouse to be 0.0073 m^2 and a 60-kg woman to be 1.62 m^2. A mouse inoculum of 4.5×10^6 particles will be dose-equivalent to 10^9 vector particles in the patient. Because our current tiers are about 10^8 per mL, a small volume of vector will be required for the initial dose. The vector was collected in AIM V but will be diluted with injection-grade normal saline with added polybrene to achieve a polybrene concentration of 8 µg/mL. Escalation will proceed as follows with three patients at each dose level.

Level 1: $10^8 \times 4$
Level 2: $3.3 \times 10^8 \times 4$
Level 3: $10^9 \times 4$
Level 4: $3.3 \times 10^9 \times 4$
Level 5: $10^{10} \times 4$

We do not expect infusion of 0.1 to 2 L of volume to be a problem because we will routinely remove an excess volume of patient's effusate prior to injection of LXSN-BRCA1sv. This amount of fluid is traditionally given with ip chemotherapy.

LXSN-BRCA1sv will be administered intraperitoneally in 0.1 to 2.0 L of normal saline (based on the amount of ascites present) through an implantable peritoneal catheter (Port-A-Cath). Surgical placement of the catheter is described in **Note 3**.

We estimate the MOI (multiplicity of infection) to be in excess of 1:1 although admittedly, this is difficult to predict because of our inability to accurately measure tumor burden in a host. The total dose of LXSN-BRCA1sv will vary between 4×10^8 to 4×10^{10} vector particles per 4-d treatment. It is calculated that a burden of approximately 10^{12} tumor cells is about the maximal compatible with life. Because in this Phase I trial we will be treating peritoneal effusions with peritoneal tumor, it is likely that the number of tumor cells treated by our intervention, based on the aforementioned total doses, will be sizably under 10^{12} cells.

3.3.2. Dose Escalation and MTD (Maximum Toxicity Dose)

Three patients will be treated with 10^8 viral particles $\times 4$. Once they have all recovered from all grade 2 or less toxicities (except alopecia) and as long as grade 3–4 toxicity is not encountered, a subsequent dose level will be initiated in three additional patients. If one grade 3 or 4 toxicity occurs at a given dose level, a minimum of six patients will be enrolled at that level. If only 1 of 6 patients has grade 3 or 4 toxicity, dose escalation will continue. The MTD of LXSN-BRCA1sv will be defined as the dose where 2 of 6 patients experience grade 3 or 4 toxicity. If 2 of 3 or 3 of 6 patients experience grade 3 or 4 toxicity, the MTD will be defined as the immediately lower dose level.

The volume of infusate may become a limiting factor at some point. Because of the theoretically predicted cell type-specific integration and expression of the antisense, it may well be that little to none host tissue toxicity is detected by this trial and/or that infusate volume (rather than toxicity) ultimately becomes the dose-limiting factor in this study. Therefore, an alternative end point will be expression of LXSN-BRCA1sv in ≥90% of tumor cells in the ascitic fluid, conditions under which we would expect local efficacy since *BRCA1* is secreted and an in vivo growth inhibitor.

3.3.3. Studies of Retroviremia

Our preclinical data indicate that infusion of relatively large quantities of vector into the peritoneal space results in detectable amounts of vector in the peripheral blood of nude mice. Because of the small volumes of blood that can be obtained from nude mice, we have been technically unable to determine whether the detectable vector is within the serum or the cells of the blood, and whether the detected vector is still capable of transduction (although a large body of literature indicates that human serum destroys retroviral particles). We propose answering these questions in patients by obtaining 20 mL of blood during each of the 4 d that the patients are present in the Clinical Research Center, separating the blood into serum and cellular components for PCR detection. If vector is detected within the serum component, then we will perform the following assay to identify the existence of transduction-capable viral vector. Serum will be incubated with OK3 target cells, and DNA will be obtained from OK3 cells before and after attempted transduction. We will use our previously employed vector primers for this assay, which has been published *(5)*.

3.3.4. Criteria for Clinical Response

Although this is a Phase I trial, patients with measurable disease will be evaluated for a clinical response to LXSN-BRCA1sv especially those that do not undergo a palliative intervention immediately after retroviral vector therapy. In general, malignant ascites is difficult to evaluate. We will follow fluid cytology, abdominal girth, CT scans of the abdomen, and local symptoms. For other sites of disease, conventional response criteria will be used as follows:

Complete Response (CR). Complete disappearance of all measurable lesions and of all signs and symptoms of disease for at least 4 wk.

Partial Response (PR). Decrease of at least 50% of the sum of the products of the two largest perpendicular diameters of all measurable lesions as determined by two observations not less than 4 wk apart. To be considered a PR, no new lesions should have appeared during this period and none should have increased in size.

Stable Disease. Less than 25% change in tumor volume from previous evaluations.

Progressive Disease. Greater than 25% increase in tumor measurements from prior evaluations.

The result of this Phase I clinical trial including observable vector stability and partial responses in patients has been published *(8)*.

4. Notes

1. The Vanderbilt Cancer Center Vector Production Facility is a dedicated facility which is used to produce viral vectors for Phase I and Phase II clinical trials of Cancer Gene Therapy approaches. The Vanderbilt Cancer Center is an NCI-designated Clinical Cancer Center that is located at Vanderbilt University Medical School in Nashville, TN. The vector-production facility is located in 468 square feet of laboratory space on the sixth floor of the new Medical Research Building II, which opened in April 1995. The goal of our research is to attempt a true "genetic correction" gene therapy approach for cancer, by altering the expression of oncogenes or replacing missing tumor suppressor genes in cancer cells. We have already used the facility to produce several batches of clinical grade retroviral vector for clinical trials. We also used the facility for producing clinical grade retroviral vector for this Phase I trial (LXSN-BRCA1sv for ovarian cancer), and plan to use it as well for Phase II studies. Because our studies are designed for the genetic alteration of cancer cells and are not vaccine studies, we will perform in vivo transductions with high titer retroviral stocks and have no intention of performing ex vivo transduction experiments.

2. Our facilities will never produce more than one product at a time. Therefore, the products will always be segregated and personnel will never work on two vectors at the same time. We use all new Cell Cube plating chamber and replaceable plastic/silicone parts, and autoclave all nondisposable pieces such as the bubble oxygenator. We validate cleaning by documentation of autoclave temperatures and procedures, and by both PCR testing for the presence of residual vector and tests for RCR.

3. a. Select site several centimeters below and lateral to the umbilicus and make a transverse incision through the skin, subcutaneous tissue, fascia, rectus muscle, and peritoneum.

   b. Introduce the distal end of the catheter to the desired infusion site.

   c. A sc pocket superior to the incision is fashioned slightly larger than the port.

   d. Prepare a sc tunnel from the catheter entry point to the portal pocket and draw the catheter through the tunnel using a long clamp.

   e. Attach catheter to port and suture port to fascia.

   f. Flush catheter to confirm placement at desired site.

References

1. Holt, J. T., Thompson, M. E., Szabo, C., Robinson-Benion, C., Arteaga, C. L., King, M-C., and Jensen, R. A. (1996) Growth retardation and tumor inhibition by BRCA1. *Nature Genet.* **12**, 298–302.
2. Steeg, P. (1996) Granin expectations in breast cancer? *Nature Genet.* **12**, 223–225.
3. Jensen, R. A., Thompson, M. E., Szabo, C., Jetton, T., van der Meer, R., Helou, B., et al. (1996) BRCA1 is secreted and exhibits properties of a granin. *Nature Genet.* **12**, 303–308.
4. Holt, J. T., et al. (1998) Growth retardation and tumor inhibition by BRCA1 (correction). *Nature Genet.* **19**, 102.
5. Arteaga, C. L. and Holt, J. T. (1996) Tissue-targeted antisense anti-fos retroviral vector inhibits established breast cancer xenografts in nude mice. *Cancer Res.* **56**, 1098–1103.
6. Thompson, M. E., Jensen, R. A., Obermiller, P. S., Page, D. L., and Holt, J. T. (1995) Decreased expression of BRCA1 accelerates growth and is frequently present during sporadic breast cancer progression. *Nature Genet.* **9**, 444–450.
7. Obermiller, P. S., Pilaro, A. M., Arteaga, C. L., and Holt, J. T. (1997) Inflammation alters distribution of antifos retroviral vector after murine intracavitary delivery, in *Clinical Trials of Genetic Therapy with Antisense DNA and DNA Vectors* (Wickstrom, E., ed.), Marcel Dekker, New York.
8. Tait, D. L., Obermiler, P. S., Redlin-Frazier, S., Jensen, R. A., Welcsh, P., Dann, J., et al. (1997) Phase I trial of BRCA1 retroviral gene therapy for ovarian cancer. *Clin. Cancer Res.* **3**, 1959–1968.

39

Methods for Chemoprotection and Chemosensitization

MDR-1 For Chemoprotection Using Retroviruses to Modify Hematopoietic Cells and Cytosine Deaminase for Chemosensitization Using Adenoviral Vectors to Modify Epithelian Neoplastic Cells

Shrlnavassan Shrimdkandada, Si Qing Fu, Lian Hua Yin, Xiang Yang David Guo, Thong Nanakorn, Xue Yan Peng, Don Dizon, Debbie Lin, Matthew Cooperberg, Jong Ho Won, and Albert Deisseroth

1. Introduction

Surgery, radiation therapy, and chemotherapy have been applied to the curative therapy of 50% of cancer patients in the United States during the past 100 years. It is clear that the chemotherapeutic agents used to develop curative therapy for leukemias, lymphomas, gestational malignancy, and testicular cancer are not as active in the more numerous epithelial neoplasms, perhaps because of the complexity of genetic change in these latter neoplasms.

The advent of molecular biology and genetics to medicine has resulted in the discovery of changes in neoplastic cells that are exerting a dominant effect on clinically relevant phenotypes (survival, remission induction percentage, and remission duration) and changes that are promoting disease progression. Now that the molecular targets are known, investigators are trying to apply this information to new directions in therapy. This chapter summarizes two new directions in genetic therapy: retroviral vectors carrying MDR-1 transcription units for chemoprotection of normal hematopoietic cells, and adenoviral

From: *Methods in Molecular Medicine, Vol. 35: Gene Therapy: Methods and Protocols*
Edited by: W. Walther and U. Stein © Humana Press, Inc., Totowa, NJ

vectors carrying cytosine deaminase transcription units for chemotherapy sensitization of neoplastic epithelial cells.

The therapy of solid tumors and hematopoietic neoplasms had its origins in ancient civilizations, at which time extracts of plants (tree bark, leaves, and roots) were used for treatment of all of human disease. Since the middle of the twentieth century, the active ingredients of these ancient extracts have been purified and introduced into therapy, singly and in combinations, for the treatment of cancer. Systematic study of these therapies has led to the discovery of curative combinations of chemotherapy for diseases, such as Hodgkins Disease by DeVita et al. *(1)*.

1.1. Chemotherapy Protection

More recently, retroviral vectors have been used for the transfer of chemotherapy resistance genes into the normal sensitive cells of the marrow and peripheral blood of patients with carcinomas of the breast and ovary, that are recurrent following surgery, prone to relapse, and have proven to be incompletely responsive to chemotherapy.

This has been done to make safe the delivery of chemotherapy immediately following an autologous transplant after intensive systemic chemotherapy for their disease.

1.2. Chemotherapy Sensitization

Adenoviral vectors carrying prodrug activation transcription units are being used for the chemotherapy and radiation therapy sensitization of solid tumor neoplasms.

2. Materials
2.1. Retroviral Vector-Mediated Transduction

Retroviral vectors are produced by collecting supernatant medium from producer cell lines. The producer cell line contains the replication cassette (*Gag, Pol,* and *Env* genes) from the virus, integrated into its chromosomal DNA, either in one or two separate locations. The recombinant plasmid is then transfected into the producer cell line. The structure of the transgene is characterized by restriction endonuclease digestion and then by total sequencing. The titer of the infectious particles that are released from the cell line is then determined. The supernatant is checked for transduction capability and the phenotype of the transduced cells is characterized. Although it was customary to collect this vector in serum-containing medium, it is now recognized that there are two reasons for collecting the retroviral particles in a serum-free medium: (1) the ligand from the retroviral envelope proteins, which engages the amphtrophic receptor on the mammian cells, is subject to complement-mediated degradation; and (2) the hematopoietic cells to be transduced can be induced to differentiate (and therefore to lose their replicative capability), by being incubated in serum-containing medium, especially in the presence of IL3 and stem-cell factor (SCF).

The transduction can be carried out by mixing the cells to be transduced with the target cells for varying periods of time. Eventually, the number of integration sites per cell is measured. In the past, it was customary to incubate the vector and the cells under conditions in which the target cells would undergo a cellular replication event. This is necessary because the cDNA produced by the action of the reverse transcriptase of the vector and the viral RNA cannot cross the nuclear membrane of the nondividing cell. Because the integration of the vector cDNA is required for there to be expression, it is necessary for the target cell to divide.

2.2. Adenoviral Vector-Mediated Infection

The adenoviral vector is stable in solution in the presence of serum, and can be physically purified using cesium density grandient centrifugation. The titers of this vector are very high, and by increasing the ratio of the plaque-forming units to the nucleated cell count, the percentage of infectivity of the target cells can be increased to 100%, providing the target cells have (1) the receptor for the fibrillar protein, which is necessary for binding; and (2) have the alpha V beta 3 integrin receptor, which is necessary for uptake of the vector into the cells and for the release from the postuptake endosome. Once released, the DNA of the vector is carried across the intact nuclear membrane of the nondividing cell into the nucleus, where it can be expressed as an episome.

Once the vector is titered, the target cells and the vector are mixed in serum-free medium for only 90 min to prevent infection. The unincorporated vector is then rinsed away. Following this, the cells can be incubated in serum-free or serum-containing medium. The transgene of the adenoviral vector may be expressed for up to 10–14 d.

3. Methods
3.1. Chemotherapy Protection

During the past 20 years, various forms of exogenous hematopoietic reconstitution have been used to rescue patients from the irreversible suppression of hematopoietic function generated by intensive systemic therapy. Although a small fraction of advanced disease patients appear to have derived some disease-free survival benefit from these intensive therapeutic interventions, the exposure of epithelial neoplastic cells to a single course of intensive therapy may not be sufficient to eradicate all disease, because most of these cells are nondividing and therefore resistant even to intensive alkylating agent therapy. Although all of the neoplastic cells are damaged by the intensive therapy, only a fraction of these cells die before the transplant. Since most therapists worry that the delivery of posttransplant chemotherapy might destroy the newly engrafted hematopoietic cells, a long interval between the intensive pre-transplant therapy and the next exposure to posttransplant therapy is a long one, during which any residual tumor cells are free to repair the DNA damage generated by the pretransplant therapy and then to regrow.

Many workers have proposed modifying the engrafting autologous cells used to rescue patients following intensive therapy with chemotherapy resistance genes. This would make safe the posttransplant delivery of chemotherapy, at a time when the damaged epithelial cells that remain after intensive therapy are most vulnerable to additional chemotherapy. These considerations led to the initiation of trials involving the use of retroviral vectors for the introduction of the Multidrug Resistance Gene (MDR-1) into the hematopoietic cells used to strengthen transplant patients following intensive chemotherapy.

These MRD-1 trials were based on animal models *(2–5)* in which it was shown that the introduction of the MDR-1 cDNA, under the governance of a promoter (which in contrast to the endogenous MDR-1 promoter, does not downregulate during differentiation), increased the resistance of the hematopoietic cells to the toxic effects of posttransplant chemotherapy. The endogenous MDR-1 promoter is downregulated during hematopoietic differentiation, such that only 1/10,000 of the cells in the marrow express sufficient levels of the protein product of MDR-1 (p-glycoprotein) to protect these cells from even conventional doses of chemotherapy *(6)*. These studies showed not only that the frequency of the vector MDR-1 modified cells increased during the delivery of post ransplant therapy *(3–4)*—implying that they were more resistant to the posttransplant chemotherapy than were the unmodified cells—but that these transcription units were active for up to 17 mo posttransplant and had sufficient self-renewal capability to sequentially repopulate six successive cohorts of lethally irradiated recipient mice *(5)*.

3.2. Notes on Chemotherapy Protection

The goals of the clinical trials *(7–8)* were:

1. To test the toxicity of the genetic modification procedure, used to introduce the MDR-1 transcription units into the target cells on their ability to repopulate rapidly in an intensively treated recipient;
2. To test for resistant phenotypes;

3. To test whether the posttransplant therapy contributed to the overall response of the tumor to therapy; and
4. To determine how long the vector MDR-1 positive cells could be detected posttransplant.

These studies *(7–8)* showed that:

1. The hematopoietic recovery was rapid, suggesting that vector modification did not damage the short-term reconstitution ability of the hematopoietic cells;
2. Resistant phenotypes appeared, but most of these may have been caused by the activation of the endogenous MDR-1 gene expression;
3. The delivery of posttransplant chemotherapy (12 cycles of taxol in a dose-escalating program up to 275 mg/M2/course) generated responses above and beyond those resulting from exposure to the pretransplant therapy;
4. MDR-1 vector modified cells were detectable post transplant, but these cells persisted only for a short period of time *(7–8)*.

Newer vectors used to promote the modification of the early long-term repopulating cells are being used to generate longer-term engraftment of the MDR-1 vector modified cells.

3.3. Genetic Chemotherapy Sensitization

The sensitivity of normal cells to the toxic effects of chemotherapy have limited both the doses of chemotherapy and the duration of therapy that can be safely administered. One way of increasing the concentration of drug and the duration of the exposure period (called the "concentration X time product," which is possible to safely administer without damaging the normal cells of the body), is to introduce into the target cells a gene coding for a prodrug activation transcription unit, the protein product of which codes for an enzyme that converts a nontoxic precursor drug into a cytotoxic molecule. In this way, levels of the toxic drug can be generated specifically within the tumor cells, which are not possible to achieve by systemic administration of the toxic drug.

We have chosen to use this approach in two clinical settings:

1. The ex vivo purging of breast cancer cells from collections of hematopoietic cells, used for autologous transplants following intensive systemic therapy in patients with advanced conditions, in whom the breast cancer cells grossly involve the marrow.
2. The sensitization of prostatic carcinoma cells to the effects of radiation therapy.

We have chosen to use the bacterial cytosine deaminase gene, a product which catalyzes the nontoxic precursor, 5-FC, into the cytotoxic drug, 5-FU.

5-FU is an ideal therapeutic approach to the purging because although it is usually thought to kill cells through a cycle-dependent mechanism, at the doses usually administered and if the intracellular levels of the 5-FU can be increased, it is incorporated extensively into mRNA, thereby disrupting its processing and translation. This kills the cells through protein starvation. The prodrug can be administered without causing toxicity to the normal cells of the body, and the tumor cells, once infected with an adenoviral vector carrying the cytosine deaminse transcription unit, can be destroyed by the doses and duration of exposure to the cytotoxic drug 5-FU.

3.4. Notes on Genetic Chemotherapy Sensitization

In the case of the purging of breast cancer cells from collections of autologous hematopoietic cells, our group has shown that the use of the adenoviral vector with the cytosine deaminase gene can reduce the level of the breast cancer cells by over one million-fold *(9)*. We plan to collect peripheral blood mononuclear cells from the patients, early in the recovery phase from conventional dose chemotherapy-induced myelosuppression, CD34 select cells, expose them to the adenoviral cytosine deaminase vector, transplant these cells into intensively treated patients, and then administer the nontoxic prodrug for 14 d following the transplant.

Since we have shown that the early CD34 selected hematopoietic cells are resistant to infection by the adenoviral vector, the hematopoietic cells are spared from the toxicity that arises from conversion of the 5-FC administered systemically into 5-FU. Because 100% of the breast cancer cells are infected by the cytosine deaminase adenoviral vector, the breast cancer cells are selectively killed.

We are also planning to inject the cytosine deaminase adenoviral vector percutaneously into the prostate glands of patients with localized disease who are destined to undergo external beam radiation therapy for this disease. The prostatic cancer cells have been shown to be 100% infectable by the cytosine deaminase adenoviral vector. Thus, the cells will be exposed to the combined effects of the 5-FU, which is a potent radiation sensitizer, and the external beam radiation therapy. We have shown that prostatic cancer cells lines, which are relatively resistant to 5-FU or to radiation, are much more sensitive to the combination.

Finally, we have introduced a tumor-specific transcriptional promoter into an adenovirus and shown that it is specifically active in ovarian cancer cells but not in normal mesotheial cells *(10)*. We will use this in the intraperitoneal vector chemosensitization therapy of ovarian cancer.

4. Summary and Conclusions

Cancer gene therapy is in its infancy. At this stage, our laboratory is using replication incompetent adenoviral vectors to sensitize tumor cells to prepare for and protect against radiation therapy and chemotherapy. In the future, we will attempt to use replication competent adenoviral vectors on a conditional basis to directly destroy or suppress the tumor cells. In that way, cancer gene therapy may one day become a systemic therapy for cancer.

Acknowledgments

The authors wish to acknowledge the support of to A. Deisseroth from the Hull Development Fund of the Yale Cancer Center, the Ensign Professorship of Medicine at the Yale University School of Medicine, the Anderson Chair for Cancer Treatment and Research, and the Bush Leukemia Research Fund at the UT MD Anderson Cancer Center. They also wish to express appreciation to Ingenex, Inc. and to the Donaghue Foundation, as well as for US Army Breast Cancer Research Program BC980260 grant, and for the NIH P01 CA 49639 and NIH P01 CA 55164 grants.

References

1. DeVita, V. T. Jr., Simon, R. M., Hubbard, S. M., et al. (1980) Curability of advanced Hodgkin's disease with chemotherapy: long term follow up of MOPP treated patients at NCI. *Ann. Intern. Med.* **92,** 587.
2. Mickisch, G. H., Licht, T., Merlino, G. T., Gottesman, M. M., and Pastan, I. (1991) Chemotherapy of transgenic mice which express the human multidrug resistance gene in bone marrow: efficacy, potency and toxicity. *Cancer Res.* **51P,** 5417.
3. Sorrentino, B. P., Brandt, S. J., Bodine, D., Gottesman, M., Pastan, I., Cline, A., and Nienhuis, A. (1992) Selection of drug resistant bone marrow cells in vivo after retroviral transfer of human MDR-1. *Science* **257,** 99.
4. Podda, S., Ward, M., Himelstein, A., Richardson, C., DelaFlor-Weiss, E., Smith, L., Gottesman, M., Pastan, I., and Bank, A. (1992) Transfer and expression of the human multiple drug resistance gene into live mice. *Proc. Natl. Acad. Sci. USA* **9L,** 9676.
5. Hanania, E. G., Fu, S., Roninson, I., Zu, Z., and Deisseroth, A. B. (1995) Resistance to taxol chemotherapy produced in mouse marrow cells by safety-modified retroviruses containing a human MDR-1 transcription unit. *Gene Therapy* **2,** 279.
6. Chaudhary, P. M. and Roninson, I. (1991) Expression and activity of p-glycoprotein, a multidrug efflux pump, in human hematopoietic stem cells. *Cell* **66,** 85.
7. Hanania, E. G., Giles, R. E., Kavanagh, J., Ellerson, D., Zu, Z., Wanhg, T., Su, Y., Kudelka, A., et al. (1996) Results of MDR-1 modification trial indicate that granulocyte/macrophage colony-forming unit cells do not contribute to post transplant

hematopoietic recovery following intensive systemic therapy. *Proc. Natl. Acad. Sci. USA* **93,** 15,346–15,351.

8. Rahman, Z., Kavanagh, J., Hortobagyi, G., Claxton, D., Holmes, F., Burtness, B., Hamer, J., Kadulka, A., et al. (1998) Post transplantation paclitaxel converts parital to complete responses in advanced breast cancer patients. *Clin. Cancer Res.* **4,** 2717–2722.

9. Garcia-Sanchez, F., Pizzorno, G., Krause, D., Liang, J., Adams, E., Loeffert, J., Fu, S. Q., Hanania, E., et al. (1998) A cytosine deaminase adenoviral vector to selectively purge breast cancer cells from hematopoietic cells. *Blood* **92,** 672–682.

10. Chung, I., Crystal, R. G., and Deisseroth, A. (1999) Adenoviral system which confers transgene expression specific for neoplastic cells. *Cancer Gene Ther.* **6,** 99–106.

Index